D1536248

THE
HEALTHY LIVING SPACE

Books by Richard Leviton

Seven Steps to Better Vision

*The Imagination of Pentecost: Rudolf Steiner and
    Contemporary Spirituality*

Brain Builders

Weddings by Design

Looking for Arthur: A Once and Future Travelogue

*Physician: Medicine and the Unsuspected
    Battle for Human Freedom*

THE
HEALTHY
LIVING SPACE

70 Practical Ways to Detoxify the Body and Home

RICHARD LEVITON

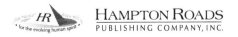
HAMPTON ROADS
PUBLISHING COMPANY, INC.

Cover design by Steve Amarillo
Cover art by Index Stock Imagery
For information write:

Hampton Roads Publishing Company, Inc.
1125 Stoney Ridge Road
Charlottesville, VA 22902

434-296-2772
fax: 434-296-5096
e-mail: hrpc@hrpub.com
www.hrpub.com

If you are unable to order this book from your local
bookseller, you may order directly from the publisher.
Call 1-800-766-8009, toll-free.

Library of Congress Catalog Card Number: 00-105253
ISBN 1-57174-209-3
10 9 8 7 6 5 4 3 2 1
Printed on acid-free paper in Canada

Dedication

To Judith A. Lewis—
visionary artist, sculptor,
healer, and partner.

Table of Contents

Acknowledgments   xiii

**The 70 Healthy Living Space
Detoxifiers at a Glance**   xiv

Notes on Products, Services, and Organizations   xix

Introduction
Why Toxicity Should Concern Us   xxi

**PART ONE
The Health Perils of the Toxic Body and Home**

CHAPTER 1 **Toxicity and Illness:**   **1**
How Your Body and Home Became Toxic
250 Chemical Contaminants in Every Human Body •
Healthy Living Space Detoxifier #1: Fill Out Your Toxicity
Self-Assessment Questionnaire • How Unrelieved Toxicity
Can Compromise Your Health • Being Slowly Poisoned
Throughout a Lifetime • Healthy Living Space Detoxifier
#2: Maintain a Household Toxic Exposure Inventory • How
Toxic Is Our Living Space, Both Body and World? •
Drinking Water Contaminated with Pesticides and Toxic
Residues • When Prozac, Viagra, and Sunscreen Flow
through Your Kitchen Tap • Air Pollution—Trigger for
Allergies, Asthma, and Respiratory Symptoms • Organo-
chlorines—Toxic Chlorine Blankets the Planet • A Radio-
active Cloud Enshrouds an Entire Generation • Tainted
Food—Glutamates, Additives, Antibiotics, and POPs •
The Toxic Living Space and You—What It All Means

CHAPTER 2 **Why You Need to Detoxify:**   **58**
Augmenting the Body's Natural Detoxification System
The Body's Burden—Total Toxic Load and Toxic Stress •
The Oxidation-Reduction Cycle at the Heart of Detoxification • The Body's Two-Phase Natural Process of Detoxification • Immunotoxicity and How the Detoxification Pathways Get Blocked • Neurological and Endocrinal Damage from Environmental Toxins • Damaging Synergistic Effects Extending into the Next Generation • Previewing the Scope and Advantages of Deliberate Detoxification • The Spiritual and Global Implications of Detoxification

PART TWO
Creating the Healthy *Body* Living Space

CHAPTER 3 **How Toxic Are You?**   **103**
Testing for Toxicity and Detoxification Ability
The Healthy Living Space Expert Interview: Peter Holyk, M.D., Contemporary Health Innovations • Healthy Living Space Detoxifier #3: Get a Clear Idea of Your Nutritional Status • Healthy Living Space Detoxifier #4: Assess Your System's Ability to Detoxify • Healthy Living Space Detoxifier #5: Determine Your Body's Total Toxic Load • Healthy Living Space Detoxifier #6: Find Out if You're Suffering from Hidden Food Allergies

CHAPTER 4 **Detoxification Preliminaries:**   **136**
Start Your Internal Cleansing with Dietary Changes and by Minimizing Your Exposure
Healthy Living Space Detoxifier #7: Rehydrate Your Body with Nature's Best Detoxifying Substance • Healthy Living Space Detoxifier #8: Get the Chlorine Out of Your Drinking and Shower Water • Healthy Living Space Detoxifier #9: Don't Fluoridate Your Teeth—Your Body Doesn't Need Fluorides • Healthy Living Space Detoxifier #10: Cleanse Your Produce of Toxic Chemicals • Healthy Living Space Detoxifier #11: Whenever Possible, Eat Organic Foods • Healthy Living Space Detoxifier #12: Minimize Your Consumption of Foods Containing Trans-fatty Acids • Healthy Living Space Detoxifier #13: Do a 3-Day Water or

Juice Fast to Rest and Regenerate Your Cells • Healthy Living Space Detoxifier #14: Do a Media/Image Fast to Cleanse Your Mind and Energy Field • Healthy Living Space Detoxifier #15: Make a Lifestyle Out of Nonstop Stress Reduction with Healing Hot Water Soaks • Healthy Living Space Detoxifier #16: Enhance Your Relaxation by Floating in 800 Pounds of Epsom Salt • Healthy Living Space Detoxifier #17: Use Music Therapy to Deepen Your Sense of Melting Relaxation

CHAPTER 5 **Safe and Effective Cleansing Programs for the Liver and Intestines** **207**

The Healthy Living Space Expert Interview: Jacob Farin, N.D., Naturopathic Physician • Healthy Living Space Detoxifier #18: Do a One-Week Elimination Diet and Liver Cleansing Program • Healthy Living Space Detoxifier #19: Use Natural Foods and Herbs to Aid Your Liver in Cleansing Itself • Healthy Living Space Detoxifier #20: Do a Natural Liver Flush to Improve Your Internal "Plumbing" • Intestinal Cleansing: Emptying Out a Storage Space the Size of a Tennis Court • Healthy Living Space Detoxifier #21: Use Six Natural Substances to Help Cleanse Your Intestines • Healthy Living Space Detoxifier #22: Remove the 50+ Feet of False Mucoid Lining from Your Intestines • Healthy Living Space Detoxifier #23: Purge the Parasites from Your Intestines • Healthy Living Space Detoxifier #24: Get Proactive with Probiotics—Plant Food for the Intestines • Healthy Living Space Detoxifier #25: Fertilize Your Bifidobacteria with Prebiotics

CHAPTER 6 **Whole-Body Cleansing Routines:** **267**
Extending the Detoxification into Everyday Activities
Healthy Living Space Detoxifier #26: Bounce on a Trampoline to Improve Your Lymphatic Drainage • Healthy Living Space Detoxifier #27: Dry Skin Brushing—Tone Up Your Body's Largest Elimination Organ • Healthy Living Space Detoxifier #28: Exercise Regularly to Enhance Blood Circulation and Toxin Removal • Healthy Living Space Detoxifier #29: Sauna Detox: How Heat Therapy Can Help Your Body Release Toxins • Healthy Living Space Detoxifier #30: A Purifying Bath: Whole-Body Detoxifying Soaks in Herbs, Salts, Oils, and Other Natural Substances

CHAPTER 7 **The Poisons in Your Mouth:**   **287**
Specialized Dental Detoxification Programs
A Gallery of Possible Toxic Consequences of Modern Dentistry • Healthy Living Space Detoxifier #31: Make Your Mouth a Mercury-Free Zone by Having Your Mercury Fillings Correctly Replaced • Healthy Living Space Detoxifier #32: Have Your Cavitations Cleaned Out and Reduce Possible Jawbone Infections • Healthy Living Space Detoxifier #33: Think Twice before Digging Another Root Canal in Your Mouth • Healthy Living Space Detoxifier #34: Determine Your Biocompatibility with Dental Materials before Putting Any More in Your Mouth

CHAPTER 8 **Guidelines for Emotional Detoxification:**   **325**
Unresolved Emotional Issues Can Become Toxic to the Body
How Unresolved Emotions Can Contribute to Illness • The Healthy Living Space Expert Interview: Patricia Kaminski, Flower Essence Practitioner • Healthy Living Space Detoxifier #35: Remedying the Four Basic States of Emotional Toxicity with Flower Essences

CHAPTER 9 **Guidelines for Spiritual Detoxification:**   **353**
Cleansing the Space around the Body
Poisons in Our Invisible Atmosphere • The Outer and Inner Aura in Disease • Healthy Living Space Detoxifier #36: Salting Your Energy Centers • Charting the Subconscious Mind in the Aura • Healthy Living Space Detoxifier #37: Request a Cleansing from Above • The Healthy Living Space Expert Interview: Rev. Leon S. LeGant, Psychic Healer • Healthy Living Space Detoxifier #38: Do a 30-Minute Spirit-Detoxifying Bath • Healthy Living Space Detoxifier #39: Shake Yourself Free of Toxic Energies • Healthy Living Space Detoxifier #40: Scrub Your Aura Clean with a Golden Sponge • Healthy Living Space Detoxifier #41: Turn Your Body into Transparent Glass • Healthy Living Space Detoxifier #42: Cutting the Cords and Ties That Bind—Psychic Plumbing • Healthy Living Space Detoxifier #43: Ground Yourself to the Center of the Earth

• Healthy Living Space Detoxifier #44: Protect Your Space by Connecting to a Higher Source • Healthy Living Space Detoxifier #45: Cleanse and Protect Your Aura with Pomanders and "Air Conditioners" • Spiritual Detoxification Is a Lifelong Activity

PART THREE
Creating the Healthy *Home* Living Space

CHAPTER 10 **Cleaning Up the Home's Indoor Environment:**   **399**
Overcoming the Effects of Sick Building Syndrome
Sick Building Syndrome: The Disease of Modern Architecture • Indoor Pollutants—A Matter of "Genuine Concern" • The Healthy Living Space Expert Interview: Michael Riversong, Design Ecologist and Environmental Assessor • Healthy Living Space Detoxifier #46: Get the Electropollution Out of Your Home • Healthy Living Space Detoxifier #47: Benefits of Nontoxic Carpets—Don't Let Your Carpets Kill You Softly • The Trouble with Indoor Air—Worse Pollution Indoors than Out • Healthy Living Space Detoxifier #48: Filter Your Home's Indoor Air to Remove Toxins and Allergens • Healthy Living Space Detoxifier #49: Install an "Indoor Waterfall" to Add Negative Ions to Your Air • Healthy Living Space Detoxifier #50: Use Houseplants to Filter Out Toxins from Your Indoor Air • Healthy Living Space Detoxifier #51: Get the Radon Out of Your Basement • Healthy Living Space Detoxifier #52: Take the SADness Out of Your Indoor Space with Full Spectrum Lighting • Healthy Living Space Detoxifier #53: Go Green with Your Household Products

CHAPTER 11 **The Feng Shui of a Healthy Home:**   **475**
Detoxifying the Energy Aspects of Your Living Space
Charting the Movement of Life Force Energy • Healthy Living Space Detoxifier #54: Evaluate the Energy Flow in Your Home with the *Ba-Gua* • The Healthy Living Space Expert Interview: Stanley Aaga Bartlett, Feng Shui Master • Healthy Living Space Detoxifier #55: Tidy Up All the Cluttered Areas in Your Home • Healthy Living Space Detoxifier #56: Repaint All the Interior Walls with Your

Color of Happiness • Healthy Living Space Detoxifier #57: Clear Your Space of All Predecessor Energy • Healthy Living Space Detoxifier #58: The Health Benefits of Ghost-Busting • Healthy Living Space Detoxifier #59: Eliminate Poison Arrows and Cutting *Qi* • Healthy Living Space Detoxifier #60: Pacify Your Neighborhood with Feng Shui Mirrors • Healthy Living Space Detoxifier #61: Optimizing the Mouth of *Qi* at Your Front Door • Healthy Living Space Detoxifier #62: Setting Up a Feng Shui-Friendly Bedroom • Healthy Living Space Detoxifier #63: Setting Up a Feng Shui-Friendly Bathroom • The Health Costs of Having an Energy-Imbalanced Home

CHAPTER 12 Cleansing the Home's Exterior Environment: **518**
Neutralizing the Effects of Geopathic Stress
Disease Can Be a Problem of Location • Healthy Living Space Detoxifier #64: When Nothing Else Heals, Try Moving Your Bed • Healthy Living Space Detoxifier #65: Scan Your Home and Environment for Signs of Geopathic Stress • The Healthy Living Space Expert Interview: Patrick MacManaway, M.D., Ch.B., Geomancer • Healthy Living Space Detoxifier #66: Take Your Energy Body Out of the Curry-Hartmann Grid • Healthy Living Space Detoxifier #67: Five Simple Techniques for Detoxifying a Room or Environment • Healthy Living Space Detoxifier #68: Put in an Energy Drainage Pipe from Your House to the Center of the Earth • Healthy Living Space Detoxifier #69: How to Take the Stress Out of a Geopathic Zone • Healthy Living Space Detoxifier #70: Selecting Energy Wells in a Geography of Enlightenment

Afterword
Life in a Healthy Living Space   **557**

Endnotes   **561**

Index   **620**

Acknowledgments

The author wishes to thank the generous contribution of time, insights, and protocols from the following experts in detoxification: Peter Holyk, M.D., Jacob Farin, N.D., Patricia Kaminski, Rev. Leon S. LeGant, Michael Riversong, Stanley Aaga Bartlett, and Patrick MacManaway, M.D. Thanks to Stephanie Marohn for her excellent editing.

The 70 Healthy Living Space

1 Fill Out Your Toxicity
Self-Assessment
Questionnaire *6*

2 Maintain a Household Toxic
Exposure Inventory *21*

3 Get a Clear Idea of Your
Nutritional Status *113*

4 Assess Your System's
Ability to Detoxify *120*

5 Determine Your Body's
Total Toxic Load *122*

6 Find Out if You're Suffering
from Hidden Food
Allergies *131*

7 Rehydrate Your Body with Nature's
Best Detoxifying Substance *137*

8 Get the Chlorine Out of Your
Drinking and Shower Water *140*

9 Don't Fluoridate Your Teeth—
Your Body Doesn't Need
Fluorides *156*

10 Cleanse Your Produce of
Toxic Chemicals *164*

11 Whenever Possible, Eat
Organic Foods *168*

12 Minimize Your Consumption
of Foods Containing
Trans-fatty Acids *184*

13 Do a 3-Day Water or Juice Fast
to Rest and Regenerate
Your Cells *189*

14 Do a Media/Image Fast to
Cleanse Your Mind and
Energy Field *193*

15 Make a Lifestyle Out of
Nonstop Stress Reduction with
Healing Hot Water Soaks *197*

16 Enhance Your Relaxation by
Floating in 800 Pounds of
Epsom Salt *201*

17 Use Music Therapy to Deepen
Your Sense of Melting
Relaxation *204*

Detoxifiers at a Glance

18 Do a One-Week Elimination Diet and Liver Cleansing Program *211*

19 Use Natural Foods and Herbs to Aid Your Liver in Cleansing Itself *216*

20 Do a Natural Liver Flush to Improve Your Internal "Plumbing" *222*

21 Use Six Natural Substances to Help Cleanse Your Intestines *232*

22 Remove the 50+ Feet of False Mucoid Lining from Your Intestines *247*

23 Purge the Parasites from Your Intestines *251*

24 Get Proactive with Probiotics— Plant Food for the Intestines *261*

25 Fertilize Your Bifidobacteria with Prebiotics *265*

26 Bounce on a Trampoline to Improve Your Lymphatic Drainage *268*

27 Dry Skin Brushing—Tone Up Your Body's Largest Elimination Organ *273*

28 Exercise Regularly to Enhance Blood Circulation and Toxin Removal *275*

29 Sauna Detox: How Heat Therapy Can Help Your Body Release Toxins *278*

30 A Purifying Bath: Whole-Body Detoxifying Soaks in Herbs, Salts, Oils, and Other Natural Substances *284*

31 Make Your Mouth a Mercury-Free Zone by Having Your Mercury Fillings Correctly Replaced *295*

32 Have Your Cavitations Cleaned Out and Reduce Possible Jawbone Infections *313*

33 Think Twice before Digging Another Root Canal in Your Mouth *318*

The 70 Healthy Living Space

34 Determine Your Biocompatibility with Dental Materials before Putting Any More in Your Mouth *321*

35 Remedying the Four Basic States of Emotional Toxicity with Flower Essences *341*

36 Salting Your Energy Centers *359*

37 Request a Cleansing from Above *369*

38 Do a 30-Minute Spirit-Detoxifying Bath *377*

39 Shake Yourself Free of Toxic Energies *380*

40 Scrub Your Aura Clean with a Golden Sponge *381*

41 Turn Your Body into Transparent Glass *382*

42 Cutting the Cords and Ties That Bind—Psychic Plumbing *384*

43 Ground Yourself to the Center of the Earth *387*

44 Protect Your Space by Connecting to a Higher Source *389*

45 Cleanse and Protect Your Aura with Pomanders and "Air Conditioners" *391*

46 Get the Electropollution Out of Your Home *417*

47 Benefits of Nontoxic Carpets—Don't Let Your Carpets Kill You Softly *426*

48 Filter Your Home's Indoor Air to Remove Toxins and Allergens *443*

49 Install an "Indoor Waterfall" to Add Negative Ions to Your Air *449*

50 Use Houseplants to Filter Out Toxins from Your Indoor Air *453*

51 Get the Radon Out of Your Basement *459*

Detoxifiers at a Glance

52 Take the SADness Out of Your Indoor Space with Full Spectrum Lighting *462*

53 Go Green with Your Household Products *468*

54 Evaluate the Energy Flow in Your Home with the *Ba-Gua* *479*

55 Tidy Up All the Cluttered Areas in Your Home *486*

56 Repaint All the Interior Walls with Your Color of Happiness *488*

57 Clear Your Space of All Predecessor Energy *490*

58 The Health Benefits of Ghost-Busting *495*

59 Eliminate Poison Arrows and Cutting *Qi* *499*

60 Pacify Your Neighborhood with Feng Shui Mirrors *504*

61 Optimizing the Mouth of *Qi* at Your Front Door *506*

62 Setting up a Feng Shui-Friendly Bedroom *509*

63 Setting up a Feng Shui-Friendly Bathroom *512*

64 When Nothing Else Heals, Try Moving Your Bed *523*

65 Scan Your Home and Environment for Signs of Geopathic Stress *528*

66 Take Your Energy Body Out of the Curry-Hartmann Grid *540*

67 Five Simple Techniques for Detoxifying a Room or Environment *546*

68 Put in an Energy Drainage Pipe from Your House to the Center of the Earth *548*

69 How to Take the Stress Out of a Geopathic Zone *551*

70 Selecting Energy Wells in a Geography of Enlightenment *555*

Note on Products, Services, and Organizations

There are many products, services, and organizations listed in this book. Their inclusion in the text does not constitute an endorsement by the author. In some cases, the author has personally tested or used the products or services, but in other cases, not. Further, the author has no financial or business connections with any of the products, services, or organizations listed.

The inclusion of this information is meant solely to help the reader find a point of orientation in what is perhaps a new and overly large field. References to specific products, such as water or air filters, for example, are only meant to serve as a starting point from which readers can launch their own more extended research and vetting. They are not meant to be the result of exhaustive research into these specific categories; rather, they are the results of a preliminary and provisional research of the field, principally through the Internet.

All health information in this book is based on sound medical and scientific research and/or the clinical protocols of credentialed health care practitioners. However, this is no substitute for qualified medical guidance and advice if there is any question about the appropriateness or applicability of any recommendation in this book to individual readers and their unique health conditions. Readers concerned about the suitability of specific techniques or substances to their specific health condition should consult a qualifed health care practitioner before undertaking any of the detoxification steps.

INTRODUCTION

Why Toxicity Should Concern Us

Ever since Rachel Carson's shocking indictment of industrial pollution in *Silent Spring*, the concept of poisons in the environment has been with us. Carson gave us the basic idea: too many toxic substances in the environment sicken, even kill, wildlife and natural systems, and they eventually make us sick too. As a society we haven't forgotten the concept of toxicity introduced by her book in 1962, yet to a large measure it has remained a concept and not a living reality, not something we know to be true in our own lives.

In other words, we don't quite see how toxicity is the order of the day for most of the world, in terms both of the landscape and the body, the planet and the home. Yet as this book will show, toxicity—the long-term health impact of long-term exposure to toxic substances—has crept up on us and now to a large extent *defines* our physical reality.

What is our physical reality? One way to describe it is to call it a living space. We, as conscious human beings, live in a body and in a home, be it studio apartment, condominium, house, or mansion. The body *and* home are our living space. Both should be considered together in any discussion of health, toxicity, or illness because they exist in a remarkable feedback system; both can make us well and both can sicken us. If we want to be healthy, we need to concern ourselves with both. A healthy living space is a body and home free of toxins.

But most of us don't have a healthy living space. We live in a toxic world, and it is steadily sickening us; in fact, so pervasive is its toxic effect that we almost don't see it. Yet scientific studies now show that nearly every corner of the planet is toxic and every human being carries residues of dozens of toxic chemicals in their cells. Every element of our physical world—air, water, earth—carries a toxic burden, is poisoned, and is poisoning us.

As we well know, the incidence of chronic and degenerative diseases, including cancer, is ever increasing. Toxicity is slowly draining the life out of us, yet so pervasive and effective is this systematic poisoning that we are barely, if at all, aware of it in our everyday living. We think the way we feel is "normal," the way a human is supposed to feel, even though we may suspect we're a little off.

We may not personally feel "sick" and we may not have been officially diagnosed as having a "condition," but we vaguely sense a degree of dysfunction in our body. We don't quite have the energy we used to; we get colds more often than before; allergies seem more prevalent; we're bothered by various minor symptoms that come and go but never really leave; our sense of vitality and immunity seem off, a bit compromised.

Increasingly, our homes have become toxic too. This is a sad and shocking idea to contemplate: the home is supposed to be the heart of our domestic life, a refuge, a haven—how can such a place designed to nourish life make us sick? Yet it does. Scientific studies show that most of our modern building and home furnishing materials—paints, plywood, glues, varnishes, carpets, upholstery, household cleaning products, bedding materials, even our clothes—are laced with toxic chemicals that are slowly released from the products into the indoor air of our increasingly airtight or inadequately ventilated homes. Headaches, rashes, allergies, respiratory problems, frequent colds, irritability, depression, immune system problems—these are among the numerous documented symptoms attributed to the effect of our exposure to toxic building materials in our homes.

So how do you get a healthy living space? You detoxify. Detoxification is a term generally understood in reference to substance abuse treatment programs, but it actually refers to a much more generalized process of ridding the body of all toxic substances, not just freeing it from dependency on alcohol or other addictive substances. Detoxification is a natural, routine activity of the body, carried out every day by the liver, lymphatic system, kidneys, and intestines. The body can handle a fair degree of toxic materials and survive, and in fact remain healthy.

But there is a limit, and for many of us, we reached that limit, and surpassed it, years ago. Now our natural detoxification processes are hindered; they don't work at full capacity; they have a tremendous backlog of toxic substances to process, and without our help at this point, they may never catch up. Not catching up with its detoxification load means the body will start to get poisoned by its ever-increasing reservoir of unprocessed toxins, and it will start to show signs of impaired health.

In many traditional societies, regular detoxification was part of the lifestyle. Once or twice a year, individuals would deliberately take steps to help their body rid itself of the toxic burden of the preceding months. People would fast, drink copious amounts of water, do a sweatlodge, take special herbs, practice specific exercises, and give their bodies a chance to cleanse themselves.

Even in healthy times, when people lived in a relatively toxic-free environment, it was a good idea to periodically give the body a break from the endless routine of eating, digesting, assimilating, and eliminating, and let it fully catch up and "clean house." With a clean house—a healthy living space—people felt better in themselves; their emotions were clearer, their minds were more unfettered, and they felt more attuned with the world.

In our day, with the environment and the body intensely polluted, the need for regular detoxification is acute. The only way to survive and *flourish* in such an environment is to undertake a comprehensive program of internal *and* external cleansing. The abiding assumption in this book is that detoxification, the basis of true and lasting health, must address both aspects of one's living environment—the body and the home. Body and home are reflections of each other and must be addressed simultaneously.

It is essential that we detoxify *both* expressions of our living space at the same time: our body and our home. If you cleanse your body but live in a toxic living space, your home will eventually sicken you; if you detoxify your home but do nothing to purge your body of its toxic burden, the healthy home will not prevent the health consequences of bodily toxicity. Your internal toxins will gradually sicken you.

A clean (detoxified) house and a clean (detoxified) body complement each other, leading to a state of harmony, balance, and deep health. The goal is a healthy body and home—a healthy living space—and the means to get there are the seventy practical steps presented in this book. *The Healthy Living Space* provides instructions on how to regain a healthy body and home based on safe, proven, nontoxic, noninvasive methods from the field of alternative medicine.

This is a how-to book on alternative medicine applications for better health through systematic detoxification, or cleansing, of both our internal and external living environments. The essence of this book is self-care: you can do it yourself. All of the procedures recommended in the book can be done by the average nonmedically trained person, although in some cases professional consultation is recommended as a complement to one's own informed initiative.

The procedures—I call them Healthy Living Space Detoxifiers—are supported by scientific research and the clinical experience of numerous physicians, health-care practitioners, and detoxification experts, seven of whom I interviewed specifically for this book. For each of the seventy Detoxifiers, I explain the reason for doing them—that is, the nature of the toxicity addressed—and the steps to follow to do them. In many cases, information about practitioners, and sources of products, services, or more information are provided to help you get started on detoxification.

Do you need to do all seventy steps? Yes, if you want a thorough detoxification of body and home. No, if you're willing to settle for less. Regarding the detoxification of the body, as a minimum it is advisable to do the steps that address the liver and intestines, in the order they're presented in chapter 5. But the steps described in chapters 4 and 6 complement the approach that focuses on the liver and intestines, as a kind of before and after framework.

You not only want to purge your body of its accumulation of toxic substances (chapter 5), but you should reduce as much as possible your further intake of toxic substances through food, air, water, and your exposure to toxic products and environments (chapters 4 and 6). If you don't change some of the aspects of your lifestyle that put you in contact with toxic substances, you may end up replenishing the supply of poisons, even though you removed them from your body with liver and intestinal detoxification.

At a bare minimum, you should seriously consider trying the steps in chapter 10 which address the sources of toxicity in your physical indoor environment. But as this book emphasizes, toxicity is a broad spectrum of pollution. It affects not only the body and our physical living space, but our emotions, mind, and energy field—all the aspects of being human.

Similarly, toxicity in the home can affect it, as a living space, in all aspects, which in turn affects your experience of the space—how it feels to be in it, what its energy is like. You will see that, remarkably, placing your bed in the wrong spot in your bedroom can be just as toxic to you as breathing the outgassed fumes from a new synthetic carpet. It poisons you on a different level.

The 70 Healthy Living Space Detoxifiers work from the more obvious physical aspects of our individual being and living environment into the more interior aspects (emotions and thoughts) and beyond this into the energy field in which our body and home reside. Ultimately, the *healthy* living space is one that is healthy for consciousness, for our lives as awake, aware human beings living in a body that dwells in an indoor living space set in a living external environment.

We don't know what it feels like to be truly healthy; our great grandparents might have, but we don't. How much of our view of the world and ourselves is conditioned by being filled with toxic substances from our industrialized world? It's a question we can answer only from the inside, after we have detoxified and taken a fresh look around at things, at our body, home, and world—a prospect that might serve as an inducement to start detoxifying.

Detoxification is not merely a medical issue, a route to better health. It isn't something to do only if you're "into" being healthy. Whether we are toxic or nontoxic defines every aspect of our physical existence, our feelings, thoughts, how our body works, how we see the world, how consciousness lives in matter. Toxicity deals with the foundations of our life, with how every cell, molecule, and organ functions, or dysfunctions. With how we think, or don't think; how we feel, or don't feel. With how our thinking and feeling are distorted or compromised or not fully available to us. A great deal is at stake.

The extent of toxicity in our environment today—body, home, and world—is shocking and distressing, but the situation is not hopeless. There is *much* an individual person can do to reverse this, both at home and in the world. Individual actions and choices count; they have an impact globally. If you start detoxifying and change your consumer habits, this starts to send little shock waves through the marketplace. You start thinking, feeling, and acting differently; you no longer are conditioned or weighed down by toxicity, and you see your responsibility in the world in a new light, or perhaps for the first time. Life after detoxification can be refreshing, even liberating.

Here is a brief survey of the ground we'll be covering in *The Healthy Living Space*, a roadmap for the way to detoxification. The book is divided into three parts. Part one, "The Health Perils of the Toxic Body and Home," discusses the nature of toxicity, defining a wide range of toxins from chemicals to energy influences (chapter 1). It documents the injurious biological effect of toxins, their prevalence in the world, and how they compromise immunity and produce illness. The biochemical processes of detoxification (through the liver, kidneys, and intestines) are explained in chapter 2, showing how you can work with your internal detoxification system.

The toxins discussed range from estrogen-mimicking industrial chemicals and irradiated and genetically modified foods to radon, stagnant life force energy, electromagnetic pollution, and harmful energies from the Earth itself, among many others. The book also explores the effects of two levels of toxins not ordinarily considered in this kind of discussion: unresolved emotional toxicity and auric toxicity, which means deleterious energies in the field surrounding the human body (the aura).

Part two, "Creating the Healthy *Body* Living Space," addresses the safe, systematic detoxification of the body using natural remedies and alternative medicine practices. First, nineteen laboratory tests are outlined in chapter 3, each of which provides essential (and low-cost) information about your specific level of toxicity and biochemical ability to withstand toxicity and disease.

Next, in chapter 4, we look at practices and lifestyle changes for internal cleansing, such as dietary modifications, the need for pure water, the avoidance of contaminated foods and beverages, and the benefits of short-term fasting, among others. It isn't all avoidance. There are some positive things to do, such as taking healing baths to reduce stress, using music to melt your tension, bouncing on a trampoline to move your lymph, or sitting in a sauna, as explained in chapters 4 and 6. These are the before and after aspects of detoxification, how to prepare for it, how to sustain the benefits.

In chapter 5, you'll get detailed instructions on how to detoxify your liver, kidneys, lymphatic system, and intestines, and information on why you should regard your teeth (and what dentists have done to them) as potential sources of toxicity. Chapter 7 will tell you how to address and resolve that dental toxicity.

Traumatic emotional experiences act as toxins when left unresolved in the system and have been shown by medical research to significantly contribute to illness. So in chapter 8, the effective role of flower remedies is discussed in conjunction with a leading practitioner. In a similar manner, unsuspected injurious energies and presences in the energy field, or aura, surrounding the human act as toxins, contributing to states of ill health and numerous physical and mental symptoms. In chapter 9, you'll find techniques for diagnosing and removing auric pollution, as well as a fascinating explanation of where it comes from.

Part three, "Creating the Healthy *Home* Living Space," looks at the layers of toxicity in the typical indoor living environment, and how to remove them or minimize their negative health effects. Chapter 10 discusses what is called "sick building syndrome," a field of research that documents the numerous ways in which structures and contents of a house or apartment contribute to ill health. The emerging discipline of Baubiologie (the "biological, living house") is detailed, along with its many practical tips on detoxifying the physical aspects of one's home. Some of the tips include the use of pollution-absorbing houseplants, negative ionization, nontoxic cleaning products, air filtration, and full spectrum lighting.

Building on this, the book moves to the next level of household toxicity, the realm described by feng shui, the increasingly popular Chinese art of placement. The shapes of rooms, the orientation of a house, the placement of furniture in a room, and many other similar factors affect the flow of energy through the house. This flow, in turn, either supports or hinders the health of the occupants. In chapter 11, feng shui experts provide numerous practical tips for improving energy flow and removing the places of stagnation or energy toxicity in the house that contribute to ill health.

In chapter 12, we look at how harmful energies from the Earth itself or the land around the house can permeate your home and make you toxic. Such energies include aberrant electromagnetic fields, deriving from electrical power lines and/or underground water currents.

The Healthy Living Space will show you how your body and home form a living system in constant interaction, feedback, and communication. Lasting health can be had when you consider both in the health equation and when you address the toxic burden of both at the same time. You live in two places: your body and your home. Both can be toxic, both can be healthy, but given the current state of the world, neither are likely to be healthy without your active participation. You already know what a toxic living space feels like; all of us in the Western industrialized part of the world know this today. But what might a detoxified living space feel like?

Part One

The Health Perils of the Toxic Body and Home

CHAPTER 1

Toxicity and Illness:

How Your Body and Home Became Toxic

It is an unfortunate fact that most of us living in the industrialized world today are toxic. We have been poisoned by the chemicals in our environment, and our bodies have become a limited toxic waste dump, a contaminated landfill, a biohazard zone. This is not an exaggeration to make a point: it *is* the point, and there is sufficient data now available to substantiate what might otherwise be viewed as a hysterical assertion.

Our bodies are overfull of poisons, not the kind that immediately make you ill, but the slow-acting kind, the ones that sicken, and even kill, you over time. They have a cumulative effect such that the more you amass in your body and the older you get without removing them, the more likely it is they will interfere with your health. Allergies, frequent colds and flus, unexplained headaches and muscle cramps, immune system disorders, hyperactivity, attention deficit disorder, chronic fatigue, environmental illness, multiple chemical sensitivities, asthma, infertility, arthritis, Alzheimer's, multiple sclerosis, heart disease, cancer—all can be attributed in large measure to unrelieved toxicity. Many more health conditions could be added to this list of toxin-generated discomfort and disease.

In fact, the spectrum of health effects ranges from chronic minor problems, such as allergies, to persistent major problems, degenerative disease, cancer, and shortened life span. The alarming fact is that there is a near certainty that right now both your body and your home are toxic. Your body is loaded with toxic substances, and your home and its furnishings, from carpets to cleaning agents, acts as a source for your continuous toxic exposure.

They're called xenobiotics— industrially produced foreign chemicals, synthetic organic chemicals that are not native to our natural environment, either within our bodies or in nature, hence the appropriate term, "xeno." As foreign substances in our natural ecosystems, most xenobiotics confound the ability of nature or our bodies to get rid of them, or even to neutralize them.

250 Chemical Contaminants in Every Human Body

They're called xenobiotics— industrially produced foreign chemicals, synthetic organic chemicals that are not native to our natural environment, either within our bodies or in nature, hence the appropriate term, "xeno." Think of plastics, pesticides, preservatives, aluminum, and thousands of other modern substances and products you take for granted, or don't even know about. That's where you'll find xenobiotics. They're in your foods and in your home. As foreign substances in our natural ecosystems, most xenobiotics confound the ability of nature or our bodies to get rid of them, or even to neutralize them.

Though they may seem to make our world run more efficiently, their hidden cost is that they unfailingly make us sick. And this buildup of toxins in our external and bodily environment has been steadily expanding since about 1800 and the onset of the Industrial Revolution.

Xenobiotics do not observe national borders. It is not only Americans or Canadians who are growing steadily more toxic. Toxicity is global. "Virtually anyone willing to put up the $2,000 for the tests will find at least 250 chemical contaminants in his or her body fat, regardless of whether he or she lives in Gary, Indiana, or on a remote island in the South Pacific."[1]

This sweeping—and alarming—statement was made only a few years ago by Theo Colborn and her colleagues in *Our Stolen Future*, a startling documentation of our toxic environment and its ramifications for worldwide health. Synthetic chemicals are everywhere and you cannot escape them, Colborn concludes.

They are in the Arctic and Polynesia, the Swiss Alps and mother's milk. In just six months of breast-feeding, an infant in the United States or Europe gets "the maximum recommended lifetime dose of dioxin," one of the world's most toxic substances, a byproduct of pesticides. This killer chemical "rides through the food web" from plants to animals to humans and can end up anywhere on the planet.

In fact, the Arctic, says Colborn, may be the most polluted environment on the planet in terms of its concentration of volatile persistent chemicals, such as PCBs, or polychlorinated biphenyls. Canadian researchers found that residents on a remote Arctic island had the highest observed levels of PCBs of any human population excepting those specifically exposed through an industrial accident. PCBs, created as coolants and insulators for electrical equipment, are world travelers, migrating through ecosystems and over great distances, lodging in the fat cells of all kinds of living organisms, Colborn observes.

Persistent chemicals such as PCBs are characterized by "extreme stability, volatility, and a particular affinity for fat." That means they persist, do not easily decay or biodegrade into nontoxic forms, are easily excited or activated and vaporized, and tend to lodge in fat cells of living biological organisms (such as humans) from which they are hard to remove. Because they lodge in fat cells, they are almost exempt from the body's natural detoxification system, which requires toxins to be water-soluble, and cannot easily deal with fat-soluble toxins.

Introduced in 1929, PCBs were banned in the United States in 1976, but by then an estimated 3.4 billion pounds of PCBs had been produced worldwide and released into the global environment. And they're still there, in the body fat of almost every living creature in the world, states Colborn. PCBs are only one class of *many* synthetic organic chemicals produced and unleashed into the global environment during the period from 1900 to 2000, which in retrospect surely ought to be called the toxic century.

One name for this global family of industrial synthetic chemicals is POPs, persistent organic pollutants.[2] These are carbon-based chemical compounds—such as PCBs, DDT, chlordane, dieldrin, HCB, aldrin, dioxins—that persist in the environment (resisting degradation), are semi-volatile (evaporating easily), and have a low water solubility (preferring fat cells). As POPs move up the food chain, from fish to human, their concentrations can increase by factors of thousands or even millions.

Here's another rivetting example. You would think living mostly outdoors and close to nature in ultra-rural Greenland amidst vast amounts of snow and no industry would be a healthy lifestyle. The opposite is true. Researchers at a major hospital in Quebec City, Quebec, found that the Inuits of Greenland (a people native to the country) had the world's highest body burden of organochlorines (toxic chlorine-derived compounds) due to environmental exposure. The Inuits depend largely on sea mammal fat for their food supply; unfortunately, the sea mammals are intensely polluted with fat-loving POPs. The researchers found evidence of twenty-five different pesticides and POPs in the fatty tissues of the Inuits examined, and they found that the native Greenlanders had concentrations that were three to thirty-four times higher than found in a population in urban, industrialized Quebec City.[3]

Although neither Greenland nor the Arctic are still pristine, surely the rarefied peaks of high mountain ranges, such as the Swiss Alps must still be relatively toxin free. Not so, says Roland Psenner, a professor at Innsbruck University in Innsbruck, Austria. Ironically, the Alps act as a magnet for toxic pollutants in the atmosphere, Psenner reports. In lakes above the tree line (typically at 8,000 feet) the fish are contaminated with DDT applied in the tropics against malaria. "We found that fish in the most contaminated lakes have 1,000 times more DDT than lower-lying lakes," Psenner states.[4]

How can toxins used in the tropics end up on an alpine snow peak? Ecologists call it global distillation, to denote a kind of "chemical nomadism." The subzero temperatures around peaks in the Alps cause atmospheric DDT, collected over Africa and India as evaporation, to humidify and fall as precipitation on the peaks. Chemicals used in Southeast Asian rice paddies vaporize and drift across the planet and condense on the bark of Arctic trees. Global distillation explains why "the bodies of seals in Siberia's Lake Baikal—the world's oldest and deepest lake—contain the same two contaminants as the alpine soil of New Hampshire's Mount Moosilauke."[5]

"There is no safe, uncontaminated place," Colborn concludes. Our body, home, neighborhood, state, nation, planet—all have become toxic, an unhealthy living space. All are contaminated with numerous xenobiotics that are capable of making us sick, and are in the process of doing so.

The concept of global distillation gives us an image of the planet uniformly blanketed in poisons—globally toxified. Organochlorines do not observe national boundaries; hydrocarbons do not stay put; pesticides hunger for the entire world. The use of a single toxic substance has planetary repercussions. When you spray dandelions in your front yard with a convenient pesticide dispenser you bought at the hardware store, you are potentially sending toxics to the far ends of the planet. You could be poisoning polar bears at the North Pole.

But once you *get* the relationship between local and global toxics,[6] you get something bigger, better. When you realize that your actions have global effects, you start thinking globally. It may be a shocking moment when you see the reciprocity, the mirroring, that exists between you and the planet—both overflowing with toxins. You see that you and your home are embedded in the planet's own body, its life, which we call its ecosystem. The load of toxins you and the planet share is the negative aspect; the positive aspect is that your willingness to detoxify also has world consequences. You can start saving the polar bears from your garage. If you can't tolerate dandelions in your lawn, it is a global act to reach for the weeding spade instead of the herbicide.

The volume of toxic substances regularly added to the world environment is staggering to contemplate. In one year alone: 550 million pounds of industrial chemicals were dumped into public sewage; 1 billion pounds of chemicals were released into the ground; 188 million pounds of chemicals were discharged into surface waters; 2.4 billion pounds of particulates were sent into the air. The estimated total of toxic chemical pollutants released into the environment in one year (1989) was 5.7 billion pounds. "That is enough to fill a line of semi-trailers parked bumper to bumper, and having a cargo capacity of 45,000 pounds each, stretching from downtown Los Angeles to Des Moines, Iowa."[7]

The purpose of this chapter is not to scare, however, but to inform and motivate. It is necessary to fully grasp the *fact* of toxicity and the degree to which it has permeated our environment, our bodies and home living spaces, not to mention the planet's ecosystem itself. It is vital to understand what unchecked toxicity is doing to our bodies and our world. But this alarming knowledge should become the *foundation* upon which we build practical, effective steps to detoxify ourselves, to deliberately remove the myriad toxins from our bodies and homes, and eventually, from the world as well.

When we start detoxifying, we inevitably become more aware—grippingly so, usually—of the state of the global body, our planetary living space. We see how it, too, is toxic. We become aware of what we're buying, using, consuming, ingesting, and, with shock, realize we have been steadily, if unknowingly, poisoning ourselves—and the environment—for years. As our consumer choices change, as our lifestyle puts a premium on health, and as our political priorities shift as a result, our personal commitment to detoxification starts to have global ramifications. But first, let's get a visceral sense of what being toxic feels like. Are we toxic and don't know it?

HEALTHY LIVING SPACE DETOXIFIER #1
Fill Out Your Toxicity Self-Assessment Questionnaire

Unless we are obviously, uncomfortably sick, ill to the extent that we are conspicuously disabled, it seems unlikely—even illogical—to think we might be toxic. If I'm so toxic, why aren't all these terrible poisons making me really ill, laying me low with a serious health problem, we reason. While it may seem logical, the reasoning is flawed.

The truth is that we are all being slowly poisoned, because although the toxins are potent, we are rarely exposed to a lethal or even sublethal, but dangerous, dose. We are instead *routinely* exposed to very small doses of many toxic chemicals, which together overwhelm our body's natural detoxification system. Notice the key words here: routinely, small doses, many. It's the *frequent* exposure to *microdoses* of *multiple* toxic chemicals that sickens us slowly. Very few of us are seriously poisoned through a single toxic exposure to a large amount of one chemical.

Over time, these many toxic chemicals to which we are routinely exposed in the *normal* course of living sicken us, at first generating dozens of "hidden" symptoms, then creating serious debilitating illnesses that conventional medical analysis does not link to a lifetime of toxic exposure. The symptoms are "hidden" only because we are not trained to look for them. Once you know what they are, toxicity becomes fairly easy to spot. Various laboratory tests, detailed in chapter 3, can confirm presumed toxicity and document its extent and nature. It may seem overwhelming to open this Pandora's box, but the guidelines presented throughout the rest of the book will show you how to deal with this toxicity effectively on your own.

You don't have to be a physician to deal with detoxification; in fact, don't expect your doctor necessarily to be on the same page as you once you wake up to the toxicity factor. Conventional doctors are still resistant to this concept and are often not even especially well educated in its intricacies and seemingly indirect causal links. On the other hand, practitioners of alternative medicine, who base diagnosis on a careful observation of the whole person, on all the body's systems and their interactions, are much more likely to credit unrelieved systemic toxicity as a prime contributing factor in numerous health conditions.

Practitioners of alternative medicine, who base diagnosis on a careful observation of the whole person, on all the body's systems and their interactions, are much more likely to credit unrelieved systemic toxicity as a prime contributing factor in numerous health conditions.

"Most people who think they are tired are actually toxic," observes Sherry Rogers, M.D., a physician based in Syracuse, New York, who for several decades has been an outspoken and well-informed advocate of the systemic toxicity hypothesis of illness. An alarming number of people, says Dr. Rogers, are "not functioning with all oars in the water."

They pass their annual physicals yet cannot deny they feel "dreadful" a fair amount of the time. They have lots of vague symptoms and never feel quite well, but it's not enough to constitute a diagnostic category, so they're dismissed as hypochondriacs. They do not wake up energized and vivacious in the morning. They rely on stimulants or relaxants to suppress the strange, persistent signals coming from their body, as if the body, in its own baffling language, is *insisting* that something is not quite right.

"Because environmental illnesses are apparently characterized by patterns of multiple symptoms in many parts of the body, including the central nervous system, it is understandable that such patients have often received diagnoses of neurasthenia, hysteria, somatization disorder, and various other psychosomatic disorders," explains Iris Bell, M.D., a psychiatrist at the University of California-San Francisco School of Medicine, and author of *Clinical Ecology: A New Approach to Environmental Illness*.[8]

But there is no such thing as a hypochondriac, asserts Dr. Rogers. When a doctor fails to understand that the clinical picture presented by a patient with multiple, vague, or ill-defined symptoms adds up to systemic toxicity, it teaches the patient to ignore or tune out the various body symptoms until they become much worse, unbearable, or even dangerous, says Dr. Rogers. Yet these same persistent, wide-ranging, "soft, subtle symptoms" have a biological function: they're meant to serve as "early warnings of worse symptoms to come if we ignore or mask (cover them up) them with medications."[9]

Consider then how many of the following soft, subtle symptoms you have experienced in the last thirty to sixty days, listed according to the particular body system or organ involved. If you get any of these symptoms at a rate between occasionally and frequently, it will be worth your while to start thinking about your health in terms of possible toxicity:

• *Brain*: Headaches, faintness, dizziness, insomnia.

• *Digestive Tract:* Nausea, vomiting, diarrhea, constipation, indigestion, bad breath, bloated after eating, belching, passing gas, heartburn, intestinal or stomach pain, unusually smelly stools, offensive smelling urine.

• *Eyes:* Itchy, bloodshot, or watery eyes, swollen, reddened, or sticky eyelids, dark circles or bags under the eyes, blurred or tunnel vision, poor night vision, inflamed or swollen eyelids.

• *Muscles and Joints:* Aches and pains in the joints, arthritis, stiffness, movement limitations, muscle aches and pains, sense of weakness or tiredness, tight or stiff neck, backaches, joints sore upon waking, joint pain after minor exertion or after eating certain foods, numbness or tingling.

- *Ears*: Itchiness, infections or aches, drainage, ringing, hearing loss.

- *Nose*: Sinus congestion, stuffiness, hay fever, sneezing attacks, unusual amount of mucus, runny nose.

- *Weight*: Overweight, underweight, anorexia, food cravings, compulsive or binge eating, water retention.

- *Mouth and Throat:* Persistent coughing; frequent need to clear the throat; sore throat; hoarseness; voice loss; discoloration or swelling in tongue, lips, and gums; canker sores; swollen lymph glands; diminished sense of taste; tongue with a grayish-white, yellow, or thick film; or tongue that is shiny, swollen, or shrunken.

- *Skin:* Acne; dry skin; scaly skin; boils; rashes; hives; hair loss; flushing; unusual amount of perspiration; bruise easily; slow or incomplete wound healing; pale, sallow, greyish, or slightly yellow skin color; loose or flabby skin; skin with a sharp, sour odor; facial blemishes; too many wrinkles or too much skin sagging for your age.

- *Heart:* Irregular, rapid, missed, or pounding heartbeat; circulatory deficits; angina pectoris or other forms of chest pain.

- *Lungs:* Shortness of breath, chest congestion, asthma, bronchitis, wheezing.

- *Mind:* Memory deficits, confusion, poor comprehension, difficulty concentrating, learning disabilities, slurred speech, stuttering, stammering, indecisiveness, mental fogginess, unusually slow or fuzzy mental processes.

- *Energy Level:* Fatigue (persistent or extreme), sluggish feeling, apathy or lethargy, hyperactivity, restlessness, sleepiness, exhausted after ordinary activities, tired after a long night's sleep, feeling hung-over without having consumed alcohol.

- *Emotions:* Sudden, uncontrollable mood swings, unaccountable anger, irritability, aggressiveness, nervousness, fear, anxiety, or depression, persistent negativity in outlook.

- *Other Problems:* Frequent or urgent urination; frequent colds, flus, and other short-term illnesses; a generalized itchiness; pronounced environmental sensitivity (unpleasant reaction to substances around you); unrelieved, intense allergies; immune weakness; unaccountable fever or chills; strange mucus discharges from eyes, ears, nose, and/or throat; general feeling of congestion, even long after a cold or flu is over; tendency to get a cold or flu when the seasons change.[10]

You can also assess your possible toxicity level by evaluating your lifestyle for evidence of certain traits or behaviors known to lead to toxicity:

- *Medical Care:* Do you have a history of antibiotic use? Do you frequently or continuously use prescription medicines? Take pain-killers and/or anti-inflammatory drugs such as aspirin, cortisone, and ibuprofen? Do you rely on allergy shots to get through allergy season? Do you have a dozen or more mercury-silver amalgam dental fillings? Several root-canalled teeth?

- *Dietary:* Do you drink more than two strong cups of caffeinated coffee per day? More than one glass of wine, beer, or spirits per day? Smoke cigarettes or get routinely exposed to secondhand tobacco smoke? Consume very little fresh fruits and vegetables or whole grains? Eat a lot of fried, fast, junk, or processed foods? Depend on sugary, high-fat, high-calorie foods? Eat irradiated foods?

- *Environment:.* Do you work or live in a brand new facility with poor indoor air circulation and windows that do not open? Are you exposed to new synthetic carpets or wood products that contain formaldehyde? Do you routinely apply garden pesticides or indoor insect fumigants? Do you work or live under conventional fluorescent lights? Do you drink chlorinated, fluoridated water? Do you live or work near high-tension electrical utility poles?

If any of these lifestyle practices (among the many that could be listed and which are discussed later in the book) characterize your situation, this may indicate that you are toxic to some degree. What kinds of effects can unchecked chronic toxicity have on us? That's the next subject we need to examine.

How Unrelieved Toxicity Can Compromise Your Health

The shocking fact is that toxicity may already be interfering with the health of millions. A University of California study in 1996 reported that an estimated 100 million Americans have a chronic illness or disability. Of this vast number, only a few (1.5 million) were sufficiently sick to require treatment in a nursing home or personal care facility. That means the other 98.5 million were among those "not functioning with all oars in the water," as Dr. Rogers pithily commented above. They are in the world, perhaps working, perhaps taking a lot of time off, not well, but not acutely sick either, suffering from a condition that does not get better or heal, but which persists and gradually worsens—the definition of chronic.

The study further documented that the 100 million chronically ill—this is more than one-third of the U.S. population—took eighty-three percent of the prescriptions written and comprised eighty percent of the hospitalizations recommended, sixty-six percent of consultations with doctors, fifty-five percent of emergency room calls, and ninety-six percent of professional home care. It's not just elderly men and women who have chronic illnesses. The study demonstrated that twenty-five percent of men and women under eighteen have at least one chronic health complaint, while thirty-three percent of those between eighteen and forty-four and sixty-six percent of those between forty-five and sixty-four have a chronic condition. In other words, the elderly account for only about one-quarter of the number of people with chronic health conditions, while the non-elderly (those aged eighteen to sixty-four and presumed to be in the prime of their lives) represent sixty percent of the cases.[11]

When you say chronic illness, you might as well say chronic toxicity. The links between the two are becoming increasingly obvious and empirically documented in the field of alternative medicine where this kind of etiology is understood and expected. One of the prime long-term results of unrelieved toxicity is the formation of a debilitating or degenerative condition. Not only is the link between chronic exposure to toxic substances and the incidence of chronic and degenerative disease becoming ever more evident, but in many respects the typical symptom picture for these illnesses match the list of symptoms associated with chronic toxicity. Perhaps there is only one disease, at the root of all others, and that disease is toxicity.

For instance, some alternative medicine physicians now speak in terms of "toxic triggers" for common and serious health problems. Along these lines: Alzheimer's can be triggered by aluminum, lead, and pesticides; allergies by formaldehyde and various common foods; anemia by lead poisoning and alcohol consumption; arthritis by allergenic foods; asthma by lead, milk products, allergenic foods (foods that produce allergic reactions), and exposure to mildew; autoimmune disease by mercury and silicone breast implants; cancer by pesticides, radiation, and low-frequency electromagnetic fields; cataracts by steroids and industrial pollutants; fibromyalgia (chronic muscle pain) by pesticides; headaches by mercury and allergenic foods; hypertension by lead, cadmium, and mercury; Parkinson's by pesticides and tobacco smoke.[12]

Further, in a well-regarded book on cancer and alternative medicine treatments, of the thirty-three documented contributing causes to all cancers listed by the two physician authors, about half were directly related to toxicity.[13]

Many toxic substances are more than toxic; they are carcinogens, capable of starting a cancer process in a human body.

The term carcinogen is an important one in any discussion of toxicity. A carcinogen is something you should avoid whenever possible. Due to the ubiquity of toxic substances in our contemporary environment, you will probably never succeed in avoiding exposure to all carcinogens; your goal should be rigorous minimization of your contact. A fair number of carcinogens have been studied and characterized by health authorities, including the U.S. government, but a larger number remain unstudied and at large in the environment.

As part of the National Toxicology Program, the Environmental Health Information Service (EHIS, part of the

United States Department of Health and Human Services) published "Substance Profiles" for forty-one "agents, substances, mixtures, or exposure circumstances known to be human carcinogens" in their *9th Report on Carcinogens, 2000*. On this list you will find aflatoxins, asbestos, benzene, dyes, environmental tobacco smoke, radon, tamoxifen, vinyl chloride, and other substances you may have heard of. The EHIS also profiled 146 substances (or categories of substances) "reasonably anticipated" to be carcinogenic. Among these poisons you will find chloroform, diesel exhaust particles, formaldehyde, urethane, and a great number of other unfamiliar agents with long, chemical names.[14]

That's 187 chemical substances you should avoid, which is not as easy as it sounds, because these agents and mixtures are used throughout the industrial world in thousands of products. And 187 toxic substances represent only a fraction of the poisons out there—what about the hundreds that remain unstudied, not yet officially tagged as carcinogens?

It's estimated that eighty percent (or 48,000) of the 60,000 industrial chemicals in use have been untested for their carcinogenicity, or their ability to damage the immune or central nervous system (CNS).[15] As a variation on this statistic, another report says only ten percent of 70,000 commercially used chemicals have been tested for their toxic effects on the nervous system.[16] Further, at least 50,000 deaths per year are due to toxic exposures in the workplace, while another 350,000 new cases of illness occur as a result of workplace-related exposures every year.

These deaths and illnesses include lung cancers from asbestos; bladder cancer from dye exposure; leukemia and lymphoma in workers exposed to benzene and ionizing radiation; chronic bronchitis from dust exposure; numerous CNS disorders from exposure to pesticides and solvents; and cardiovascular disease from carbon monoxide exposure. Bear in mind, these are conservative figures, based on 1992 data, so you can safely assume the numbers are now higher.

You can make the case for the health-damaging effects of long-term unchecked toxicity by looking at the change in morbidity (disease prevalence) and mortality statistics since 1980. Between 1980 and 1992, the United States death rate due to infectious diseases increased by fifty-eight percent. A fair amount of this was due to AIDS-related deaths, but there was also a measured increase in the death rate from respiratory infections (up twenty percent) and from blood poisoning (septicemia, up eighty-three percent); and mortality from infections increased by twenty-five percent among the elderly (sixty-five and older). In 1980, death by infectious disease was not even in the list of the top four killers, but by 1992, it had become number three.[17] Why?

Conventional doctors point to the failure of standard antibiotics to kill the old germs, now known as antibiotic-resistant microbes. Perhaps. But the more astute medical researchers are pointing to sustained damage to the human immune system due to our constant exposure to toxic chemicals. For example, cases of asthma increased by fifty-eight percent between 1970 and 1992, a trend that led the National Academy of Sciences to state that the various known common air pollutants (nitrogen dioxide and ozone) "interact with allergens to increase the frequency and severity of asthma attacks."[18]

In other words, pollutants plus a predisposition to allergenicity equals more asthma. Once you damage or compromise the function of the immune system, you become vulnerable to more illness, more infectious disease. When the immune system is damaged by chemical exposure, this can result in heightened allergic reactions to specific or, in many cases, to any chemicals.

The more pronounced chronic illnesses, such as chronic fatigue syndrome (CFS), environmental illness (EI), and multiple chemical sensitivities (MCS), point acutely, even dramatically, to the way unrelieved toxicity can generate a host of unpleasant, debilitating, *seemingly* unrelated symptoms sufficient to seriously incapacitate a person. But the symptoms *are* related: they are the "fruit" of unchecked toxicity. But this is, without qualification, poisoned fruit.

Of these three major conditions, EI and MCS tend to be ignored, denied, misdiagnosed, or willfully marginalized by conventional physicians. At the same time, worldwide membership in MCS support groups increases at an average of 132% per year, while a 1995 survey by the Chemical Injury Information Network of White Sulpher Springs, Montana, revealed that MCS is reported (by patients) as a health problem in 36 countries, including France, South Africa, Brazil, and Croatia.

One recent study showed that sixty-seven percent of patients diagnosed with CFS and fibromyalgia (chronic muscle pain) also had MCS; while medical professionals estimate 0.5% to 1% of the total population suffers from MCS, MCS support groups place that figure higher, at 10% to 15%. Among the top three chemical offenders most commonly listed in MCS cases are pesticides, formaldehyde, and solvents.[19] (For more on MCS, see chapter 10.)

Consider the typical or composite symptom list for a person suffering from environmental illness (EI). The symptoms run the gamut of neurologic, immunologic, respiratory, endocrine, cardiovascular, and genitourinary dysfunction. EI symptomatology is staggering (see figure 1-1).[20]

It doesn't take too much imagination to see that the symptom picture of EI (or CFS, MCS, or even, to some extent, fibromyalgia) is highly similar to the standard list for toxicity symptoms. The symptom lists for chronic fatigue, multiple chemical sensitivities, and fibromyalgia are also suggestively similar. In these intensely debilitating conditions, you can see the body-wide effects of unchecked toxicity.

Figure 1-1. The Staggering List of Symptoms for Environmental Illness

Many of these are also symptoms of chronic toxicity

headaches, often migraine	cold intolerance	congenital anomalies
loss of short-term memory	depression	genitourinary tract disease
forgetfulness	carbohydrate intolerance	requiring hysterectomy
tension	increased sensitivity to body	frequent colds
sleepiness	molds	bronchitis
cognitive dulling	adrenal depletion	congestion
confused thinking	immune system	asthma
learning disabilities	dysregulation	shortness of breath
spaciness	menstrual cramps	joint and muscle pains
visual anomalies	hyperactivity	spasms
falling accidents	laryngitis	backaches
clumsiness	increased pulse rate	sinus infections
bladder and bowel	heart pounding	hypothyroidism
incontinence	skipped heart beats	nasal stuffiness
bloating	faintness	dizziness
diarrhea	chronic nausea	earaches
indigestion	skin rashes	watery eyes
constipation	eczema	blurred vision
alcohol intolerance	sore throats	
fatigue	miscarriages	

The body's natural detoxification systems—liver, kidneys, intestines, and lymph and immune systems—are overwhelmed by the toxic load. They are so swamped by the poisons they can barely function and the body falls apart, system by system, leaving the person vulnerable and reactive to nearly everything. For good reason, the popular press has dubbed environmental illness "20th century disease," and characterized its sufferers as being "allergic to the 20th century."

The body's natural detoxification systems—liver, kidneys, intestines, and lymph and immune system—are overwhelmed by the toxic load. They are so swamped by the poisons they can barely function and the body falls apart, system by system, leaving the person vulnerable and reactive to nearly everything.

Being Slowly Poisoned Throughout a Lifetime

Some people are so toxic they are "an entire organic chemistry lab" in themselves, says William J. Rea, M.D., president of the Environmental Health Center in Dallas, Texas, which he founded in 1974 as a facility to detoxify patients of chemical toxicity. Like Dr. Rogers, Dr. Rea is one of the leading medical authorities in forwarding this new understanding of systemic toxicity and its relationship to chronic illness.

Early on, Dr. Rea's research showed that our industrial chemical pharmacy is evident even in the newborn. When he analyzed the blood of new mothers, and the chemical composition of the umbilical cord blood of their infants, he found numerous chemicals present in both, including toxins such as acetone, benzene, styrene, carbon tetrachloride, and methopropyl-ketone. Often the levels were higher in the babies than in their mothers, suggesting "bioconcentration in the newborn."

In another study, Rea tested the blood levels of pesticides in 200 chemically sensitive patients. Among the highest concentrations of chemicals, Rea found DDT and DDE in sixty-two percent of the samples, Hexachlorobenzene in fifty-seven percent, Heptachlor epoxide in fifty-four percent, Beta-BHC in thirty-four percent, and Endosulfan 1 in twenty-four percent. In another study of volatile organic chemicals in 114 patients, Rea found tetrachloroethylene in eighty-three percent, toluene in sixty-three percent, xylene in fifty-nine percent, and six other major chemicals in a range of twenty-two to fifty percent of patients tested. Rea next tested for aliphatic hydrocarbon solvents (found in glue, cement, adhesives, paint thinner, plastics, gasoline) in eighty-five chemically sensitive patients. He also discovered seventy-two patients had detectable blood levels of solvents, and eighty-five percent had at least three solvents present.

In a different test of 200 patients Rea found that ninety-nine percent had residues at or above 0.05 parts per billion of chlorinated hydrocarbon pesticides, while the mean was 3.4 pesticides per patient. "These data suggest that chlorinated hydrocarbon pesticides are extremely common in the patient population investigated . . . (any) of which may be capable of inducing a variety of biochemical changes at low levels."[21]

Not only can multiple toxic chemicals present in the body produce numerous physiologically based symptoms, they can also generate many of the symptoms normally associated with "mental illness." In a clinical study of forty-two subjects under a month's treatment for hypersensitivities and allergies, Rea found that a variety of psychological states—depression, mental blankness, anger, a sense of physical detachment, anxiety, psychotic behavior, emotional disruption, fatigue, and concentration deficits—have been linked to allergic exposures to chemical substances, fumes, and industrial products.

He also proved the case in reverse. When these chemically toxic patients were detoxified, they showed "a significant measure of relief from such states as depression, alienation, suspiciousness, and misspent emotional/physical energy, and an increase in effortful cognitive processing." They also had "substantial gains in essentially all spheres of activity." Depression is one of the cardinal signs of an adverse reaction to environmental toxins, Rea stated.[22]

Sometimes it's easier to understand how long-term, low-dose toxicity works and what effects it has on the body by considering what happens when a person has an acute reaction to a larger than typical exposure to common toxic elements such as paint or dry-cleaning materials. Study a case of pronounced, short-term clinical toxicity and you'll see a condensed version of what it's like to be slowly poisoned throughout a lifetime. It's the slowness that makes us often miss the body's indications that a toxic state exists.

"Most persons 'enjoy' good health, and have a tendency to dismiss 'minor' symptoms, attributing them to a 'cold,' the 'flu,' or some temporary inconvenience," observes Janette D. Sherman, M.D., a physician based in Alexandria, Virginia, who specializes in toxicology. Because of this masking and misinterpretation of body symptoms, illness gets established and is often far advanced before a person typically seeks medical help.

Most people, says Dr. Sherman, ignore the early symptoms—a change in bowel, sexual, or bladder function; shortness of breath during mild exercise; confusion and memory loss—but when their inconvenient symptoms become too significant to discount, *then* they seek a physician. If they're lucky, they might find one who understands the links between toxicity and symptoms. Here are some cases from Dr. Sherman's practice that illustrate these links:[23]

- **Case: Toxicity from Paint Exposure**. A man worked in the paint industry as a mixer for almost thirty years. He routinely handled heavy leaky bags of pigments and was exposed to urethane acid and vinyl paints; he also handled various toxic chemicals such as toluene, benzene, and others, and said his shoes and socks were often soaked from having absorbed the floor spills of these chemicals. When he was fifty-two, he reported chest pain and soon after developed cancer. In the next three years, he became so short of breath he had to use an oxygen mask when he slept. By the time he was fifty-five, he was "permanently and totally disabled," says Dr. Sherman. Thirty years of daily toxic exposure had nearly killed him, and what life was left him he would spend as a cripple.

- **Case: Toxicity from Dry-Cleaning Solvent Exposure**. A teenager worked in a dry-cleaning shop. One day she had to mop up some thirty gallons of dry-cleaning solvent that had leaked all over the floor. Two days later she was in the hospital, complaining of headache, shortness of breath, and dizziness. Five days after this, she was back in the emergency room reporting chills, fever, and nausea. A year later, she was still having headaches, as well as vision problems, memory deficits, and a lack of interest in socializing. An examination revealed other neurological problems, including lack of muscle coordination, emotional disturbances, and mental deterioration. She was so sick that at eighteen, she was unable to remain in school. Her exposure to the dry-cleaning solvent—most likely 1,1,1-trichloroethane, says Dr. Sherman—produced "undoubtedly irreversible" brain damage.

- **Case: Toxicity from Coffee Filter Exposure**. This case involved a man who worked in a factory that made paper coffee filters. One day he went to his doctor complaining of headaches over his right eye and ghost images; he said he'd been suffering daily with the ghost images for six months, but from the headaches for two years. Various clinical tests (X-rays, CAT scans, and others) were performed, but the results came back normal. Over the next few years, as his symptoms did not abate, the man was put on a roster of different drugs, and received more tests and procedures. After five years of headaches, by then age forty-five, he was no better, and he was given even stronger drugs. Within the next year, he sustained three heart attacks and was sicker than ever.

  This unfortunate man became "a walking pharmacopoeia and suffered an irreversible side effect from his medication, while the *cause* of his illness went unquestioned and unrecognized," comments Dr. Sherman. The medical mystery of this man's case was that no doctor had thought to ask him about his work history and possible exposure to toxic substances. Instead, they chased after his symptoms with various medical "magic bullets," failing to help him because they never understood the cause of his sickness. It turned out the coffee filters were permeated with a resin containing formaldehyde, the vapors of which were released in the process. The man inhaled this gas every day. Formaldehyde is a well-known and widely documented toxic substance, capable of producing a great number of symptoms.

- **Case: Toxic Effects on the Central Nervous System**. A healthy, vigorous woman, sixty-eight, worked part-time doing lawn maintenance, a seemingly innocuous employment. One day she mowed the lawn, raked the clippings, and bagged them, as she usually did. About ten days later, she had a persistent headache and a prickly sensation in her legs. Two weeks later, her legs had become so weak she couldn't climb the stairs in her house, and she tended to lose her balance and fall backwards. Two months after the original incident, she was unable to work at all. She was experiencing intense pain and numbness in her legs and had a chronic rash on her upper torso. A clinical evaluation showed she had an acute case of nerve toxicity.

It turned out the lawn she had been maintaining had been sprayed with herbicides to kill the weeds. The specific chemicals in the pesticide formula have been linked with neurotoxicity, cancer, skin disorders, and birth defects. In mowing, raking, and bagging the grass clippings, the woman inhaled a strong dose of these killer chemicals.

- **Case: Toxic Effects on the Respiratory System.** A man, aged thirty-three, was in good health and physically fit. One weekend a pesticide was sprayed inside the office building where he worked, but during its application, the ventilation system was not running, which meant the pesticide fumes remained inside the building. When he reported to work on Monday, the man detected an offensive odor in the building, and soon noticed dizziness and burning sensation in his chest. He began to feel listless. In a few days, he ended up in the hospital with a respiratory infection and remained there for almost two weeks. Nine months later, the office building was sprayed again. This time, within three hours of being exposed to its indoor air, the man developed cold symptoms; a few days later at work, he got nausea and chills, then fainted. He lost six weeks of work from a chest obstruction; when he returned to work, he got sick immediately, with the same symptoms.

His was a case of acute pesticide toxicity, says Dr. Sherman. The specific pesticide used (a semisynthetic pyrethroid mixed with aromatic hydrocarbons) is known to be an allergenic chemical. It is also known that once you are exposed to it and manifest allergic symptoms, the next time it will take a much smaller dose to produce the same, or worse, reaction. You may also start reacting to products chemically similar to the original offending substance.

These cases represent a problem of increasing prevalence, says Dr. Sherman; she calls it "chemical assault." A healthy, previously nonreactive person is exposed to a toxic pesticide or other chemical agent without his or her knowledge or consent, and sickens immediately. Worse, a previous ability to tolerate some degree of toxic exposure is now removed. Once the chemical sensitivity has been induced, the person becomes "symptomatic after exposure to levels of agents that previously would not have bothered him." The chemical assaults are often not minor or temporary, Dr. Sherman adds. They can result in "life-long adverse effects."

The discerning reader may query: But most of us are never exposed to such high or prolonged doses, so how can this be relevant? These cases of acute toxicity are a kind of time-lapse photograph of the toxic process. It's true, their effects are exaggerated in terms of what most people are likely to experience, but the symptoms and consequences are right on point for what unrelieved toxicity will eventually produce in anyone over a lifetime, or sooner. These people were sickened fairly quickly and noticeably; the rest of us just have weaker doses of the same poisons, so we will grow ill more slowly. But the life-long adverse effects and induced chemical sensitivity are still the outcome, and they are what we must contend with as a result of merely living in the industrialized world today.

HEALTHY LIVING SPACE DETOXIFIER #2
Maintain a Household Toxic Exposure Inventory

The life of the typical North American routinely exposes one to a stunning variety of toxic substances (in the guise of familiar, presumed "safe" consumer products) that can slowly poison us. But we assume their safety at our peril. Among the familiar consumer products that we must now regard as potentially toxic are: solvents for cleaning carpets, furniture, and clothing; caustic cleaning agents for the bathroom and kitchen; household or garden pesticides; aerosol spray cans (they can leak other chemicals besides the intended ones, such as the chemicals used to pressurize the cans); cosmetics (hair sprays, dyes, shampoos, nail polish); detergent soaps; and plastic food and prescription drug containers.

Consider the matter of household pesticides. It is estimated that eighty percent of U.S. homes have an average of three to four pesticide products in use, such as pest strips, bug bombs, bait boxes, flea collars, pesticidal pet shampoos, and others. It is further estimated that about 70 million U.S. households perform

4 billion pesticide applications per year—in other words, putting on a new flea collar, applying anti-cockroach material, or spraying bugs directly. This averages out to fifty-seven pesticide applications annually per household.

Seen from a different angle, the non-agricultural use of pesticides is burgeoning and, with it, the release of ever more toxic substances into the environment and human body. The global market for home and garden pesticides is worth $7 billion annually, and is growing by four percent a year, with U.S. householders accounting for forty percent of the market for household pesticides. To get the full picture, you have to add to this staggering data the amount of pesticides used as "turf care," for lawns and golf courses. In 1999, for example, 125 new golf courses were created in Europe and 40 in Japan; Japanese golf courses now account for about 33% of all commercially applied non-agricultural pesticides in the world.[24]

The United States Environmental Protection Agency (EPA) reports that about thirty-nine percent of households use insecticides because bugs are a major problem, but thirty-seven percent of households use them even when there is no major infestation other than perhaps a few ants strolling through the kitchen. There are lots of consumer choices when it comes to household pesticides: about 20,000 different pesticide products for the homeowner, bearing 300 active ingredients and 1,700 inert ingredients (these are not listed on the labels nor are they regulated). Are the inert ingredients worth worrying about? Yes, according to the EPA, which stated in 1991 that 300 inert ingredients were "generally recognized as safe," 68 were "potentially toxic," 56 were definitely toxic, and as to the possible toxicity of another 1,300, they didn't know.[25]

Given the fact that the majority of conventional physicians still do not recognize—or understand, perhaps—the link between toxic exposure and symptom manifestation, Dr. Sherman recommends that individuals keep a log of their toxic exposures. In effect, she says, pretend you are an industrial worker in your own home and wherever you go, and maintain a daily inventory of toxic substances you are exposed to, including all household items (as indicated in the partial list cited above) with which you are routinely in contact. Dr. Sherman calls it a Consumer Product Use Record.

Here's how to do it. In one column, record the name of the product, including its manufacturer; for example, dog flea powder, irethane pillows, hair spray, carbon paper. In the middle column, record the date you used it. If you can't remember the day and month, at least record the year. In the third column, on the right, keep a log of any symptoms observed as a result of using the product.

For example, under oven cleaner, which you use monthly, you might be recording coughing in user and wheezing in young child who observed the oven cleaning; or for vinyl paint to which you were exposed ten years ago, you remember you got skin and eye redness soon after using the product; or after using carbon paper over a period of four years as part of a job, you developed itching on your face and hands; or the diarrhea and wheezing that came on after you used that insect spray.

As you gain in knowledge regarding the great number of potentially toxic substances, you will find yourself adding more items to your list, such as prepared foods, nonorganic foods (ones produced with synthetic fertilizers and sprayed with pesticides), synthetic clothing, furniture, fluorescent lights (non-full-spectrum)—indeed, *many* things you always took for granted to be harmless.

The inventory of toxic exposures should include substances you are exposed to on the job as well as in your home, or in any public facility you might visit.[26] There are several benefits to this simple task. First, as you record your own reactions to familiar products you realize how slow-acting, low-dose poisons actually affect your system. Your cough, headache, mild little skin rash—suddenly they have a traceable cause. Second, if you develop anomalous symptoms (such as allergies, headaches, rashes, aches and pains) for which your conventional doctor cannot find a satisfactory cause, you can present this list as evidence of prolonged, low-dose toxic exposure.

Third, as you maintain the list on a daily basis, you become more *aware* of the consumer products with which you surround yourself, and you begin to realize that maybe some substitutions with less toxic products might be a good idea. You begin to gradually lessen your exposure to toxic substances. This is a very important element of detoxification: reduce your exposure, and minimize your toxic dose.

Fourth, you become a more discerning, ecologically sensitive, "green" consumer, less easily swayed by the claims of advertising and custom. Convenience often has a toxic price—your health. Green always has a consumer benefit—your health. "A bland acceptance of advertising and failure to appreciate the ramifications of chemical manufacture, use, and disposal allow unecological and unhealthy practices to be promoted and to flourish without critical assessment," comments Dr. Sherman.[27]

How Toxic Is Our Living Space, Both Body and World?

The answer is straightforward: intensely toxic. In 1986, the Environmental Protection Agency gave the scientific world a preliminary glimpse at the degree to which xenobiotics had infiltrated the tissues of most Americans. As part of their National Human Adipose Tissue Survey launched in 1976, EPA studied human tissue samples for residues of fifty-four different environmental chemical toxins, or xenobiotics.

They found that 5 of these were present in 100% of the samples, 9 ranged between 91% and 98% percent of samples, and 6 were present in between 76% and 89% of samples. Not only were a wide range of industrial chemicals present in human tissue, but their concentrations in those tissue cells were high, sufficient to give every person a total toxic burden of between 57.4 to 6,350ng (ng = 1 nanogram) of toxins per gram of fat. Benzene, a widely used industrial solvent, was present in ninety-six percent of samples; toluene, a chemical used widely in industrial processes, was found in ninety-one percent of samples; PCBs in eighty-three percent. In total, twenty different toxic compounds were detected in seventy-six percent of human tissue cells tested. Further, seventy-six percent of the people tested carried 25,704ng of total toxic compounds per gram of fat.[28]

Another U.S. government study from the late 1980s examined 5,994 people aged 12-74 for toxic residues and found that 99.5% had blood levels of p,p-DDE (derived from a pesticide) equal to or greater than 1 part per billion (ppb), with a range of 1 ppb to 379 ppb.[29] Autopsies of deceased elderly Texas residents showed traces of five pesticides or pesticide breakdown products in 100% of the tissue samples studied.[30] Another study of Michigan school children aged four showed that seventy percent had residues of DDT, fifty percent of PCBs, and twenty-one percent of PBBs.[31] "These ongoing assessments have shown quite clearly it is not a question of if we are carrying a burden of toxic xenobiotic compounds; it is a question of how much and how they affect our health."[32]

Often contamination comes from common, everyday products we take most for granted, such as cosmetics, solvents, detergents, plastics, lubricating oils, and wood finishes. Scientists at the Centers for Disease Control (CDC) and Prevention's National Center for Environmental Health examined urine samples of 289 adults, aged 20-60 years, for traces of metabolites of seven toxic substances called phthalates. This chemical family represents yet another toxic substance commonly contaminating humans at this time.

These are chemicals commonly used in the products mentioned above (although mainly as plasticizers in PVC products); as a result, they are described as "ubiquitous industrial chemicals" with "multiple exposure routes" for humans, according to the scientists at CDC. Humans may be exposed to these chemicals orally, through the skin, through breathing, or intravenously. When these substances are broken down in the body, their presence can be traced by way of their metabolites, the new chemical form in which they exist and can exert toxic effects inside the body.

All seven of the phthalates have a wide range of chemical and toxic characteristics, the CDC scientists noted. They are suspected to be cancer-causing and they are associated with reproductive disorders based on animal studies. Not only were all the test subjects found to be contaminated with residues of these chemical substances, but the levels detected of each of the seven were high. The highest levels of exposure were to diethyl phthalate, dibutyl phthalate, and benzyl butyl phthalate, ranging from 137 to 3,750 parts per billion.

More troubling still was the discovery that women of childbearing age (20-40) had "significantly higher levels" of monobutyl phthalate, known to be a reproductive toxicant to laboratory rodents. The levels of this chemical in women of this age were higher than in any other age or gender group. Further, most of the highest exposure levels to monobutyl phthalate were found in women of the twenty to forty age group, portending possible future damage to their reproductive capacities.[33]

The release of toxic chemicals into the world environment has certainly not abated since the 1980s. So we can reasonably expect the general level of toxicity, in terms of toxic compound residues detectable in human fat cells, to be most likely higher today. In many respects, our bodies and the planet's ecosystem have been forced to deal with many toxic substances not formerly present in either context.

Thousands of new, synthesized organic chemicals—hydrocarbons (from petroleum), chlorine-based chemicals, and other potentially injurious substances such as heavy metals (mercury, aluminum, cadmium)—have been applied in every aspect of our world and its industries.

We also have to contend with nuclear radiation residues in our air and soil, left over from atomic blasts in the 1950s, and in our foods irradiated without our consent for longer supermarket shelf life. Our municipal water supplies are laced with chlorine and fluorine, both of which have toxic resumes, and our air and soil are contaminated with multiple toxic agents. The toxic world is too much with us; we have ingested it; its poisons live within us.

The *fact* of pollution is so deeply entrenched in public awareness that we almost screen it out, figuring our body will deal with it somehow. It does deal with it, as best it can, and for as long as it can. But eventually, our body's detoxification system gets overwhelmed, perhaps a little at first, then gradually more so, until the load of toxins outstrips our body's ability to eliminate them.

"One reason that so many people are walking toxic dumps is that we humans are at the top of the food chain," comments one physician.[34] Toxins bioaccumulate in the food chain, from plants, to animals, to humans. Eat a plant and you may get pesticides and synthetic fertilizer residues; eat a chicken that ate the plant and that has also been fed hormones, antibiotics, and other additives, and you get all these toxins as well in your herb-grilled chicken breast.

Drinking Water Contaminated with Pesticides and Toxic Residues

Consider the matter of pesticide and herbicide residues potentially found in fruits and vegetables in the United States. In terms of sales, pesticides are a $30 billion industry, with 62% of sales in the United States so it's not the kind of toxic substance you can easily legislate off the market.

Currently about 400 pesticides are licensed for use on America's agricultural crops, and in 1995, 1.2 billion pounds were applied to farm lands, forests, lawns, and fields—a 100 million pound increase from 1993. It is estimated that about half of pesticide use is for nonagricultural purposes—on golf courses, as previously discussed, but also in parks, on roadsides, on school grounds and in the buildings, along railroad tracks and under utility lines, in airplanes, in hospitals, in mass transit areas, in swimming pools and hot tubs, in hotels, in paper mills, and in building materials and food containers.

Here is a graphic way to conceive of the enormous volume of pesticides released into the world environment every year, which is estimated to be one billion pounds. "If put in 100-pound sacks and laid end to end, they would encircle the planet."[35] Further consider the fact that since the 1940s, approximately 15,000 different chemical compounds and 35,000 different chemical formulations have been used as pesticides. Add to this the fact that there are about 630 active ingredients present in pesticides, but that these can be combined with other chemicals present in the formulas—the inert ingredients—to make several thousand more toxic formulations.[36]

The Environmental Protection Agency has not tested all the pesticides in commercial use to determine their safety levels and maximum exposure recommendations for humans. Many may have been discontinued but their residues are long-lived and remain in the environment and possibly in human fat cells. Just because a seriously toxic pesticide such as DDT is banned in the United States does not mean another country will not use it on vegetables, fruits, and even coffee it ships to U.S. markets.[37]

When it comes to pesticides, as California goes, so goes the nation, except in this case the trend is to increasing application of toxic pesticides. California agriculture accounts for twenty-five percent of total U.S. pesticide use (and five percent of world use) such that 6.5 pounds of pesticides are used per person each year in California, about double the national rate of 3.1 pounds per capita. And total pesticide application in California is rising, up 31% between 1991 and 1995 to 212 million pounds; pesticides used only for agriculture increased by 37% during this same period.

Further, the use of the most toxic pesticides, ones known to produce cancer, increased by 129%, so that this type of supertoxic pesticide accounts for 11% of California agricultural pesticide use. Use of pesticides known to be acute toxic nerve poisons increased by fifty-two percent, and use of supposedly restricted pesticides climbed by thirty-four percent. It was as if there was a frenzy to use ever more toxic sprays to insure the California crops. "The total volume of carcinogens, reproductive hazards, endocrine disruptors, Category I highly acute systemic poisons, Category II nerve toxins, and restricted use pesticides increased 32% between 1991 and 1995, and now comprise 72 million pounds, or 34% of total reported pesticide use in the state."[38]

It's not that Californian farmers are planting more acreage; acres devoted to agriculture remained constant during this period, but the amount of pesticides dumped on each acre grew by thirty-five percent, from eighteen to twenty-five pounds per acre. Which California crops got the biggest dose of poison? Strawberries and grapes.

In 1995 alone, 59 million pounds of pesticides were sprayed on California grapes, while their strawberries were doused with 300 pounds of pesticide per acre. California fruits and nuts are dosed with seven times the amount of pesticides per acre as other crops; vegetables and melons get four times the pesticide per acre as other crops; and carrots are the seventh most heavily treated crop, receiving a disproportionately high amount of total pesticides as well as some of the most toxic. Also high on the pesticide list are tomatoes (fresh and for processing), almonds, oranges, dates, pears, lemons, and cabbage.

So if you're buying "fresh" fruits and vegetables in the winter, you might wish to keep these figures in mind because every grape, strawberry, and most vegetables will enter your kitchen bearing residues of this vast volume of pesticides. From the toxic fields of California to your overworked liver.

If you live in California, your potential toxic exposure to pesticides is even greater. Consider first the ramifications of "pesticide drift." When a pesticide is applied to a field, a certain portion of it drifts off in the air currents and is blown elsewhere. But something else happens, and that is even more troublesome. After application, pesticides emit a large amount of gas. This is a reactive organic gas, the components of which are known collectively as volatile organic chemicals, or VOCs, and which contribute to smog. These VOCs can cause cancer, birth defects, and damage to the nerves, heart, and kidneys. Pesticide use—and drift—in California represents "the tip of a 100-million pound iceberg of hazardous chemicals emitted statewide each year," according to the Environmental Working Group (EWG), an ecological advocacy group in Washington, D.C.

During a two-year period, from 1996 to 1998, EWG collected 100 air samples from eight agricultural counties in central California. About two thirds of the samples contained toxic pesticides. In another test of fifty-five air samples, EWG found that fifty-three percent tested positive for traces of carcinogenic pesticides or ones known to produce birth defects and/or damage the brain. In a test of thirty-nine air samples, eighty percent had traces of methyl bromide, a fumigant that causes nerve damage. EWG estimated that statewide about 98.9 million pounds of VOCs are emitted from pesticides applied for agricultural land in California. In the San Joaquin Valley, one of the state's prime farming regions, 34 million pounds of VOCs are emitted each year from pesticides, representing 13% of VOCs from all possible sources in that region.[39]

Consider the data published by the World Resources Institute in 1996 on the public health risks of pesticides and their effects on the human immune system.[40] "Hundreds of millions of people are significantly exposed to pesticides every day, either directly in farm and garden use or in residues in water, air, and food." Children in rural areas and breastfeeding infants whose mothers have been exposed can receive "substantial doses" of pesticides. Insofar as pesticides can suppress the immune system, the risk is greatest with infants and children, as well as the elderly or those chronically ill or malnourished.

In fact, the Institute reported that based on studies from Canada and Russia, children and adults exposed to pesticides "suffer similar immune system alterations and higher rates of infectious disease" than the general population. A study in Moldova showed that eighty percent of children living in agricultural districts, where pesticide application was heavy, had suppressed immunity as a result of pesticide toxicity. They were also three times more likely to have an infectious disease of the digestive tract, and two to five times more likely to be ill with a respiratory illness than children living in non-farming districts. Even more striking was the data from India showing that Indian factory workers chronically exposed to pesticides registered a sixty-six percent decline in white blood cell counts; after three months' vacation away from the offending factory, their white blood cell counts returned to a normal level.

Exposure to pesticides is now being linked to Parkinson's disease, according to a new study from Stanford University's School of Medicine. Researchers interviewed 496 patients diagnosed with Parkinson's regarding their pesticide exposure (through home and garden pesticide use). They found that people exposed to in-home insecticides were seventy percent more likely to develop Parkinson's than those who had not been exposed. The average amount of time for exposure was about seventy-seven days. The study concluded that exposure to garden insecticides brought a fifty percent increased risk of developing Parkinson's. The amount of time people spent using pesticides was directly related to their disease risk. People who handle herbicides for up to thirty days (total exposure) had a 40% increased risk; people who were exposed for 160 days, had a 70% heightened risk.[41]

Yet another source of toxicity through agriculture is the practice of incorporating industrial toxic waste materials into fertilizer used by farmers. Among the most prevalent toxic substances found in hazardous-waste-derived fertilizers are lead, cadmium, chromium, nickel, zinc, copper, sulfuric acid, and dioxin. According EWG, each year millions of pounds of toxic waste materials are used to make agricultural fertilizers. The toxic sludge is typically laden with metal and chemical impurities, steelmill smokestack ash, air pollution scrubber brine, and other industrial byproducts. These byproducts become basic materials for "a substantial portion" of all fertilizers used in U.S. agriculture.

EWG states that more than 600 companies in 44 states shipped 270 million pounds of toxic wastes to farms and fertilizer companies between 1990 and 1995. California was in the top three both for states that shipped hazardous wastes and for those that received them for fertilizer material.

Although, in *theory*, says EWG, fertilizers are subject to federal toxic chemical contamination standards, in *practice* "there is almost no monitoring of fertilizer or soil contamination levels" and they may be "much higher" than the allowable limits.[42] The implications are obvious and upsetting: the toxic substances get absorbed by the plants, which get consumed by either people or animals.

Further, one of the chief hazards of this intense and wide-spread use of pesticides and herbicides is that invariably some portion of the volume applied runs off into public water supplies. World Resources Institute states that eighty-five percent to ninety percent of agriculturally applied pesticides get dispersed into the air, soil, and water, and not on the intended plants, thereby guaranteeing environmental pollution.

For example, municipal and private well water sources in farming states tend to have high levels of pesticide residues. Traces of at least one pesticide were detected in forty percent of wells tested in Minnesota; twenty-eight out of seventy wells had one or more pesticides in Iowa; and in northeast Iowa alone, at least seventy percent of the wells tested had pesticide contamination. In thirty-eight states, traces of as many as seventy-four different agricultural pesticides were detected in groundwater sources.[43]

One of the chief hazards of this intense and widespread use of pesticides and herbicides is that invariably some portion of the volume applied runs off into public water supplies.

In California alone, researchers found evidence of fifty different pesticides in the groundwater. As of late 1999, more than one million residents of the state's Central Valley (where much of the agriculture happens) were consuming water contaminated with DBCP, a pesticide regarded as one of the most potent carcinogens (it produces testicular cancer) presently available. DBCP contaminates were found in the tap water of 38 communities in nine counties and at amounts far above the recommended safety level. In 19 communities, bottle-fed babies, by the time they turned one year old, had already received a lifetime's "safe" dose of DBCP through the infant formula mixed with tap water. The fact that DBCP was banned nationwide in 1979 has not stopped the toxic substance from showing up in the tap water of California's Central Valley twenty years later.[44]

In the farming-intensive American Midwest, one of the most toxic pesticides, atrazine, is now showing up in the tap water of nearly 800 communities. Approximately 10.5 million people are affected by this atrazine-polluted tap water. "Some tap water is so contaminated that infants get their lifetime limit of atrazine before they are four months old," and in forty midwestern towns, they get it by their first birthdays.[45]

EPA data indicates that 34 million Americans in 6,900 communities drink tap water contaminated with arsenic[46] at levels that pose a health risk. Several national surveys found arsenic traces in three percent to thirty-nine percent of all drinking water samples studied, with concentrations averaging 10 ppb (parts per billion) or less. What's a safe level for arsenic? The World Health Organization (WHO) says 10 ppb, EPA says 50 ppb, but the Natural Resources Defense Council (NRDC) says it should be only 3 ppb. NRDC is contemplating a lawsuit against EPA to force the agency to revise the 58-year-old arsenic standard.[47] A different study conducted by the U.S. Geological Survey showed that 10% of the 18,850 samples tested (private wells and public water supplies) had arsenic at levels that exceeded WHO's safety standards of 10 ppb.[48]

So what happens if you drink arsenic-tainted water for a fair bit of time? You could get heart disease or prostate cancer, and/or die sooner than expected. Researchers for the EPA studied the relationship between various arsenic levels in public and private drinking water (wells) in towns in one county in Utah. The arsenic levels ranged from 14 to 166 ppb—in other words, from well under the EPA's safety limit to more than three times it. EPA researchers found that sustained arsenic ingestion led to a higher rate of deaths from heart disease, prostate cancer, and kidney inflammation in men; in women, more died from all forms of heart disease.[49]

Finnish researchers found that even very low exposure levels of arsenic were associated with an increase in bladder and kidney cancer. They studied the water consumption patterns of 275 subjects over a 14-year period as well as 61 cases of bladder cancer and 49 cases of kidney cancer.[50] The lesson here is that *low* exposures to a *single* toxic substance *sustained* over time can still produce serious health consequences.

Toxic substances also enter public drinking water sources from nonagricultural sources, such as heavy industry. In May 2000, the EPA reported that U.S. total toxic pollution was three times worse than previously estimated. The EPA stated that in 1998, 7.3 billion pounds of toxic materials were dumped into the environment, an amount three times higher than the previous measure, obtained a few years earlier. According to the EPA, sixty-three percent of the increase in toxics comes from the mining and electric utility industries. The mining industry alone dumped 3.5 billion pounds of toxics in 1998, mostly in the form of heavy metals and caustic materials applied to ores to leech out minerals. U.S. electric utilities dumped 1.1 billion pounds of toxic substances (including hydrochloric acid, sulfuric acid, and hydrogen fluoride, all emitted as airborne pollutants) into the U.S. environment in 1998.[51] Bear in mind, this data describes toxic releases for only one year from only two sources of pollution.

When you talk about contaminated water, inevitably the subject of chlorine comes up. If you are a public health official, your attitude about chlorine is that it's a chemical hero; but if you're versed in nutrition, biochemistry, and toxicology, you think of chlorine as a substance to avoid. Ever since 1908 when the first public water supply was chlorinated (in Boonton, New Jersey), Americans have been drinking, cooking with, showering, and bathing in chlorinated water such that today the water of seventy percent of Americans is chlorinated. The subject of chlorinated water and how to minimize your exposure to it is discussed in detail in chapter 4, but there is an interesting observation to make here.

You would logically think drinking chlorinated tap water, versus bathing or showering in it, would be the less healthy of the two activities. But it's not. "The simple, relaxing act of taking a bath turns out to be a significant route of exposure to volatile organics," as Sandra Steingraber commented in *Living Downstream*.[52] Volatile organics are carbon-based compounds that vaporize more readily than water. Chlorine is one. A recent study showed that elevated levels of volatile organic compounds, including chlorine, can be detected in the exhaled breath of people who have just showered. From the shower spout to your cells, as it were.

Taking a ten-minute shower or thirty-minute bath can give you a higher internal dose of volatile compounds (including chlorine) than drinking a half-gallon of chlorinated tap water. One reason a bath chlorinates you more fully than a glass of tap water is that the latter goes essentially from your mouth to your liver, where it is broken down (metabolized) before its components enter the bloodstream. But when you shower or bathe, your skin is enveloped in the subtle chlorinated fumes, your lungs get a direct infusion through your inhalations, and still more volatile-compounded water may enter your system through your body's orifices.

Consider this strange yet revealing example. A 1984 study in Illinois showed that 150 private wells and one municipal well were intensely polluted with volatile organochlorine solvents. Five years later, a follow-up study of the indoor air quality of the homes serviced or affected by those same toxic wells found elevated levels of the organochlorines in the blood of the residents. However, their blood levels were more in accord with the organochlorine level found in the indoor air rather than in the contaminated water.

Researchers found that the air levels were more or less matched with "shower run times"—how long the residents ran a shower. These studies "support the notion that inhalation contributes more significantly to overall body burden of volatile organic compounds than drinking—even when water contamination is dramatic," said Steingraber.

When Prozac, Viagra, and Sunscreen Flow through Your Kitchen Tap

There is another reason to be circumspect about wells and public water supplies. Evidence is increasingly accumulating that groundwater and municipal water supplies may be contaminated with a new class of pollutants: residues of pharmaceutical drugs given to humans and animals. Traces of substances such as antibiotics, hormones, pain killers, tranquilizers, and even chemotherapy agents are being measured in drinking water. German researchers announced in 1998 that they had discerned thirty to sixty drugs in a typical water sample, some of which were at concentrations comparable to the level at which pesticides are found in water (parts per billion).

The German researchers specifically detected clofibric acid, a drug used to reduce blood cholesterol levels. It wasn't only German water that was polluted with this prescription drug. It turns out the entire North Sea contains a measurable quantity of this drug, specifically, one to two parts per trillion (ppt). It doesn't sound like much until you calculate that this means the sea contains forty-eight to ninety-six tons of clofibric acid. Tap water in Berlin was found to have 165 ppt, and both the Danube and Po Rivers had traces of the drug.

How did all this cholesterol-reducing drug get into the public water? Through human excretion, then seepage into the groundwater through sewage sludge. It seems that for humans and animals, anywhere from fifty percent to ninety percent of most drugs are excreted without any chemical change.[53]

The danger of clofibric water pollution is just one example out of many that could be cited. It's more instructive to take the larger view. Two scientists—Christian G. Daughton, an environmental chemist with EPA, and Thomas A. Ternes, an environmental chemist with the ESWE-Institute for Water Research and Water Technology in Wiesbaden-Schierstein, Germany—provided just such a view in a landmark article in *Environmental Health Perspectives* in 1999.

First, they state that the quantity of pharmaceuticals (prescription drugs, diagnostic agents) and personal care products (fragrances, sunscreen agents, and others) entering the environment each year is about equal to the amount of pesticides used in a year. A large portion of a given drug and residues of the personal care products enter the environment unused or unmetabolized (not chemically broken down and neutralized) by the human body. More crucially, they continuously enter the environment; there is no seasonality to their discharge, as with agricultural pollutants.

They get excreted through the urine or feces, enter the sewage system, and eventually find their way into the waterways, and still later, into the bodies of animals and people drinking that water. Or they might get collected in toxic sludge used for fertilizer and eventually be absorbed by plants fed to animals or humans.

The trouble is that the biochemical action of these substances is at best only poorly understood at this point. What happens when they combine unnaturally by virtue of their proximity in a given water source is unknown. Further, most drugs and personal care products were never tested for their environmental impact, only for their effects on the human user. This is highly risky because the number of pharmaceuticals and personal care products is escalating, "adding exponentially to the already large array of chemical classes" that can potentially pollute the environment.

Daughton and Ternes list sixty-six classes of pharmaceuticals (which include 200 of the most popular prescription drugs), all of which are designed to have powerful, deep-set biological effects on living organisms. In fact, the drugs are designed to change the functioning of the immune, endocrine, or nerve signalling systems in the body. That is acceptable if you are the intended receiver—it's your prescription. But with the presence of these pharmaceuticals in our environment, most of us are ingesting samplers from an "enormous array" of prescription drugs that were not meant for us.

So consider this, state Daughton and Ternes. "A major unaddressed issue regarding human health is the long-term effects of ingesting via potable waters very low subtherapeutic doses of numerous pharmaceuticals multiple times a day for many decades." Put differently, when you pour a glass of water from the tap for your young children, you could be feeding them low levels of birth control pills, athlete's foot remedies, sunburn creams, Viagra, Prozac, Valium, and any of dozens more prescription drugs or personal care product residues. Bear in mind that low and very low do not mean inactive. For almost all of these substances, a very low dose is all that's needed to produce the intended result.

The residues of the drugs and products remain in the water for a long time, as most of them are highly persistent and resistant to breakdown. The profound danger here is not necessarily obvious, however. There is a high possibility of "continual but undetectable or unnoticed effects" on the various life forms living in the water, and the effects produced could "accumulate so slowly that major change goes undetected" until suddenly it starts to "cascade to irreversible damage." This damage can include human disease, even genetic mutation. You can't get much more toxic than that.

Even that is not the end of the problem. It is likely to get worse. The "enormous array" of pharmaceuticals will continue to diversify and grow as the human genetic blueprint (the human genome) is completed, observe Daughton and Ternes. Currently, prescription drugs work because they are targeted at some 500 distinct biochemical receptors, but as the human genome is mapped, many more receptors will be identified, such that the total number could grow by twenty times, yielding 3,000 to 10,000 drug targets. This means of course that hundreds of more drugs will be available to potentially pollute the environment and toxify animal and plant life and humans.[54]

Air Pollution—Trigger for Allergies, Asthma, and Respiratory Symptoms

Air pollution is a matter so often discussed as to be almost taken for granted or accepted as an inconvenience of modern urban life in especially toxic air zones such as Los Angeles and Mexico City. We've heard the term "smog" so often we tend to become oblivious to its meaning. Yet it remains a vital concern and is a source of heavy toxicity.

By now, each of the six major air pollutants (primarily released from automotive emissions) has its own well-researched toxic resume. The six are ozone, lead, carbon monoxide, sulfur dioxide, nitrogen dioxide, and particulate matter.[55]

Ozone is a respiratory irritant and allergen and can produce coughing, shortness of breath, chest tightness, mucus membrane irritation, allergies, asthma, and respiratory infections. Lead can cause behavioral problems and lowered IQ in children. Carbon monoxide reduces the blood's ability to transport oxygen to the body's cells, thereby affecting breathing, producing dizziness and headaches, and causing strokes or heart attacks. The two dioxides seriously irritate the lungs, producing coughs, chest tightness, respiratory illness, or even respiratory paralysis in high doses.

Particulate matter, found in smog, gets inhaled into the deepest part of the lungs where it produces lung problems. With the exception of lead, all of these air pollutants interfere with oxygen delivery. If a person is already asthmatic, exposure to any of these pollutants will worsen the condition, making them a serious health risk.[56]

Let's be sure we understand what smog is. It is defined as a sickening photochemical mixture produced in the lower atmosphere when sunlight strikes various pollutants in the air, most notably, industrial pollutants and particulates from automotive exhaust. The largest component of smog is ground-level ozone (a form of oxygen). Compounds called nitrogen oxides (produced when fuels are burned) mix with volatile organic compounds (VOCs, including organochlorines, released when liquid solvents, fuels, and organic chemicals evaporate) in the atmosphere. As most people who have been to Los Angeles know, smog is at its worst on hot, sunny summer days because smog formation is dependent on temperature and sunlight. Just about any kind of combustion-driven vehicle contributes to smog, from motor scooters to jumbo jets.

Smog is bad news because it is a strong and irritating pollutant—irritating to the mucus membranes of the respiratory tract, especially the lungs. Ironically, on a high smog day, if you're out exercising, thinking you're doing your mind and body some good by stretching the muscles and inhaling deeper, you may get these benefits, but at the cost of an increased ingestion of smog pollutants. Typical symptoms of smog toxicity include aching lungs, wheezing, eye irritation, shortness of breath, nausea, coughing, and headache.

Public health estimates state that about 15 million residents of the South Coast Basin, a 12,000-square-mile area that includes Los Angeles and three neighboring counties—it's the nation's second most populous urban area—inhale dirty air about 33% of the time. And when the smog index is high, it's not unusual to find hospital admissions higher than usual. Researchers at the Rancho Los Amigos National Rehabilitation Center in Downey, California, found that between the years 1992 and 1995, regardless of type of patient (such as age or ethnic group, excepting those older than sixty-five), atmospheric stagnation with a high degree of air pollution increased the risk and incidence of hospitalization for lung and heart problems (see figure 1-2).[57]

Even if you don't experience the obvious symptoms of the "smog complex," as it's called, you may still have smog residues in your body. Medical researchers at the University of Southern California examined the bodies of 152 deceased young people aged fifteen to twenty-five who had died from accidents or homicide. In lung autopsies of 100 of these subjects, seventy-five percent had a slight degree of lung inflammation while twenty-seven percent had signs of severe lung tissue damage. All of the bodies autopsied showed some degree of airway inflammation, thirty-nine percent had severe illness lodged in the bronchial glands, and

Figure 1-2. The 33 Top Toxic Substances Found in Urban Air
According to data provided by the Environmental Protection Agency, 2000

acetaldehyde	ethylene oxide
acrolein	formaldehyde
acrylonitrile	hexachlorobenzene
arsenic compounds	hydrazine
benzene	lead compounds
beryllium compounds	manganese compounds
1, 3-butadiene	mercury compounds
cadmium compounds	methylene chloride
carbon tetrachloride	nickel compounds
chloroform	polychlorinated biphenyls (PCBs)
chromium compounds	polycyclic organic matter (POM)
coke oven emissions	quinoline
dioxin	1,1,2, 2-tetrachloroethane
ethylene dibromide	perchloroethylene
propylene dichloride	trichloroethylene
1, 3-dichloropropene	vinyl chloride
ethylene dichloride	

twenty-nine percent had disease in the bronchial linings. In all, fifty-four percent of the youths—more than half of a group of young people randomly examined—had signs of at least one severe lung illness.[58]

Particulate matter, which in large cities is comprised of thirty-five percent to eighty percent diesel exhaust particulates, may be a trigger for allergies. Japanese scientists noted that allergic diseases are more prevalent in polluted areas and speculated this higher incidence must be due to environmental factors. They found that exposure to diesel exhaust particulates in the air produces allergic reactions in the immune system such that they felt confident in attributing some of the increase in allergies and allergic diseases to this air pollutant.[59] It gets even stranger because the airborne pollutants can make natural allergenic materials, such as plant pollens, even more irritating to the human nervous system and lungs, producing a greater degree of inflammation.[60]

Further, if you already have asthma, exposure to air pollution is likely to make your symptoms worse. A study of almost 4,000 Southern California school children (fourth to tenth grade) from twelve different communities showed that children with asthma were more likely to develop "persistent" lower respiratory tract symptoms (including bronchitis) when exposed to air pollution. Among the rest of the children, exposure to air pollution resulted in a significant increase in phlegm production (mucus in the nose and throat). Among the air pollutants, exposure to nitrogen dioxide produced the greatest number of respiratory symptoms.[61]

Particulate matter, which in large cities is comprised of thirty-five to eighty percent diesel exhaust particulates, may be a trigger for allergies. Japanese scientists noted that allergic diseases are more prevalent in polluted areas and speculated this higher incidence must be due to environmental factors.

Researchers in the former East Germany obtained similar results when they studied the respiratory health of 2,470 school children, aged 5 to 14. Some had lived in one of two industrially polluted counties (from mining and smelting), and others came from a neighboring county without any sources of industrial pollution. The health differences were striking. Children in the polluted county had a fifty percent increased lifetime prevalence for developing allergies, eczema, and bronchitis, and fifty percent more respiratory symptoms, such as wheezing, shortness of breath, and coughing than those in the pollution-free county. Further, children from the toxic counties had a lifetime higher rate of sensitization (a chronic allergic response, such that you react to increasingly smaller doses of an allergen) and respiratory disorders.[62]

Very young children seem to be especially sensitive to airborne pollutants, especially particulate matter. A study of medical visits by children to physicians in Santiago, Chile, over a two-year period showed that as the particulate concentration in the air increased, so did the doctor visits. For children under two, respiratory symptoms requiring medical visits increased by four percent to twelve percent as the air pollution increased, and for children three to fifteen years old, the rate of respiratory tract symptoms rose by three percent to nine percent.[63]

Air polluted with fine particulate matter may shorten a person's lifespan. A sixteen-year study conducted by scientists at Harvard University involving 8,111 residents of six U.S. cities showed that air pollution (specifically particulate matter content) was strongly associated with an unusual number of deaths from lung cancer and heart disease, even in people who did not smoke. The researchers also concluded that sustained exposure to particulate air pollution can reduce your lifespan by two years. Incidentally, all six cities had air pollution levels *lower* than the federal health permissible standard—in other words, the air pollution was at a supposedly safe level.[64]

A study from Central Europe found similar results, namely, more deaths as the air pollution index rose. German researchers studied mortality rates in a highly polluted region of the Czech Republic for the years 1982 to 1994. They found a 3.8% increase in the number of deaths in association with measurable increases in particulate air pollution. They also found that for each day the particulate matter concentration increased by 100 micrograms per cubic meter (1µg = 0.000001g), there was a 9.8% rise in deaths. However, the researchers found "no evidence for an association" between the number of deaths and particulate air pollution in the rural nonindustrialized area in Germany near the Czech border used for a comparison.[65]

Organochlorines—Toxic
Chlorine Blankets the Planet

Air pollution and its toxic effects are increasingly a global health concern, as numerous scientific studies show. We could also focus on a single family of chemicals to deepen our impression of the extent of environmental pollution: organochlorines.

These are synthetic compounds composed of chlorine and organic substances—chlorinated organic substances, to put it simply. According to Joe Thornton, a biologist at Columbia University's Center for Environmental Research and Conservation in New York City, and author of the landmark study, *Pandora's Poison: Chlorine, Health, and a New Environmental Strategy*, "Everyone on Earth now eats, drinks, and breathes a constantly changing and poorly characterized soup of organochlorines, including dozens of compounds that cause severe health damage at low doses."[66]

They're found everywhere, but in plastics especially; anytime you burn some plastic, you release chlorine gas that can form new organochlorines. In fact, disposing of plastic waste without producing organochlorines is regarded as nearly impossible. Ever since the large-scale manufacture of plastics began in the 1940s, "a witch's brew of toxic, persistent pollutants has come to blanket the entire planet, from suburban backyards to the deep oceans, from our own bodies to snow at the North Pole."[67]

We have reached the state of universal exposure, says Thornton. Laboratory analysis of samples of human fat cells, blood, breath, semen, urine, and mother's milk all bear traces of organochlorines; you don't have to have been living near a site of conspicuous contamination to be organochlorinated. Anywhere you check in the Northern Hemisphere, according to Thornton, you will find the air contains a baseline concentration of 200 parts per trillion of trichloroethane, an organochlorine.

The term organochlorines refers to a chemical family with some 11,000 different forms now commercially produced, not to mention the thousands more formed as byproducts.[68] When chlorine gas produced by the chemical industry meets organic matter in industrial processes it forms an organochlorine. When chlorine gas is employed in the manufacture of plastics, paper, pesticides, solvents, bleach, sewage disinfectants, and numerous industrial chemicals, or in the treatment of water, the combination generates organochlorines, such as dioxins, PCBs, and thousands of other lesser-known though seriously toxic substances. You will find organochlorines in chlorinated public water, in solvents and dry-cleaning solutions, PVC plastics, and bleached paper, among many other items.

The trouble is that almost none of the 11,000 organochlorines are native to the natural world. It is true that nature produces a small number—estimates vary from several hundreds to one thousand—mainly through algae, fungi, sponges, coral, and microorganisms. But no organochlorines are known to occur naturally in animal and human tissue as a result of this generation; they don't get deposited in the fat cells of living organisms. Organochlorines, says Thornton, appear to be "completely foreign" to all vertebrates, including humans, mammals, birds, reptiles, and amphibians.

Organochlorines may have excellent chemical and industrial properties, but these same qualities make them toxic to the environment and all living organisms. Chlorine gas is highly reactive, combining quickly, indiscriminately, even *randomly*, with any organic matter it encounters, leading to numerous *inciden-*

tal byproducts of unknown but presumed toxicity. For example, chlorinating public water supplies leads to at least seventy identified organochlorine byproducts, a fair number of which are known carcinogens. This number, says Thornton, represents only twenty-five percent to fifty percent of all the organochlorines present in the water; the rest simply have not been characterized yet.

Organochlorines are highly stable, which means they persist in the environment for a long time, in some cases for centuries, it is speculated.[69] Nearly all of the world's persistent organic pollutants (POPs, discussed previously) are organochlorines. Thus their concentration in the air, water, and soil progressively accumulates over time.

Industry likes organochlorines because they enable organic chemicals to dissolve in oil, but this same trait makes organochlorines favor the fatty tissues of biological organisms, including people. Fat-soluble toxic substances are much harder for the body's natural detoxification mechanisms to flush out than those that dissolve readily in water. Further, organochlorines, as they move up the food chain to humans, can reach tissue concentrations "many millions of times greater" than those found in the outside environment, says Thornton. A 1990 Japanese study showed that striped dolphins had PCB levels 13 million times higher than the levels found in their ambient environment, the North Pacific Ocean, and DDT residues 37 million times higher.

In the 1990s, several hundred organochlorines were finally subjected to toxicology studies and were found to have serious health effects on almost every aspect of human biological functioning, including disruption of the endocrine system with effects across the generations. Even more alarming, some of these chemicals can produce effects at extremely tiny doses, in the parts per trillion range. How small a dose is this? It's a ratio "equivalent to one drop in a train of railroad tank cars ten miles long," says Thornton.

At least 190 different organochlorines (including dioxins, PCBs, and DDT) have been detected in the fatty tissues (as well as mother's milk, blood, breath, semen, saliva, and urine) of people living in the United States and Canada, and now comprise a considerable portion of their total toxic load. "Absolutely everyone" now carries a toxic body burden of these 190 organochlorines, says Thornton; since humans are at the top of the food chain, "our own bodies have become the ultimate dumps" for the products of the chlorine chemistry industry. Ironically, one way of getting some of these organochlorines out of the body is through breast milk.

The breast milk of women in the United States and Canada has been found to contain sixteen different pesticides, eighteen dioxins and furans, sixty-five types of PCBs, and thirty other toxic, industrially derived substances. The obvious consequence is that nursing infants are exposed to excessive amounts of toxic substances virtually at birth and, in many cases, even before birth as many of these substances are known to cross the placental barrier. In the case of dioxin, for example, one study showed that in one year an infant was likely to receive a dose of dioxin representing a lifetime cancer risk 187 times above the government's "acceptable" level.

At least 100 organochlorines are carcinogens, and many others are believed to be mutagenic, that is, capable of causing DNA to mutate.

Organochlorines are known to suppress the immune system, reduce sperm count, produce infertility, contribute to cancer, create learning disabilities in children, and cause many other serious conditions. They are regarded as neurotoxins (poisons to nerve and brain cells) and reproductive toxicants (poisons to the male and female reproductive systems).

For example, chlorinated hydrocarbons (CHCs) may be responsible for some miscarriages. Researchers found that twenty percent of eighty-nine women who had sustained repeated miscarriages had traces of at least one CHC in their blood at a range that exceeded the acceptable level.[70] As another example of reproductive poisoning, exposure to dioxins may contribute to endometriosis in women. When scientists examined the blood of forty-four women with endometriosis (a menstrual disorder in which monthly bleeding occurs from multiple sites outside the uterus), they found they were eight times more likely to have measurable levels of dioxin than women of the same age without endometriosis.[71]

Organochlorines disrupt the basic mechanisms by which the body regulates itself, making them "incompatible with basic physiological functions," says Thornton. For example, the level of dioxin the average human bears in his fatty tissues (clinically called the average body burden) already is enough to generate reproductive, developmental, and immunological problems in laboratory animals. In many cases, it's proven to be enough to produce those problems in people, too.

So pervasive and toxic are organochlorines that Thornton likens chlorine chemistry, the industrial process that spawned the entire class of chlorine-based chemicals, to splitting the atom.[72] Like nuclear power, chlorine chemistry is "an inherently dangerous technology of great power," an unprecedented "human intervention in the structure of matter," he says, warning that we may harness it, but we will never be able to completely control it. In fact, organochlorines may be a major contributing factor to the "global toxic pollution" under way, which is contributing to "a slow, worldwide erosion" of human health, Thornton concludes.

A Radioactive Cloud
Enshrouds an Entire Generation

Another toxic element that is so widespread in North America as to be judged ubiquitous is nuclear radiation. You can be exposed by living near a nuclear reactor or through contact with the residual fallout from atomic testing in the 1950s in the continental United States. Of the 3,053 counties in the United States, 1,321 (or more than 33%) are nuclear counties. This means the residents in those counties live within 100 miles of a reactor and are regularly exposed to radiation through the air and water.

Research by Jay Gould, a former EPA scientist and author of *The Enemy Within*, indicates that the 1,321 nuclear counties account for fifty percent of all deaths from breast cancer; that four more women per 100,000 die of breast cancer in nuclear counties than in non-nuclear ones; and that in the 14 U.S. counties that house the seven oldest reactors, there was a 37% increase in breast cancer deaths between 1950 and 1989 compared to a 1% rise everywhere else.[73]

Nearly all of the continental United States has been irradiated with nuclear fallout. Bear in mind, 184 atomic bombs have been exploded in the air over Nevada since 1945, and their fallout drifted east across the country. In fact, the combined fallout from all nuclear testing performed above ground by the United States and former Soviet Union is equivalent to 40,000 Hiroshima bombs. It doesn't matter where you live in the United States. Your soil has been visited by toxic nuclear fallout in the last fifty years.

The radioactive clouds from the earliest atomic blasts in Nevada in 1951 were tracked as they drifted across the United States, heading out over the Atlantic Ocean after passing over New England. In some instances, due to the speed with which the radioactive clouds were blown by the prevailing easterly winds, various northeastern cities "reported levels of radioactivity as high as those reported close to the test site," observes Gould. As everyone knows, many radioactive isotopes take a very long time to decay; their half-lives are reckoned in the thousands of years.

The Baby Boomers are the first U.S. population group to have been uniformly poisoned with nuclear radiation, uniformly exposed in utero to strontium-90 (a radioactive isotope generated by nuclear weapons testing) in the atmosphere making them toxic even before birth.

Medical research shows that radiation tends to affect the immune system and the activity of the thyroid gland, an important endocrine gland in the neck.[74] Nuclear radiation is also linked to low birth weights in newborns as well as breast cancer. In fact, depressed thyroid gland function, fairly widespread already in the general adult population, is now showing up more in newborns.

According to Gould's research, in fifteen states (accounting for forty-four percent of the U.S. population), the number of hypothyroid live births (babies born with underactive thyroid glands) increased by seven percent from 1986 to 1992. This was linked with releases of radioactive iodine and strontium into the environment during that time (such as by the Chernobyl nuclear reactor accident in 1986). "Hypothyroidism among newborns indicates damage to the fetal thyroid from radioactive iodine (I-131) ingested by the mother," says Gould. Between 1986 and 1987 (the year after Chernobyl), the incidence of people having underactive thyroid function rose by 8.4% in 31 states.

Seen in another way, an entire generation—the Baby Boomers, born between 1945 and 1964—are the first U.S. population group to have been uniformly poisoned with nuclear radiation. Baby Boomers were uniformly exposed *in utero* to strontium-90 (a radioactive isotope generated by nuclear weapons testing) in the atmosphere making them toxic even before birth. During that twenty-year span, says Gould, atmospheric levels of strontium-90 increased fiftyfold; at the same time, there was a fifty percent increase in the percentage of underweight newborns.

Gould observes that the true cost of victory in World War II—achieved by the atomic blasts in Japan—was "an uncontrollable epidemic rise in radiation-induced illnesses." In fact, Gould contends that Baby Boomers reaching the age of forty-five in 1995, were "contracting and dying of both breast and prostate cancer at rates unprecedented in medical records going back to 1935."[75] Among the major reasons for this increase in cancer rates, Gould says, were the toxic effects of the Three Mile Island (1979) and Chernobyl (1986) nuclear disasters, compounded by continuing radioactive emissions from the numerous nuclear power reactors online throughout the United States.

Evidence supportive of this last supposition was provided in a recent study. Between 1987 and 1998, twelve nuclear power reactors in the United States were closed down. One of them was at Rancho Seco, a densely populated area near Sacramento, California. After the reactor ceased operations, public health officials observed "significant decreases" in mortality and cancer incidence in fetuses, infants, and small children. This data contrasted with the worsening of infant health after the Rancho Seco plant opened in 1974 and started releasing low levels of radionuclides into the local environment.

"The data suggest that a relationship between nuclear emissions and adverse health effects exists, especially since fetuses and newborns are most sensitive to radiation," concluded Joseph J. Mangano, director of the Radiation and Public Health Project in Brooklyn, New York, and author of the study. The plant's closing reduced local levels of dietary radioactivity, as measured in the local pasteurized milk supply, added Mangano.[76]

Gould also provides evidence to support the point. Why are cancer rates so high in the Hamptons, the tony eastern end of Long Island, New York? Rates for breast and prostate cancer were twenty percent higher from 1978 to 1987 in the Hamptons than in the rest of Long Island, according to the New York

Cancer Registry. The reason, says Gould, is probably that for fifty years that end of Long Island has received sustained toxic doses of both pesticides from agriculture and strontium-90 from nuclear reactors (one on Long Island, and three in Connecticut, a few miles across the Long Island Sound), both of which made their way into the public water and food supply. In particular, cancer rates in five towns, just south of the four nuclear reactors, had cancer rates thirty percent higher than the county average (sixty-two towns in total).[77]

Tainted Food—Glutamates, Additives, Antibiotics, and POPs

You will encounter yet another family of toxic substances in foods. Not foods as they originate in nature, but as they have been processed by the food industry. This family is known as excitotoxins, and includes the food additives MSG (monosodium glutamate, often added to Chinese food to amplify its flavor), hydrolyzed vegetable protein (HVP, concentrated soybean protein, both an additive and a processed food), and aspartame (the artificial sweetener found in NutraSweet), all of which have been called into question in recent years. These three substances are everywhere in our prepared food system, present in almost all processed foods: as natural flavorings, flavor enhancers, spices, yeast extracts, textured protein, soy protein extracts, and in soups, gravies, and diet soft drinks.

According to neurosurgeon Russell L. Blaylock, M.D., these excitotoxins are best avoided. Ingested in prepared foods or beverages, they stimulate a body's neurons. More specifically, they excite nerve and brain cells (neurons) because of their chemical similarity to neurotransmitters, whose job is to excite (or inhibit) neuronal cell activity. But this neural stimulation by a foreign substance is not a desirable occurrence. Excitotoxins, present in the brain at unnaturally and therefore dangerously high concentrations are "neurological time bombs," says Blaylock.[78]

Research suggests excitotoxins can play a critical role in the development of neurological disorders including migraines, strokes, seizures, hypoglycemia, infections, abnormal neural development, learning disorders, Alzheimer's, Parkinson's, and possibly another eight serious health conditions.

Part of the problem has to do with glutamate, a natural amino acid. It is the glutamate in monosodium glutamate and other excitotoxins that is the toxic substance. This at first seems strange since glutamate is a naturally occurring amino acid (a protein building block) found in many foods. In whole foods, glutamate is not dangerous at all; but when it becomes free—isolated from its natural context—and used on its own as a chemical substance, then it becomes a risk. When bound in foods, it is slowly digested and absorbed by the tissues, especially muscles, before it can build up to a toxic concentration. But when you take it straight, in MSG, HVP, or any of the other excitotoxin forms, its effects are more pronounced and it becomes toxic.

Normally, glutamate is found in large but appropriate concentrations in the human brain. In fact, it is the most commonly used brain neurotransmitter, but it exists in the extracellular fluid in very small concentrations. When the body takes in additional—or excessive—amounts of glutamate through food additives and taste enhancers, the brain's natural and correct balance of neurochemicals that excite and inhibit activity is disturbed. In effect, the brain gets overstimulated, or too excited—toxically so. When the brain's concentration of glutamate rises above a certain specific level, brain cells start to fire abnormally. The brain cells start a process of slow, delayed death called excitotoxicity—they are excited (overstimulated) to death. Excitotoxins entering the body through prepared foods thus set in motion "a cascade of destruction" that leads to "serious distortions" of the nervous system.

The effects of excitotoxicity are not always immediate or obvious, but play out over time, and can easily be missed or misdiagnosed by clinicians, or attributed to other causes. While excitotoxins may not *cause* neurodegenerative conditions such as Alzheimer's, Parkinson's, and ALS (amyotrophic lateral sclerosis), they are believed to *precipitate* these disorders and probably *worsen* their pathology, says Blaylock. As mentioned earlier in this chapter, they can serve as triggers. Exposure to excitotoxins in prepared foods might be what it takes to push a person with a propensity to develop a neurodegenerative disease into progressing to a full-blown disorder.

The problem of glutamates and excitotoxins is actually a subset of a much larger problem, namely, that of food additives in general. Additives and their potential dangers have been topics of discussion since the 1970s in some circles in the United States, but today, additives and processed foods are virtually a fact of life that we've come to take for granted. While the natural foods and organic agriculture industry continue to grow, the bulk of the American food supply is still adulterated with some 3,000 additives and other chemical substances added to foods for various reasons.

What is a food additive? Think sulfites, nitrates, nitrites, salicylates, food colors and dyes, monoglycerides and diglycerides, sugar substitutes (aspartame, acesulfame K, saccharin), BHA, BHT, polysorbate 60, olestra, emulsifiers, thickening agents, calcium (or sodium) propionate, citric acid, EDTA, and many more.[79]

Nearly all food additives have a toxic resumé to some degree. For example, the yellow dye known as tartrazine and the preservative benzoate are known to cause hives in people of all ages, and hyperactivity and abnormal behavior in children. On its own, tartrazine can generate symptoms within ninety minutes of ingestion, including asthma, generalized swelling, headaches, and behavioral changes. Nitrites (in the form of sodium salts, used as preservatives) can combine with amino acids in the body and produce nitrosamines, which are potentially carcinogenic. Olestra, the notorious "fake fat" introduced into the U.S. food supply in the mid-1990s, can cause diarrhea and loose stools, abdominal cramps, and flatulence. Cochineal extract (or carmine dye), a colorant derived from insects and used in fruit drinks, candy, yogurt, and other foods, can produce life-threatening allergic reactions, from mild hives and itchy skin to dangerous anaphylaxis (toxic allergic shock).[80]

Nutritionist and food researcher Carol Simontacchi takes the subject of neurotoxins and toxic food additives a step further, declaring that our modern Western diet of prepared and processed foods is "quite literally, driving us crazy." They are "crazy makers," she explains in a new book of the same title, destroying our brains and the neurochemical foundations of our intelligence. The bulk of the foods most Americans regularly eat are devoid of essential nutrients and loaded with too many toxic chemicals, notably pesticides, says Simontacchi. They have too few of the essential organ-building nutrients and too many of the organ-damaging industrial chemicals.

The result is a near epidemic of nutrition-related illnesses such as anorexia nervosa, bulimia, deficient cognition, depression, panic and anxiety attacks, mood imbalances, various forms of mental dysfunction or illness, and antisocial, even violent behavior, among others. Our host of new, manufactured foods, Simontacchi argues, have changed our bodies and brains, altered the brain's ability to think, and even altered the structure and function of the brain itself. "When the brain malfunctions, sending bizarre messages to our mouths or limbs, we never wonder if the toxic thought is the product of a toxic lunch."

Forget proper nutrition; forget even poor nutrition. Simontacchi says our dietary approach is an expression of "anti-nutrition." Through our ill-advised food choices—either nutrient-deficient or neurotoxic—we accelerate the damage to our brains and nervous systems with the "very foods (or nonfoods) that we are stuffing into our mouths." We dig our graves with our forks, she says. We poison ourselves with nearly every mouthful.

Simontacchi argues that infants, adolescents, and adults alike consume diets that lead directly to diminished brain capacity because the necessary brain-building nutrients are lacking and toxic additional elements are present. For example, she reports that ninety percent of children under age five are routinely exposed to thirteen different neurotoxic insecticides in their food; that for infants aged six to twelve months, commercial baby food is the primary source of unsafe levels of organophosphates; and that laboratory tests of eight brands of baby food (in 1995) showed residues of sixteen different pesticides. This is no way to build a healthy, optimally functioning young brain, says Simontacchi.[81]

One class of food additives that we should be especially concerned about are antibiotics given to "factory farm" animals. These are cattle, chicken, and pigs raised in large lots and intended for human ingestion. Some 750 different drug products are approved for use in food animals, and fifty percent of the total antibiotic use in the United States is on food animals. The farm animals who receive this infusion of antibiotics are not necessarily sick. In many cases, "farmers feed livestock a low-level diet of antibiotics to attack bacteria that might require the animals' body to expend energy to kill off." Farmers would rather the animals use that energy to fatten up quickly.[82]

The farmers may make their quick profit return, but the rest of us pay the price. The antibiotic residues are passed on to humans who consume the animals; aside from the additional toxicity this presents to the human liver, antibiotic drug use in food animals actually contributes to the development of multiple drug-resistant bacteria and thereby a failure of antibiotics to work when administered to humans. In fact, the connection between factory farm antibiotic use and the failure of antibiotics to work in humans is becoming increasingly evident.

In 1974, an antibiotic called Virginiamycin was approved for livestock use. In 1999, a closely related antibiotic called Synercid was approved for human use. Soon after, researchers started to find bacteria that were resistant to Virginiamycin (it didn't kill them anymore) in fifty percent of chicken, turkey, and pork found in the supermarket. Since the two antibiotics are closely related, concern was raised that the effectiveness of Synercid might now be seriously diminished.

The Synercid-Virginiamycin example is only one among many. A medical report published in May 1999 stated that infections by antibiotic-resistant bacteria increased eightfold between 1992 and 1997.[83] Further, the resistance of one strain of the bacteria salmonella (a microorganism that produces food poisoning) to five different antibiotics grew by thirty-four percent between 1980 and 1996. In other words, in about one third of the cases, five different antibiotics will have no effect against this bacteria.[84] Chickens are a prime source for two types of food poisoning bacteria: an estimated twenty percent of U.S. broiler chickens are contaminated with salmonella and eighty percent with campylobacter.[85]

It's all insidious: you eat some supermarket-bought chicken (laced with antibiotics); some months later you develop a serious respiratory infection and are given antibiotics to save your life, and they don't—because they can't. Ironically, the antibiotics, when overused, also become less effective on the farm animals. As one commentator quipped, "Low doses don't kill bacteria—they just make them mad."[86]

Further, the introduction of yet more antibiotics into the human system (most people have antibiotic residues in their cells and intestines from various medical treatments earlier in their life) gives the liver, the body's prime detoxifying organ, yet more work, and it disrupts the delicate balance of microflora in the intestines, tipping the scale towards the toxic microorganisms. This in turn provides a "seed bed" for the development of numerous forms of bodily discomfort and disease.

Factory-farmed food animals are also laced with hormones (six are approved for use), growth hormone (bovine somatotropin growth hormone, BGH), and other toxic substances that make their way into the human body when we consume the meat, eggs, or dairy products from these animals.

Earlier in this chapter, I mentioned the term persistent organic pollutants, or POPs, the toxic "family" of industrial chemicals found almost everywhere in the modern environment, including our foods. In fact, "the major route of exposure to POPs in humans is through consumption of food," most notably, high-fat foods such as meat, fish, and dairy products, although POPs are also found in vegetables, fruits, and cereals. Ironically, once POPs enter the human intestinal tract, ninety percent of them are absorbed, which is a rate higher than a fair number of other nutrients and natural foodstuffs. Further, with infants, absorption is "nearly complete."[87]

The United States Food and Drug Administration (FDA) conducted an analysis of 155 various common foods found in the U.S. marketplace during the years 1991 to 1997 for traces of the top twelve POPs. The so-called "Dirty Dozen" include eight insecticides (aldrin, chlordane, DDT, dieldrin, endrin, heptachlor, toxaphene, and mirex), one fungicide (hexachlorobenzene), two byproducts of organochlorine production (dioxins and furans), and PCBs.

Of the twelve POPs, FDA found evidence of seven of them in the various foods tested. They found DDT residues in 136 food items, dieldrin in 100, and 14 to 34 foods contaminated with chlordane, heptachlor, hexachlorobenzene, or toxaphene.[88] Consider this carefully: 136 out of 155 foods were contaminated with DDT (remember, this was banned in the United States years ago), and 100 with dieldrin. This means that about eight out of ten foods you are likely to buy in the supermarket will have traces of DDT, and six out of ten will be contaminated with dieldrin.

A Greenpeace study on POPs in our food supply revealed that the average daily dietary intake (ADI) of organochlorines in the United States is as follows, based on 1990 statistics: 1.56 µg/person/day of DDTs; 0.12 µg of HCH (hexachlorocyclohexane); 0.1 µg of dieldrin. It's worse in other countries, such as China. There the ADI is 20.47 µg for DDTs and 5.04 µg for HCH. Vietnam is pretty toxic too: intake of DDTs is 19 µg and for HCH, 5.4 µg. India has by far the worst intake averages, with ADI of 48 µg for DDTs, 155 µg for HCH, and 19 µg for aldrin and dieldrin.[89]

Research by the FDA and the United States Department of Agriculture also showed that pregnant and nursing women tend to eat "many" more POP-contaminated foods than men. For example: both butter and pickles have been found to contain chlordane residues; DDT has been found in butter, American and cheddar cheese, sour cream, hamburger, peanut butter, and milk; dieldrin in dill pickles, pumpkin pie, butter, peanut butter, and American and cheddar cheese; heptachlor in plain bagels and cracked wheat bread. Further, according to the Environmental Working Group (EWG), which presented the government data on their website,[90] a pregnant or nursing woman tends to eat sixteen of the fifty most POP-contaminated foods, a rate much higher than for the typical U.S. male. Among the top sixteen most POP-toxic foods, EWG lists: American cheese, butter, cheddar cheese, cheeseburgers, dill pickles, hamburgers, lasagna with meat, peanut butter, peanuts, pepperoni pizza, potato chips, pumpkin pie, raisins, sour cream, vanilla ice cream, and whole milk.[91]

Yet another term used to describe these ubiquitous environment chemicals is PBTs, or persistent, bioaccumulative, and toxic pollutants, according to a report released by the EPA in September 2000. With all of these terms—VOCs, POPs, PBTs—there is a fair amount of overlap, but at the same time, they provide confirmation and public—in this case, governmental—recognition that toxic substances in the environment are a serious human health problem. Chief among the PBTs, according to the EPA, are methylmercury (mainly from tainted fish and hospital waste incineration), polychlorinated biphenyls, or PCBs, and dioxin (from pesticides).

In a report on their new initiatives to control and reduce levels of PBTs in the environment, the EPA acknowledged that PBTs concentrate in the food chain to toxic levels, and have an uncanny ability to travel long distances and to linger for generations in people and the environment. They noted that dioxin levels have now reached the level associated with adverse non-cancer effects, which is probably one-step away from being a widespread carcinogen; and that twenty-five percent of children and nine percent of adults in the United States are exposed to unacceptable levels of methylmercury. Levels of PBTs in the Arctic are expected to rise significantly due to the distribution phenomenon called global distillation (described previously) as a result of "increased local and southeast Asian industrialization."[92]

The Toxic Living Space and You—What It All Means

It is not the intent of this chapter to provide complete documentation of every source of environmental pollution and bodily toxicity. To do this subject justice would take a book in itself. It is more important here to gain an understanding of the extent of pollution and its health consequences. You have gotten a sense of the players—POPs, VOCs, PBTs, pesticides, phthalates, organochlorines, nuclear radiation, excitotoxins, "crazy-maker" foods—and how they permeate our bodies and the modern environment. And you have come to see that to some extent everyone has toxic substances within their fatty tissues and that every corner of the planet carries toxics in its soil, water, plant, and animal life.

This knowledge can seem at first overwhelming, intimidating, even depressing. Part of the reason it might seem too much to know is that, as a culture, we have known so little, and have never been encouraged to ask. So it is shocking to suddenly expand our awareness, to start digesting the awesome details of global toxicity and its permeation of our living space, both body and home. But what else would motivate us to take the needed steps to start detoxifying ourselves and to start petitioning for ecological awareness and pollution reform in society? Taking a long hard look at the extent of the damage, and the risk of still more damage, is sobering, but it gives us a sound information base upon which to build a practical program of detoxification and minimization of further exposure to toxic substances.

As discussed throughout this chapter, many of the persistent organic pollutants are very stable, very persistent, and very deeply entrenched in human flesh. It is unlikely that even the most comprehensive detoxification program will flush them all out of your system.[93] It is also unlikely that you will be able to live in such a way that you avoid all contact with toxic sources.

What is likely and therefore prudent is to *reduce* your exposure, *minimize* your contact, and *maximize* your body's excretion of the toxic substances you can't avoid. The goal of this book is to show you how (and why) to adopt many practical ways of helping your body detoxify itself of as much of its toxic load as it can and at the same time to build up your body's natural resistance to toxic substances.

One of the chief tools you need in this effort to clean up your living space is awareness. Pollutants are so prevalent, so taken for granted, so invisible in our world today that it is very easy to get exposed many times during a single day without being aware of it. Here are a few examples:

I visited some friends in another state recently. One of their neighbors was an avid gardener, and had an acre devoted to a lovely flower garden, with statuary, fountains, a fish pond, contemplation benches, and many flowering bushes and plants. On the day of my visit, she was using a small bottle with a pump to spray pesticide on dandelions growing by the roadside at the edge of her garden. The device hardly made a sound, and the liquid looked like water, but it was a poison and it was emitting little molecular clouds of toxins. I stepped back so as not to breathe these pesticide fumes, but my friend showed no such concern.

What is likely and therefore prudent is to reduce your exposure, minimize your contact, and maximize your body's excretion of the toxic substances you can't avoid.

Another friend works in an art gallery and reported this incident to me. The gallery is a small, rectangular space with no cross ventilation from front door to back door. An artist supervising the installation of his show asked if anyone on the staff—there were five people present—minded if he sprayed a "fairly nasty paint" on the wall behind his sculptures. Nobody minded, except my friend, who opened the front door and stood outside while the toxic paint was sprayed on the walls. Everyone else regarded the paint as if it were as routine as secondhand tobacco smoke, and therefore to be viewed as benign (an erroneous conclusion in both cases).

A third friend made a routine shopping visit to a small mall in a medium-size college town. When she arrived in the parking lot, she noticed a few police blocking entry of traffic at the far end, while others ran around, shouting and waving things. She parked, walked a few paces, and was about to enter a store when she smelled the foulest chemical odor she had ever experienced. She had no idea what it was, but noticed that already some of her throat muscles felt stiff, as if they had turned to wood. She left the mall and drove home.

When she called one of the stores in the mall, she was told a medical waste truck had leaked diesel and this had combined with recent acid rain to produce the smell. She was also told that officials from the Environmental Protection Agency had been called in. No diesel she had ever encountered had smelled like that, so she didn't believe the story. It took a day for her neck to feel normal again, and for all numbness to go away. But as to the health effects on all the store personnel and shoppers who were exposed to those obviously toxic fumes all that day and who were not kept from the mall one can only guess.

You can see from these three simple examples—presented to me in the space of five days—how crucial is awareness, being alert to when you are about to get a low-dose toxic exposure and avoiding it or minimizing your exposure time.

Some of the toxic agents mentioned in this chapter will be discussed in greater detail in later chapters, along with practical steps for detoxification and lifestyle arrangement to help you avoid or minimize further exposure to them. In the next chapter, we look at the body's natural detoxification system and see what happens when it gets overwhelmed by environmental toxins and can no longer rid the body of toxic substances.

CHAPTER 2

Why You Need to Detoxify:

Augmenting the Body's Natural Detoxification System

The essential point in this chapter is that while your body has innate detoxification mechanisms, the degree to which the average person is now toxic often limits the ability of these systems to work. In other words, your body may be so overloaded with toxins that it cannot do its naturally appointed job of toxin removal, of detoxification. This failure leaves you less than optimally fit, sluggish, tired, allergic, aching, sore, subject to any of dozens of symptoms, and eventually suffering a chronic health problem, or worse, a degenerative condition, such as cancer.

While the solution is straightforward—deliberately, responsibly detoxifying to unclog and catalyze the body's own internal cleansing systems—the question that must be answered is this: why is the body's natural detoxification system ineffective? What are the consequences of being toxic and unable to fully detoxify ourselves of poisons we get from our environment? How should the detoxification system work if it is in top condition? Why should we strive to return it to optimal efficiency? These are the questions we'll consider in this chapter.

The Body's Burden—Total Toxic Load and Toxic Stress

Physicians who are alerted to the necessities of healthy detoxification often speak of the body in terms of toxic overload.

They may use clinical terms such as total toxic burden, total toxic load, and toxic stress to indicate a condition of dysfunctional, inefficient, even incompetent detoxification. In nonmedical, layperson's terms, this is like a drain that is so clogged with debris it lets only ten percent of the grey water flow down, trapping the other ninety percent and creating a stagnant pool of toxic water.

Naturopaths Peter Bennett, N.D., and Stephen Barrie, N.D., have come up with an amusing yet accurate term for our life under the influence of toxins: we are in-*toxin*-cated, they declare.[1] It's like being inebriated, except it isn't alcohol we consumed, but a long list of toxins from substances in our environment; even worse, we don't even remember the "party" at which we imbibed the poisons. Drs. Bennett and Barrie, like many alternative-minded practitioners sensitive to the importance of detoxification, use the image of an overflowing barrel—a perhaps more apt analogy than the clogged drain.

Think of your body and its organs and systems as a barrel into which there is a slow, steady drip of toxic water. Eventually, unless you drain the barrel (detoxify), the barrel will overflow, and toxic water will spill over everything, will permeate parts of your body ill-equipped to handle the deluge.

Think of your body and its organs and systems as a barrel into which there is a slow, steady drip of toxic water. Eventually, unless you drain the barrel (detoxify), the barrel will overflow, and toxic water will spill over everything, will permeate parts of your body ill-equipped to handle the deluge. "That toxic overflow is the beginning of disease and disability," explain Bennett and Barrie. They add that if your detoxification system (your liver, kidneys, intestines, and immune and lymphatic systems) is overworked (which includes being nutritionally depleted or deficient, as explained below), any new exposure to toxins from foods or environmental substances and products is even harder to handle and creates an even greater toxic problem for the components of that system—your liver, intestines, and immune system. In other words, if your "barrel" is full, even a minimal toxic exposure can have the health impact of a large one.

Where does the excess toxicity go when it overflows into other parts of your body? A great deal of it accumulates in the spaces between the cells, in a place called the extracellular connective tissue matrix. "It is, in a sense, a living matrix—a place where many systems intersect and are coordinated," explains Rudolf Ballentine, M.D., in *Radical Healing*. This space between the cells is the background, the field or ground supporting the major organs; for this reason, conventional medicine tends to overlook this area as a focal point for toxicity, says Dr. Ballentine. But they shouldn't. It is crucial to the body's functioning.

This matrix is an all-purpose dump site and part of the drainage system within the body. It takes cellular and lymphatic system waste and holds it in temporary storage. The fluids in this space can get saturated with toxins and start to leak the excess into neighboring connective tissue. When the storage capacity of this extracellular space is exceeded and leakage occurs, you begin to develop signs of toxicity. For example, you may feel stiffness or pain in the body; these symptoms result from the irritation produced by these deposits in the connective tissues.

The extracellular matrix also comprises "an intricate communications network" running alongside that of the nervous and endocrine system. But if the matrix is overburdened with toxic storage, the communications don't work properly and the energy channels get compromised. At that point, you will start feeling ill, with symptoms such as general tiredness, dullness of the mind and senses, bad breath, heaviness, lack of strength, indigestion, constipation, coated tongue, and foul-smelling urine and/or feces, says Dr. Ballentine. Then you start moving "from congestion to disease."[2]

Here is another analogy by which to appreciate an overburdened detoxification system. Think of your immune system as a kettle, suggests Kenneth Bock, M.D., an alternative-minded physician who directs the Rhinebeck Health Center in New York State. Like a barrel, a kettle can hold only a finite amount of toxins. But there are many categories of toxins that can get into our immune system kettle, explains Dr. Bock.

These include psychosocial factors (such as emotional stress); environmental pollution (toxins and heavy metals out in the world); tobacco smoke; radiation and electromagnetic field exposure; prescription and recreational drugs; hormonal imbalances; infectious agents (microorganisms); allergies and other sensitivities (to chemicals, foods, plant substances); dietary stresses (excesses or deficiencies in nutrients, too many synthetic chemicals); and our genetic blueprint, which is to say, the balance of strengths and weaknesses and our general predisposition to certain types of health problems.

"Any one part of our immune system load can put us 'over the top' of the kettle if our accumulated burden is high," says Dr. Bock. In other words, we can tolerate perhaps six categories of toxins or toxic loads, but the seventh will make the immune system kettle overflow, and we get sick from the spillage. (Note that individual tolerance varies; some people might experience overflow at four, or even fewer, toxic categories.)

Here is a vivid example provided by Dr. Bock, citing a case originally described in *The Wall Street Journal*.[3] A man who was vigorous and athletic mowed his lawn and collected the grass clippings, then almost fell down dead. He got dizzy, nauseous, and developed a terrible headache. Ten days later he was just as sick, and getting worse, and five months later, he got testicular cancer. As the years passed, he had seizures, walking difficulties, and other health deficits. What had happened?

The man was poisoned by a lawn pesticide sprayed on his grass; he inhaled the fumes and they sickened him. His liver was unable to detoxify the chemical because it was already burdened with detoxifying the components of Tagamet, a drug for peptic ulcers, on top of the environmental pollutants to which we are all exposed. The constant demand to detoxify the Tagamet left him vulnerable to carcinogens and defenseless against their effects once they entered his body.

"How many of us have toxins accumulating in our bodies?" queries Dr. Bock. "The scary truth is, we all do." Many of us, shockingly, are "walking toxic dumps," he adds. It is almost impossible for anyone in the Western world today (and perhaps anywhere in the world at all now) to avoid building up some degree of immune toxic load, Dr. Bock explains, but he adds that the problem is also the doorway to the solution. Anyone can purposefully lower their immune load—drain the kettle—by a careful program of detoxification.[4]

The Oxidation-Reduction Cycle
at the Heart of Detoxification

Before we look at how we can clear our detoxification system—empty the kettle or at least pour out some of the water—it's important to get a picture of the biochemical struggle constantly under way in the human body, and meet its players: the toxins, called free radicals; and the anti-toxins, called antioxidants.

First, there are two types of toxins, or free radicals. *Exotoxins* are those that enter the body from the environment, from products, substances, medicines, additives, foods, the air and water we consume. *Endotoxins* are produced inside us, as natural byproducts of digestive activity or through illness. Sources of free radicals include pesticides, industrial pollutants, smoking, alcohol, viruses, most infections, allergies, stress, even certain foods and excessive exercise. Toxins of either type can bioaccumulate by being stored in the body's fatty tissues, including cell membranes; once the toxins are fat-soluble (as opposed to water-soluble), it is harder for the body to detoxify them.

Second, there is a natural chemical process that takes place continuously inside the body that is the key to the toxicity-detoxification situation. It's called oxidation and refers to the way oxygen combines with a substance to release energy. A fire is "fueled" or driven by oxidation, and so are the body's digestive and metabolic processes. The body uses oxygen, drawn from the outer environment, to "burn" fats and carbohydrates from ingested foods to generate energy to run a myriad of cellular processes. The body generates energy for itself by oxidizing the foods we consume in a controlled way. That's why we eat food in the first place: to provide this cellular fuel released by the chemical processes known as metabolism.

However, this process of cellular oxidation has some natural byproducts—smoke, so to speak, if this were wood we were burning—including carbon dioxide and water, which are harmless, and free radicals, which are harmful, highly reactive molecules—"molecular marauders," says Dr. Bock. All chemical reactions in the body involve the transfer of electrons, as a kind of "currency" exchange. In this case, the exchange is for energy to run the body. The metabolism of food, or oxidation, removes electrons one by one from the foods. Think of oxidation as a controlled fire that releases energy but also sends off sparks. In this analogy, the sparks are free radicals, or unpaired, unstable, chemically reactive electrons.

A free radical is a toxic molecule of oxygen with an unpaired electron.[5] A free radical tries to remedy its instability by stealing an electron from another molecule; when it does, a new free radical is produced, and this leads to a chain reaction of ever multiplying free radicals and unstable molecules. In a sense, it's the instability—the unpairedness—that creates all the damage. The proliferation of free radicals as a result of oxidation is called oxidative stress. The degree of oxidative stress can be taken as a measure of the body's capacity, or incapacity, to handle toxins and perform its own detoxification (see chapter 3).

Free radicals are formed when molecules within cells react with oxygen (oxidize) as part of normal metabolic processes. Free radicals then begin to break down cells, especially the cell membranes, often in a matter of minutes to an hour. A single free radical can destroy a cell. Their work is enhanced if there are not enough free-radical quenching nutrients, such as vitamins C and E, which are normally present in the cell. A free radical attacks the cell's membranes, eventually rupturing it; this allows the egress of bacteria, viruses, and other pathogenic microorganisms into the cell and the leakage of essential nutrients out of the cell.

Once inside the cells, free radicals can change the cell's physical structure, making it rigid and inflexible. Free radicals harmfully alter important molecules, such as proteins, enzymes, fats, even DNA. They can commandeer the cell's genetic apparatus, as it were, rewriting or destroying essential genetic programming. This in turn can lead to cellular mutations, which is only one step away from cancer.

Fat cells (the unsaturated lipid molecules, specifically) are especially vulnerable to free radical disturbance. When the fat components of cells are damaged by free radicals, lipid peroxides result. The quantity of lipid peroxides in your blood can be taken as an index of your risk for what's called oxygen free radical pathology and the chance of developing a degenerative disease as a result of widespread and continuous cell damage. High blood levels of lipid peroxides mean your system has *already* been damaged by free radicals.

Free radical pathology in many ways is the cornerstone of the model that explains how toxins make you sick. The means by which other toxic substances or procedures, such as irradiation, heavy metals, solvents, pesticides, and prescription drugs, produce pathology is by generating free radicals in the body. As free radicals can potentially damage every aspect of cell function including the integrity of its membrane, a long list of degenerative illnesses can be set in motion once free radicals start damaging your cells.

So central to the dynamics of health is the concept of free radical damage that practitioners of alternative medicine now speak in terms of free radical pathology as "a unified cause of chronic illness."[6] The term mentioned above, oxidative stress, is pivotal to this discussion of toxicity and illness. A person's degree of oxidative stress depends on the balance between the rate at which free radicals produce damage and antioxidants repair it, or the rate at which free radicals proliferate and the antioxidants quench them. If free radicals predominate, the degree of oxidative stress increases, and eventually you get sick, and still later, start to develop degenerative disease.

"Unfortunately, many people run an abnormally high level of oxidative stress that could increase their probability of early incidence of age-related diseases," states a consumer information booklet from Genox Corporation, a clinical laboratory in Baltimore, Maryland, that tests for oxidative stress. Evidence now suggests that even individuals who seem healthy may have a much higher than average (and therefore undesirable) level of oxidative stress and may already be "well on their way towards developing an oxidative stress-related disease," states Genox.

According to Genox, oxidative-stress-induced dysfunctions and diseases are many but can include accelerated aging processes; heart disease (stroke, heart attack); disorders in the gastrointestinal tract (including diabetes and pancreatitis); macular degeneration, cataracts, and other eye problems; kidney and skin disorders; nervous system problems (Parkinson's, Alzheimer's, muscular dystrophy, multiple sclerosis); lung cancer and emphysema; and serious problems with red blood cells, the liver, and immune system (rheumatoid arthritis).[7] As early as 1988, scientists were prepared to attribute at least sixty disorders to free radical damage, and one expert in the field declared that few people reach their maximum life span but rather die prematurely from diseases, the vast majority of which are free-radical-related diseases.

The theory connecting free radical toxicity with aging and disease was formulated in 1954, however, and one of its leading proponents since then has been Denham Harman, M.D., of the University of Nebraska College of Medicine in Omaha. After age twenty-eight, says Dr. Harman, "the inborn aging process" is the major risk factor for disease and death; this inborn aging process is strongly (but not exclusively) determined by free radical reactions in the body and the body's ability to neutralize them. Such free radical reactions, a growing consensus maintains, "are a major cause of aging, possibly the only one," states Dr. Harman. He adds that average life expectancy at birth can be increased by five to ten years and a "healthy active life span" obtained "by nutritious low caloric diets supplemented with one or more free radical reaction inhibitors [antioxidants]."[8]

Harman's research makes it clear that *early* detection of high levels of oxidative stress (through laboratory testing, as explained in chapter 3) gives you the chance to stop the progression of oxidative stress to disease. The earlier you can find out if you are oxidatively stressed, the sooner you can take corrective action in the form of a carefully planned detoxification program and antioxidant supplementation.

Early detection of high levels of oxidative stress gives you the chance to stop the progression of oxidative stress to disease. The earlier you can find out if you are oxidatively stressed, the sooner you can take corrective action in the form of a carefully planned detoxification program and antioxidant supplementation.

On the other side of the toxicity picture are the antioxidants, the natural elements that work against oxidative free radicals. An antioxidant (meaning "against oxidation") is a natural biochemical substance that protects living cells against damage from harmful free radicals. Antioxidants work against the process of oxidation—the robbing of electrons from substances. Antioxidants in the body react readily with oxygen breakdown products and free radicals, and neutralize them before they can damage the body. Dr. Bock uses the analogy of an indoor fireplace spewing sparks that could ignite the carpet; the sparks are free radicals, and the screen that you place preventively before the burning logs comprises the antioxidants.

The antioxidants render free radicals harmless by a process known as reduction: they add back the missing electron by giving up a molecule from themselves to the unpaired electron in the free radical. Thus oxidation and reduction form a system (sometimes referred to by the abbreviation "redox"). In oxidation, an electron is lost, producing a free radical; in reduction, the electron is given back by an antioxidant; even simpler: oxidation=electron loss; reduction=electron gain. When the redox system runs in balance, you stay healthy because your natural detoxification system works efficiently; when it runs in a state of imbalance, you get toxic and eventually, you get sick.

Adequate nutrient intake is vital to your body having the biochemicals it needs to run the antioxidant-reduction pole of the redox cycle. Antioxidant nutrients include vitamins A, C, and E, beta carotene, selenium, coenzyme Q10, pycnogenol (pine bark extract), L-glutathione, superoxide dismutase, and bioflavonoids. Plant antioxidants include *Ginkgo biloba* and garlic. When antioxidants are taken in combination, the effect is stronger than when they are used individually.

The Body's Two-Phase Natural Process of Detoxification

The human body is well equipped to handle a normal load of toxins and to neutralize and remove them from its interior. Of course in this discussion, the key term is "normal load" because, as discussed in chapter 1 and earlier in this chapter, most of us no longer carry a normal toxic burden, able to be handled by the body's innate detoxification system. Rather, many of us have far too many toxins in our bodies, a situation that tends to compromise and limit the body's natural ability to detoxify itself.

In effect, many of us are too toxic for our bodies' detoxification mechanisms to work properly, and we end up depositing toxins in various fatty tissues as "seeds" for imminent health problems. To understand how our natural detoxification pathways get blocked and dysfunctional, let's first study how the healthy body is meant to deal with toxicity through what physiologists call the liver's two phases of detoxification.

The liver is the prime receptacle of and processing center for all the toxins our body ingests or produces internally as part of its standard biological processes. As noted earlier, the kidneys and intestines are the other principal players in detoxification, but only about twenty-five percent takes place in the intestines; the rest happens in the liver. In brief, in Phase I detoxification various toxic biochemicals are modified to make them an easier mark for the detoxification enzymes that will neutralize them in Phase II. The key concept is that liver-mobilized enzymes neutralize toxic chemicals so the body can excrete them, and this process depends on adequate body reserves of key nutrients.

Phase I Detoxification

The goal of this phase, which scientists label "biotransformation," is to chemically alter in the liver any substances the liver identifies as toxins ("xenobiotics," or foreign life) and to change them into an intermediate form. You might say this is like taking the stinger out of the bee without killing it.

Generally speaking, the liver has to deal with toxins that have a preference for fat (lipophilic, or "fat-loving") and that are not water soluble, that is, they don't mix with or dissolve in water. These fat-soluble toxins also are nonpolar, which means they have no electrical charge. Phase I detoxification will make them water-soluble and electrically charged, both of which changes favor easier excretion from the body. This biotransformation is accomplished in part by the addition of an atom (or several) to the toxin, such that it loses electrons (oxidation) or gains electrons (reduction), and the removal of a specific component of its makeup, such as taking away a group of sulfur or halogen molecules.

The toxins can include pollutants that enter the body through the air, water, and foods we consume, or through medicines and drugs. They also include toxic chemicals produced naturally—that is, for a biological reason—but which, if allowed to build up internally, are toxic to the body. These include various hormones and inflammatory chemicals such as histamine, involved in the allergic reaction.

Various enzymes are required to perform Phase I detoxification, and these are known as mixed function oxidative enzymes, collectively called cytochrome P450. It's estimated that about 50-100 enzymes comprise this group. But let's stop for a moment: What is an enzyme?

An enzyme is a specialized living protein fundamental to all living processes in the body, necessary for every chemical reaction and the normal activity of our organs, tissues, fluids, and cells. Enzymes, of which there are hundreds of thousands, are essential for the production of energy required to run all the functions of cells. Enzymes enable the body to digest and assimilate food. There are special enzymes for digesting proteins, carbohydrates, fats, and plant fibers. Enzymes also assist in clearing the body of toxins and cellular debris, in addition to assisting the liver in its detoxification processes.

The competence of the cytochrome P450 system can vary considerably among individuals, due apparently to genetics, one's level of toxic exposure, and one's nutritional status. For example, it is known that, to work optimally, cytochrome P450 requires vitamins C, B2, B3, B6, and B12; copper; magnesium; zinc; folic acid; and flavonoids. If your diet has been nutritionally inadequate and you are exposed to a high degree of toxins—say air pollution in a big city such as Los Angeles—your detoxification capabilities are already set a notch or two lower than ideal. An Italian study of chemical plant factory workers, for example, showed that those with an underactive cytochrome P450 system were more vulnerable to carcinogens (substances known or suspected to contribute to the emergence and spread of cancer).[9]

What happens when the liver's enzyme team encounters a xenobiotic, or toxin? It tries to 1) change the substance into a less toxic form; 2) neutralize it by rendering it water-soluble so it can be easily excreted in the urine; or 3) convert it to a more chemically active form, making it an easier target for the Phase II detoxification (this process is called bioactivation). It is ironic that the very process of changing, neutralizing, and converting toxins itself produces free radicals, which also must be neutralized or removed from the system. Every time a foreign toxin is metabolized (chemically acted upon—"digested" in a sense), a free radical results. Each new free radical generated during detoxification can in turn harm the liver and compromise its continuing detoxification abilities. Incidentally, eating foods to which we have allergies also produces free radicals as well as the histamine and other inflammatory products related to an allergic reaction. All of these further strains the liver's detoxifying capacity.

Normally, the liver is able to handle the temporary increase in free radicals via its highly competent antioxidant protein, glutathione, which comes into play in Phase II detoxification. However, if the liver is flooded with toxins in Phase I and has to work overtime to neutralize the free radicals, this uses up the glutathione reserves, leaving none for Phase II. This highlights a tricky part of Phase I. In converting toxins to make them easier targets for Phase II, the new forms, known as "activated intermediates," can be much more toxic than the originals.

The goal is to get these activated intermediates dealt with as quickly as possible in Phase II and removed from the body. In a balanced detoxification process, the activated intermediates are generated at a rate that Phase II can keep up with; in an unbalanced process, Phase II gets overloaded with the activated intermediates and your detoxification ends up being pathological, itself producing poisons. People with this problem are known clinically as "pathological detoxifiers," and they tend to be excessively reactive to externally contacted poisons because their total toxic burden has already been reached and their Phase II abilities are dangerously compromised.

Biologists have discovered that certain foods, herbs, nutrients, and industrial or human-made substances can activate Phase I while others can inhibit its action. Among those that can trigger Phase I are alcohol, nicotine (tobacco smoke), phenobarbital, steroids, niacin, riboflavin, vitamin C, sassafras, caraway and dill seeds, oranges, tangerines, cabbage, broccoli, Brussels sprouts, and charcoal-broiled meats.

In a complementary way, specific nutrients can help the Phase I process: choline, fatty acids, lecithin, methionine (an amino acid), milk thistle (an herb), beta-carotene (a vitamin A precursor), vitamin B1, vitamins C and E, copper, iron, magnesium, manganese, molybdenum, sulfur, and zinc.

The practical aspect of this information is immediate: if you are deficient in any of these nutrients, your Phase I detoxification may be hindered; if you are undergoing a deliberate detoxification program and you supplement with these nutrients, the process may proceed at a far better rate of competence than otherwise.

But there is an equally long list of substances that can block Phase I from getting started, and these include various antidepressants, antihistamines, and other drugs; chemicals found in grapefruit juice; turmeric; red chili pepper; and clove oil. Scientists found that naringenin, a substance naturally occurring in grapefruit juice, can decrease your levels of cytochrome P450 by thirty percent.[10]

Phase II Detoxification

Chemically speaking, what happens in this second part of your body's natural detoxification process is called conjugation. This means various liver enzymes affix chemicals to the toxin, which has been oxidized or partially changed from Phase I activity, either to neutralize it or to make it easily excreted through the urine or bile. The goal is to prepare (alter) the toxic substance so it can be excreted from the body. There are six pathways in Phase II, each involving specific ways of neutralizing toxins; we might say that each of these six detoxification pathways specializes in dealing with a certain family or type of toxin.

One of the main pathways is glutathione conjugation. A liver enzyme called glutathione S-transferase (glutathione is made of three amino acids, the building blocks of proteins) combines (or conjugates) sulfur with the toxic substance making it water soluble and easily excreted. Glutathione is the body's main defense against free radicals and a key neutralizer of the free radicals generated during Phase I. "The combination of detoxification and free radical protection results in glutathione being one of the most important anticarcinogens and antioxidants in our cells, which means that a deficiency is devastating," comments naturopathic educator and physician Joseph Pizzorno, N.D., former president of Bastyr University in Seattle, Washington.[11]

The glutathione detoxification (or conjugation) pathway generates up to sixty percent of the toxins that get excreted in the bile. These include industrial toxins such as PCBs and a fair number of carcinogenic substances. Glutathione is also a potent antioxidant, collecting and neutralizing free radicals in the blood. The trouble is if your system gets overloaded by deadly toxins—by an intense one-time or prolonged exposure to toxins, such as in a chemical plant or nuclear power plant—your glutathione reserves get used up and you become essentially defenseless against the powerful free radicals. You then become more susceptible to serious illnesses including cancer because your immune defenses have been dangerously weakened.

Another important detoxification pathway is called amino acid conjugation, which involves five amino acids that combine with and neutralize specific targeted poisons. These poisons include at least four classes of drugs and five types of xenobiotics, or foreign toxic chemicals. Let's stop for a moment to be sure we understand the essential term, amino acid.

Amino acids are the basic building blocks of the 40,000 different proteins in the body, including enzymes, hormones, and the key brain chemical messenger molecules called neurotransmitters. Eight amino acids cannot be made by the body and must be obtained through the diet; others are produced in the body but not always in sufficient amounts. The body's main "amino acid pool" consists of: alanine, arginine, aspargine, aspartic acid, carnitine, citrulline, cysteine, cystine, GABA, glutamic acid, glutamine, glycine, histidine, isoleucine, leucine, lysine, methionine, ornithine, phenylalanine, proline, serine, taurine, threonine, tryptophan, tyrosine, and valine. The amino acids involved in amino acid conjugation are glycine, taurine, glutamine, arginine, and ornithine.

Here is an interesting fact about one aspect of the amino acid conjugation pathway. If you consume a lot of soft drinks (sodas) that contain benzoates, this substance binds with your body's reserve of glycine, one of the five conjugation amino acids, and makes it unavailable to the body. This then makes it hard for your system to detoxifiy toluene, an organic solvent found in many industrial products and substances one encounters on an almost daily basis.[12] Similarly, aspirin can grab up glycine reserves in the liver, thereby slowing down the glycine detoxification pathway. These limitations in glycine detoxification are of course reversible by supplementing with glycine, along with the other amino acids.

Another Phase II detoxification pathway is called glucuronidation, which entails the binding of glucuronic acid with foreign toxins. This pathway is responsible for neutralizing at least fifteen known types of prescription drugs, five xenobiotics, and various substances of dietary origin (free radicals naturally generated in the body during the metabolism of foods).

Sulfation, still another detoxification pathway, is often defective in people due to inadequate intake of dietary sulfate. This means if you are exposed to toxins that are supposed to be detoxified by the sulfation pathway and you are deficient in sulfate, your system will be unable to neutralize these substances and they remain free to produce illness and various health problems such as Alzheimer's, Parkinson's, autism, rheumatoid arthritis, food sensitivity, and multiple chemical sensitivity, among others.

When it's working optimally, the sulfation pathway will use sulfur-containing compounds to handle the neutralization of neurotransmitters, steroid hormones (including excess thyroid and estrogen), drugs, industrial chemicals, various compounds derived from benzene (as used in plastics, disinfectants, and drugs), and toxins from the environment and our own intestines. According to naturopathic educators Peter Bennett, N.D., and Stephen Barrie, N.D., this is often "the weakest pathway in most people, from a dietary standpoint."[13]

The preceding examples make it clear how important satisfactory nutrition is to successful and efficient detoxification, and show what happens when you are deficient in only one element, such as glutathione or sulfate. These facts also make a strong case for undergoing some kind of diagnostic screening and testing, as described in the next chapter, to document your actual biochemical status and degree of detoxification competency.

After the liver finishes its two-phase detoxification process, the bile carries the toxic metabolites (the neutralized residues or converted substances) to the intestines for excretion. The liver produces about one quart of bile every day as a carrier for toxins to be excreted from the intestines (to which it is sent), but also as a way of emulsifying fats and fat-soluble vitamins in the intestines, and as the primary excretion pathway for cholesterol and unneeded calcium.

As with Phase I, this second aspect of the liver's detoxification process requires sufficient internal levels of key nutrients or can be enhanced by the ingestion of specific substances, including cysteine, glycine, and taurine, garlic, L-glutathione, N-acetyl-cysteine (NAC, a cysteine precursor), folic acid, vitamins B 1, 2, 3, 5, 6, and 12, germanium, magnesium, manganese, molybdenum, selenium, sulfur, and zinc.

Immunotoxicity and How the
Detoxification Pathways Get Blocked

We have just reviewed the liver's two-phase detoxification system as it is meant to work, but for many people, this optimum operation is only a physiological ideal and not a bodily reality. For many, certain elements of the detoxification pathway are blocked, compromised, or dysfunctional, leading to a state of chronic internal stagnation and immunotoxicity.

When the detoxification pathways in the liver are blocked or inefficient, the toxic products build up in the bloodstream and intestines, producing an extra load of "foreign" substances the immune system must deal with. The immune system may get overloaded and overstimulated; it will start to show signs of this condition in allergies, headaches, chronic sinus conditions, inflammatory states (muscle soreness and intestinal irritation), infections (colds and flus) that keep coming back, swollen lymph glands, and from here on to more serious disorders. In other words, through your system's inability to completely detoxify itself, you are slowly but definitely "growing" illness from within. Eventually, assuming you do not actively detoxify, the toxicity will have "sprouted" some noxious growth inside your body and you will be sick in one form or another.

Through your system's inability to completely detoxify itself, you are slowly but definitely "growing" illness from within. Eventually, assuming you do not actively detoxify, the toxicity will have "sprouted" some noxious growth inside your body and you will be sick in one form or another.

In addition to considering the state of the liver's detoxification pathways, we must also pay attention to the intestines. While the issue of chronic constipation and colon cleansing is discussed thoroughly in chapter 4, a quick overview is worthwhile here. You must appreciate the astonishing fact that the human intestines, large and small, comprise a twenty-six-foot-long internal organ. That leaves a lot of room for storage; daily bowel motions do not indicate that a person is not chronically constipated. Most people are, because the intestines are so, literally, accommodating. Early signs of intestinal toxicity include headaches, sinus problems, allergies, sluggishness, mental torpor, irritation, mood swings, concentration problems, weight gain, and others.

If unrelieved, these symptoms provide a platform for the next layer of complications to arise. The intestinal wall might start to "leak," producing a symptom physicians call "leaky gut syndrome" or intestinal permeability. Intestinal toxins migrate out of the intestines into the bloodstream and into general systemic circulation. This is not desirable. The immune system goes on alert and soon will become hyperstimulated. It tags all the toxins floating in the blood as foreign proteins and has to work overtime to deal with them.

The immune system treats these foreign substances or antigens as invaders, causing antibodies to form and couple with them. This antigen and antibody combination is known as a circulating immune complex, or CIC. In a healthy person, CICs are neutralized, but in someone with a compromised immune system, they tend to accumulate in the blood where they burden the detoxification pathways or initiate an allergic reaction. If too many CICs accumulate, the kidneys cannot excrete enough of them through the urine. The CICs are then stored in soft tissues, causing inflammation and bringing stress to the immune system. The overload can lead to a variety of chronic health conditions, including autoimmune disorders and cancer.

When environmental pollutants and our own internally generated free radicals are not neutralized and removed from the body, they start having serious adverse effects inside us. They become toxic to the immune system—hence, immunotoxins. Numerous symptoms can result, but among those related to unrelieved toxicity is the strange cluster of symptoms that began to show up in people in the 1990s. This cluster was subsequently labeled environmental illness. In a sense, environmental illness represents the exaggerated, almost surreal result of unrelieved toxicity, demonstrating how it affects numerous body functions, throws out multiple symptoms, and generally baffles conventional medical thinking. However, the thinking in the world of alternative, natural medicine is that conditions like EI are the result of aggravated systemic toxicity.

As discussed in chapter 1, EI is similar in many respects to multiple chemical sensitivity (detailed in chapter 10) and chronic fatigue syndrome. It is a multispectrum dysfunctional state believed to be produced by excessive exposure to environmental pollutants and a corresponding inability of the body to detoxify them. Dismissed as an imaginary illness and given other pejorative labels by conventional medicine, EI found confirmation initially among the ranks of practitioners of environmental medicine, formerly called clinical ecology.

In fact, it was in the late 1940s when pioneering clinical ecologist Theron Randolph, M.D., first identified the health deteriorating effect of environmental toxins and promulgated the medical understanding that many conditions, such as allergies and other chronic problems, could be produced by the glut of unprocessed toxins in the human body.

Dr. Randolph had been building on earlier work that linked food allergies with chronic diseases of unknown origin (rheumatoid arthritis, ulcerative colitis, migraines) and common symptoms (headache, fatigue, hyperactivity, depression). He proposed that synthetic environmental chemicals (particularly in air pollution) could cause the same allergic symptoms as did reactions to food. Randolph reported 1,000 cases of patients who showed psychotic behavior directly related to exposures to specific toxic substances.

The prime "cause" of this growing list of illnesses was the "relatively new chemical environment," Dr. Randolph claimed. This environment itself is ill, he said, and the aim of clinical ecology is to "identify, minimize, or neutralize the impingement of specific environmental exposures." In the 1980s, other progressive physicians, such as William J. Rea, M.D., of the Environmental Health Center, in Dallas, Texas, extended and further documented Randolph's model of toxicity-mediated illness and developed clinical protocols for detoxifying patients who were dangerously toxic. Today his center is one of the nation's prime detoxification facilities, offering a pollution-free environment in which chemically toxic patients can flush the poisons out of their systems under medical supervision.[14]

Among its other contributions, Dr. Rea's ongoing research has dissolved the dismissive label of "hypochondriasis" from the complaints of numerous patients that they have been poisoned by their environment. It's not in their minds; they are not making it up, says Dr. Rea. "Susceptibility to environmental inciters such as air, food and water components is becoming an increasingly recognized health problem," he observed in 1991. The adverse reactions patients sustain can include "a spectrum of symptoms" that affect the smooth muscles, mucus membranes, and collagen in various body systems to do with breathing, digesting, and excreting. Their sensitivities and allergic reactions are "actually due to reactions to foods and chemicals found in the patient's home and work environments," says Dr. Rea.[15] (See chapter 10 for more details.)

Dr. Rea based this conclusion on solid laboratory work. He took fifty patients aged twenty-one to sixty-one who reported chemical sensitivities and who had various symptoms including asthma and arthritis, and partially detoxified—that is, desensitized—them in a less chemically polluted indoor environment. They went on a partial fast for three to four days, staying clear of all suspected allergens. Then Dr. Rea tested them, challenging their systems with small doses of inhaled toxic chemicals to see if they produced the same toxic symptoms again. They did. He used phenol, petroleum-derived ethyl alcohol, formaldehyde, chlorine, and a pesticide in doses they were likely to encounter in the outside environment. This study demonstrated that chemical sensitivity "clearly does exist" and may be blamed for a considerable number of symptoms.[16]

As the discipline of clinical ecology, or environmental medicine, developed in North America, its essential principles became clarified. The first is the concept of total environmental load, or total toxic burden, as mentioned previously. This states that the sum of all toxic exposures—all potential stressors, such as food intolerances, inhalant allergies, and psychosocial stress, all of which are cross-reactive—is predictive of health. Second, chronic low-level exposure produces damage to the immune system and initiates flawed physiological adaptation. Third, because many toxic chemicals are lipophilic (fat-soluble and stored in body fat) and remain in the body for decades, low-level chemical exposures have a cumulative effect.

Another prominent physician practicing environmental medicine in the spirit of Randolph and Rea is Sherry Rogers, M.D., a Diplomate of the American Academy of Environmental Medicine, the author of ten patient-centered medical books linking toxicity to health conditions, and director of the Northeast Center for Environmental Medicine in Syracuse, New York.

Since 1977, she has specialized in otherwise baffling medical conditions like environmental illness and has written extensively about the blocked detoxification pathways involved in conditions like EI. Her own debilitating bout with chemical sensitivity—for years she had arthritis-like chronic back pain due to unrelieved chemical exposure, including formaldehyde; she called herself "a severe universal reactor"—led her to investigate the biochemistry of detoxification and the factors that blocked it.

As we learned above, there are complex biochemical processes in the human organism whereby, under conditions of good health, foreign toxic substances are filtered out, neutralized, and removed from the body. EI patients, for example, do not operate under conditions of normal health; their detoxification pathways are blocked. EI patients of course are the extreme example of faulty detoxification, but the extremity of this dysfunction helps us understand how problems in detoxification can affect us at lesser levels of blockage and how these blockages can become major problems.

Due to toxic overload or nutritional deficit, or both, many people have "a maladaptation of the detoxification system," explains Dr. Rogers. We are the first generation to be exposed to a tremendous number of toxic chemicals, and the process by which the body tries to detoxify our contact with these pollutants produces enormous stress and nutrient deficiencies. The maladaptation of the detoxification system that results helps generate numerous chronic and serious health problems, explains Dr. Rogers.

To illustrate the concept of maladaptation, let's look at the aldehyde detoxification pathway. Aldehydes (the basis of formaldehyde) are extremely toxic to humans; if the aldehyde pathway is bottlenecked, aldehydes accumulate dangerously in the system. The blocked aldehyde detoxification pathway can explain the whole "spreading phenomenon" of chemical sensitivity (the expanding web of interlinked, multiple symptoms, in which symptoms multiply and everything worsens) including "toxic brain syndrome."

When chemicals like aldehydes can't be degraded, they get metabolized into chloral hydrate in the brain. Chloral hydrate was once infamous as the prime ingredient in the "Mickey Finn" knockout drops used by gangsters wanting to dispatch uncooperative colleagues. When somebody slipped you a Mickey, you were out for hours. In the brain, chloral hydrate produces "bizarre fluctuating cerebral symptoms—feeling spacey, dopey, dizzy, an inability to concentrate, mood swings, irritability, exhaustion, numbness, depression," says Dr. Rogers. The average physician could easily misdiagnose multiple chemical sensitivity as mental illness at this point.

What worsens the impact of the environmentally overloaded detoxification system is nutritional deficiency. Most people aren't detoxifying with "a full deck" of nutrients, says Rogers. Nutritionally poor diets and depleted agricultural soil fail to provide adequate supplies; meanwhile, the detoxification process itself depletes vital stores of minerals and vitamins (notably, glutathione). Even health-conscious adults may be nutrient-deficient. Magnesium, for example, is a component of over 300 enzymes and metabolic pathways, present in nearly every phase of the detoxification pathways; it is also the focus of the most under-recognized electrolyte disorder in the United States, claims Dr. Rogers.[17]

Unrelieved toxicity may proceed to other categories of symptoms besides allergies, environmental illness, and multiple chemical sensitivity. Immunotoxicity can lead to autoimmune disease and cancer. First, the capacity of your immune system to withstand infections and the constant creation of individual cancer cells (which happens even in healthy individuals) diminishes. At the same time, your sensitivity (or reactivity) to allergens (substances producing allergies) intensifies, and you react to a greater number of substances than ever before. You may eventually develop autoimmunity, in which your immune system reacts against itself—against your body—somehow now perceiving it as foreign. Various autoimmune diseases such as rheumatoid arthritis and lupus erythematosus may result.

The documentation of immune damage produced by the pesticide DDT is extensive. Even though it was banned in the United States decades ago, it is present in the environment in

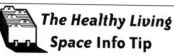

The Healthy Living Space Info Tip

For Sherry Rogers, M.D., contact: Northeast Center for Environmental Medicine, P.O. Box 2716 2800 West Genessee Street, Syracuse, NY 13220; tel: 315-488-2856.

For her books and a medically referenced monthly newsletter, *Total Wellness*, contact: Prestige Publishing, P.O. Box 3068, Syracuse, NY 13220; tel: 800-846-6687 or 315-455-7862.

For William J. Rea., M.D.: Environmental Health Center— Dallas, 8345 Walnut Hill Lane, Suite 220, Dallas, TX 75231; tel: 214-368-4132; fax: 214-691-8432; website: www.ehcd.com.

For Walter J. Crinnion, N.D., 13401 NE Bel-Red Road, #A4, Suite A-4, Bellevue, WA 98005; tel: 206-747-9200; fax: 206-747-7567.

residual amounts and in agricultural products deriving from countries in which the poison has not been banned. DDT toxicity was linked with numerous functional changes in the immune system and its key cells, and in damaging changes in various immune-related organs such as the spleen, thymus, and lymph glands. Serious health effects of a similar nature have been noted with human exposure to chlordanes (once used in termite pesticides, then banned, but still found in certain crops and seed treatment) and HCBs (hexachlorobenzene, a chlorinated pesticide, found in fungicides and dry-cleaning solvents).

Studies conducted at Dr. Rea's Environmental Health Center showed that people with two or more OCCs (organochlorine compounds) in their blood have some degree of immunotoxicity. As naturopath and detoxification expert Walter J. Crinnion, N.D., of Bellevue, Washington, comments, we are now struggling under a burden of multiple environmental toxins. "Some individuals appear to be less able to clear the daily chemical exposure from the body than others, leading to a total load of toxins that exceeds the ability of the body to adapt."

When this happens, the organ systems typically affected are the immune, neurological, and endocrine systems, Dr. Crinnion says. Further, the resulting immunotoxicity may be the prime cause of the increasing incidence of asthma, allergies, cancers, and chronic viral infections. A great number of symptoms can result from this toxic residue, including mood and cognitive disorders as well as problems with reproduction, libido, menstruation, metabolism, and the ability to cope with stress.[18] Dr. Crinnion cites research in which blood analysis revealed at least four major immune cell imbalances in 298 patients who had been exposed to industrial chemicals.

Chronic fatigue syndrome (CFS), like environmental illness and multiple chemical sensitivity, is a baffling illness that starts to make sense when you figure environmental toxicity as a probable contributing cause, says Dr. Crinnion. In 1998, he tested this idea by taking a group of people with CFS through a detoxification program, "designed to reduce their body burden of environmental toxins." Ninety-three reported "good or great improvement" as a result of the program.[19]

It is becoming more apparent that a variety of industrial chemicals can produce many of the chief CFS symptoms, adds

Dr. Crinnion. Exposure to any one of at least sixty-six different chemical compounds can produce fatigue, and trichloroethylene, a common airborne solvent found in urban air, can produce excessive fatigue. Chlorinated pesticides, lead toxicity, and tissue residues of DDE (the breakdown product of DDT), hexachlorobenzene, and organophosphates have been associated with CFS. In fact, organophosphates cause "an identical set" of symptoms to that of CFS, as well as similar disturbances in the nervous and endocrine systems, says Dr. Crinnion.

The correlation of unrelieved toxicity and the presence of specific carcinogens with the onset of cancer is well-documented. For example, women with breast cancer have been shown to have elevated levels of OCCs compared to women who are free of cancer. Among the specific chemicals found in the fatty tissue of the breast cancer patients were traces of DDT, DDE, PCBs, and lindane (also known as HCH or BHC, used to kill lice). Further, levels of these chemicals were found to be higher in the malignant tissues than elsewhere in the cancer patient's body. Researchers reporting in the *Journal of the National Cancer Institute* estimated that higher than average levels of DDE and PCB in the blood can represent a *fourfold* increase in the risk of breast cancer.[20]

Correlations have also been reported between exposure to toxic chemicals found in household pesticide products and the onset of childhood cancers, such as brain cancer. Specifically, these products included pesticide "bombs," treatments for termites, flea collars for pets, and various pesticide sprays for the garden.[21] Other common household pesticide products or weed killers have been associated with soft tissue sarcomas (a form of cancer) and leukemia in children, while among adults, the use of 2,4-D herbicides have been linked to higher rates of lung and stomach cancer, leukemia, and both Hodgkin's lymphoma and non-Hodgkin's lymphoma. The risk of developing soft tissue sarcomas due to exposure to 2,4-D can be as much as five to seven times higher, and even, according to one study, forty times higher.[22]

Exposure to polyvinyl chloride (PVC) has also been linked with the development of a form of testicular cancer. In a study of 148 cases of cancer of the testicles and 314 healthy men, scientists at the Orebro Medical Center in Sweden correlated the patients' work history and lifetime toxic exposure. They found a sixfold increase in the risk for seminoma, a type of testicular cancer, among workers in the plastics industry who were exposed to PVC.[23]

Neurological and Endocrinal Damage from Environmental Toxins

The neurological effects of toxicity are evident in a rising incidence of childhood behavior and cognitive function disorders as well as development delays. A report by the Greater Boston Physicians for Social Responsibility published in May 2000 put the matter of childhood and toxic effects in bold relief. The intent was to study the various toxic environmental threats to child development, specifically in the areas of learning, behavioral, and developmental disabilities.

The report, entitled *In Harm's Way: Toxic Threats to Child Development*, documents the "epidemic" of developmental, learning, and behavioral disabilities now evident in the United States. For example, seventeen percent of children under age eighteen suffer from one of these above-mentioned problems; attention deficit hyperactivity disorder affects an estimated three percent to six percent of schoolchildren, but the percentage may be as high as seventeen percent; learning disabilities affect five percent to ten percent of children in school; between 1977 and 1994, the number of children in special education programs for learning disabilities increased by 191%; autism exists in 2 out of 1,000 children, with a doubling of its prevalence from 1966 to 1997.

Next, the report demonstrates the proven relationship between exposures and body levels of certain toxic substances and cognitive defects. These toxic chemicals include lead, mercury, manganese, nicotine, dioxins, PCBs, pesticides, and solvents. The scientific research now available makes a strong case for a link between exposure to each of these substances (or categories of substances) and specific developmental or learning disabilities, including hyperactivity; impaired stamina, coordination, and memory; reduced IQ; impulsive behavior; decreased social adaptability; attention deficits; impaired speech and language skills; mental retardation; gait and visual disturbances; aggression and delinquent behavior, and others.[24]

Consider what lead can do to a child. A 1998 estimate proposed that nearly one million American children younger than age five are believed to suffer from low-level lead poisoning, derived mostly from leaded gasoline residues (as a fine toxic dust in the soil and air) and lead paint in old buildings (which also flakes, peels, and disintegrates into a fine powder). Low-level lead toxicity can cause permanent cognitive problems, such as learning disabilities, hyperactivity, reduced IQ, poor motor coordination, hearing loss, and diminished stature (failure to grow). Lead-toxic children may also have a hard time paying attention and controlling their impulses, and in some cases, may be prone to delinquency and violence.

Lead is rightly blamed for the "dumbing down" of schoolchildren. A 1993 study concluded that lead exposure diminishes a child's mental abilities and that the relationship between lead levels and IQ deficits was "remarkably consistent."

These negative results have been observed from exposures to lead considerably below the so-called "acceptable" exposure level put forth by the U.S. government. The developing nervous system of a child is especially vulnerable to lead toxicity, even at the "low" and "acceptable" exposure (or ingestion) rate of ten micrograms (mcg/dL) per day. There is so much lead in the environment today—an estimated 10 million metric tonnes were introduced into the environment during the twentieth century—that there is now "an almost unbelievably large 'sink' of toxic powder available in soil and in house dust, waiting to cause brain damage in toddlers."[25] Even more alarming is the estimate by the National Research Council in 1993 that the average American has a typical body burden of lead 300 to 500 times higher than that found in our prehistoric ancestors.[26]

Lead is rightly blamed for the "dumbing down" of schoolchildren. A 1993 analysis by the American Academy of Pediatrics of eighteen medical studies on lead toxicity concluded that lead exposure diminishes a child's mental abilities and that the relationship between lead levels and IQ deficits was "remarkably consistent." They further reported that for every increase in blood lead levels of 10 mcg/dL there was an average lowering of IQ in children by 4 to 7 points. The effect of losing five IQ points means that fifty percent more children fall into the IQ 80 category, which is barely in the realm of normal intelligence.[27]

Lead may also be a key factor in the outbreak of violence among children and adolescents, reveals research from Dartmouth College. According to the "neurotoxicity hypothesis of violent crime," lead and manganese toxicity can result in loss of control over impulsive, antisocial, and/or violent, aggressive behavior. It is believed these elements can alter brain chemistry (their inevitable action as neurotoxins) in such a way that there is a breakdown in the "inhibition mechanism" that normally holds us back from becoming assaultive.[28]

A 1996 report from the University of Pittsburgh showed that young boys—the study examined 301 males, aged 7 and 11—with more lead in their bones than the expected average "consistently" had more incidents of aggressive and delinquent behavior. The leaded boys exhibited ever more aggressive, delinquent behavior as they moved through adolescence.[29] Studies linking lead and aggressive behavior have been appearing since the 1970s such that the case against lead is very persuasive.

Roger D. Masters, who headed the Dartmouth College research, also showed a correlation between high lead rates, criminal behavior, and the use of silicofluoride to fluoridate public water supplies. He noted that there was a doubling of the crime rate in areas where silicofluoride was in the water. This substance appears to increase the amount of toxins that enter the bloodstream from the intestines. In places where the public water contained silicofluoride, five times as many children had high lead levels compared to other communities. One clear effect is that toxic chemicals can destroy inhibitory systems and cause violence, Masters stated.[30]

This is only a précis of a small portion of the available research on lead toxicity and child development. Similar documented cases can be made against numerous other toxic industrial chemicals regarding their injurious effect on intelligence, development, and other aspects of growing up.

This makes it clear why substances such as lead and the others cited above are labeled "developmental neurotoxicants," according to the authors of *In Harm's Way*. They use this term to indicate how the toxic chemicals poison the nerve cells to such an extent that they impair the normal growth processes in a child. "These chemicals, which the child ingests through foods, environmental exposures, and in utero from the mother, may be directly toxic to cells or interfere with hormones (endocrine disruptors), neurotransmitters, or other growth factors." The authors further state that our scientific understanding of the effect on humans of toxic exposures is not advanced enough to "accurately predict the impact of toxicants" and thereby protect children from unhealthy exposures and their long-term effects.

The most chilling consequence of toxicity—acting as it does deep within the body's core life systems and even spanning generations—is the way it disrupts the endocrine system. Evidence now exists that chemicals can disturb the endocrine system on both a short- and long-term basis (see figure 2-1).

Here is a review of some aspects of the short-term side of endocrine disruption due to environmental chemicals. According to Dr. Walter Crinnion, there are five principal ways in which toxins can damage the endocrine system. This system consists of the various endocrine glands: the testicles, ovaries, pancreas, adrenals, thyroid, parathyroid, and pituitary. All of these glands and their hormones are central to the regulation and normalization of the body's complex, interconnected systems, from metabolism and heat production to spermatogenesis and uterine preparations for pregnancy.

The endocrine glands accomplish these important functions by virtue of the numerous critical but highly sensitive hormones they secrete. Hormones—at least 100 different ones have been identified—are the chemical messengers of the endocrine system that impose order through an intricate communication system among the body's estimated 50 trillion cells. Central among the body's hormones are the "male" sex hormone (testosterone), the "female" sex hormones (estrogen and progesterone), melatonin (produced by the pineal gland), growth hormone (by the pituitary gland), thyroxin (by the thyroid gland), and DHEA (by the adrenal glands).

Toxic damage to the endocrine system, says Dr. Crinnion, shows up in sleep disturbances, shifts in energy level or mood; changes in weight, appetite, or intestinal function; a change in sexual interest and function, and for women, in menstrual changes; alterations in how we sense temperature and the degree to which we flush or perspire; and unaccountable changes in skin texture and hair growth. These symptoms, with the exception of the reproductive ones, typically manifest after problems in the immune and neurological systems are already evident, Dr. Crinnion says.[31]

One endocrine organ that is especially sensitive to toxicity is the thyroid gland, located in the front of the neck.[32] It is not surprising to find that a growing number of North Americans have imbalanced thyroids, being either underactive (hypothyroidism, the more common problem) or overactive (hyperthyroidism). At least seven industrial chemicals, including calcium-channel blockers, steroids, and chlorinated hydrocarbons, have been shown to reduce the secretion of a key thyroid hormone called T4.

Figure 2-1. The Endocrine System

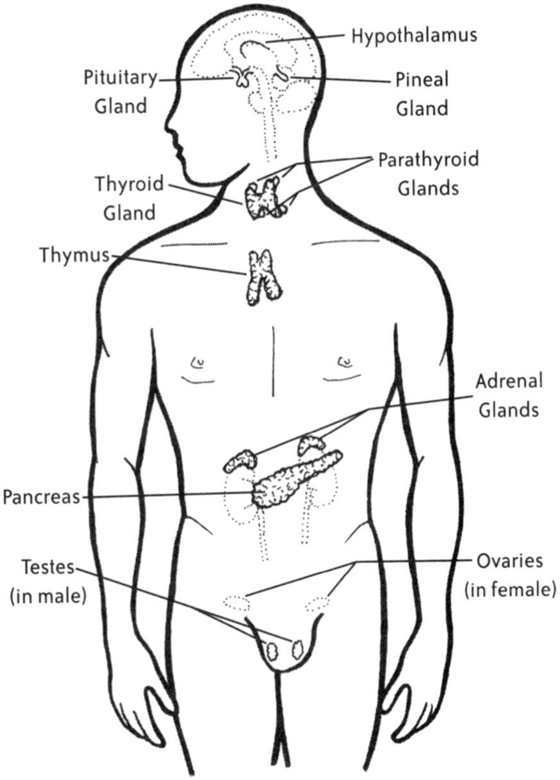

In a laboratory experiment, when rats were exposed to soil, dust, and air extracts taken from a toxic landfill known to harbor at least three dangerous pollutants including PCBs, their levels of thyroid hormone dropped;[33] and when laboratory animals were fed fish harvested from the toxic, polluted Great Lakes, their thyroid's ability to regulate body functions became compromised.[34] Thyroid function is also weakened when the system is exposed to lead, carbon disulfide, and polybrominated biphenyls, or PBBs (used as fire retardants, in plastic parts subject to heating, and in equipment such as televisions, radios, business machines, and hand tools). Research published in 1994 showed that exposure to even very low levels of PCBs and dioxin could damage thyroid function in the mother and her developing fetus and result in neurological damage to the child, producing learning disabilities, hyperactivity, and problems with attention.[35]

Polychlorinated biphenyls, or PCBs, a toxic compound related to PBBs, are structurally similar to a thyroid hormone (an example of the hormone mimicking effect of environmental toxins). PCBs are used for insulating and cooling electrical equipment, in hydraulic fluids, as plasticizers, and in inks, dyes, adhesives, and certain pesticides. Because they mimic a thyroid hormone, once inside the human body, PCBs can either help or hinder thyroid regulation and thus all the body processes that the thyroid controls, which include body temperature and metabolism. They can further damage the way a thyroid hormone (in this case, T3) is moved through the bloodstream and how it is produced within the cells. If an infant is exposed to PCBs, "this can have a devastating effect on neurological and anatomical development," observes Dr. Crinnion.

The long-term endocrine disruption is especially accomplished by what are known as environmental estrogens. These are industrial, human-made chemicals (often petrochemicals, made with a petroleum base) that are widely distributed throughout the environment, having permeated the water and plant and animal foods.[36] They enter the human system from the environment as pollutants; once inside the body, they mimic estrogen, naturally present in both women and men, and overload the system with this one hormone.

It is alarming to realize that the body, so competent and well-designed, can be overwhelmed by environmental chemicals and *mistake* a human-made chemical for a natural, essential hormone. It also highlights how serious the matters of environmental pollution and human physiological toxicity have become. Not only can the body no longer keep up with the toxic burden, it can no longer distinguish, in some instances, an unwanted toxin from a desired hormone.

Let's have a closer look at this subject. Environmental estrogens, also called xenoestrogens, are present primarily in "greenhouse gases," herbicides, and pesticides such as DDT, and industrial byproducts from the manufacture of plastics and paper, as well as from the incineration of hazardous wastes.

Environmental estrogens often cause an imbalance of estrogen relative to progesterone, another key "female" hormone. When a woman's body has too much estrogen (a condition called estrogen dominance), a variety of health problems can result, including breast cancer, fibroids, and endometriosis. According to some researchers, environmental estrogens also affect men, and may contribute to testicular cancer, urinary tract disorders, and low sperm count, or infertility.

Researchers in the past decade have been studying links between environmental estrogens and prostate and testicular cancer, reduced sperm counts and sperm volume, undescended testes in newborn males, urinary tract abnormalities, a 400% increase in ectopic pregnancies (the fetus forms outside the uterus), and a serious rise in breast cancer. Hormone-disrupting chemicals are also linked with miscarriages and endometriosis. One type of breast cancer that is on the rise is occurring in women past the age of menopause in the form of estrogen-responsive tumors. This means the cancerous tissue in the breast is rich in estrogen receptors and will grow when exposed to additional estrogen.

Research now supports the theory that exposure to estrogenic organochlorines (found in pesticides) may increase the risk and incidence of breast cancer. Tissue samples from 240 women who developed breast cancer between 1976 and 1993 were studied along with samples from 477 cancer-free controls. Scientists found that one organochlorine in particular, dieldrin[37]—they also looked for traces of DDT and polychlorinated biphenyls—was associated with a "significantly increased dose-related risk" of breast cancer, meaning, the more dieldrin the woman was exposed to, the greater the chances she had breast cancer.[38]

Endocrine-disrupting chemicals may have a special preference for women, new research suggests. It is often noted that women are more prone to autoimmune diseases, such as lupus erythematosus and rheumatoid arthritis. Why is that? One theory, backed by preliminary research, is that estrogens promote autoimmune diseases mediated by certain immune cells. Male sex hormones, called androgens, tend to inhibit the onset of these conditions. In other words, it seems that estrogens regulate autoimmunity, so if women have more than their fair share of toxic exposure to environmental estrogens, they will be more prone to develop estrogen-related health problems.[39]

Toxic exposures can also upset other hormone-dependent processes. Here is an example, substantiated by scientific research, of what pesticide residues can do to sexual maturation in children. Scientists at the University of Granada School of Medicine in Spain took tissue fat samples from children living in farm areas in southeastern Spain. They found traces of 14 pesticides, and of the 113 samples studied, 43 had traces of at least one pesticide, such as lindane, heptachlor, aldrin, or dieldrin. Some of the chemicals have estrogenic activity. The scientists also found a correlation between exposure to estrogenic chemicals in pesticides and sexual maturation problems in boys, specifically, a failure for testicles to descend in some cases.

Given the fact that estrogenic chemicals are found not only in pesticides, but are used in the food industry, in plasticizers, and in dental sealants, "concerns are warranted." Even more so because "the number of new substances that mimic the action of endogenous [within the body] estrogens is increasing rapidly."[40]

"Unequivocal evidence" now exists, state researchers at Brunel University in Uxbridge, England, that the waters of the world contain a wide variety of endocrine-disrupting chemicals. So extensive is this pollution and so unknown the results that "this makes predicting possible effects difficult." Scientists do know that strange sexual changes and other "adverse effects" are happening to marine life living in the chemically polluted waters: female mollusks are becoming masculinized, and male fish are getting feminized. In other words, basic gender differentiation is starting to blur in marine life under the influence of environmental estrogens.[41]

Another alarming fact about hormone-disrupting chemicals is how little it takes to produce biological damage. Hormones are powerful, which means the body deals with them in very small, even infinitesimal, doses. Estrogen is biologically active even at only a few parts per trillion. While most environmental estrogens are less powerful than the hormone estrogen, they tend to be present in body tissues in concentrations of several parts per billion, or million—in other words, they are more pervasive in the body than natural estrogen.

Further, synthetic estrogens may be much more active in the body than natural estrogen because they do not bind to proteins as carrier molecules and are therefore more mobile. The result is that because the human body is used to dealing with only tiny amounts of hormones, high doses of synthetic estrogen "can swamp the receptors and actually shut down any response."[42]

There is yet another factor showing how environmental estrogens can easily damage the body and disrupt its endocrine system, especially during fetal and infant development. There are "windows of extreme susceptibility" during the development of the fetus or baby. Get exposed to a synthetic estrogen during these small windows and your system is in serious trouble. For example, only those girls who as fetuses were exposed to the toxin DES during the first sixteen weeks of gestation developed clear cell cancer. Girls exposed to DES after the sixteenth week did not develop this disease.

One toxin can do a lot of damage to the endocrine system, but we are rarely exposed to only one environmental estrogen. Since 1991, fifty different synthetic industrial chemicals capable of disrupting the human endocrine system have been identified; they can also interfere with hormonal activities in birds, fish, mammals, and other species.[43] These hormone-disrupting chemicals are found in common, frequently encountered products, such as plastics, detergents, and pesticides. Dr. Crinnion notes that when you factor the *combined* estrogenic effect of the organochlorines[44] we are likely to be exposed to, it *increases* our exposure rate by a factor of 1,600 times. This has been demonstrated in the case of exposure to two or three common pesticides at low levels.

One toxin can do a lot of damage to the endocrine system, but we are rarely exposed to only one environmental estrogen. Since 1991, fifty different synthetic industrial chemicals capable of disrupting the human endocrine system have been identified.

Further, estrogenicity (the state in which nonestrogen chemicals act *as* estrogen, thereby multiplying the body's reserves of this one hormone) can activate other compounds, not normally acting like estrogens, to become estrogenic, thereby adding to the total. It produces a synergistic effect, yielding toxic results greater than the sum of individual chemical actions. Chlordane, which on its own does not disrupt human hormones, greatly enhances the estrogenic effect of other chemicals already present, thus magnifying the total hormone disruption.[45]

Damaging Synergistic Effects Extending into the Next Generation

To say that fifty chemicals have been identified as estrogenic, or hormonally disruptive, must be measured against the staggering number of chemicals now in use: 70,000, plus the

1,000 or so new ones introduced every year. Most of these haven't been tested to see if they interfere with hormonal activity, so the consequences of our routine or occasional exposure is unknown. However, based on the evidence accumulating for the first fifty, the chance that many of these chemicals are hormone-disrupters is high.

But that's only part of the picture. To accurately assess their potential effect, you would have to test what happens when any number of these chemicals are combined in a human physiology; the number of possible permutations is sufficient to stagger the statistical imagination. If you wanted to test the 1,000 most common toxic chemicals in unique combinations of three, this would take 166 million different experiments; if each experiment took an hour and 100 laboratories worked 24/7, it would take 180 years to finish the work.[46] Meanwhile, millions more men, women, and children are being slowly poisoned by exposure to toxic environmental chemicals, the health impacts of which have never been adequately tested.[47]

This is especially unfortunate because children are particularly sensitive to pesticide exposure and are routinely exposed to them in their school environment, both indoors and outdoors. Given their smaller size, a single exposure to pesticides results in a larger dose of toxins than for adults. Children's internal organs, still developing, are more vulnerable to toxins, and their systems generally are less competent at detoxifying than an adult system is. "Low levels of pesticide exposure can adversely affect a child's neurological, respiratory, immune, and endocrine system," noted Kagan Owens and Jay Feldman in a comprehensive review article on the problem, "The Schooling of State Pesticide Laws," in 1998.

They report that chloropyrifos (brand name: Dursban) is one of the insecticides most widely used in schools. It "poisons" children by diminishing the body's output of cholinesterase, an enzyme needed to transmit nerve impulses. This enzyme deficit in turn produces various symptoms including nausea, dizziness, headaches, aching joints, disorientation, and concentration problems, state Owens and Feldman. Another widely used class of insecticide, synthetic pyrethroids, overstimulates nerves producing hypersensitivity and asthma; still others are known to negatively affect the immune system, resulting in an increased incidence of allergies, asthma, hypersensitivity to chemicals, and a generally reduced immune defense against infections and cancer. While about thirty states have taken some action to limit pesticide exposure of children while at school, the combined regulatory (and preventative) action is still "limited."[48]

Of considerable concern in this matter is the way environmental estrogens present in a mother can be transferred to and produce health damage in her offspring. According to the World Resources Institute of Washington, D.C., an advocacy group that monitors environmental toxins and their health impact, these chemicals interfere with the development of babies before (prenatally) or soon after birth. "Estrogen mimics are extremely potent in part because unlike most natural estrogen, they cross the placental barrier, exposing the fetus to greater than normal levels of hormone." These exposures in turn can disturb the fetus' hormonal balances, thereby throwing potentially everything biological in its young life into jeopardy, "from fertility to gender itself."[49]

Research shows that in most cases the effects of environmental estrogen exposure are more pronounced in the offspring than in the exposed parents, although the extent of the effects on the latter should not be minimized by any means. In other words, if you, as a female, are toxic with environmental estrogens and do not detoxify before pregnancy, you may be inadvertently passing these poisons on to your baby in the womb. You may also transmit them through your milk if you breastfeed your infant. It has further been noted that the effects of exposure in many cases are delayed in the next generation, such that they do not fully manifest until the offspring is an adult.

It is not only the fact that hormone-disrupting chemicals have a long-term, multi-generational impact. They interfere with deep-set, essential life processes, with the way chemical messages are transmitted throughout the body. In many respects, this is more serious than the fact that they are carcinogens as well, capable of initiating a cancer process. According to Theo Colborn and her co-authors in *Our Stolen Future*, an excellent review of the health consequences of environmental estrogens, hormonally active synthetic chemicals are "thugs on the biological information highway that sabotage vital communication."

They jam and scramble the messages; they spread biochemical disinformation; they seriously damage the endocrine system at its critical level of development, says Colborn, including sexual differentiation and brain organization. It is a "toxic assault" that reaches into the unborn generation and poisons its members even before they're born. Colborn also says that hormone-disrupting chemicals, when they affect the fetus, "can diminish individuals without making them sick," producing "impaired function" but not necessarily overt disease.

Development can be derailed; cognitive unfolding can be stunted; and the toxic etiology can be hard to trace using conventional medical models. For example, says Colborn, a boy who gets exposed to toxic estrogenic chemicals in utero (from his mother) could have health problems throughout his life. As a child his testicles do not descend; at puberty, he has a low sperm count; at middle age, he gets cancer of the testicles. The fact of "hand-me-down" poisons means potentially three generations receive the negative health impact of environmental estrogens, says Colborn. In other words, the grandchildren of a toxic grandmother can also be poisoned by her toxic exposures, transmitted across two generations.[50]

Previewing the Scope and Advantages of Deliberate Detoxification

A great deal more evidence could be marshaled to make the case for an alarming degree of widespread toxicity among humans in our time. But the facts and extrapolations reviewed here should be enough to motivate us to think about detoxification, that is, voluntarily assisting our internal detoxification system to catch up on processing its toxic burden and ridding our bodies of a lifetime accumulation of toxins. Getting yourself involved in a carefully planned and responsibly staged detoxification program could be one of the smartest things you ever do for your health and well-being.

A chemical detoxification program capable of ridding the body of its toxic burden must address five key physiological functions of the body, states Stephen B. Edelson, M.D., director of the Edelson Center for Environmental and Preventive Medicine in Atlanta, Georgia. Dr. Edelson has for many years been a leading proponent of and expert in the means of chemical detoxification as a way of treating numerous serious health conditions, including cancer. He has formulated a multidisciplinary medical approach he calls clinical molecular medicine as an effective way of treating and preventing disease.[51]

Dr. Edelson says you must correct the functioning of the liver (help its two phases to work optimally); the blood circulation (it must be "free flowing" so it can carry and adequate oxygen supply to the cells); the adrenal and thyroid glands (their hormones influence enzyme activities and metabolism); the kidneys (so they can flush out toxins through the urine); and the intestines (accelerated "transit time" so that old and new fecal matter as well as neutralized toxins and bile are excreted frequently). So how do you do this?

According to Dr. Edelson, a detoxification program should include a reduction in your body's burden of environmental chemicals and toxins, a lowering of its overall stress, and an enhancement of its antioxidant mechanisms. Some of the ways these goals can be accomplished include eating a wholesome nontoxic diet, normalizing your nutritional status, exercising, "upregulating" liver detoxification (giving the liver all it needs to run its two-phased detoxification), and using sauna and/or heat treatment to sweat toxins through the skin.[52]

For cases of serious heavy metal toxicity, a process called biodetoxification is required, says Dr. Edelson; here a chelating (binding up) substance is infused intravenously into the patient's blood to gather up heavy metals such as mercury from within the body and enable the system to excrete it through the urine. In another process called heat depuration, you get into a sauna that can produce an indoor temperature of 150°F, a level of heat judged necessary to mobilize chemicals stored deep in body tissues. For biodetoxification and heat depuration you need to resort to a clinic (Edelson offers a Biodetoxification Center as part of his medical offices), but the recommendations cited above can be undertaken at home or on your own. These will be taken up in practical detail in various chapters in this book.

Detoxification is a medical term that refers to a wide range of practices, from the simple to the complex. "Anything that supports our elimination can be said to help us detoxify," comments detoxification authority Elson M. Haas, M.D., director of the

Preventive Medical Center of Marin in San Rafael, California. "Doing nothing more than drinking an extra quart of water a day will usually help us eliminate more toxins."

As a therapy, Dr. Haas regards detoxification (including fasting and internal cleansing) as "one of the most powerful" healing approaches he has encountered in his more than twenty-five years of medical practice. In fact, detoxification is "the missing link in Western medicine and a key to the health and vitality of our civilization," he states.[53] The detoxification program reduces your body's intake of toxins and enhances its removal of those already present. A detoxification program, says Dr. Haas, should help the body's five cleansing systems to work better: these are the respiratory (lungs, throat, sinuses, nose), gastrointestinal (liver, gallbladder, colon), urinary (kidneys, bladder), skin (sweat and tear glands), and lymphatic (the lymph glands, channels, and organs, such as the spleen).

Dr. Haas also defines toxins broadly. They include any substance that "creates irritating and/or harmful effects" in the body such that these effects undermine our health or put stress on our biochemical processes. As such, toxins can include the obvious physical poisons from our environment, but they can also include more subtle influences. "Negative 'ethers,' psychic and spiritual influences, thought patterns, and negative emotions, all can be toxins as well, both as stressors and by changing the normal physiology of the body and possibly producing specific symptoms." (See chapter 9 for more information about these subtler toxins.)

As to *why* we should detoxify, Dr. Haas groups the answers into two categories. First, in terms of disease prevention and treatment, internal cleansing can reduce symptoms, treat existing disease, help the internal organs rest, purify, and rejuvenate all the body's systems, facilitate weight loss, improve skin quality, slow the aging process, improve flexibility, and enhance fertility. Second, in terms of gaining new benefits, detoxification can help us become more organized, creative, motivated, relaxed, energized, clear in the head, inwardly focused, environmentally attuned, and can generally fine-tune the senses, says Dr. Haas.[54]

These last two benefits of detoxification tend to be under-acknowledged by most medical practitioners but should be given much more attention. Once the body is relatively purified and freed to conduct its physiological processes of digestion, assimilation, detoxification, and elimination *unimpeded* by a toxic overload, it can actually support our awareness. It can support our state of mind, our processes of consciousness, even the degree to which we are conscious, or shall we say, freely aware of our inner and outer environment.

The Spiritual and Global Implications of Detoxification

Let's put it simply: detoxification can enable us to have more *sustained awareness* at our disposal. Dr. Haas explains that during detoxification, clarity of mind, emotional cleansing, and profound spiritual awareness may result. "We are more sensitive to subtle vibrations of people, situations, emotions, and nature."[55]

The processes of detoxification, including the three levels of physiology, emotions, and energy field can teach us a lot about ourselves. All we have to do is observe. Detoxification is an excellent way to gain self-knowledge.

The processes of detoxification, including the three levels of physiology, emotions, and energy field (the realm of Dr. Haas' "psychic and spiritual influences") can teach us a lot about ourselves. All we have to do is observe. Detoxification is an excellent way to gain self-knowledge.

We can see, for example, the effect of a lifetime of dietary neglect, inattention, or abuse as we purge our intestines and liver. We may find ourselves saying: Who would have ever thought my colon could hold that much old matter and in such a toxic state? We may observe with a small measure of awe as we unravel buried emotional patterns, untie very old emotional knots, and see our physical and psychological symptoms start to ease up and go away. Again we may marvel to ourselves: I never would have thought my childhood or adolescent feelings (or whatever: you fill in the appropriate time period and content) could have had that kind of powerful effect on my body.

Finally, as we discern the effects of subtle psychic and spiritual influences on our bodies and energy fields (or auras), derived from other people, toxic environments, and energy imbalances in our homes or work spaces, we may step back and reflect. How could I have gone these many years oblivious to this realm of influence, when now I can see what a mess it can make of my mind, emotions, and body? "I cleanse because it makes me feel more vital, creative, and open to emotional and spiritual energies," comments Dr. Haas.

In an unexpected but tangible sense, detoxification is a spiritual activity. Certainly it can produce numerous physical benefits, such as increased energy, reduced allergies and congestion, and a cessation of many negative health symptoms, and it can lead to heightened mental focus, sharpness, and performance as well as emotional clarity and stability. But there is more.

Detoxification enables you to get into a new, wakeful, conscious relationship with your body, your prime living space in the material world. Most of the time we take our physical bodies for granted; in fact, we take our existence for granted—the fact of our existence, the fact that we are awake and aware inside biological human forms. Illness can rivet our attention, for a while, on this sheer physical fact, but most of the time we try to avoid this awareness.

During detoxification, you can *watch* the changes in how you feel, think, and feel as you live in your body, as you purify your bodily living space. You realize—you see the irrefutable proof—that what you eat affects how your body runs, how it is, how you are. You come to understand that healthy, organic, wholesome foods and substances produce one kind of biological result, and fast foods, junk foods, and processed, toxic foods and substances produce another, and that this other kind of result is unpleasant, undesirable, and sickening.

You come to see that where you live, what you surround yourself with, in terms of furnishings and architectural shapes and energies, also have marked effects on all aspects of your body, mind, and spirit. You begin to see your body and home as one environment, as one extended living space that is either healthy or toxic. You begin to consciously inhabit your body and home and to appreciate how both are nested in the larger world. Even better, you see that it's your choice whether you reside in a healthy or a toxic living space.

Here is the practical payoff from this growing environmental awareness. If you choose to have a healthy living space, start a detoxification program, and develop a lifelong detoxification aware-ness, all of your consumer choices start to shift. Coming to terms with the elements in your diet and home that either support or destroy your health, you form a new relationship to your body, your home, and to the world—to the planet itself, as the ultimate source of nutrients and furnishings. You see your body and home as a sin-gle living space, as a place for you as a conscious being to reside in, but which is dependent on the "outside" world for supplies.

As you eliminate the toxic substances and reach for organic, wholesome, "green" products, your choices have an effect in the marketplace. They have *global* implications because through your consumer choices in service of your detoxification (itself in service of your desire to have a healthy living space, both body and home), you are energizing the nontoxic world economy and removing your support from the toxic world economy.

Consider one example. Say you choose to buy only organi-cally grown soybeans and soybean products as part of your detoxification dietary change. What are the global implications of this single consumer choice?

First, you are saying no to the input of numerous pesticides routinely sprayed on soybeans, which are absorbed to an extent by the beans themselves and which eventually enter the human food chain.

Second, you are saying no to the use of genetically modified (GM) soybeans with their resident pesticide and to the interests of world agribusiness concerns that want to convert the world to GM foods using seed stocks they own.

Third, you are saying no to the standard use of synthetic agricultural fertilizers, which deplete the soil and run off into public water systems, residues of which eventually enter the body through municipal water.

Fourth, you are saying no to the soil-depleting practices of monocropping or the single crop rotation farming cycle of soy-beans and corn, a process that in part has reduced the total number of farms and farmers and concentrated food production in the hands of agribusiness.

Fifth, you are saying no to the use of soybeans as a food additive in the form of concentrates, isolates, and hydrolyzed vegetable protein, products widely found in processed, fast, and junk foods that contribute to toxicity and intestinal stagnation.

Sixth, you are saying no to the mass distribution of processed foods through conventional supermarkets that lack ecological awareness and support the interests of world agribusiness and its steady despoliation of the environment.

Seventh, you are saying no to the use of hormones and antibiotics in the meat industry (which get into human bodies through ingestion of the animal) and to the squandering of plant resources in raising animal protein versus consuming plant proteins directly.

These are some of the global implications of your decision to buy only organically raised soybeans. What are the implications of saying yes to only organically grown beans?

First, you are affirming the ecologically sound practices of organic agriculture, with its emphasis on soil husbandry and abstention from pesticides and synthetic fertilizers.

Second, you are saying yes to all the green initiatives under way around the planet, in support of the environment and its responsible stewards.

Third, you are saying yes to the decentralization of food production, to the resurgence of regional and community agriculture, and to the preservation of natural seed stocks and the natural delineation between species. (Genetically modified foods mix genes from different species.)

Fourth, you are saying yes to foods that are relatively easy to digest and which, due to their purity, can contribute to a calmer, clearer state of mind.[56]

Fifth, you are contributing to a rise in the general level of awareness about the relationship between health, food, consciousness, and the environment—expressed in part by the Green movement. Spread across the Western industrialized nations, this awareness could eventually produce a radical shift in culture and industry.

Sixth, you are saying yes to a nutritionally based, dietary approach to health maintenance, symptom reduction, and, in some cases, to disease treatment. This in turn has ramifications for drug-based conventional medicine and its health-care infrastructure.

Seventh, you are assisting in reducing global warming insofar as it is due in part to deforestation, especially in the rain forests, clearcut for grazing of cattle required by the world animal protein market.

All of this may seem far removed from the benefits you reasonably expect from a few days of colon cleansing, liver flushing, and a couple of hours sweating in a sauna. Yet it is true and will probably become evident to you upon reflection, especially *after* you have detoxified. In any event, now that we have identified the numerous toxins in our environment, seen what they can do to our health, and appreciated the need to deliberately support the body's natural but probably overburdened detoxification system, the next step is to assess your individual level of toxicity. The best and most reliable way to do this is through a laboratory test of your blood, urine, feces, saliva, or breath, a topic we explore in the next chapter.

Part Two

Creating the Healthy
Body Living Space

CHAPTER 3

How Toxic Are You?

Testing for Toxicity and Detoxification Ability

At this point, we are sufficiently alerted to the possibility of toxicity in our bodies and homes and what it can do to our health. But how can we tell if we are toxic, if our bodies actually harbor a fair share of the toxic residues known to exist—unnaturally—in the human body in the twenty-first century. Being sick is one kind of feedback, though not an ideal one. Having a chronic problem, such as frequent colds, susceptibility to the flu, or chronic fatigue, multiple chemical sensitivity, or environmental illness, is another indication, but still imprecise.

The most reliable way to find out if your body is unduly toxic, meaning so toxic your body can no longer naturally cope with the toxic load, is to have one or more laboratory tests on your blood, urine, stool, or hair, looking for *traces* of toxic materials, such as heavy metals, and looking for *absences* of key nutrients necessary for the body's natural detoxification processes. You will observe here a definite interactive system: the more toxins your body carries, the less likely it is to have the detoxification nutrients required to purify itself, *and* the more deficient your system is in detoxification nutrients, the easier it is for toxins to accumulate and place an almost unbearable toxic burden on the body.

Gradually, as real and true medical knowledge of the human system develops, more health-care practitioners are including laboratory testing of patients for toxic burden and nutrient status as a routine part of their initial diagnosis and case workup. I say "real and true" because in recent decades conventional medicine's dependence on powerful drugs and procedures that mask, suppress, or eradicate symptoms has tended to eclipse an accurate understanding of the real complexity of human physiology.

But before you detoxify, in many cases it is helpful to have a clear idea of what toxins you're dealing with and what the body's detoxification capabilities are.

The concept of broadscale toxicity as a primary causative factor for many states of illness is not a new idea, only one Western medicine has forgotten. Toxicity has always been the conceptual foundation of all natural medical practices, especially naturopathy, which developed and flourished in the nineteenth century and is experiencing a resurgence today—for the same reason it was successful when it first appeared on the medical scene. It understands the role of toxicity and it knows how to remove it. But before you detoxify, in many cases it is helpful to have a clear idea of what toxins you're dealing with and what the body's detoxification capabilities are. This is where laboratory tests come into the picture, the focus of the present chapter.

The Healthy Living Space Expert Interview: Peter Holyk, M.D., Contemporary Health Innovations

A good example of the new trend to focus on general toxicity as a primary factor in illness is the medical practice of Peter Holyk, M.D., a board certified ophthamologist and founder of Contemporary Health Innovations, P.A., in Sebastian, Florida. Founded in 1997, Dr. Holyk's clinic offers a variety of toxicity-oriented services including testing for heavy metals, toxins, and micronutrient status; nutritional supplementation programs; allergy elimination techniques; diet and lifestyle counseling; hormonal rebalancing; and EDTA chelation.

Dr. Holyk, originally trained in conventional medicine, was "converted" to the more broadly focused toxicity-conscious viewpoint by direct experience. His wife got very sick; in fact, so did he. In dealing with both illnesses and finding ways to reverse them, Dr. Holyk came to appreciate the importance of toxicity in health and illness.

His illness was about as bad as it gets: brain cancer. When he was thirty-five, his physician discovered a tumor in his brain the size of a baseball. Forecasts of lifelong quadriplegia were handed him; doubts were cast on whether he would even survive the brain surgery. In other words, he got the usual "doom and gloom" world view of conventional medicine in the face of an extreme example of unchecked toxicity. Surgery was successful in reducing the size of the tumor to that of a thimble. Since chemotherapy and radiation were offered him with only limited hope of success after surgery, he refused them. Dr. Holyk got his life back, but as the months passed, he began to suspect "something was missing" from the medical world view in which he been trained and treated.

How come conventional medicine had had so few options to offer him for the cancer, he wondered. And what had produced the cancer in the first place? "*Now* I've figured out why that problem occurred," says Dr. Holyk, fifteen years later. "I didn't get a brain tumor because the sun was on the wrong side of the moon. I got a tumor because I was exposed to enough toxins and did not have the right micronutrients to help support my immune system to keep the cancer at bay."

Every day, every person has at least one cancer cell arise in their body in the natural course of cell division, but in most people, the immune system is alert and strong enough to neutralize these rogue cells before they can do any damage. "This is why 100% of the population does not get terminal cancer—because their body is strong enough to kill the cancer cells."

Now Dr. Holyk knows that what makes this immune vigilance possible is a high essential nutrient status, yet this nutrition-supported immune vitality is decreasingly present in Westerners, says Dr. Holyk. One of the key immune agents that deals with cancer as well as other "foreign" proteins and materials in the body is a group of cells called natural killer cells.[i] Unfortunately, research suggests that across the general population, natural killer cell function is declining at "an alarming rate" because "we don't have the nutrition to support it." Dr. Holyk adds, "You may be exposed to the same level of toxins as the next person who doesn't get sick, but you do. That's because if you're deficient in your immune defenses, you are going to get more sick."

As we saw in chapter 2, toxicity is not only prevalent, it is ubiquitous, around us and inside us. The average person in a Western industrialized nation is now routinely exposed to potentially 70,000 different chemicals every day, and the average person carries trace amounts in their body of an estimated 500 different toxins at one time, explains Dr. Holyk. "If your immune defenses aren't good, you're in deep trouble." Further, the average person is typically deficient in vital micronutrients, certain trace elements such as vanadium or lithium, among others, whose presence, however minute, is essential for other biochemical processes necessary to health.

But Dr. Holyk didn't appreciate this all at once. The picture of toxicity, immune response, and nutrient status emerged over a period of years as he delved into the subject. In fact, for many years, despite his experience with the brain tumor, he remained in a state of "absolute skepticism" about the role of toxicity and nutrition, as he admits today. "I was so busy being a doctor that I didn't pay attention to the facts in front of me." He would read reports and scientific studies attesting to the interplay of toxins and nutrients, but discard it as "nonsense." "I dismissed a lot of it, but then, all of a sudden, I couldn't dismiss it anymore. I had to start paying attention to it."

His wife's long illness—gallbladder removal followed by chronic fatigue—shook him out of his skepticism. First she had her gallbladder removed when she was only in her late twenties, an unusually young age to develop a dysfunctional gallbladder. Then she developed chronic fatigue syndrome, such that she was unable to get out of bed at all on some days. Eventually the possibility of severe toxicity became apparent to Dr. Holyk, and his wife underwent laboratory testing for heavy metals. They were specifically looking for mercury and lead, two of the most prevalent toxic heavy metals to show up in the human body.

Their hunch was sound because it turned out she had severe lead and mercury poisoning and that these toxic metals were contributing mightily to her chronic illness. Where did the lead and mercury come from? Toxic residues of lead are almost ubiquitous in the modern environment, from old water pipes and lead-based paint to leaded gasoline residues in the dirt by the roadsides. The chief source of mercury, besides contaminated fish and pesticides, is dental amalgam fillings in which mercury typically comprises about fifty percent of the different components of the filling.

A growing body of research shows that not only can mercury leach from a dental filling, but it can migrate throughout the body, producing (or contributing to) a long list of mild to serious health problems, including chronic fatigue. Mercury is released from the fillings as a vapor that is absorbed through the nasal cavity and then lungs, then transported through the bloodstream to be deposited in fatty tissues, including in the brain and nervous system, says Dr. Holyk.

In both cases, lead and mercury toxicity can be a cumulative development; you usually don't have a single, intense exposure to a heavy metal with resulting obvious signs of poisoning. Rather, you get poisoned slowly, in tiny doses that steadily accrete within your system, continuously polluting your internal environment and contributing to its dysfunction. In his wife's case, carefully removing the mercury and lead from her system (in that order) helped restore her to health and productivity. It also counselled Dr. Holyk in the vital importance of screening patients for toxicity, such as in the following case history he offers from his medical files.

A woman in her mid-forties, named Penelope, developed sudden blindness in one eye. Her conventional physician forecast that she might develop multiple sclerosis (MS), as this kind of seemingly inexplicable blindness is a precursor of MS in twenty percent of cases. Penelope easily could have slipped into the MS diagnosis had she not had the good fortune to contact Dr. Holyk. In taking Penelope's health history, he learned that three weeks before the sudden onset of blindness, she had sustained a major break in one of her mercury-based dental fillings. Instead of having the tooth capped, she had the amalgam filling replaced.

This dental procedure actually doubled her mercury exposure: first, the broken mercury filling meant that mercury vapors and tiny particles of the metal were free to enter her bloodstream; second, removing the broken tooth (without specialized dental precautions required for *safe* mercury removal) further mobilized free mercury so it could enter her system; then installing another mercury filling introduced more mercury that could potentially leach into her blood, along with that amount steadily liberated from the other numerous mercury-based fillings in Penelope's mouth.

Regrettably, it is still the case that the majority of American physicians and dentists do not make this well-proven connection between mercury fillings and mercury toxicity—to their patients' peril.[2] Ironically, "studies performed on dentists who have occupational exposure to mercury have shown diminished fine motor coordination and slowed response time to various stimuli," states Dr. Holyk.

Dr. Holyk, with good evidential grounds for suspecting mercury toxicity as the prime cause of Penelope's blindness, had her go through two simple medical tests: a hair analysis, which has a good reputation for revealing heavy metal toxicity (described below), and a DMPS challenge.[3] This latter procedure involves the introduction by injection of a nontoxic substance (DMPS) that binds up mercury in the system, which is then excreted in the urine; the urine is then evaluated for mercury levels. Both tests confirmed that Penelope had a high level of mercury toxicity.

Based on this accurate medical information, Dr. Holyk next laid out a treatment program. He prescribed an intensive two-week supplemental program of nutrients and micronutrients (minerals needed in minute or trace levels) and he arranged to have Penelope's mercury-based dental fillings removed by a *qualified* dentist. Qualified here means that the dentist understands the extreme need to protect the patient from mercury mobilization and migration once the fillings are in the process of being removed. (See chapter 7 for more on mercury toxicity and safe amalgam removal.)

If done inexpertly, a person can end up far sicker after amalgam removal than before, because the procedure itself liberates a comparatively vast amount of mercury into the bloodstream, compared to the much smaller, though toxic, amounts slowly released with the fillings in place. "It's very dangerous to take out amalgams if you don't know how to do it correctly," comments Dr. Holyk. "I've had people walk into my office after an amalgam removal with partial paralysis, partial blindness—you name it. So beware."

Penelope had her mercury amalgams removed under carefully controlled conditions and Dr. Holyk continued to boost her nutritional status for several weeks. She also received DMPS (by injection) to clear free mercury from her bloodstream, enabling it to pass out of her body in her urine. Her visual acuity now became a kind of daily feedback report on the ongoing state of detoxification. In the troubled eye, her eyesight had diminished from an original 20/20 to 20/60, and from there to perceiving only light, but no detail or color in that eye. Yet twenty-four hours after receiving a DMPS injection, that eye registered 20/25, the abatement of symptoms showing the dramatic effect of mercury removal.

Over the next weeks, Penelope's visual acuity fluctuated a bit, dropping off to 20/40, then coming back to 20/25 with another DMPS injection, says Dr. Holyk. While Penelope continued with the nutrients and DMPS detoxification, her eyesight stayed at around 20/25 for a year; after a while, she let some of the elements slide, and her eyesight dropped back to around 20/70. These fluctuations reflected ongoing detoxification. The amount of time it takes for complete mercury removal and health improvement can vary considerably among patients. "Sometimes we see improvement in patients right away; other patients have so much mercury in their system that we're still pulling out large amounts after a year of treatment," says Dr. Holyk.

"Mercury toxicity is one of the very biggest problems that I encounter, followed by lead," says Dr. Holyk. But that's only the start of the list. Generally, Dr. Holyk tests for fifteen toxins, following a startling report by the Environmental Protection Agency in the 1980s stating that five heavy metals (mercury, cadmium, lead, antimony, and beryllium) showed up in 100% of the human fat samples tested in the study. "I can tell you if you routinely tested *all* patients for heavy metals, you would find almost everyone has a problem," confides Dr. Holyk.

When he says "all" patients, Dr. Holyk doesn't mean only those who crawl into a medical practice chronically ill, fatigued, or hypersensitive to numerous chemicals, but also people who are not obviously sick, who may not even suspect toxicity, yet who perhaps notice a vague sense of sluggishness or compromised function or ability. The thing about toxicity is that there is only a quantitative difference between "a vague sense" and full-blown toxicity.

This is why for Dr. Holyk two matters come immediately to mind in assessing a new patient's symptoms: micronutrient status and toxicity. Is this person deficient in key vitamins or minerals necessary for normal detoxification processes, and is this patient carrying a toxic burden of cumulative heavy metal, solvent, or pesticide poisoning?

The relationship between mercury toxicity and nutrient status is even more interwoven, says Dr. Holyk. There are two ways of making this point. First, certain substances such as mercury can be mistaken for magnesium by the body. "If you don't have enough magnesium in your body, your body will suck in a molecule of mercury to take its place." With the magnesium slots filled with the impostor, mercury, there is now no room for real magnesium, and you become magnesium deficient. The toxin now blocks your system from absorbing the required real nutrient, explains Dr. Holyk. You may want to fortify yourself nutritionally, but your body cannot absorb the desired nutrients because mercury molecules are taking their rightful place in your cell chemistry. That's the first complication.

For Dr. Holyk two matters come immediately to mind in assessing a new patient's symptoms: micronutrient status and toxicity. Is this person deficient in key vitamins or minerals necessary for normal detoxification processes, and is this patient carrying a toxic burden of cumulative heavy metal, solvent, or pesticide poisoning?

The second problem is that with all this mercury now in place in the cells, the body's natural detoxification processes are compromised, even blocked. As discussed in chapter 2, the liver has a two-phase detoxification procedure. Phase I involves a group of enzymes called cytochrome P450, a key to successful liver detoxification. "Yet if you get mercury in your system, it will bind to specific sites of the cytochrome P450 system and shut it down. This phase of the liver's detoxification will not work. Your liver cannot detoxify because mercury has shut down your detoxification system." It doesn't end there, either, adds Dr. Holyk.

Cytochrome P450 is crucial to the formation of hormones, such as testosterone and progesterone, the male and female "sex" hormones, respectively. "If mercury binds into the cytochrome P450 system, you cannot make your own hormones any more. You have a real problem. You can see when one toxin binds one specific chemical how much biochemical havoc it creates. What about the effects of all the other toxins we're exposed to? We're lucky we function as well as we do considering the degree to which I find toxic levels and deficient micronutrient status in patients."

At this point in the evolution of enlightened medical practice in the United States, there are many inexpensive but reliable testing options available to both physician and patient. Many of them do not require a physician's prescription other than for the initial drawing of a blood sample. When it comes to tests for toxicity, Dr. Holyk tends to rely on hair analyses, the DMPS challenge for mercury levels, certain specialized forms of blood assays, and kinesiological muscle testing.

"The best way in my opinion to find out about micronutrients is to look for intracellular nutrients," explains Dr. Holyk. By "intracellular" he means nutrients found inside blood cells. For this information, he relies on a blood test called a packed red blood cell intracellular analysis. It's a bit complicated, but the idea is this: normally, a blood sample is spun in a centrifuge and the serum (the watery portion of the blood) is examined for a specific nutrient, say magnesium. But magnesium exists mostly *inside* the cells—it's an *intra*cellular nutrient. Since the plug of red blood cells was discarded in the centrifuge, the test will not indicate the true level of magnesium in this patient, explains Dr. Holyk. The packed red blood cell intracellular analysis looks at what's inside the cells and therefore provides a more accurate result, he adds.

As for kinesiological muscle testing, Dr. Holyk asserts that he has found its results to be comparable and consistent with those obtained from blood assays and another diagnostic approach called electrodermal screening (EDS). Chiropractors, for example, often use kinesiological muscle testing to determine if a person is allergic to a substance, will respond well or poorly to a proposed substance, and ask other medical questions necessary to form a clear diagnosis. The principle behind muscle testing is simple: a muscle's strength noticeably wanes in the presence of a toxic or nondesired substance.

In the case of electrodermal screening, specific surface points on the hands and feet (associated with acupuncture meridians) are probed with a device hooked up to a computer; a single patient can be tested for the suitability of hundreds of substances in a short time using this approach. Specific toxins can be ascertained along with the appropriateness, or not, of proposed remedies.[4]

Dr. Holyk also reports good results from a testing method called Biological Terrain Assessment, another computer-assisted evaluation of a patient's cellular environment. It studies the biochemical condition of the blood, urine, and/or saliva in terms of pH (the ratio of acidity to alkalinity, a general indication of chemical balance or imbalance), oxidation-reduction potential (how much "oxidation stress" the body is carrying, a measure of cellular toxicity), and resistivity (a tissue's resistance to the flow of electrical current).

Insofar as food and substance allergies play a large role in toxicity, Dr. Holyk often uses Nambudripad Allergy Elimination Technique (NAET), a system of both diagnosis and treatment that uses acupressure, acupuncture, and allergy desensitization techniques to neutralize the allergenic effect of numerous substances. "I've almost not found a person who did not have a toxic problem or did not have an allergy problem, or both," he states. "To some degree they may be interdependent, although I think they actually are two independent variables—but they are both extremely common."

The essential point, Dr. Holyk emphasizes, is to *know* your patient's nutritional status, immune defense capabilities, and level of toxicity. Then you can unravel their health problems, initiate a successful detoxification program, and start rebuilding, or maintaining, optimal health. In other words, reliable nutritional and physiological *information* is the key to successful detoxification and creating a healthy living space. Reliable diagnostic information about your biochemical and physiological status provides answers not only as to why you may be already sick, but it can also highlight vulnerable areas and tendencies toward developing future illnesses or imbalances. Even better, diagnostic tests such as these can equip you with enough advance information to *prevent* most future health problems and in effect to treat disease before it ever happens.

While you most likely will not need to do all of the laboratory tests outlined in this chapter (see figure 3-1), a selection may illuminate certain otherwise baffling aspects of your

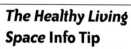

The Healthy Living Space Info Tip
To contact Peter Holyk, M.D.: Contemporary Health Innovations, PA, 600 Schumann Drive, Sebastian, FL 32958; tel: 561-388-5554; fax: 561-388-2410; website: www.chimed.com.

Figure 3-1. 19 Reliable Tests to Measure Your Possible Toxicity

Packed Blood Cell Elements Profile	Detoxification Profile
Whole Blood Elements Profile	Hair Analysis
CellMate Blood Test Report	Urine Elements Profiles—Essentials and Toxics
Individualized Optimal Nutrition (ION)	Special Provocative Mercury Test
Functional Intracellular Analysis (FIA)	Oral Toxicity Testing
Total Antioxidant Status	Comprehensive Digestive Stool Analysis
Pantox Profile	Comprehensive Parasitology Profile
Biological Terrain Assessment	Immuno 1 Bloodprint
Oxidative Protection Screen	Nambudripad Allergy Elimination Technique
Oxidative Stress Profile	(NAET)

---

health condition. Some tests you can order on your own; others require a physician's prescription; and most yield their best results if you work with a qualified health-care practitioner who can interpret the data.

HEALTHY LIVING SPACE DETOXIFIER #3
Get a Clear Idea of Your Nutritional Status

As Dr. Holyk explains, your nutritional status—the levels of specific major nutrients and micronutrients in your body, especially those involved in detoxification—is a key element to both your health and your system's ability to detoxify and mount a strong immune defense.

You may think you have good, satisfactory, or even excellent nutritional status, yet it is often the case that a person is deficient, or even seriously lacking in a few key elements. It's only when you get sick that this unchecked deficiency reveals itself and hinders your recovery process. The *only* way to know in advance if you are lacking in a few or many essential elements is to have good testing (such as urine, stool, and hair, described below) before you get sick, or at the start of a deliberate detoxification program. Below are brief overviews of a number of well-known and widely used laboratory tests to determine nutrient status.

Packed Blood Cell Elements Profile

This is the test referred to by Dr. Holyk above as "packed red blood cell intracellular analysis." Offered by Doctor's Data, an independent reference laboratory that specializes in tests to measure levels of toxic and essential elements in the blood and urine, this test assesses the status of nutrients inside blood cells or in blood cell membranes. According to Doctor's Data, this test is "an excellent diagnostic tool" to measure anti-inflammatory processes (your body's ability to withstand inflammations, especially internal ones that could lead to arthritis or fibromyalgia), immune function, and problems associated with zinc deficiency (such as poor wound healing and attention deficit disorder).

Specifically, this test looks for levels of thirteen nutrients, major players such as calcium, magnesium, potassium, phosphorus, zinc, and iron; and several key micronutrients such as vanadium, molybdenum, and boron. It contrasts the results against an established reference range—levels generally considered optimal for health and statistically prevalent in healthy people.

For example, in a sample laboratory report, a male, aged thirty-five, had calcium at 13 µg/g (which means parts per million); the reference range for calcium is 8-31 µg/g, which means he was at the very low end of "acceptable," and probably on the verge of being deficient. His iron came in at 968 µg/g compared to the reference range for iron of 745-1050 µg/g, placing him well within the acceptable, well-fortified range for this nutrient. The test also measures blood levels for five toxic elements: antimony, arsenic, cadmium, lead, and mercury. This man tested 0.076 µg/g for mercury compared to the reference range of less than 0.01 µg/g; this meant that he had some mercury toxicity in his system as his numbers for mercury were higher than the acceptable range.

Whole Blood Elements Profile

This is also offered by Doctor's Data and is designed to measure circulating blood levels of toxic and nutrient elements. It is particularly recommended by Doctor's Data to be used before and during a detoxification treatment, and is well suited to identify dietary inadequacies (in terms of nutrient intake) and the function of the gastrointestinal, endocrine, and kidney systems. The test measures levels of twelve nutrients (many of the same nutrients measured in the Packed Blood Cell Elements Profile) and six toxic elements (including bismuth, nickel, and uranium) based on their levels in the whole blood (the watery portion, or plasma, plus the red blood cells). The results are not necessarily the same as in the previous test because the test measures nutrient and toxic status in a larger, more diffuse volume than only packed red blood cells.

CellMate Blood Test Report

The manufacturer of this test describes it as an "extension" to standard blood tests because it compares a person's blood chemistry to a database of medical research. The results for concentrations of individual nutrients are presented in terms of a percent status, that is, how much above or below the normal range they deviate. The report also matches results against tabulated symptom correlations for numerous illnesses; this is called disease pattern matching and enables the physician to make quick recognition of similar patterns. For example, a person may have five results that give them an eighty-three percent match for the blood conditions typically observed in someone with hypersplenism (overactive spleen).

The Basic Status Report presents your lows and highs in over fifty categories (including key immune cells) as a bar graph, making it easy to see at a glance where your nutrient excesses and deficiencies lie. And the test indicates nutrients that would be useful to take as supplements, drugs and drug interactions to avoid, and supplements to avoid based on your specific biochemistry. The value of this test is that it puts the biochemical information in the context of normal ranges for excesses and deficiencies and with respect to known matching disease patterns.

Individualized Optimal Nutrition (ION)

The ION test measures your specific nutritional status and provides a specific supplemental program to restore deficiencies. The test studies blood and/or urine samples to uncover nutritional status and "metabolic trends," by which MetaMetrix, ION's provider, means how well your body processes foods to extract the necessary nutrients.

A blood or urine test, says MetaMetrix, is like taking a "snapshot in time" of your nutrient status, showing the effects of what you have been eating, the degree of stress your system has been under (which can result from nutrient deficiencies), and the impact of supplementation. It is very hard to know if you have optimal nutritional status without a test. You may assume you are healthy, or you may feel normal or "okay," but you may still have a suboptimal nutritional state.

The ION program has five subprofiles including amino acid, B-vitamin/mineral, antioxidant, fatty acid, and disease risk status. Let's look at each of these and see why this knowledge is valuable for a detoxification program.

Amino acids, which are the building blocks of proteins, have to do with energy, endurance, concentration, mood, and alertness, and play key roles in brain function, immune system operation, tissue repair, regulation of blood sugar levels, and general energy levels. If your diet lacks sufficient amino acids, any of these vital functions may be impaired, providing the foundation for toxicity and the body's inability to detoxify, as well as the development of dysfunction and eventual illness.

Similarly, B-vitamins and minerals are essential for numerous bodily functions and are, in the words of MetaMetrix, "the spark plugs necessary for your metabolic engine." For example, the mineral magnesium is required for at least 300 different enzyme reactions in the body, but studies show that in fifty percent of hospitalized patients, magnesium levels are low, which suggests the magnesium deficiency might be linked to numerous health problems that lead to hospitalization.

As discussed in chapter 2, antioxidants are specific nutrients (such as vitamins A, C, and E) that protect your system against toxins (free radicals) that can lead to disease. As MetaMetrix puts it: "Normal biological processes and environmental pollutants produce unstable molecules called free radicals that wreak havoc on tissues by setting tiny 'fires' of oxidation."

The unbalanced state of oxidative stress (see below, for another test) can lead to many physiological problems; in this analogy, antioxidants are the "indispensable molecular fire extinguishers." When free radicals damage the fat (lipid) portion of cell membranes, toxic products called lipid peroxides are formed. These are associated with the development of numerous physical problems including heart disease, arthritis, liver disorders, allergic inflammation, and others. Therefore, this component of the ION test measures your level of free radical activity (and oxidative stress) and the defense status of selected antioxidants.

Certain fatty acids—the test measures levels of twenty-five—are essential to optimal body function because, among other things, they are a source of essential hormones and regulate inflammation, which, if unchecked, can lead to arthritis and chronic muscle pain, among other conditions.[5] Typically, we get too many of the wrong kinds of fats from our diet (hydrogenated and trans-fatty acids), which contribute to cellular degeneration and illness, and too little of the "good" fats, such as those found in fish, flaxseed, and various oils from vegetables and nuts. An imbalanced fat intake is directly linked with many serious illnesses, including stroke, heart attack, and cancer. If you are deficient in any of the essential fatty acids, various metabolic mechanisms that require them may no longer work properly.

The last component of the ION test screens the various organs (especially the liver and kidneys) for risk of developing disease, based on levels of certain biochemicals interpreted as disease risk indicators.

Functional Intracellular Analysis (FIA)

This test of nutrient status is based on examining a sample of the person's white blood cells, called lymphocytes. The test looks inside your white blood cells to see how well nineteen nutrients and antioxidant systems are functioning based on their level of cell growth. According to SpectraCell Laboratories, providers of the test, the FIA uncovers deficiencies usually missed by serum-based tests.

FIA is called "functional" for a good reason. White blood cells are isolated and removed from the blood sample, then grown in culture media, being given the optimal nutrients for cell growth. Then specific nutrients are removed, one at a time from the media, requiring the white blood cells to replenish these nutrients from their own reserves. "If there are no deficiencies in a particular vitamin, the cells will still grow adequately," explains SpectraCell. "If, however, the cells do not grow adequately, it represents a deficiency of that vitamin." In other words, you get an accurate report on your body's functional nutritional status, on how well it performs its job for *your* system specifically based on the nutrients and nutrient levels available to it.

Total Antioxidant Status

This test measures levels of all the antioxidants present in a blood sample according to their ability to stop a particular oxidation reaction, which is to say, a targeted free-radical-initiated activity. The test, developed by King James Medical Laboratory, looks at three antioxidant defense systems: primary antioxidants (superoxide dismutase, glutathione peroxidase, and metal-binding proteins), which prevent new free radical groups from arising; secondary antioxidants (vitamins E and C, beta-carotene, uric acid, bilirubin, and albumin), which collect free radicals, preventing them from working together to produce toxic chain reactions; and third-level antioxidants (DNA repair enzymes), which repair "biomolecules" that have been damaged by free radicals.

Pantox Profile

Pantox Laboratories provides a blood test called the Pantox Profile, which "interprets the biochemical defense system" by measuring the blood concentration of twenty-five substances central to the body's antioxidant response and compares these results with values obtained from other people of the same gender and age. Each substance analyzed for a given person is then plotted as a percentile, expressed as a vertical bar graph for easy comprehension. When the blood concentrations of these twenty-five substances are interpreted, they serve as "very early indicators" of potential health problems. The test results don't show the presence of disease; rather they demonstrate your ability to resist it.

The key point here is that early recognition of nutritional deficiencies or imbalances known to be associated with various illnesses leads to correction and prevention. This is why Pantox recommends this test as a "regular biochemical checkup." Pantox emphasizes that aging and age-dependent degenerative disease (which encompasses a great number of illnesses) are the "byproducts of normal metabolism."

Technically, "normal" metabolism involves the production of free radicals; it should also include their deactivation by antioxidants, but when this doesn't happen, your imbalanced metabolism slowly sickens you. A test of this type is useful in terms when a person needs to know if their nutritional defense systems are in optimal shape.

Biological Terrain Assessment

This test provides an in-depth view of the elements of an individual's chemistry and the underlying causes of an imbalance, thereby enabling the practitioner to determine an individualized program for the patient. The test looks at biochemical conditions within the cells, specifically in three categories. These are pH (the balance between acidity and alkalinity), oxidative stress (oxidation-reduction potential, or redox, indicating electron potential and enzymatic activity), and resistivity (molecular ion movement and gross mineral concentration).

These three factors largely determine what is now being called the cell's internal environment, milieu, or terrain—its overall quality of (cellular) life. You could even think of it as the "soil" of the cell; just as in gardening, healthy soil with the right balance of microorganisms and nutrients produces the healthiest, most nourishing vegetables. The "vegetables" in this analogy are the biochemical activities of cell life and function. The idea of terrain actually originated with the early nineteenth century physiologist, Claude Bernard, who stated that the cell's environment determines its function and integrity, and thereby the vitality of the entire body.

The key point here is that early recognition of nutritional deficiencies or imbalances known to be associated with various illnesses leads to correction and prevention. This is why Pantox likes to recommend this test as a "regular biochemical checkup."

Biological terrain is assessed with the help of a computerized device called the BTA S-2000, which displays the results—information on "the body's internal biochemical markers," explains the manufacturer—in various charts and graphs on a computer screen, based on its analysis of a sample of the patient's blood, urine, and saliva. "Many patients who initially undergo Biological Terrain Assessment come into their practitioner's office with reports of 'normal' laboratory values and yet display illness both objectively and subjectively," explains Robert C. Greenberg, M.D., the inventor of the BTA S-2000. "After analyzing their bodily fluids for pH, redox, and resistivity, important data begins to emerge."[6]

Dr. Greenberg explains that "often very subtle yet potent influences" are under way in a person's biochemistry, but are not

The Healthy Living Space Info Tip

For Packed Blood Cell Elements Profile, Whole Blood Elements Profile:
Doctor's Data,
P.O. Box 111,
West Chicago, IL 60186;
tel: 800-323-2784 or 630-377-8139;
fax: 630-587-7860;
e-mail: inquiries@doctorsdata.com;
website: www.doctorsdata.com (see website for sample laboratory reports for these tests).

For CellMate Blood Test Report:
Carbon Based Corporation,
P.O. Box 4549,
Incline Village, NV 89450;
tel: 775-832-8485 or 800-908-0000;
fax: 775-832-8488;
website: www.carbonbased.com.

For ION: MetaMetrix Clinical Laboratory, Inc.,
5000 Peachtree Industrial Boulevard,
Norcross, GA 30071;
tel: 800-221-4640;
fax: 770-441-2237;
e-mail: nutrition@metametrix.com;
website: www.metametrix.com.

For FIA: SpectraCell Laboratories, Inc.,
515 Post Oak Boulevard, Suite 830,
Houston, TX 77027;
tel: 800-227-5227;
website: www.spectracell.com.

For Total Antioxidant Status: King James Medical Laboratory, Inc., 24700 Center Ridge Road, Cleveland, OH 44145;
tel: 800-437-1404;
fax: 440-835-2177;
e-mail: CustomerService@kingjamesomegatech-lab.com;
website: www.kingjamesomegatech-lab.com.

necessarily detected by standard laboratory tests. Some of these toxic influences can include parasites, viruses, fungi, pollutants, free radicals, nutritional deficiencies, oxygen depletion, and the body's inability to excrete carbon dioxide. If standard tests cannot measure these factors, many patients may remain toxic or sick and their doctors confused as to the true medical condition.

HEALTHY LIVING SPACE DETOXIFIER #4
Assess Your System's Ability to Detoxify

The preceding tests will give you a clear idea about your system's nutrient levels and its overall ability to provide the nutritional elements essential for a strong immune defense. Now you need to find out how capable your natural detoxification system is and to what degree its detoxification ability may be already compromised by an excess of toxins.

Oxidative Protection Screen

This test is offered as a functional assessment of oxidative protection, according to its provider, AAL Reference Laboratories. It looks at the extent of oxidative damage (from free radicals) and your body's ability to protect itself against free radical onslaughts. Free radicals not only come from substances brought into the body, but they are the natural byproducts of metabolic processes and the liver's own detoxification program. As explained in chapter 2, if your liver detoxifies the body too quickly (as in Phase I) or has blocked pathways for toxin elimination (Phase II), free radicals accumulate.

Oxidative stress therefore is a reliable measure of how well your body can handle the stress of free radical oxidation—too many poisons in the system.

The test generates a Total Oxidative Protection (TOP) Index for each client, which is a measure of your system's total antioxidant ability—in other words, it tells you how well protected you are. The higher the TOP Index, the stronger your immune defense is.

The test also measures levels of lipid peroxides, which indicate the degree to which your system is suffering oxidative stress, or the overall impact of too many free radicals, especially those acting on the fatty acids in cells. According to AAL Reference Laboratories, the higher the lipid peroxide levels, the greater the degree your system has been negatively affected by free radicals, or toxins. A healthy individual will have very low levels of lipid peroxides. Therefore, this assay provides information on your level of toxicity.

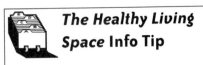

The Healthy Living Space Info Tip

For Pantox Profile:
Pantox Laboratories,
4622 Santa Fe Street,
San Diego, CA 92109;
tel: 888-PANTOX-8, or 888-726-8698,
or 858-272-3885;
fax: 858-272-1621;
website: www.pantox.com.

For Biological Terrain Assessment:
Biological Technologies International, Inc., P.O. Box 560, Payson, AZ 85547;
tel: 520-474-4181;
fax: 520-474-1501;
website: www.bioterrain.com.

The two results—TOP Index and lipid peroxides levels—are correlated and interpreted together. For example, if the test indicates you have normal lipid peroxides but low TOP Index, it means you are losing your antioxidant protection reserve. If unchecked, this may progress to a loss of oxidative protection. If the test indicates you have high lipid peroxides and normal TOP Index, this means your system is producing free radicals faster than your antioxidant system can cope with. This may be happening because of excess tobacco smoke inhalation, too much exercise, being obese, or having a diet with too many polyunsaturated fats or oils. If you have increased lipid peroxides levels and a low TOP Index, this indicates a state of poor oxidative protection.

Oxidative Stress Profile

Genox Corporation of Baltimore, Maryland, offers an analysis of oxidative stress with four components. The test measures the rate of generation of free radicals; the levels of antioxidants ("scavengers of reactive oxygen species") and the rate at which lipid peroxides are reduced; the level of oxidative damage already sustained by the person; and the rate at which oxidative repair is accomplished and the rate of removal of free radicals. Genox obtains these measures by assaying a sample of blood, urine, or breath, although in special cases, a tissue or cell sample from the mouth or bladder may be used.

The Healthy Living Space Info Tip

For Oxidative Protection Screen:
AAL Reference Laboratories, Inc.,
1715 E. Wilshire, #715,
Santa Ana, CA 92705;
tel: 714-972-9979 or 800-522-2611;
fax: 714-543-2034;
e-mail: inquire@aalrl.com;
website: www.antibodyassay.com.

For Oxidative Stress Profile:
Genox Corporation,
1414 Key Highway,
Baltimore, MD 21230;
tel: 410-347-7616 or 800-810-5450;
lab: 410-347-7637;
fax: 410-347-7617;
e-mail: info@genox.com;
website: www.genox.com.

For Detoxification Profile:
Great Smokies Diagnostic Laboratory,
63 Zillicoa Street,
Asheville, NC 28801;
tel: 800-522-4762;
fax: 828-252-9303;
e-mail: cs@gsdl.com;
website: www.gsdl.com.

Detoxification Profile

In this test, certain "challenge" substances, such as caffeine, acetaminophen, and salicylate (aspirin), are given in tablet form to see how well the body performs each stage of the detoxification process related to these substances. In other words, the test studies how well your body can "clear" these substances, passing them out through the urine. The results, as analyzed in the urine and saliva, and sometimes blood, shed light on your system's detoxification ability, in both its Phase I and Phase II stages. As explained in chapter 2, in liver detoxification, the body's enzymes collect and "activate" (alter or neutralize) toxic substances, such that other enzymes can convert these toxins into water-soluble forms that can be eliminated through the urine and stool.

In effect, this test highlights your liver's ability to detoxify. The test studies the metabolites (organic compounds produced by breaking down the challenge substances), the byproducts of detoxification (such as glutathione, a key detoxifying substance found in the liver), and the toxins (in various changed forms) one would expect to be excreted during a detoxification, such as lipid peroxides. The information provided by this test is valuable because both Phase I and Phase II of your liver's detoxification system must function adequately so that toxins can be neutralized and excreted, and because the two phases must work in balance with each other.

HEALTHY LIVING SPACE DETOXIFIER #5
Determine Your Body's Total Toxic Load

The preceding set of tests provides information on the functional status of your liver and its two-phase detoxification system.

Now it's time to get specific: what is your total toxic load? Which toxic substances is your body storing? Do you have heavy metal toxicity, intestinal imbalances, or parasites? The matter of intestinal balances and parasitic infestation will be discussed at greater length later in the book (chapter 5), but both are the focus of important laboratory tests. Imbalances in the microbial population of the intestines can result from prolonged, unrelieved toxicity and they also further contribute to this toxicity. Parasites (living microscopic organisms such as various species of worms that don't belong in the human body) can enter the intestines through our food and water and contribute to intestinal imbalance, rob us of crucial nutrients, and generally sicken us.

Simple laboratory tests involving samples of hair, urine, and/or stool can provide clinically valuable information on your toxic load and possible intestinal imbalances or parasitic involvement.

Hair Analysis

Although hair analysis got its start in the 1930s, progressive physicians have turned increasingly to it in recent decades. In fact, over 1,500 peer-reviewed scientific papers have been published on hair analysis. An analysis of a patient's hair sample is considered a reliable window into the level of toxicity present, specifically, heavy metals. A hair analysis typically evaluates the amount (parts per million) in the body of twenty-two elements such as aluminum, mercury, cobalt, cadmium, arsenic, nickel, and others.

The hair seems to have a remarkable ability to register the concentration of various metals in the body. Typically about one gram of hair is selected, or about two teaspoons, taken from the first one and one-half inches of hair closest to the scalp at the nape of the neck. In fact, the deposition of metals in strands of hair is somewhat like tree rings, which form in accordance with growth spurts. In the case of hair, as a strand grows, its biochemical composition reflects the various metals the individual has been exposed to or ingested. In fact, in the case of some toxic metals, "hair more closely reflects the body's mineral stores than blood or urine," states King James Medical Laboratory, which offers the Omegatech Hair Analysis.

The Laboratory further explains that "the hair becomes a stable time record of the exposure and circulation of metals. The metal content of the hair varies along its length relative to the type and amount of each metal the hair cells are exposed to during their growth."[7]

If for example you submitted a hair sample today and compared the analysis results with one you obtained a year earlier, the results could be quite different. They would depend on which metals you were exposed to during the time that hair strand was growing. If you worked around lead paint or had a mercury filling replaced (perhaps not expertly) a year ago but since then had stayed away entirely from all paints and never seen a dentist, your hair analysis would yield different results for lead and mercury.

Doctor's Data, which offers a Hair Elemental Profile, explains that the hair analysis offers a "temporal record of metabolism"—how well your digestion and absorption of nutrients are going right now—as well as an exposure index to various toxic metals. The company emphasizes that this test is useful for the early detection of "elemental aberrations, because deviations often appear in hair prior to overt symptoms." Not only do you get information about possible heavy metal toxicity, but you can potentially get this information early enough to serve as an advance warning of possible future (or imminent) health problems.

According to Trace Mineral Systems, a testing company in Alexandria, Virginia, which also offers a hair analysis, hair is "the ideal biopsy material" and hair analysis is now "an extremely precise analytical test." A blood mineral analysis will show which substances are circulating extracellularly (outside and between the cells), and a urine test will tell you which elements have been excreted, but a hair analysis will highlight a person's individualized mineral absorption during a specified time period, explains Trace Mineral Systems.

Urine Elements Profiles—Essentials and Toxics

The value of the hair analysis is that it provides an initial mineral screening of your system. If it indicates significant metal toxicity, you might need a more comprehensive test called a urine analysis to give diagnostic information about various heavy metals based on their presence in the urine. The better urine analyses will collect a patient's urine from a 24-hour period, with samples taken at regular intervals. This gives a more balanced and thereby accurate picture of urine composition, as its contents may vary by the hour according to circadian hormonal secretions, dietary intake, and fluctuating stress levels.

A urine test reveals information about elements both essential to the body's operation and those regarded as toxic. For example, a typical urine test will assess the levels of eighteen "expected elements" such as sodium, potassium, calcium, magnesium, and various other key nutrients, and compare their excretion levels against optimal norms and reference ranges. Then a twenty-four-hour urine toxic metals test can show the amounts present of at least fifteen undesirable toxic metals, including mercury, tin, uranium, cadmium, and others, again, comparing them against reference ranges.

For example, in a sample urine toxic metals test report supplied by Doctor's Data (available on their website) a male, aged 65, tested with 4.7 µg/g (parts per million) of cadmium, a toxic metal found in tobacco smoke. The reference range (the safe level) for cadmium is less than 2 µg/g , meaning this man had cadmium toxicity. He also had high levels of mercury at 2.4 µg/g (reference range: 3.0 µg/g) and lead at 13 µg/g (reference range: 15 µg/g). His levels for mercury and lead may not have exceeded the reference range, but they were close, indicating an excess of both metals in his system and a potential for heavy-metal-mediated illness.

This same patient had notable imbalances in his essential elements, namely, in calcium, magnesium, sulfur, zinc, and iron, all of which considerably exceeded the reference range. Recall Dr. Peter Holyk's observation, cited earlier, that mercury can be mistaken for magnesium by the body. "If you don't have enough magnesium in your body, your body will suck in a molecule of mercury to take its place," he commented. This patient had significant mercury in his urine and a magnesium level of 261 µg/g, compared to the reference range for magnesium of 46-200 µg/g.

Was there a magnesium-mercury feedback loop happening in this man? A health-care practitioner, skilled in interpreting this data and understanding that heavy metal toxicity can lead to essential nutrient imbalances, and vice versa, could assemble a useful diagnostic picture of this client, using the data from both aspects of the urine test.

Special Provocative Mercury Test

The situation may arise in which you or your physician may wish to gather more specific data on suspected high mercury levels in your system. The man referred to above, whose mercury was 2.4 µg/g as against the reference range of 3.0 µg/g, is a good example of someone who would probably want to quantify his mercury load more precisely.

Using a metal chelator called DMSA (2,3-dimercaptosuccinic acid), the body is challenged to release some of its mercury store through the urine; DMSA, as a chelator, binds up the mercury stored in tissues and removes it from the body. The DMSA challenge also measures urine levels of lead, cadmium, arsenic, and nickel. You take a 500-mg capsule of DMSA, then collect all your urine during the next six hours, after which you mail the specimen to the laboratory. Analysis of the mercury in the urine gives an indication of the "mercury burden" of the body. As a substance, DMSA is an FDA-approved drug used for the treatment of lead toxicity in children, and is widely regarded as a capable binding agent (chelator) for removing mercury from the body, even from the brain.

There is some disagreement among practitioners on the utility of this test, however. "According to Dr. David Quegg of Doctor's Data," says Dr. Holyk, "DMSA is a very poor way to do a mercury challenge. I only use (and he only suggests using) DMPS."

Oral Toxicity Testing

Mercury is not the only toxic element associated with your teeth. Various standard dental procedures, such as root canals and extractions, can generate toxic products over time that gradually sicken the individual and generally remain undetected because physicians aren't looking in the right place for them. This test seeks to identify these somewhat hidden toxins by analyzing what the layperson would regard as saliva samples. As you will learn in chapter 7, dental toxicity from mercury fillings, root canals, and cavitations, is potentially as major a factor in total toxic body load as that produced by the intestines. "According to some authorities, it is even worse," notes Dr. Holyk.

"Studies have shown that pathogenic [disease-producing] oral bacteria produce extremely high levels of toxins at sites of active infection," states Affinity Labeling Technologies of Lexington, Kentucky, a biotechnology company founded by Boyd Haley, Ph.D., chairman of the chemistry department at the University of Kentucky, and Curt Pendergrass, Ph.D. Their test is called the ALT, Inc., Four Part in Vitro Toxicity Testing of Oral Samples.

The test analyzes extracts from a patient's oral samples including gingival crevicular fluid, extracted teeth (such as those that bear root canals), and materials from cavitations ("cavities" in the jawbones, located underneath the areas where extracted teeth were once set in the jaw) for the presence of bacterial toxins, human inflammatory proteins (such as antibodies and serum albumin), and other undesired toxic elements.[8]

The company also offers a seven-minute chairside test called TOPAS (Toxicity Prescreening Assay), which dentists can perform (painlessly) on patients during a dental checkup. For this, a specially treated swab is placed against a given tooth at the gumline, and it turns one color or another, depending on the degree of periodontal toxicity present. The test measures levels of protein in the gingival fluid, based on the understanding that dental bacterial infection increases these levels.

Comprehensive Digestive Stool Analysis

A diagnostic tool whose use is steadily becoming more widespread is the stool analysis, or the biochemical evaluation of a sample of the patient's feces. This test shows how well (or poorly) your digestive system handles the foods you eat, how well the wastes and toxins are eliminated in the stool, and the general state of intestinal microbial balance or imbalance. The technical term for this latter state is intestinal dysbiosis.[9]

The human intestines form an ecosystem with temperature, food source, and moisture at near ideal conditions for the growth of simple life forms, explains Richard S. Lord, Ph.D., of MetaMetrix Clinical Laboratory. "The human gut has been

"The human gut has been described as a continuous flow microbial growth chamber," explains Richard S. Lord, Ph.D., of MetaMetrix Clinical Laboratory, adding that a healthy intestine hatches about three pounds of viable microorganisms every day.

described as a continuous flow microbial growth chamber," he says, adding that a healthy intestine hatches about three pounds of viable microorganisms every day.[10] In other words, *many* microorganisms are *supposed* to be resident in the intestinal tract; most are benign and beneficial, but a few are not. Even so, in a healthy person, there is a balanced ecology in which the beneficial and undesirable organisms live together in a specific balance or ratio. When this balance is disturbed, intestinal dysbiosis results, and this sets the stage for numerous gastrointestinal-mediated illnesses and health problems.

Dysbiosis leads to an excess of bacterial toxins which in turn irritate the mucosal tissues of the gastrointestinal tract; if their buildup is excessive, they may "leak" into the bloodstream and put a significant burden on the liver and immune system. Intestinal dysbiosis favors the overgrowth of yeast, specifically *Candida albicans*, which causes numerous health problems, including allergies. Dysbiosis also favors (or can be the result of) parasitic infestation—the prevalence of tiny worms and other parasitic organisms in the gastrointestinal tract that leach nutrients and disturb digestive processes.

According to Great Smokies Diagnostic Laboratory, which provides the Comprehensive Digestive Stool Analysis (CDSA), this noninvasive tool for analyzing the digestive tract "helps pinpoint imbalances, provides clues about current symptoms, and warns of potential problems should the imbalances progress." The CDSA can identify "critical imbalances previously unsuspected," as well as hidden yeast or bacterial infections, intestinal flora balance, dietary fiber intake, and intestinal immune function. It does this by studying the levels of various marker substances including certain fats (triglycerides), vegetable and meat fibers, various fatty acids, and others (twenty-five markers in all).

Doctor's Data offers a Fecal Metals test to assess the levels of thirteen toxic heavy metals. In a sample report (available at their website) on a woman, aged forty-six, it was shown that many of her heavy metal levels exceeded the reference range. For example, her mercury was high at 0.321 mg/kg, compared to a reference range of less than 0.05 (for someone without dental amalgams); her antimony was 0.254 mg/kg against a reference range of less than 0.08; lead was 1.26 mg/kg (reference range: less than 0.5 mg/kg); tungsten 0.185 mg/kg (reference range: less than 0.09 mg/kg); copper was 90 mg/kg (reference range: 60 mg/kg); and bismuth was 0.417 mg/kg (reference range: less than 0.05 mg/kg).

Basically, this woman was seriously high in about half the toxic metals tested, and she had significant levels of the other heavy metals. Her overall health status (or presenting symptoms) was not provided with the sample report, but one can assume she had (or will soon have) some significant health problems given this level of heavy metal toxicity. "For several toxic elements such as mercury, cadmium, lead, antimony, and uranium, biliary excretion of metals into the feces is the primary natural route of elimination from the body," says Doctor's Data.

Comprehensive Parasitology Profile

Mention parasites in the intestines and most people assume you have to travel in exotic lands before this is something to worry about. However, the medical reality is far different. Many people get infested with gastrointestinal parasites merely from the foods they consume while living in North America. We also get exposed to parasites through raw and undercooked food, treated and untreated water, insects, and household pets, as well as through contact with people who have poor hygiene. Microscopic parasites—protozoa, roundworms, pinworms, hookworms, tapeworms, and flukes—can get transmitted through fecally contaminated foods, water, or other materials.

Undetected, intestinal parasites begin destabilizing the microfloral ecology of the intestines, an imbalance that then leads to numerous other health problems, including generalized toxicity. A parasite growing inside your body, leaching all your nutrients and energy, can weaken your immune system and leave you vulnerable to many diseases. Further, a long-term parasitic infection can alter the mucosal lining of the intestines, leading to "leaky gut" or intestinal permeability. Toxins leak through the gut wall into the blood and get distributed throughout the body, producing, at a minimum, allergies and digestive problems. If parasites are present, your body's ability to detoxify its toxic burden is further compromised, and environmental toxins can gain a deeper foothold on your body's systems.

Here's a vivid example of how this works, as related by Gary Kaplan, D.O., an osteopath practicing in Arlington, Virginia. Dr. Kaplan explains that he has observed in a number of patients that parasitic infestation produces symptoms of arthritis and fibromyalgia, or generalized muscle pain, and sometimes asthma. The parasites trigger the immune system, which dispatches antibodies (specialized immune cells that neutralize specific toxins) to deal with the foreign protein in its midst.

The parasites generate an "antigenic reaction," which is not unlike an intense allergic attack, only in this case, it's prolonged. An antigen is a foreign protein or particle that does not belong in the body and which is tagged as a toxin by the immune system, and to which an antibody is assigned. It is often the case that as the parasitic infestation proceeds without medical resolution, the person's digestion suffers. One of Dr. Kaplan's patients developed asthma after being infected with a strain of *Giardia lamblia*, a microscopic organism. Not only did this indicate an antigenic reaction, "the antigenic reaction manifested as asthma," says Dr. Kaplan. After he treated the patient for *Giardia* infestation, all the asthma symptoms cleared up.[11]

Testing for parasites is often indicated when other more obvious sources and sites for toxicity are not forthcoming in terms of explaining a chronic health problem. The more overt symptoms of parasite infestation are diarrhea and abdominal pain, but many other symptoms have been noted: nausea, vomiting, gas, bloating, foul-smelling stools, anorexia or weight loss, gastritis, fever, chills, headache, constipation, and fatigue. Add to this list other, seemingly unrelated problems including joint and muscle aches, anemia, allergies, chronic fatigue, sleep disturbances, and depression, according to Great Smokies Diagnostic Laboratory.

Their Comprehensive Parasitology Profile examines stool specimens for a wide range of protozoal parasites, including amoebae, flagellates, ciliates, coccidia, and microsporidia. If parasites are identified, this makes it easier for a qualified health-care practitioner to put together an effective parasite detoxification program.

HEALTHY LIVING SPACE DETOXIFIER #6
Find Out if You're Suffering from Hidden Food Allergies

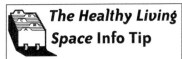

When people think of allergies, more often than not it's in terms of pollen and substance allergies and their characteristic symptoms of stuffy nose; itchy, red, and teary eyes; sneezing; face reddening; and the rest. However, just as serious and widespread a health problem is the matter of food allergies, most commonly to wheat, corn, dairy products, eggs, and chocolate. However, the list of possible allergenic foods—that is, foods that trigger an allergic reaction—is enormous, and given the ubiquity of the five substances just mentioned within the hundreds of processed foods available in North America, your chances of encountering a food to which you are allergic are very high.

According to James Braly, M.D., an expert in allergies and allergy testing and medical director of Immuno Laboratories in Fort Lauderdale, Florida, a recent poll of 722 U.S. physicians quoted them as estimating that between 8% and 19% of the general population and 8.8% and 21% of infants have food allergies. Dr. Braly contends those numbers, in reality, are probably higher. In fact, he says that along with undernutrition, undiagnosed, or hidden, food allergies are a major health problem in the United States today. For many people, the continuous exposure to environmental toxins either creates or worsens their allergies. The allergies in turn, in the way they provoke the immune system into a state of perpetual alert, add to the body's toxic load and eventually weaken the immune system.

How can you tell if you have a hidden food allergy? There are many symptoms that typically occur in one who is chronically reactive, and these can be taken as reliable indicators of probable food allergies, according to a questionnaire developed by Immuno Laboratories. Consider whether you have any of the following symptoms: digestive (diarrhea, constipation, bloating, gas, belching); joints and muscles (pain, aches, weakness, stiffness); mouth and throat (coughing, clearing throat, sore throat, canker sores); weight (cravings, binge eating, water retention); energy levels (fatigue, apathy, hyperactivity); ears (itchiness, aches, infections, ringing, draining); eyes (watery, itchy, swollen, blurred vision); emotions (mood swings, anxiety, irritability, depression); mental (confusion, impaired memory and concentration); head (headaches, dizziness); hives, rashes, hair loss, shortness of breath, irregular heartbeat, and many others.

The problem in identifying food allergies is that in most cases they involve a *delayed* reaction, taking several days—up to seventy-two hours—for symptoms to appear, whereas substance and pollen allergies typically produce immediate reactions with obvious, characteristic signs appearing within a few hours after contact or ingestion. Not only can food allergies produce delayed reactions, but the symptoms that manifest are not necessarily obviously related to foods.

It all has to do with immunoglobulins, which are activated as part of the allergic reaction. An immunoglobulin is one of a class of five specially designed antibody proteins produced in the spleen, bone marrow, or lymph tissue and involved in the immune system's defense response to foreign substances. The main types of immunoglobulins, grouped according to their concentration in the blood, are: IgG (80%), IgA (10-15%), IgM (5-10%), IgD (less than 0.1%), and IgE (less than 0.01%).

Food allergies that produce immediate reactions are mediated through IgE, but those that are delayed pertain to IgG, and in some cases, IgA, explains Dr. Braly. Usually with an IgE allergic reaction, only one food is involved, but with delayed IgG-mediated allergies, there can be multiple foods involved, even as many as ten. "Up to 80 medical conditions—from arthritis, asthma, and autism to insomnia, psoriasis, and insulin-dependent diabetes—have been clinically associated with IgG food allergy reactions," says Dr. Braly. Ironically, often the foods that produce the most serious food allergies are those we are most drawn to or for which we feel the strongest craving—the one to which we are addicted, if you will.

Immuno 1 Bloodprint

The diagnostic problem lies in the fact that the standard blood test or skin prick test for food allergies will not indicate a delayed food sensitivity, or one working through IgG. You have to test a person for IgG activity to accurately pinpoint a delayed food allergy, says Dr. Braly. That is why his company, Immuno Laboratories, developed the Immuno 1 Bloodprint to monitor for levels of IgG antibodies that get activated after a person ingests any of 102 suspected allergenic foods. If these antibodies are detected in the blood, it means the immune system is reacting to food allergens, regarding them as hostile to the body's internal environment.

"Up to 80 medical conditions—from arthritis, asthma, and autism to insomnia, psoriasis, and insulin-dependent diabetes—have been clinically associated with IgG food allergy reactions," says Dr. Braly.

In fact, this test looks for evidence of antibodies to IgG's subsets, which include IgG1, IgG2, IgG3, and IgG4. Testing for this degree of specificity is important, Dr. Braly stresses, because fifty percent of IgG-mediated food allergies work through IgG1, but forty percent come through IgG4, while ten percent are with IgG2 and IgG3. Unless you test for all these variations, you may still miss a delayed food sensitivity. By not screening for all the subclasses of the IgG immunoglobulin, the resulting allergy treatment could be only sixty percent effective, says Dr. Braly.

It pays to be specific when it comes to the top five allergenic foods, too. For example, the prime allergen in wheat is gluten, but the component that drives that allergenicity is a protein called gliadin; scientific studies have identified at least eighteen medical conditions directly linked to gliadin sensitivity. In other words wheat (and eggs and dairy protein) have "subfractions" that can produce equal, if not worse, allergic reactions than the whole food. This means that to accurately pinpoint food allergies, you need to test the whole and subfractions of the prime allergenic foods, according to Dr. Braly. Dairy milk has twenty-five different proteins, of which five have been consistently linked with allergies.[12]

The Immuno 1 Bloodprint exposes a sample of the patient's drawn blood to a series of vials containing one of 102 test allergens, reactions are observed, and delayed food allergies are identified. The following are results from a sample report. This patient tested reactive (allergic) to fourteen foods: banana, barley, cheese, clam, egg, oats, oyster, pineapple, rice, rye, sugar cane, wheat, baker's yeast, and brewer's yeast. Of these, she had the strongest reactions to rye, wheat, and baker's yeast (registering a "three" out of possible "four," which is the most severe allergic reaction).

Based on the test results, the next step is dietary change, such as only eating the offending foods once every four days (or never, not for a long while, or not for one to four weeks) to reduce the body's "habit" of reacting to them as allergens and to give it time to clear out the allergy "products" from its system.

Dr. Braly cites another case history, this time involving a woman, aged thirty-nine, who was always bloated and cramped and endured other intestinal misery after every meal, even simple ones. This had been her lot for many years. She also had chronic sinus and ear problems, pain in her joints and muscles, mood swings, and hyperactivity, and just before seeing Dr. Braly and immediately after taking some cold medicine with orange juice, she developed rectal bleeding and esophageal reflux (severe heartburn).

The Immuno 1 Bloodprint showed that she was allergic to 17 foods, or 16.6% of the items on the test list; it also demonstrated she had a serious overgrowth of the yeast-like fungus *Candida albicans* in her intestines. With the allergens identified, the woman stayed away from the seventeen allergenic foods and all foods containing yeasts, so as not to support further growth of the *Candida*. After implementing these steps, she regained her health in the next few months, even losing twenty-two pounds.[13]

Nambudripad Allergy Elimination Technique (NAET)

While the Immuno 1 Bloodprint can identify the various types of hidden food allergies, the standard food allergy treatment essentially involves avoiding the offending foods for a long time, then gradually rotating them with foods better tolerated.

However, back in 1984, a California chiropractor named Devi S. Nambudripad, D.C., figured out a way to use acupuncture, chiropractic, and kinesiology to not only diagnose food and substance allergies, but to eliminate them as well. She then publicized her results in a popular book called *Say Goodbye to Illness*. Today Dr. Nambudripad's success is attested to by the fact that there is now a nationwide network of 3,000 NAET-trained physicians and health-care practitioners offering it to their patients (see her website for practitioner referrals).

Using kinesiology (muscle testing), the NAET practitioner is able to first ascertain if the patient is allergic to a specific substance. Allergens weaken the muscles, which makes it fairly easy to judge allergenicity by using a test muscle, such as the arm. The list of possible allergenic substances is surprising, even bizarre, revealing that you can potentially be allergic to almost anything: cotton underpants, fenugreek tea, leather belts, piano keys, saliva, sewing needles, diamond rings, tap water, and computer keyboards. One woman was allergic to her husband.

The gist of the technique is that the specific allergenic substance is held by the patient close to one of the acupuncture meridians; the practitioner applies acupressure to a specific acupuncture meridian at the same time; then the substance is avoided entirely for twenty-five hours, slightly longer than the time it takes for energy in the body to cycle through all the meridians. Somehow, the nervous system is desensitized through the acupuncture meridians to no longer react allergically to the substance. The brain is taught to reinterpret its contact with the substance, now regarding it as a neutral, acceptable thing and not a poison. Dr. Nambudripad claims that often only one session is required to "permanently eliminate an allergy" and to put the person in a situation in which he or she can actually resume contact with or ingestion of the previously allergenic substance.[14]

With the laboratory testing of your blood, urine, stool, saliva, muscles, teeth, and other physiological indicators detailed in this chapter, you can get a clear, quantified picture of your nutritional and immune status and degree of toxicity. Armed with this information, you can now move confidently into the next phase of creating the healthy living body space: practical detoxification protocols that work to clear the intestines, liver, kidneys, and lymph of this residue of toxins and rebuild your cellular health and reestablish proper nutrient levels—the subject of the next four chapters.

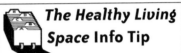

The Healthy Living Space Info Tip

For Immuno 1 Bloodprint:
Immuno Laboratories,
1620 West Oakland Park Boulevard,
Fort Lauderdale, FL 33311;
tel: 800-231-9197;
e-mail: pcssales@immuno.com;
website: www.immunolabs.com.

For NAET:
Devi Nambudripad, D.C.,
Pain Clinic,
6714 Beach Boulevard,
Buena Park, CA 90621;
tel: 714-523-3068 or 714-523-0800
or 714-523-8900;
e-mail: naet@earthlink.net;
website: www.naet.com or
www.allergy-naet.com.

CHAPTER 4

Detoxification Preliminaries:

Start Your Internal Cleansing with Dietary Changes and by Minimizing Your Exposure

As groundwork for the more organ-focused stages of detoxification, you will need to reconsider your many dietary choices, even staples as basic as water. The U.S. food supply today is considerably adulterated, either deliberately in the course of its manufacture, with additives and preservatives, or inadvertently, in the course of its preparation or packaging.

One of the simplest and most effective steps you can take as a preliminary to colon and liver cleansing is to drastically reduce your intake of toxic substances through your food and water. This in itself is a detoxification step of profound physiological impact, but it is one that will require of you a fair measure of attention and vigilance to what constitutes your daily diet.

As a complement to reducing your toxic intake, you may find it beneficial to help your mind and nervous system calm down, to step back a bit from the daily onslaught of toxic or stressful energies, thoughts, and emotions. Detoxification itself brings deep relaxation and ease to all the cells of the body. Purposefully relaxing yourself supports the detoxification effort. This chapter incudes a review of a few relaxation techniques.

HEALTHY LIVING SPACE DETOXIFIER #7
Rehydrate Your Body with Nature's
Best Detoxifying Substance

One of the most basic recommendations for detoxification is to drink a great deal of pure water, probably double the amount you presently drink. At least thirty-two ounces daily is a good start, consumed directly as water, which disqualifies the water content of teas, coffee, and other beverages. In fact, naturopathic physicians recommend that during the more advanced stages of detoxification (see chapter 5) you increase your water intake to sixty-four ounces daily, consuming it in small but regular amounts throughout the day.[1] Some say you should drink that much routinely, even if you're not doing a detoxification regimen.

It may surprise many people to learn they might be functionally dehydrated. Even though we consume a fair amount of liquid during the day—tea, coffee, sodas, beers, soups—we may still be depriving our bodies and cells of even a minimal water supply. Take coffee, for example.

You would think that the more coffee you drink in a day, the more water enters your body, thereby fulfilling your body's daily need for fresh water. It's not the case. Naturopathic educators Peter Bennett, N.D., and Stephen Barrie, N.D., observe that dehydration is "especially prevalent" in heavy coffee drinkers because coffee is a strong diuretic, which means its chemical action is to flush water out of the body (which you will experience as increased urination), more than the amount contained in each cup of coffee consumed.[2]

Chronic low-grade dehydration allows wastes to accumulate in the blood and overtaxes the kidneys, which need adequate water to mix with toxins to excrete them from the body in the urine. In fact, our bodies may be "crying out" for water and we are entirely missing the call, according to F. Batmanghelidj, M.D., a physician who practices in Falls Church, Virginia, and who, for the past eighteen years, has made the issue of unsuspected chronic low-grade dehydration the basis of a medical theory and practice. Dr. Batmanghelidj claims that a great many ailments, from indigestion to arthritis, high blood pressure to diabetes, and back pain to depression are actually due, in small or large part, to the body's unsatisfied demands for adequate water intake, that they are "dehydration-produced disorders." This also means that the "water cure," as he calls it, may be effective in reversing a number of otherwise difficult health conditions, such as angina, migraines, colitis, asthma, and high blood cholesterol, as well as the ones mentioned above.

Most bodies live in a condition of water-deprivation stress. You are not sick—you are thirsty, which is why you don't need to treat thirst with medications, but with copious amounts of fresh, pure water, Dr. Batmanghelidj says.

The simple truth, he states in his book, *Your Body's Many Cries for Water*, is that "dehydration can cause disease."[3] Every function of the body is dependent on adequate water and the continuous flow of fresh water into the body. It is important to remember that it is not dehydration alone that is the problem. Copious amounts of water are needed every day by the body to flush out toxins from the cells and to complete the body's multi-faceted detoxification process. Water is needed for each step of the process. If you are dehydrated, your detoxification processes may be stalled, or certainly compromised, and toxins accumulate in the tissues, leading to disease. Like Drs. Bennett and Barrie, Dr. Batmanghelidj points out that tea, coffee, alcohol, and prepared beverages (sodas, fruit drinks) are counterproductive in terms of hydrating the body. They contain dehydrating agents (and diuretics), so depending on them to satisfy the body's daily needs for water is "an elementary but catastrophic mistake."

Complicating matters is the fact that your body will not necessarily manifest a dry mouth symptom to let you know it is stressed for lack of water, says Dr. Batmanghelidj. This signal, when it occurs, "is the *last* outward sign of *extreme* dehydration." The damage occurs, he says, "at a level of persistent dehydration that does not necessarily demonstrate a 'dry mouth' signal."

Consider what restoring adequate water intake can do for a case of dyspepsia— indigestion based in the stomach. Dyspeptic pain (which is experienced mainly as heartburn, duodenitis, or gastritis) is the most important thirst signal the body produces, denoting dehydration, says Dr. Batmanghelidj. The sole treatment for this condition should be increased water intake, he says. He has successfully treated 3,000 cases in this way. "They all responded to an increase in their water intake, and their clinical problems associated with the pain disappeared."

He cites a dramatic case in which a patient had such severe stomach pain he had to be carried by others into Dr. Batmanghelidj's clinic. The patient experienced relief after he had consumed three glasses (twenty-four ounces) of water. On the average, says Dr. Batmanghelidj, it takes eight minutes to achieve total pain relief from dyspepsia by drinking water. "A well-regulated and constantly alert attention to daily water intake will prevent the emergence of most of the major diseases," he states.

How much water is enough to satisfy the body and prevent disease? This would be an "absolute minimum" of forty-eight to sixty-four ounces daily of fresh, pure water, says Dr. Batmanghelidj. The best times to drink water are thirty minutes before eating, and two and one-half hours after eating, and before going to bed. Another "water cure" advocate, Terry Grossman, M.D., who practices in Denver, Colorado, advises six to ten glasses of water daily, which is forty-eight to eighty ounces. His "water prescription" is that "every day you should drink that amount of water in ounces to equal one-half of your body weight in pounds." That means, if you weigh 110 pounds, you drink 55 ounces; if you weigh 200 pounds, you drink 100 ounces. Dr. Grossman says it is best to drink the water away from mealtimes so as not to dilute the digestive juices required to digest your meals.[4]

One way to monitor your intake is to examine the color and consistency of your urine. If it is dark yellow, dense or strong smelling, or even slightly orange in color, it means your body is dehydrated, says Dr. Batmanghelidj, and your kidneys are stressed. Dark yellow urine is concentrated urine, dense with toxic excretions. Ideally, if you are healthy, urine from a well-hydrated body should be almost colorless to light yellow, he says.

> *How much water is enough to satisfy the body and prevent disease? This would be an "absolute minimum" of forty-eight to sixty-four ounces daily of fresh, pure water, says Dr. Batmanghelidj. The best times to drink water are thirty minutes before eating, two and one-half hours after eating, and before going to bed.*

This is something you can observe during the day in relationship to both your food and water intake.

HEALTHY LIVING SPACE DETOXIFIER #8
Get the Chlorine Out of Your Drinking and Shower Water

A compelling reason to filter your drinking water is that your body depends on a substantial supply of fresh, pure water to accomplish its continual detoxification. In fact, water itself is an excellent detoxifying substance, flushing out toxins from cells and carrying them out of the body through the urine. During a deliberate detoxification regimen, you will most likely be at least doubling your water intake.

It is excellent advice to drink *lots* more water, but the trouble with this recommendation is that nearly all tap water is contaminated with trace amounts of pesticides, industrial pollutants, and chlorine byproducts. If you use chlorinated water with all its toxic baggage as your prime water source (especially in a detoxification program), you are continually introducing more toxic substances even though you are trying to flush others out of your body. You won't make as much progress in cleansing your cells as you will if you do not introduce more chlorinated byproducts.

It's important to remember that the cumulative *effect is the key: the more you ingest a toxic substance, the greater the chance it will have a toxic effect one day. In the same way, unilateral reduction of toxic intake is the order of the day in the field of self-care detoxification.*

It's important to remember that the *cumulative* effect is the key: the more you ingest a toxic substance, the greater the chance it will have a toxic effect one day. In the same way, unilateral *reduction* of toxic intake is the order of the day in the field of self-care detoxification. Ingest fewer toxic substances of any kind—this is one of the most practical steps you can take.

So, before you double your water intake, you need to reexamine your source of drinking water and look into nonchlorinated alternatives, such as bottled water and home filtration. First, let's look more closely at the problems with chlorinated water.

Chlorination of municipal drinking water has been a fact of life that most people have accepted routinely and uncritically for nearly the entire twentieth century, since 1908 when municipalities began adding chlorine to drinking water to disinfect it. Even though chlorine does a good job at disinfecting water, unfortunately it produces other toxic substances that, in terms of public health issues, may produce worse conditions than the original organic toxicants (mostly bacteria) found in water sources.

The problem is that chlorine produces toxic "disinfection byproducts." When chlorine is added to water, it naturally reacts with organic matter such as humic and fulvic acids, which are present in the untreated, "raw" water. This reaction creates a new category of chlorinated chemicals jointly known as trihalomethanes (THMs). It was only in the 1970s, some seventy years after water chlorination began on a large scale, that scientists discovered these toxic disinfection byproducts, and that chloroform produced cancer in laboratory rats.

There are potentially many different kinds of THMs produced when water is chlorinated, but public health officials tend to focus on only four: chloroform, bromoform, bromodichloromethane, and chlorodibromomethane. Technically, for it to be deemed "acceptable," municipal water servicing more than 10,000 people is not supposed to have any of these four THMs at levels greater than 100 parts per billion.

Unfortunately, THMs are not the only pollutants likely to be found in your drinking water and which are not removed or affected by chlorination. These others include pesticides, polycyclic aromatic hydrocarbons, volatile hydrocarbons (also known as VOCs, volatile organic chemicals), and phenols.[5] Researchers identified seventy VOCs (notably hydrocarbons—see figure 4-1) that were formed during municipal treatment of drinking water; most of the hydrocarbons passed through the entire water treatment process with "little change in concentration"—meaning they were available full strength at the typical kitchen faucet.[6]

Let's look at this more closely. What are we likely to find in our tap water if it is municipally treated, or perhaps regardless of its source? Here is a partial list: trace metals (lead, aluminum, cadmium, chromium), VOCs, THMs, organisms (coliform bacteria, worms, parasites, or protozoa, such as *Cryptosporidium* and

Figure 4-1. Toxic Contaminants Typically Found in Tapwater—A Partial List

CONTAMINANT	SOURCE	HEALTH EFFECT
Trace heavy metals		
antimony	coal/ore mining, petroleum refining	carcinogen, irritates eyes
arsenic	defoliants, soil sterilants, wood treatment	skin tumors, nervous system
asbestos	insulation, fireproofing, building materials	probable carcinogen
cadmium	fungicides, batteries, pain enamels	kidney disorders, bronchitis, anemia
chromium	leather tanning, iron/steel mfg., wood chemicals	liver/kidney disorders
copper	corroded pipes	stomach/intestinal distress
fluoride	drinking water additive	dental fluorisis, bone fractures, cancer
lead	plumbing materials, batteries, gasoline, paints and inks	hypertension, kidneys
mercury	various industrial processes	central nervous system, brain dysfunction
selenium	animal feeds, wood products/processing	nervous system, mucus membranes
Volatile organic chemicals and trihalomethanes		
aldicarb sulfone	pesticides	central nervous system, liver/kidneys, anemia, leukemia
atrazine	pesticides	nervous, reproductive, respiratory systems, probable carcinogen
benzene	petroleum	leukemia, anemia, possibly cancer
bromodichloromethane	chlorinated water	probable carcinogen
carbon tetrachloride	chlorinated water	nervous and digestive system, carcinogen
chlordane	pesticides	anemia, leukemia, probable carcinogen
1,2-dichloroethylene	chlorinated water	kidneys, liver, carcinogen
1,2-dichloropropane	chlorinated water	affects lungs, liver, kidneys
ethylene dibromide		probable carcinogen
heptachlor	pesticides	nervous, reproductive systems, liver, kidneys, probable carcinogen
lindane	pesticides	probable carcinogen, anemia, leukemia

CONTAMINANT	SOURCE	HEALTH EFFECT
nitrate	tobacco products	methmoglobinemia (Blue Baby Syndrome), carcinogen
pentachlorophenol	wood varnish, laundry spray	probable carcinogen
tetrachloroethylene	chlorinated water	probable carcinogen
toluene	paints, thinners, cosmetics	narcosis, respiratory system irritant

Microorganisms and pathogens

Campylobacter jejuni		diarrhea, affects nervous system
coliform bacteria	human fecal matter	gastrointestinal distress
Cryptosporidium parvum		diarrhea, gastrointestinal distress
Giardia lamblia		stomach cramps, intestinal distress
Salmonella		severe dysentery, chronic arthritis

Giardia[7]), and numerous chemical contaminants—at least fifty-nine identified contaminants in all. Seen from another angle, these are fifty-nine reasons to consider installing a competent water filter in your kitchen.

"There is widespread potential for human exposure to disinfection byproducts (DBPs) in drinking water because everyone drinks, bathes, cooks, and cleans with water," stated G.A. Boorman of the National Institute of Environmental Health Sciences of Research Triangle Park in North Carolina in a 1999 review of THMs.[8] Add to this flushing the toilet and washing clothes and dishes—these activities can also introduce THMs into the indoor air of your home. It doesn't stop there either.

In fact, drinking chlorinated water is not necessarily the prime route for exposure to THMs. Taiwanese researchers measured the inhalation exposure for THMs of household residents during a day. They found that the people inhaled 26.4 mcg/day during the shower, 1.56 mcg during pre- and post-cooking activities, and 3.29 mcg during cooking itself. This exposure is in addition to whatever amount the people directly ingested by drinking tap water, which the researchers estimated to be about the same amount, "indicating that inhalation is an important pathway for THM exposure from drinking water."[9]

You must additionally factor in the chlorine and chlorination disinfection products found in all the commercial beverages you drink, cups of tea or coffee you enjoy in restaurants, and the water used in hundreds of commercially prepared foods. Even though you may be filtering out the chlorine and its byproducts from your home drinking water supply (explained below), it doesn't mean the rest of the world is.

The principle becomes one of minimization; you probably will not be able to completely avoid chlorine and its byproducts in all the food and water situations you encounter, but you probably can *reduce* your exposure by a great deal. As with many slow-acting toxic substances to which we are routinely exposed at low but constant doses, they have a cumulative effect. If you cut way back on the amount regularly entering your body, you greatly improve your chances that your body's own detoxification system will be able to handle this amount. You will get even better results if you help your liver out with specific liver-cleansing herbs (see chapter 5).

There are several reasons why you should to try to minimize or eliminate your exposure to chlorinated water through drinking and from inhaling the fumes when you shower. Chlorine itself is believed to destroy polyunsaturated fatty acids and vitamin E in the body; it gets stored in the body's fatty tisues where it is slow to degrade; and it can also destroy beneficial intestinal bacteria that aid in digestion and in defense against pathogenic microorganisms. Regarding trihalomethanes, there are far more than four THMs, and they are for the most part unstudied, their toxicity unknown. At least six other THMs have been identified. It is known, however, that THMs can contribute to reproductive disorders, including miscarriage, birth defects, and various types of cancer, such as bladder and colon cancer.

Reproductive Effects

Let's look at miscarriages first. California researchers announced in 1998 that they had developed strong evidence linking the consumption of chlorinated water with an increased risk of miscarriage or spontaneous abortion, based on a study of 5,144 pregnant women drawn from three counties and serviced by 78 municipal water companies. The women, whose average age was twenty-eight, reported their water consumption patterns during their first trimester some years earlier.

Women who drank at least five cups daily of cold chlorinated tap water with more than 75 ppm of THMs had miscarriages at a rate 15.7% higher (nearly double) the national average. Women who drank less than this amount or whose tap water had less than

75 ppm of THMs had miscarriages at the rate of 9.5% higher. The study also showed that eighteen percent of the women drank tap water with much higher THM levels, up to 157 ppm. In summary, women with a high THM exposure had a likelihood of spontaneous abortion 1.8 times higher than among women with a low exposure.[10]

The results of this study reinforced conclusions published six years earlier in another evaluation of chlorination and women's health in California. In 1992, scientists at the California Department of Health Services studied 5,000 women in a single county (one of the three counties in the 1998 study). These women had a ten percent to fifty percent higher risk of spontaneous abortion than should be expected if they drank more tap water than bottled water during their first eight weeks of pregnancy. Women who drank at least six cups of chlorinated tap water per day had an average 2.17 times higher risk of miscarriage (the range of risk was 1.1 to 3.9).[11]

Three other studies published that same year (1992) confirmed the results, placing the miscarriage rate at twelve percent to fourteen percent from a four-cup daily consumption of chlorinated tap water. Researchers at the University of California at San Francisco studied pregnancies from 1980 to 1985 in four areas of one California county and found that among women who consumed no chlorinated tap water during their pregnancies (relying on bottled water), no birth defects were noted in 263 births, but for women who drank tap water, 4% of 908 births had defects. The scientists also found "an overall excess" of spontaneous abortions among women drinking chlorinated tap water during their first trimester.[12]

The California Department of Health Services concluded in 1992 that results from four out of five studies of pregnancy outcomes and water consumption patterns "suggest that women abstaining from tap water or [those] drinking bottled water during the first trimester of pregnancy may be at reduced risk of spontaneous abortion."[13]

Further correlations were demonstrated by researchers at the School of Public Health at the University of North Carolina at Chapel Hill in 1998. They looked at the records of 1,893 live births in Colorado between 1990 and 1993; all the women had consumed water containing THMs during their pregnancies. The scientists found "a weak association" between THM exposure during the third trimester and low birth weight and "a large increase in risk" for low birth weight at the highest rate of THM exposure. The data was sufficient to indicate "a potentially important relation" between a pregnant woman drinking THM-contaminated tap water and the chances of birthing a baby with some kind of defect as a result of "retarded fetal growth."[14]

A similar retrospective study in Halifax, Nova Scotia, revealed that women were 1.66 times more likely to experience stillbirths if their average THM exposure level during pregnancy was 100 mcg/liter or greater compared to women who ingested only 0-49 mcg/l during the same time. The researchers, who studied birth records from 1988 to 1995, found little evidence for birth defects, but they did note "chromosomal abnormalities," which is to say, defects in the infants' DNA.[15] When toxic effects start showing up in chromosomes and genes, you are at the molecular level where cancer (and many other serious health disorders) begins (see page 148).

Other recent research shows a connection between serious birth defects, such as neural tube defects (spina bifida, in which the spinal cord is not properly enclosed by bone), and total THMs consumed in tap water. The research, conducted in New Jersey, reported a doubled risk of neural tube defects among women with the highest THM exposure from drinking water.[16]

A study three years earlier in New Jersey showed the chance of neural tube defects was increased threefold when the pregnant woman was exposed to THMs at rates higher than 80 ppb. These researchers, part of the Agency for Toxic Substances and Disease Registry in the United States Department of Health and Human Services, looked at 80,938 live births and 594 fetal deaths during the period 1985-1988. They were able to tentatively link specific THMs with different birth defects.

For example, total THM ingestion was linked with infants born small for their gestational age, and with central nervous system and cardiac defects. Carbon tetrachloride intake was associated with low birth weight and various defects in the nervous system, heart, and mouth; benzene was linked to neural tube and cardiac defects.[17] It is possible that chloroform (one of the four main THMs) disrupts the fetus' uptake of vitamin B12, which has been linked to neural tube defects.[18]

Norwegian researchers looked at three aspects of "reproductive toxicity" with respect to pregnant women ingesting chlorinated tap water. They found that out of 141,077 births in a two-year period (1993-1995), 1.8% of infants (2,608) were born with birth defects and there was a strong likelihood these birth defects were due in part to THMs. The scientists reported that women with a high chlorination exposure were 1.4 times more at risk of having a baby delivered with some kind of malformation, 1.26 times more likely to birth a baby with a neural tube defect, and 1.99 times more likely to birth an infant with urinary tract defects.

"This study provides further evidence of the role of chlorination of humic water [raw water containing organic matter] as a potential cause of birth defects, in a country with relatively low levels of chlorination byproducts," the researchers noted. In other words, because Norway is not so heavily chlorinated as other industrialized countries, the results are more meaningful, because the average person is routinely exposed to fewer THMs there than elsewhere.[19]

Among the THMs, bromodichloromethane (BDCM) and chloroform are considered the two most prominent. In rat studies, both produced noticeable damage to the liver and kidneys twenty-four hours after ingestion. After forty-eight hours, BDCM produced "more persistent liver toxicity" than chloroform and was "slightly more toxic" to the kidneys as well.[20] Bear in mind that the liver and kidneys are two of the body's prime detoxification, filtration, and toxin excretion organs, so if THMs make these organs toxic, their ability to remove other toxic substances from the body is impaired.

Carcinogenic Effects

The scientific research linking cancer and sustained THM intake through drinking chlorinated tap water is equally strong. In fact, evidence suggesting a link between THMs and cancer was suspected as early as 1974; since that time, at least eighteen studies have appeared strengthening the link between carcinogens in chlorinated drinking water and the onset of various types of cancer, especially bladder and colon cancer.

A study by the National Cancer Institute in 1987 examined the water consumption habits of 2,805 men and women with bladder cancer and 5,258 cancer-free men and women drawn from ten different areas of the United States. They found that people who drank eight cups of chlorinated tap water for forty to fifty-nine years had a forty percent higher risk of getting bladder cancer than those who consumed less than this, or who drank unchlorinated water. Among those in the study, men and women who drank the highest volume of chlorinated tap water for sixty years had an eighty percent increased risk.

By some strange biochemical twist, nonsmokers had a far higher risk than smokers, even though tobacco smoke on its own can cause bladder cancer; nonsmokers drinking chlorinated tap water for 60 years had a 310% increased risk of bladder cancer. The researchers estimated that of the people studied, twelve percent of the bladder cancer cases could be blamed on chlorinated water; among the nonsmokers in the group, that number was twenty-seven percent.[21]

- In 1982, researchers acknowledged that studies have "clearly shown" that most, possibly all, U.S. drinking water contains chemicals that have mutagenic or carcinogenic activity, meaning they can make healthy human cells change (mutate) or become poisoned (by carcinogens), initiating a cancer.[22]

- In 1982, scientists studied cancer deaths in women from twenty-eight Wisconsin counties during the years 1972-1977 and found that colon cancer appeared to be "related significantly" to THM levels in drinking water, increasing the risk of colon cancer by 2.8 times.[23]

- In 1987, scientists injected laboratory mice regularly for two years with bromodichloromethane, a THM found in chlorinated water. There was "clear evidence" of a cancer process in both males and females after two years, particularly in the kidneys and colon of both sexes and ovarian abcesses in the females. Of the four primary THMs, bromodichloromethane caused the "widest spectrum" of cancers in rodents, researchers stated.[24]

- In 1993, researchers at the National Institutes of Health reported the results of their two-year study with laboratory rodents that had received daily amounts of three THMs, chlorine, and chloramine. They found that the THMs were carcinogenic to the liver, kidneys, and intestines of the rodents studied. They concluded that these are "the chemicals of greatest concern" in determining whether chlorinated drinking water is cancer causing.[25]

- In 1995, researchers at the Department of Family and Community Medicine at the Medical College of Wisconsin at Milwaukee stated that the byproducts of water chlorination "possibly" account for 5,000 cases of bladder cancer and 8,000 cases of rectal cancer each year in the United States.[26]

- In 1996, scientists at the Department of Community Health and Epidemiology at Queen's University in Kingston, Ontario, studied 696 cases of bladder cancer and correlated them with the patient's drinking water patterns over a thiry-five-year period. They found that those who drank chlorinated tap water regularly for thirty-five years or more had "an increased risk" of bladder cancer compared to those who consumed it for ten years or less. They also reported that those who had a THM intake of 50 mcg/liter or more for 35 years had an increased risk as well. In other words, "the risk of bladder cancer increases with both duration and concentration of exposure to chlorination byproducts." The general risk to the population of bladder cancer was thereby increased by fourteen percent to sixteen percent, making THMs "a potentially important risk factor."[27]

- In 1997, researchers at the School of Public Health at the University of Minnesota at Minneapolis announced the results of their study of 28,237 women from Iowa. Women who drank chlorinated tap water had an increased risk of colon and all types of cancers compared to women who did not drink chlorinated water.[28]

- In 1998, researchers at the National Cancer Institute found that among 1,123 cases of bladder cancer compared to 1,983 controls (people without cancer but of the same age and gender) there was an "overall association" between chlorinated water intake and the risk of bladder cancer. Specifically, among men, if they were smokers and drank chlorinated tap water, this "mutually enhanced" their risk of getting bladder cancer.[29]

- In 1998, other scientists at the National Cancer Institute studied 685 cases of colon cancer and 655 cases of rectal cancer, compared to 2,434 controls. They found an association between drinking chlorinated water over a sixty-year period and the incidence of rectal cancer, but not of colon cancer. However, they found that subjects who drank chlorinated water and had a low dietary fiber intake over a period of 40 years increased their risk of rectal cancer by 2.4 times compared to 0.9 times for those who had a high fiber intake and did not drink chlorinated water.[30]

- In 1999, ingesting chlorination byproducts was positively linked with brain cancer. A study of 375 brain cancer cases in Iowa and the patients' lifetime water consumption patterns showed an increased risk of brain cancer with exposure to THMs.[31]

The preceding brief review of some of the available scientific evidence makes it clear that it would be prudent to think about radically reducing your exposure to THMs found in chlorinated tap water. There are two practical steps you can take in your home: install a water filter for your drinking and cooking water; and install a shower and bath-faucet filter.

Obviously, using high quality bottled water is a viable solution to contaminated drinking water, an effective remedy that's easy to implement. There is a financial factor, however. Using bottled water for drinking purposes (not cooking) for a year in a two-person household (including the rental or amortized purchase of the dispenser) will cost you about the same as the one-time purchase of a mid-level water purifier for about $500. Using bottled water for cooking purposes adds to the expense. The only subsequent costs of a water purifier are cartridge replacements. In year two, you will start saving a significant amount of money on your water purification.

At any rate, since the option of using bottled water is already generally well known, there is no need to pursue it further here. Instead, we will focus on home water filtration units.

As elsewhere in this book, discussion of a specific product is not meant as an endorsement, nor is the listing of one or more products meant to be a definitive listing of what is available, or a ranking as to quality, or even an assurance of quality. Rather, specific products are mentioned to give you an idea of what is available, and a few places to begin your investigation of items best suited to your needs.

Water Filters to Remove Chlorine

There are many options here, from the inexpensive counter-top activated charcoal filter approach to expensive under-the-counter reverse osmosis units. You can spend $50 or $3000, depending on how thoroughly you want to remove tap water contaminants. Let's look at a few examples:

INEXPENSIVE FILTRATION. The Pūr line of water purifiers offers a series of pitcher, countertop, or under-sink filtration units in a modest price range, from about $25 to $100. The pitcher unit holds two gallons. The filter lasts about two months (forty gallons), and the unit removes *Giardia* and *Cryptosporidium*, and reduces the levels of lead, chlorine, copper, zinc, and asbestos. The faucet mounts reduce levels of some THMs, a broader list of VOC chemicals, and the microorganisms cited above. The countertop/under-sink units remove the same substances, but have a longer filter life (200 gallons).

CHARCOAL FILTRATION. An inexpensive countertop approach uses a charcoal (carbon) block filter and a separate spout to channel purified water. An example of this method is the TerraFlo CBLX, which uses a solid carbon cartridge (under-the-counter models are available, too) to filter out selected agricultural pollutants and reduce THMs, VOCs (forty-one different ones are cited by the manufacturer), mercury, lead, chlorine, and the levels of certain parasites. The filter lasts for 400 gallons, and the units sell for $100 or less.

MICROFILTRATION. The Seagull IV X-1 series of "microfiltration" water purifiers made by General Ecology of Exton, Pennsylvania, are countertop models (although they can be installed under the counter) that are effective against three types of water contaminants, according to the manufacturer. These include parasitic cysts, specific chemicals such as pesticides and VOCs, hazardous waste from various industries (such as iron), and THMs.

The systems employ the Structured Matrix technology that removes viruses, bacteria, protozoa, and many organic and inorganic chemicals at "the highest 'purification' micron level (0.4 microns absolute)," says the manufacturer. However, the unit does not remove fluoride (see below for a discussion of why fluoride should be filtered out of drinking water), which is a salt and part of a family not considered contaminants.

The unit accomplishes its purification through an ultrafine submicron filtration device that collects contaminants as small as 0.1 microns; the cartridge (which does not contain charcoal) needs to be replaced annually, or sooner, depending on use, but generally can handle from 1,000 to 6,000 gallons. The different Seagull models process from one to six gallons of water per minute, and weigh from four to twenty-four pounds. You can install them without a plumber, and they generally cost between $500 and $1000.

According to the company's technical reports, the Seagull units are able to remove (to the level of being not detectable) seventeen out of twenty pesticide residues, THMs, and VOCs; and drastically reduce the levels of the other three pesticides. Out of thirteen listed microbiological water contaminants (mostly bacteria), the unit reduces levels of all to nondetectable amounts; it also significantly reduces the iron, cadmium, mercury, and lead content in the finished water.

Another water purification system that uses filtration is the Everpure line, which consists of eleven different units to choose from. Two—S-200 and QC4-VOC—remove or reduce the levels of many volatile organic chemicals (such as benzene and toluene) and many THMs as well as lead, chlorine, chloramines, molds and algae, *Giardia* and *Cryptosporidium* cysts, asbestos fibers, oxidized iron, manganese, and sulfides, as well as 99.9% of all particles 0.5 microns and larger (which the other 9 units do also). The S-200 has a water flow rate of 0.5 gallons per minute and a cartridge life of 300 gallons, while the QC4-VOC has the same flow rate but a cartridge life of 500 gallons; both units are installed under the counter.

REVERSE OSMOSIS. This approach employs a semipermeable membrane that removes particles, salts, and dissolved contaminants, as if molecule by molecule, from raw tap water. In reverse osmosis (RO), water first passes through a 5-micron particle prefilter that takes out large particles of dirt and debris; then the water is squeezed under great pressure through microscopic pores to eliminate about ninety-nine percent of its impurities; finally, any remaining odors or objectionable tastes are removed by a carbon post filter.

One example of an RO device is the PPW Home Reverse Osmosis System, made by Pure-Pro Water Corporation in Mokena, Illinois. According to the manufacturer, this unit removes ninety-five percent to ninety-nine percent of all dissolved mineral and chemical contaminants from raw tap water. Specifically, the unit can remove ninety percent of the fluoride, ninety-seven percent of detergents, ninety-seven percent of herbicides, insecticides, PCBs, lead, and strontium (a radiation product), among others, including ninety-eight percent of THMs (especially chloroform) and other organic toxic chemicals. The unit can produce about fifty to seventy gallons of RO water per day, and holds three to four gallons at a time in a special tank.

The RO approach has advantages and disadvantages: it removes salts (the technology was originally designed by the U.S. Navy to remove salt from ocean water to make it drinkable) which means it catches fluoride (undesirable, see below), but also calcium, sodium, and potassium (essential nutrients); it is not always well suited to remove biological pathogens, but it is well equipped to filter out VOCs. If the RO membrane is *small* enough—that is, smaller than bacteria, viruses, or various parasites—it will remove most pathogenic microorganisms from the water it treats.

Other advantages of RO are daily volume capacity and the thoroughness with which it removes finely dissolved contaminants from the water. According to the manufacturer, once maintenance and water costs are factored in, the unit produces pure water for about five cents a gallon. However, there is a certain degree of water waste with RO. To purify one gallon of water, it will flush it with several gallons (as many as six) of raw water, and these extra gallons get sent back down the drain. So you are paying for water that gets recycled down the drain.

ULTRAVIOLET PURIFICATION. In this approach, an ultraviolet (UV) lamp sterilizes tap water and removes or reduces the levels of chlorine, THMs, VOCs, microorganisms, and selected

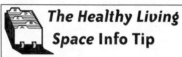
The Healthy Living Space Info Tip

For Pūr units:
Pūr Recovery Engineering, Inc.,
9300 North 75th Avenue,
Minneapolis, MN 55428;
tel: 800-787-5463;
website: www.purwater.com.

For TerraFlo CBLX:
Global Environmental
Technologies, Inc.,
P.O. Box 8839,
1001-1003 S. 10th Street,
Allentown, PA 18105;
tel: 610-821-4901;
fax: 610-821-5507;
email: getwater@terraflo.com;
website: www.terraflo.com.

Or from Real Goods,
200 Clara Street,
Ukiah, CA 95482;
tel: 800-762-7325;
website: www.realgoods.com.

For more information about
Seagull IV X-1 series, contact:
General Ecology, Inc.,
151 Sheree Blvd.,
Exton, PA 19341;
tel: 800-441-8166 or 610-363-7900;
fax: 610-363-0412;
e-mail: info@generalecology.com;
website: www.general-ecology.com.

Also available from:
Nirvana Safe Haven,
3441 Golden Rain Road, Suite 3,
Walnut Creek, CA 94595;
tel: 800-968-9355 or 925-472-8868;
fax: 925-938-9019;
e-mail: dailya@nontoxic.com;
website: www.nontoxic.com.

chemicals. For example, the Sun-Pure Water Purifier uses a five-step program to clean the water: carbon block filters remove chlorine and many THMs and VOCs; a lead sorbent matrix mixed with the carbon block filter removes heavy metals; activated tricalcium phosphate removes fluorides; granular activated carbon removes bad tastes and odors as well as chemicals; and the ultraviolet sterilization chamber deactivates the various microbial life forms that could cause disease. The filter cartridges last for 1,300 gallons, and the UV lamp needs replacement annually. The system delivers water at the rate of 30 gallons/hour (or 0.5 gallons/minute), and at a cost of $0.05/gallon daily (about $400 for the unit), according to the manufacturer.

Shower Filters to Remove Chlorine

The idea behind a shower filter is to remove a fair amount of chlorine and selected heavy metals, and sometimes radon and certain bacteria (such as *Cryptosporidium*) from the incoming water, usually by way of an activated charcoal filter. The device is installed in place of the conventional shower faucet. Shower filters do not remove THMs, only chlorine. Let's briefly review a few typical products:

The Shower Filter from Paragon Water Systems, for example, uses a five-stage filtration system, including activated carbon and a KDF filter.[32] The KDF uses an electrochemical process to reduce the water content of various organic and inorganic elements that affect the water's taste, including some pesticides, organic chemicals, and hydrogen sulfide. Water passes through very fine micron filters before coming out as a spray.

Another version of the same approach is called the Aqua-Stream Shower Filter. Using a combination of a charcoal filter and a KDF filter, this unit processes 2.2 gallons of water per minute; its cartridge lasts up to two years; and the device weighs four pounds and sells for $150 or less.

A third version, offered by Nirvana Safe Haven, is called the KDF Chlorine-free Shower Unit. The company states that one filter will filter about 45,000 gallons of water (or last about eighteen months), and will remove chlorine (converting it to nontoxic zinc chloride), eradicate algae and fungi, control bacterial growth, and reduce hydrogen sulfide and factors contributing to water hardness.

The Sprite Slim-Line Shower Filter from Ace Pump Corporation uses a noncarbon-based filtration media (called Chlorgon, specifically designed for the needs of the shower, says the company) to remove both free and combined (bonded with other elements) chlorine, as well as odors, heavy metals, dirt, and sediment from shower water. The cartridge needs to be replaced about every six months.

Get the Chlorine Out of Your Swimming Pool

Routine or long-term exposure to chlorinated water in swimming pools can be hazardous to your health. Competitive swimmers have been shown to absorb toxic levels of chlorine and THMs during their training; similar chlorine absorption patterns have been observed in recreational swimming, especially among children. "This exposure comes from breathing chloroform-laden air near the water's surface and absorbing this and other compounds through the skin."[33]

If you own a swimming pool and want an alternative to chlorine to keep the microorganisms out of your water, a device called the Floatron may be the solution. Using solar ionization, this is a small, floatable device that employs solar power to generate a low electric current; the mineral ions produced (and introduced into the water) effectively stop the growth of algae and bacteria in your swimming water. Essentially, the unit produces mineral water as a way of controlling microbial growth, and it cuts the need for any chlorine by eighty percent. The remaining twenty percent of the normal chlorine (or other oxidizers such as bromine or hydrogen peroxide) amount is required to control water clouding due to suntan lotion, body fluids, and dust accumulation in the water. The Floatron can

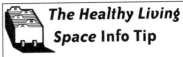

The Healthy Living Space Info Tip

For Everpure S-200 and QC4-VOC: Everpure, Inc., 660 Blackhawk Drive, Westmont, IL 60559; tel: 630-654-4000; fax: 630-654-1115; customer service: 800-942-1153; website: www.everpure.com.

For PPW Home Reverse Osmosis System: Pure-Pro USA Corporation, 19425 Everett Lane, Mokena, IL 60448; tel: 800-993-2933; e-mail: info@purepro.net; website: www.purepro.net.

For Sun-Pure Water Purifier: see Real Goods info on page 154.

handle pool volumes of up to 40,000 gallons and sells for about $300.

There are at least three other nonchlorine alternatives for cleansing your swimming pool water. These include ozonation (injecting ozone gas [a form of oxygen] into pool water; a small amount of chlorine will still be needed); ultraviolet light (supplemented with a small dose of chlorine); and biguanide, or polyhexamethylene biguanide (Baquacil), a safe and nontoxic chemical disinfectant.

HEALTHY LIVING SPACE DETOXIFIER #9
Don't Fluoridate Your Teeth— Your Body Doesn't Need Fluorides

We find another water-related toxicity issue with fluorides. The matter of adding fluoride to municipal water supplies is charged with the same controversy and lack of understanding of the biological consequences as is the chlorination issue. Water fluoridation has been touted for decades as beneficial in preventing dental caries (cavities) in children, but the research supporting this claim is spotty and not definitive. Further, a fair amount of evidence that fluoridation produces minor health consequences such as dental fluorosis (see below) and contributes to serious health disorders such as osteoporosis and cancer has received insufficient attention from medical and water authorities, and is not widely known among the public.

The recommendation here is straightforward: if possible, reduce or eliminate your intake of fluoridated tap water and fluoridated toothpaste. There is good reason to regard fluoride in the same way as chlorine—a toxic substance best avoided.

Today an estimated 250 million people worldwide and some 130 million Americans in 9,600 communities (or almost fifty percent of the U.S. population) drink fluoridated water, including residents of 41 of the country's fifty largest cities. According to the Centers for Disease Prevention and Control (CDC), 62% of the U.S. population (as of 1996) received fluoridated water, with a target of seventy-five percent set for the year 2000; the CDC planned to achieve this increase of another 30 million fluoridated Americans by way of "substantial public education and advocacy" primarily focused on the dental benefits.[34] Fluoridation is an American obsession, as only two percent of Europeans are forced to drink fluoridated water, and most of that takes place in England (ten percent of the population) and Ireland (sixty-six percent).

Some states and communities in the United States still do not routinely fluoridate their public water, so if you live in such a place, count yourself lucky. The trend, however, is to fluoridate all water sources in the United States, typically at the rate of 1 part fluoride per million parts water, or 1 ppm, although up to 4 ppm is allowed. Why such an urgency to fluoridate?

Water fluoridation in the United States began in 1945 in Grand Rapids, Michigan, when manufacturers of phosphate fertilizer[35] and aluminum[36] found a new place to dump their abundant supplies of their hazardous byproduct: fluoride. Even though a fifteen-year scientific study had been set in place to determine the safety (or not) of fluoridated water, it was suspended after only eighteen months so that widespread fluoridation could begin.

Previously, fluoride stores had been disposed of in small amounts as components in insecticides and rat poison; then scientists came up with evidence that fluoride ingestion may be related to a lower incidence of dental cavities. The first proposal that the nation's water be fluoridated (1939) came not from a dentist, however, but from a scientist employed by the aluminum industry. "Now instead of paying for the expense of disposing of their toxic waste products, companies could make money by selling them to municipal water authorities, turning the public into a highly cost-effective toxic waste dump for industry's excess fluoride."[37]

Aside from the human health impact of consuming fluoridated water, there is a negative environmental impact. To

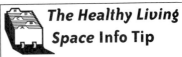

fluoridate water for 100 million people, you need to dump about 20,000 tons of fluoride into municipal water supplies each year.

The recommendation here is straightforward: if possible, reduce or eliminate your intake of fluoridated tap water and fluoridated toothpaste. There is good reason to regard fluoride in the same way as chlorine—a toxic substance best avoided.

The human body stores about fifty percent of its fluoride intake from fluoridated water in the teeth and bones. Each year, the remaining 10,000 tons of fluoride gets flushed down the toilet, and eventually enters the environment as yet another source of toxic pollution. It is quite likely we get some of this excreted fluoride back (and into our bodies again) when we drink tap water and eat conventionally raised produce and prepared foods. This recycling of fluoride was known as early as 1964, when a study of the fluoride levels in the sewage of fifty-six California cities showed levels equal to or higher than the permissible levels in fluoridated water.[38]

Is there evidence supporting the claim that fluoridated water reduces cavities in children? Yes, to some extent, the research supports in a limited sense the basic claim, but other research contradicts it and, as we will see below, other health risks associated with fluoride may far outweigh the modest benefits.

It is instructive that when fluoridation stops, dental health does not necessarily plummet. A town in Finland stopped fluoridating its water after doing so for 33 years. Scientists found, after examining the dental status of 1,325 children (age 3 to 9) before and after cessation of fluoridation, that there was no increase in dental cavities three years after cessation.[39] In Durham, North Carolina, fluoridation was halted for eleven months in 1990, enabling scientists to assess the effect of fluoride on children's teeth. Examining the dental records of 1,696 children (kindergarten to grade five), researchers found the temporary cessation of fluroidation "had little effect on caries"— in other words, there was no measurable increase in cavities.[40]

In 1990, public health officials in La Salud, Cuba, studied the effects on children's teeth of no longer fluoridating public water (at 0.8 ppm). Seven years after cessation, the level of dental caries for children six to nine was low, and had not risen; for ten to eleven year olds, the numbers had decreased; and in twelve to thirteen year olds, there was a "significant decrease," and the percentage of children this age who were free of cavities had increased from thirty-three percent (during fluoridation) to fifty-five percent, under no fluoridation. However, researchers concluded the fact that schoolchildren did a fluoride-based mouth rinse fifteen times a year at school might have contributed to the improved dental status.[41]

Fluoride Can Produce Dental Fluorosis

The evidence that ingesting fluoridated water leads to dental fluorosis is compelling. In the early stages of this condition, the enamel on teeth gets mottled, opaque, and sometimes stained. Later on, the teeth pit and get brittle, and they may chip, and develop a yellow, brown, or even black appearance.

The incidence of fluorosis increases when the concentration of fluoride in public water supplies exceeds 2 ppm; when it reaches 8 ppm, systemic fluorosis can start to appear, involving a bony overgrowth, neurological problems, and even arthritis. Researchers at the College of Dentistry at the University of Iowa concluded in 1999, "Several studies indicate that primary-tooth fluorosis can be prevalent and severe in areas of very high water fluoride concentrations."[42] Typically, the fluorosis happens on primary molars (premolars), but it can also affect incisors.

More specifically, a study by the School of Public Health at the University of Michigan at Ann Arbor found that fluoride was able to reduce dental cavities best at levels of up to 0.7 ppm, but that at these levels, 13% to 21% of schoolchildren developed dental fluorosis as a result. At fluoridation levels higher than 0.7 ppm, the incidence of dental fluorosis soared to between 29% and 41% (at 1.2 ppm fluoride).[43] Another study showed that children and teenagers (8-16 years old) who consumed fluoridated water containing from 0.3 ppm (considered a low level) to 1 ppm (considered optimal) of fluoride had fluorosis on an average of 15% of their teeth surfaces.[44]

Researchers at Harvard School of Dental Medicine in Boston, Massachusetts, found that in children aged one to seven who had been routinely exposed to fluoridated water, sixty-nine percent had at least "very mild fluorosis" while thirteen percent had "moderate to severe" fluorosis.[45] In a study of 233 "optimally fluoridated" children, aged 10-14, researchers at the University of Connecticut Health Center at Farmington found a "strong association" between the use of fluoride toothpaste, fluoride supplement, and powdered infant formula (containing fluoridated water) and mild to moderate fluorosis.[46] Norwegian scientists reported that fourteen percent of children aged five to eighteen who had been lifelong consumers of fluoridated water at a low level had dental fluorosis, while seventy-eight of those who had fluoride at a moderate to high level had the problem.[47]

The age at which the body is subjected to fluoridated water is important to the onset of fluorosis, researchers at the University of Chile at Santiago found. Children under sixteen months of age who had fluoridated water by way of powdered milk formula were twenty times more likely to develop fluorosis than those who were exposed later; children aged sixteen to twenty-four months were four times more likely.[48] Norwegian researchers came to the same conclusion, stating that "early mineralizing teeth (central incisors and first molars) are highly susceptible to dental fluorosis if exposed to fluoride" in the earliest months of life, from birth to twelve months. The fluoride apparently interferes with mineral absorption and utilization needed to produce strong enamel on the teeth.[49]

Fluoride Can Contribute to Cancer

Evidence continues to accumulate linking fluoride ingestion (through tap water, toothpaste, and supplements) with bone, skin, joint, kidney, mouth, and uterine cancer. According to one estimate, fluoride may be linked to as many as 10,000 cancer deaths annually in the United States,[50] but a former chemist with the National Cancer Institute estimated that fluoride caused 61,000 cases of cancer in 1995 and will cause 90,000 cases annually by the year 2015.[51] Researchers at the School of Medicine at the University of the Ryukyus in Okinawa, Japan, reported that, based on their study of twenty fluoridated municipalities, "a significant positive correlation" was observed between fluoride concentration in the drinking water and uterine cancer among women drinking it.[52]

Even at supposedly "safe" and "acceptable" doses of 1 ppm, fluoride can initiate a cancer process (as demonstrated in laboratory mice, whose tumor growth rate increased by twenty-five percent), and it can synergistically increase the carcinogenicity of other toxic substances. One study of cancer rates over a thirty-year period as seen in ten fluoridated cities versus ten nonfluoridated cities showed that after seventeen years of fluoridation, the cancer rate grew by ten percent, mostly in people over age forty-five.[53] At least eight other scientific studies present evidence linking fluoridated water with the onset of bone cancer.

Other Health Problems Associated with Fluoride

Fluoride exposure can disrupt the production of collagen in bones and lead to the breakdown of collagen in bones, muscles, skin, cartilage, the lungs, kidney, and trachea. Fluoride depletes the energy supplies of white blood cells, key immune system agents needed to destroy foreign cells; it can also cause premature body aging. Fluoride can also confuse the immune system and cause it to "attack" the body's own tissues. Further, it has been shown to depress the activity of the thyroid gland in the neck, an endocrine gland that regulates metabolism and the body's internal temperature.[54]

Fluoride consumption may also contribute to the risk of bone fractures in males and females of all ages, and to hip fracture in the elderly, even though, paradoxically, it seems to promote bone density. An English study of 914 cases of hip fracture among the elderly found some degree of risk associated with lifelong fluoridated water intake, at levels ranging from 0.15 to 1.79 ppm.[55]

Since 1986, eight peer-reviewed medical studies have confirmed an increase in the cases of hip fractures in fluoridated communities, ranging from 40% to 100%, depending on the age of the subjects and the fluoride concentration in their water. One study reported that for women seventy-five and older consuming fluoridated water, the risk was double that of women in nonfluoridated communities. Another study stated that the risk of hip fracture increases as the fluoride level climbs above 0.11 ppm.[56]

Scientists at the University of Technology in Sydney, Australia, stated in 1997 that their review of the scientific data "reveals a consistent pattern of evidence—hip fractures, skeletal fluorosis, the effect of fluoride on bone structure, fluoride levels in bones and osteosarcomas [bone cancers]—pointing to the existence of causal mechanisms by which fluoride damages bones." These scientists further pointed out that research supports the view that ingesting fluoride, by drinking fluoridated water, has "negligible" benefit; what benefit does accrue to the teeth comes from using fluoride lozenges and mouth rinses in which the chemical has direct contact with the teeth.[57]

Sustained fluoride ingestion can cause widespread toxicity. Laboratory rats were fed differing amounts of sodium fluoride over a period of ninety-nine weeks. Scientists observed a thirty percent drop in weight and found evidence of fluoride toxicity in the teeth, bones, and stomach; the incidence and severity of these symptoms were directly related to the dose and duration of exposure.[58]

Fluoride appears to have deleterious effects on the brain. One critic of fluoridation, referring to the fact that many children use fluoridated toothpaste, queried: "Brushing your brain with fluoride?" Evidence now links fluoride with IQ deficiencies in children, and suggests fluoride may produce nerve cell and brain damage *in utero*, as the mother passes the fluoride on to the fetus when she consumes fluoridated water. Children living in a low-fluoride area had higher IQs than comparable children in a high-fluoride area.[59] Further, low levels of fluoride given to test animals produced damages to brain tissue similar to those changes seen in the brains of humans with Alzheimer's and other forms of dementia.[60]

In fact, a study with rats showed that the presence of fluoride in the body made aluminum (in the tissues already) more available and more capable of entering the brain. Similarly, fluoride makes lead more "bioavailable" in the body, and scientists have demonstrated that children drinking fluoridated water have elevated lead levels in their blood. [61]

Varying levels of fluoride in drinking water (3-11 ppm) can affect the central nervous system and brain without producing noticeable physical malformations. Instead, it can affect functioning, producing symptoms such as attention deficit disorder when ingestion was 100 ppm from sublingual drops. This may seem like a high exposure, but it isn't an unlikely one, because toothpastes often contain 1000-1500 ppm of fluoride, and mouth rinses 230-900 ppm.

According to toxicologist Phyllis Mullenix, Ph.D., of the Forsyth Research Institute in Boston, Massachusetts, fluoride accumulates in brain tissues. The central nervous system is "vulnerable" to fluoride, and the effects on behavior depend on what age you are when exposed. In other words, not only can fluoride negatively affect mineralizing tissues (as in dental fluorosis in very young people), but it seems to negatively affect the developing brain as well.

Dr. Mullenix found evidence of a "generic behavioral pattern disruption" in rats dosed with fluoride, and that these disruptions were indicators of likely muscle and coordination problems, IQ deficits, and learning disabilities in humans due to fluoride intake. Dr. Mullenix also reported that the severity of the effect fluoride had on the brain depended on the section of the brain in which it was concentrated.[62] Should we be surprised? Sodium fluoride, which is routinely added to water supplies across the United States, is listed with the Environmental Protection Agency as a rat poison.

All you have to do is brush your teeth in fluoridated water with a fluoridated toothpaste and rinse your mouth with a fluoridated mouthwash and you will get the high exposure—every day. Plus you need to add to this fluoride ingestion from ambient sources, such as air pollution. At least 155,000 tons of industrial fluoride are released into the atmosphere every year by factories (from production of or involving iron, steel, aluminum, copper, lead, and zinc), and the level of emissions of fluoride into lakes, oceans, and rivers has been placed at 500,00 tons annually.[63] In 1991, the United States Public Health Service estimated that a 110-pound adult living in an "optimally fluoridated" city had a total daily fluoride intake, from all sources, as high as 6.6 milligrams. In 1997, the Environmental Protection Agency estimated that the typical American consumed five times more fluoride in that year than in 1971, and this was from foods and beverages only, not fluoridated tap water.[64]

STEAM DISTILLATION. One technology known to effectively remove fluoride from tap water is called steam distillation. Two others that also perform this function are reverse osmosis and deionization. According to Waterwise, a company that manufactures three types of steam water distillers, the units also remove various heavy metals, selected THMs and VOCs, radon, selected microorganisms including viruses, and most minerals.

The process is simple to describe: Water is heated in a chamber where it turns to steam; this vapor rises, leaving impurities (dissolved solids, salts, heavy metals) behind in the boiling chamber. The vapor then condenses into water in another chamber, percolating through a coconut shell carbon filter, where more of the VOCs are removed.

Steam distillation is a much slower process of preparing high-quality drinking water; it takes about four hours to produce one gallon (Model 9000) at a cost of about $0.25 per gallon, or 24 hours to make 9 gallons (Model 7000). Obviously, this approach will be suitable only if you want a limited amount of high-quality drinking water, and don't plan to use it for cooking as well.

SPECIALTY FLUORIDE FILTER. A special filter called Fluoride-X can be attached to your present drinking water inflow or can be used in conjunction with a water filter. The Fluoride-X (which sells for about $100) is a specialty cartridge containing the ABA2000 series of aluminum oxides that remove fluoride salts from the point-of-use water. According to the unit's distributor, the filter lasts for about two years' worth of household water filtration.

HEALTHY LIVING SPACE DETOXIFIER #10
Cleanse Your Produce of Toxic Chemicals

As profoundly important and as rich with impact as your choice in water consumption is your choice of food. As a consumer, you have the option, every time you buy a food, of selecting one that is conventionally produced or one that is organic and/or natural or, if a prepared food, contains organically produced ingredients. Either way, your choice makes a powerful difference, both to your physical health and to the well-being of the planet. Thinking green is good for your cells as well as for the planet's ecosystem.

If you cannot find organic produce (or cannot afford it—admittedly, it costs more to get chemically clean foods), yet wish

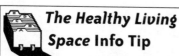

The Healthy Living Space Info Tip

For information about Steam Distillation Models 4000, 7000, and 9000:
Waterwise, Inc.,
P.O. Box 494000,
Leesburg, FL 34749;
tel: 800-874-9028 or 352-787-5008;
fax: 352-787-8123;
website: www.waterwise.com.

For Fluoride-X:
Nirvana Safe Haven,
3441 Golden Rain Road, Suite 3,
Walnut Creek, CA 94595;
tel: 800-968-9355;
fax: 925-938-9019;
e-mail: daliya@nontoxic.com;
website: www.nontoxic.com.

See also: Environmental Management, Inc. (Fluoride-X's manufacturer),
8680 Miralani Drive, Suite 121,
San Diego, CA 92126;
tel: 858-566-4522;
fax: 858-566-9521.

to eat fresh, *clean* fruits and vegetables, there are some simple measures you can take to cleanse your produce of some of their agricultural pollutants before you consume them. Even if your foods are organic, there is no assurance that tap water will be sufficient to cleanse them of any chemical contaminants they might carry on their surface, picked up in transit from organic field to your kitchen. For this reason, cleaning your produce is a good practice.

If you cannot find organic produce (or cannot afford it—admittedly, it costs more to get chemically clean foods), yet wish to eat fresh, clean fruits and vegetables, there are some simple measures you can take to cleanse your produce of some of their agricultural pollutants before you consume them.

Conceptually, using a produce rinse is like washing your hands before eating. Further, the rinse can remove germs (pathogenic bacteria, fungal spores, molds, parasites, pinworms) introduced to the produce during processing and handling, as well as chemical contaminants. Washing produce with water alone, or soap and water alone, is not sufficient to remove pesticide residues; this is largely because many pesticides are not water soluble. You need something stronger.

Be careful, however. The availability of nontoxic rinses to cleanse pesticides and residues from produce (thereby making it relatively easy to de-pollute fruits and vegetables) should not reduce our consumer pressure to have the use of pesticides in agriculture curtailed as much as possible.

Bleach Your Produce

It may surprise you, but an effective method for ridding produce of most of its surface layer of pesticide residue is washing it with conventional bleach, available as Clorox. This approach was originally publicized by Hazel Parcells, N.D., D.C., Ph.D., a natural healing expert who lived to 106 by following her own health protocols, including this one.

According to Dr. Parcells, bleach is "the most effective food cleanser." However, household bleach does not mean chlorine; it contains no more free chlorine than table salt (sodium chloride) does. The sodium hypochlorite in Clorox (present in a 5.25%

solution) acts as a natural oxygenator, capable of neutralizing fungi and bacteria and removing industrial chemicals. Dr. Parcells called her approach the Parcells Oxygen Soak, and she (and her many patients) used it successfully for forty years to cleanse and even revitalize produce.

Add one tablespoon of original Clorox bleach to a gallon of nonfluoridated and nonchlorinated water. Separate your foods into different groups, as each group will get a soak of a different length. If you have just returned from shopping, this would be a convenient time to process your produce. Immerse leafy vegetables in the Clorox bleach solution for five to ten minutes; root and heavy fiber vegetables and thick-skinned fruits get ten to fifteen minutes; thin-skinned berries, five minutes; medium-skinned fruits, ten minutes; citrus and bananas, fifteen; eggs, twenty to thirty minutes; thawed meats, ten minutes/pound; frozen meats, fifteen to twenty minutes/pound. After the Clorox rinse, place the produce or food item in a fresh water rinse for five to ten minutes; then dry and prepare for storage in the refrigerator, says Dr. Parcells. This last water rinse oxygenates the produce, giving them a new burst of vitality and color.[65]

Organiclean Fruit and Vegetable Wash

This is a nonsoap spray that comes in an eight-ounce plastic bottle and is made from natural ingredients including coconuts, bilberry, sugar cane, maple sugar, and oranges, lemons, and other citrus fruits. Using other natural cleaning agents (called "biosurfactants"), the product "creates a slippery surface and 'lifting action' for better removal of surface pesticides, chemicals, dirt, and other inorganic pollutants," says its manufacturer. All you have to do is spray and rinse off.

Fit

This is a widely advertised natural rinse solution that contains purified water, vegetable-derived oleic acid and glycerol, ethyl alcohol (from corn), potassium hydrate (from minerals), baking soda, citric acid (from corn starch and molasses), and distilled grapefruit oil. With Fit, you can either soak (broccoli, cauliflower, grapes, lettuce, snow peas) or spray (fruits, carrots, cucumbers, corn, onions, tomatoes) your produce. If you spray, you need to rub the produce for about twenty seconds, or if the produce is hard to rub, let it sit with the Fit spray on its surface for a few minutes; in either case, then rinse with fresh water. According to the manufacturer (Procter & Gamble), there is no aftertaste or smell on the cleansed produce.

Mom's Veggiewash

The product manufacturer does not provide a list of ingredients, but assures consumers it is made of safe, inert, nontoxic, biodegradable liquid surfactants that contain no animal products or petroleum derivatives. It is based on natural vegetable oils instead. According to Earth Partnership, the manufacturer, Mom's Veggiewash can remove ninety-four percent of oil-based chlorinated hydrocarbon pesticide residues, such as the organochlorines from Endosulfan. Endosulfan is found on "practically every vegetable and fruit" in the United States, according to company information sheets.

Research first published in 1965 demonstrates how washing produce with a "surfactant" can drastically reduce the pesticide residue content. Untreated green beans had 31 ppm of toxaphene; after being washed with water, the level was 24.9 ppm; after being washed with 0.1% polyether alcohol, it had dropped to 13 ppm; and after being washed in a 1% nonionic surfactant solution (functionally similar to Mom's Veggiewash, which uses a 5% nonionic surfactant solution from plant sources), the pesticide level was down to 12 ppm, or almost 2.5 times reduced. The results were even more striking with mustard greens. They started off having 233 ppm of toxaphene, then after water washing, 100 ppm; after the alcohol, 23 ppm; and after the surfactant, 20 ppm.[66]

With this product, place the produce in a colander and spray. It is recommended to treat even those fruits and vegetables which have skins you will not be eating, such as citrus, bananas, watermelon, cantaloupe, and the like, as the contaminants found on their skin can get into your body through peeling the fruit, followed by eating it without washing the hands again. After spraying, let the produce sit for a few minutes, then rinse with clean water.

Some produce may be waxed (such as cucumbers, apples, peppers, tomatoes). In that case, douse the produce in warm water, spray with Veggiewash, brush briskly with a vegetable brush,

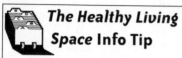

and rinse. If you see a dusty powder or scale form on the produce, this is a wax residue, and you need to repeat the cleansing.

HEALTHY LIVING SPACE DETOXIFIER #11
Whenever Possible, Eat Organic Foods

Chapter 1 acquainted you with the perils of conventionally grown food in terms of pesticide residues, industrial pollutants, processing additives, and other contaminants (see the section entitled "Tainted Food—Glutamates, Additives, Antibiotics, and POPs"). Avoiding further exposure to these toxic substances through your foods alone is sufficient reason to consider eating only organically produced foods.

However, there are three additional, perhaps even more persuasive reasons, for going organic: genetically modified foods; irradiated foods; and bovine growth hormone (BGH) in dairy products. In most cases, foods containing these substances are not labeled as such.

Thus, at present, only if you use foods that are certified and labeled organic can you avoid the health hazards of these three obnoxious, adulterative processes, which are now routinely done to foods in the American marketplace with the endorsement of U.S. government "health" authorities. By some bizarre inversion of its public health protection mandate, the FDA does not require food manufacturers (or growers) to label foods or products with the information that they contain genetically modified organisms, have been irradiated, or have traces of bovine growth hormone.

Why You Should Avoid Genetically Modified Foods

The matter of genetically engineered or modified crops and foods is one of the most intense public information scams of our time. It is as if the government, the food industry, and nearly all the media do not want the public to be aware of what is going on, or to know the health hazards posed by creating transgenic foods.

Genetically modified organisms (GMO) are plants, vegetables, fruits, and animals in which genes from other species have

Figure 4-2. Crops Containing Genetically Modified Organisms (GMOs)

Basic Food Crops Known to Contain GMOs:

FOOD ITEM	GMO
tomatoes	genes from bacteria, viruses, flounder, shellfish
potatoes	wax moth DNA, *Bacillus thuringiensis* bacteria
corn	virus, *Bacillus thuringiensis* bacteria
corn syrup and fructose	virus, *Bacillus thuringiensis* bacteria
soybeans	Roundup pesticide, bacteria genes
yellow crookneck squash	two viruses
canola oil	California bay turnip, virus and bacteria genes
cottonseed oil	bacteria and virus genes to tolerate pesticides
papaya	some strains have been genetically altered
cotton	bacteria and virus genes
Atlantic salmon	two genes from other species of fish

GMO-based foods that have been approved, are under government approval, or industry development:

apples	sunflowers	watermelons
rice	cucumbers	wheat
barley	lettuce	beans
chestnuts	melons	pineapples
strawberries	peppers	beets
sugar cane	walnuts	

been inserted to improve or alter various targeted characteristics. This is not the same as plant breeding, or manipulating gene patterns within a single species. It is called transgenic because genes (genic) are moved across (trans) species in ways that most critics of GMOs emphatically state nature never intended to have happen. Some people call them "genfoods," but others call them "frankenfoods."[67]

Scientists now regard the gene pool of many species of plants and animals as a kind of smorgasbord of genetic possibilities and desired traits. The once sacrosanct and uncrossable boundaries between species have now been broached, with experimental abandon. For examples, soybeans are crossbred with petunias; tomatoes are interlaced with genes from viruses; and corn, potatoes, soybeans, and cotton now bear pest-resistant genetic material.

The transgenic combinations are strange: antifreeze genes from flounder have been inserted in tomatoes to protect them from frost damage; chicken genes have been inserted into potatoes to bolster disease resistance; Chinese hamster genes are now in tobacco plants to increase sterol production; and human genes have been inserted in pigs, salmon, trout, and rice. Almost forty common vegetables, dairy products, and hundreds of processed foods now contain genes from all over the place: from viruses, bacteria, flowers, insects, and animals (see figure 4-2). An estimated 3,000 varieties of plants and animals now contain genes from other species, and transgenic experimentation is a burgeoning field.

Beware of potatoes. Monsanto, a major player in GMOs, recently released its New Leaf potato under the oxymoronic "NatureMark" label. This potato bears a gene intended to ward off insects. In 1997, nine million U.S. acres were planted to potatoes, corn, and cotton with seed carrying a gene from *Bacillus thuringiensis*, a synthetic version of a natural insecticide. As of 1998, GMO-based seeds accounted for twelve percent of U.S. corn acreage, thirty percent of soybeans, and forty percent of cotton.[68]

Watch out for soybeans, especially if you like soy foods such as tofu. Traces of a major pesticide used on corn and soybeans called Roundup have now been genetically inserted into the soybean seed itself, enabling the resultant plant to tolerate higher dosages of Roundup and other pesticides applied to the fields. The new GMO soybean is called Roundup Ready, and in 1997, it represented ten percent of the U.S. soybean crop. So unless your tofu or tempeh is made from certified organically grown soybeans, you have just added a little pesticide to your vegetarian stir-fry every time you use tofu.

It's not just GMO-based tofu you should be concerned about. The same problem holds with soymilk and soy-based infant formula. In fact, an estimated sixty percent of prepared, packaged foods contain GMOs, especially if there is a corn or soybean ingredient. A company called Genetic ID Inc., of Fairfield, Iowa, offers a DNA of food items to determine if GMOs are present. "With soy foods, such as tofu, soymilk, and infant formula, if it is not made from organically raised soybeans, almost always it is contaminated with genetically engineered soy," states molecular biologist John B. Fagan, who developed Genetic-ID's test. Dr. Fagan tested the top five brands of soy-based infant formula and found that four (Carnation Alsoy, Similac Neocare, Isomil, and Enfamil Prosobee; Edensoy had no GMOs) had "measurable levels" of GMOs, and that three had "very high levels."[69]

The reasonable person, upon hearing this for the first time, will probably say, yes, it sounds a bit adventurous, if not out of control, but are there any health hazards? This is the shocking part: nobody knows because no long-term studies have been done or were apparently even required. The American public is the experimental subject in this safety test, but the results won't be in for a few years, or a generation. Genetic effects from consuming GMO-based foods could well be on the order of the multigenerational damage produced by endocrine-disrupting hormones (discussed in chapter 2).

Say you have food allergies and you are carefully avoiding your known allergens, one of which is Brazil nuts. Now you consume a product that contains a Pioneer Hi-Bred GMO soybean, which contains Brazil nut genes. Suddenly you get a food reaction from a food on your nonallergenic list. This scenario is not a supposition, but a summary of a situation that actually happened. In 1996, eight individuals consuming these soybeans developed serious, potentially deadly allergic attacks because of the hidden Brazil nut genes. They reacted to the miniscule amount of Brazil nut in each soybean as if they were eating only Brazil nuts.[70] We can only await news of further outbreaks of unsuspected allergic reactions to other GMOs.

According to the Council for Responsible Genetics, a non-profit organization of scientists and public health advocates concerned with biotechnology and based in Cambridge, Massachusetts, GMOs "may cause unintended side effects that make foods hazardous for human consumption. Unpredictable gene expression may result in unanticipated toxic effects or allergies."[71] In other words, the Brazil nut allergy outbreak may have been only the proverbial "shot across the bow" presaging a much more traumatic outbreak of health problems resulting from GMOs.

Not only is the risk of sustaining surprise food allergies heightened by the advent of GMOs, but it is making it harder to guarantee that organically produced crops are truly organic, which is to say, free of GMOs. The problem is now being called transgenic pollution: pollen from a GMO crop blows across the field to an organic crop, cross-pollinating it, making it de facto another GMO crop. A small producer of tortilla chips made from organically produced grains had to throw out 87,000 bags of corn chips worth $147,000 in 1999 when a test revealed their corn contained GMOs. There was no deception involved because the organic farmer was certified, but his neighbor, who planted GMO corn, wasn't. The GMO corn cross-pollinated the organic corn. This same news report stated that GMO crops now occupy 90 million U.S. acres, or about 25% of the country's total croplands.[72]

There are at least three other identified health hazards with GMOs. That is to say, a few progressive scientists have identified potential problems, but have no idea how to extrapolate these into real-time scenarios. They just know the hazards portend serious trouble.

The first has to do with DNA uptake by human cells. At least two scientists propose that the viruses used in various GMO foods could be the most dangerous aspect of the genetic modification process itself. Typically, the virus used for gene implantation comes from the cauliflower mosaic virus (CMV), found naturally and harmlessly in many common vegetables. CMV in nature cannot enter human cells because it is biochemically specific to plants, but when it is used as the source for GMO virus genes, its protein coat is removed (which normally alerts mammalian immune systems that it is a foreign protein). This creates "naked DNA" enabling the virus to be taken into human and animal cells (because it's no longer recognized as foreign), there to become part of the organism's DNA structure.

The naked viral DNA is more infectious and thereby more dangerous than intact virus. Nobody knows what this might produce, but the speculations run to the grim type of scenario. Other research has shown that viral DNA resists digestion and can enter the bloodstream and white blood cells, the immune system's key defense agents. "Because these viruses are capable of recombining and jumping species, we must be aware that we cannot rule out the possibility of their triggering a vast range of public health disasters."[73] Because the cauliflower mosaic virus (or viral promoter) is found in almost all GMO-foods, the inclusion could be setting off bizarre, unknown, and/or hazardous biochemical reactions in the body.

The second health hazard pertains to the GMO-allergen problem, but at a deeper level. It seems GMOs produce a new allergen called the anti-idiotope allergen. When the body produces an antibody (an immune defense protein) against an allergen (a foreign protein), it also produces an antibody against this antibody, and this is called an anti-idiotope antibody. Now most GMOs contain a gene to resist the action of antibiotics, and these genes produce an enzyme that is similar to an antibiotic and is also an allergen. In other words, antibodies that are allergens get produced, which means most GMOs "are likely to be allergenic to people sensitive to antibiotics."[74] If you are already allergic to antibiotics, you will probably also be allergeric to GMOs.

The possibilities for new forms of allergic reactions to supposedly common—in truth, GMO-ed—foods could be staggering, and possibly innumerable. "The allergenic potential of these newly introduced microbial proteins is uncertain, unpredictable, and untestable," stated Marion Nestle, Ph.D., in an editorial in the *New England Journal of Medicine*.[75]

The third problem has to do with antibiotic resistance. All GMO-based foods contain antibiotic-resistant marker genes enabling them to resist getting destroyed by antibiotics. It seems that these genes survive the genetic manipulation process and remain intact and functional in the digestive tracts of mammals. They transfer horizontally from the GMO-foods to the bacteria in the digestive track of animals and humans consuming them. The result is that the consumers may be "incubating ever more virulent pathogens" as their natural defense systems are compromised.[76] Their systems may be more resistant to the effect of antibiotics given for medical reasons, and it is possible that the antibiotic resistance may be passed also to other dangerous microbes, further worsening the problem of antibiotic-resistant infections.

There is no indication that the public, to the degree it is aware of this development to include GMOs in many foods, is in favor of it. Nearly all polls since 1995, when public awareness of GMOs began (about a year after their introduction) both in the United States and internationally, register strong majority opposition to GMOs. A *Time* magazine ongoing Internet poll, which began in

---

Figure 4-3. What Is Organically Grown Produce?

Produce may be labeled organic if these conditions are fulfilled:

• Yearly verification of farmer's organic standards by any of forty-five independent, third party certifying agencies

• Nonuse of toxic pesticides, insecticides, herbicides, fungicides, and synthetic fertilizers on a field to be labeled organic for three years

• Physical barrier or buffer zone separating organic fields from neighboring farms if they use toxic pesticides and synthetic fertilizers, or minimum twenty-five-foot distance between fields

• No genetically modified or engineered seeds or crops or animals may be used anywhere on the farm certified as organic

• Conscientious soil-building program is practiced, using natural processes to enhance organic matter and optimum soil health

• Crop rotation of nonperennial crops

• No manure containing human excrement or urine may be used on the fields

• Soil nutrient sources containing highly soluble nitrate, phosphate, or chloride are prohibited

Source: "International Certification Standards, March 2000," International Crop Improvement Association, Lincoln, NE. OCIA is the world's largest organic certification organization, with 62 chapters in 20 countries, and involving 20,000 farmers.

October 1999, revealed that by February 2000, of the 154,000 respondents who had logged in to the questionnaire, 55% were "very concerned" they were consuming GMO-based foods. An MSNBC poll in January 2000 showed that eighty-one percent of Americans want GMO-foods to be labeled as such and that eighty-nine percent think the U.S. government should require premarket safety testing of GMOs. Twelve other U.S. polls registered an overwhelming majority in favor of GMO restrictions, as did most polls conducted in Europe, Australia, and New Zealand.[77]

In the meantime, U.S. consumers who wish to avoid or minimize their consumption of GMO-foods must exercise extreme market vigilance and should use certified organic foods when possible (see figure 4-3). According to BioDemocracy and Organic Consumers Association, a public advocacy group based in Little Marais, Minnesota, there are fifteen companies producing GMOs, which they dub the "Frankenfoods Fifteen": Kellogg's, Campbell Soup Company, Safeway, Nabisco, McDonald's, Frito-

Lay, Nestle, Heinz Foods, Quaker Oats, General Mills, Kraft, Hershey's, Coca-Cola, Starbucks, Procter & Gamble. The inference is that if you want to avoid GMOs, don't use any food products from any of these fifteen food companies (see figure 4-4).

There are upwards of 30,000 prepared foods now on the market that contain GMOs and must be avoided by the GMO-banning consumer. For example, consider how many products, such as sodas and beverages, including health food versions, contain corn syrup or fructose, both now made from GMO corn. Corn syrup and fructose are also found in yogurt, aspirin, and most sweet products. Then consider these GMO-rich corn-based products: nonorganic corn oil, cornstarch, cornmeal, baking soda, baking powder, and glycose syrup.

You will need to avoid soy protein in all its forms (unless it is certified organic): soy flour in baked goods, pizza, cookies, and

---

Figure 4-4. Commercially Prepared Foods Known to Contain GMOs*:

Fritos Corn Chips	Land O'Lakes Butter
Bravos Tortilla Chips	Cabot Creamery Butter
Kellogg's Corn Flakes	Fleishmann's Margarine
Total Corn Flakes	Gardenburgers
Blue Morning Cereal	Boca Burger Chef Max Favorite
Heinz 2 Baby Cereal	Morning Star Farms Better 'n Burgers
Enfamil Prosobee Soy Formula	Green Giant Harvest Burgers
Similac Isomil Soy Formula	McDonald's McVeggie Burger
Carnation Alsoy Infant Formula	McDonald's French Fries
Quaker Chewy Granola Bars	Kraft Salad Dressings
Snackwell's Granola Bars	Ovaltine Malt Powdered Mix
Ball Park Franks	Bac-Os Bacon Flavored Bits
Duncan Hines Cake Mix	Old El Paso Taco Shells
Quick Loaf Bread Mix	Jiffy Corn Muffin Mix
Ultra Slim Fast	Coca-Cola
Quaker Yellow Corn Meal	Nestle's Chocolate
Light Life Gimme Lean	NutraSweet
Aunt Jemima Pancake Mix	Karo Corn Syrup

*Source: *Non-Toxic Times*, 1:8, June 2000, published by Seventh Generation (www.seventhgen.com), which states these specific products have been independently tested and found to contain GMOs.

pasta; meat product fillers; vegetarian meat substitutes (tofu hot dogs); soymilk infant formula; diet and protein shakes; protein bars; chocolate and candy bars; margarine; ice cream; soy oil in salad dressings and snack chips; lecithin.

In the meantime, U.S. consumers who wish to avoid or minimize their consumption of GMO-foods must exercise extreme market vigilance. There are upwards of 30,000 prepared foods now on the market that contain GMOs and must be avoided by the GMO-banning consumer.

Aspartame, found in the artificial sweeteners Equal or NutraSweet, contains a GMO as do most nonorganic cheeses. Food additives such as lactase, catalase, and amylase contain GMOs; most livestock and commercially raised seafood are fed GMO-based feeds.[78] Without argument, the list is dizzying in scope. You can easily end up spending a great deal of your time merely trying to avoid getting poisoned by what you eat and drink.

Why You Should Be Wary of Nonorganic Dairy Products

The problem with conventionally produced dairy products is that there is a good chance they contain another GMO in the form of a hormone. Specifically, it is called the bovine growth hormone (BGH), or recombinant bovine somatotrophin hormone, in its more technical guise. The result is that standard dairy milk and dairy products may no longer be healthy foods.[79]

Again, thanks to the FDA in concert with Monsanto, the hormone's manufacturer, there is almost no way to tell which dairy products contain the hormone unless they are certified organic. Not only does the FDA not require dairy products to carry a BGH label, for a while, Monsanto was suing any dairy product manufacturers who labeled their products as BGH-free. Since 1993, BGH has been administered to dairy cows to increase their milk yield, but evidence is already available suggesting it might cause cancer in humans.

BGH contains a hormone called IGF-1 (insulin-like growth factor), found in both cows and people (in the saliva and blood). It causes cells to divide and grow, and this is how the hormone increases cows' milk yield. However, the hormone's penchant for stimulating cell proliferation in cows is what makes it a possible carcinogen in humans.

Research shows that pasteurization does not destroy BGH and that the human stomach does not break down BGH when it comes into the body in a dairy product; instead, the large intestine absorbs it because it already has receptor sites for IGF-1. Pasteurization actually increases the IGF-1 content of milk as does BGH itself, so when you drink BGH-produced milk, you consume higher than usual levels of this hormone.

According to research published by Samuel Epstein, M.D., chairman of the Cancer Prevention Coalition and professor at the University of Illinois Medical Center, both in Chicago, Illinois, IGF-1 promotes the transformation of normal breast tissue into cancerous tissue and the proliferation of cancer cells in the breast. "All women will now be exposed to an *additional* breast cancer risk due to milk from cows treated with recombinant growth hormone," he states.[80]

Dr. Epstein states that IGF-1 levels in BGH-produced milk can be up to ten times the levels in nontreated milk, and ten times as potent because its chemical form has been truncated. This is especially risky for infants and small children, he adds. European research showed that the amount of excreted IGF-1 in milk may be increased over non-BGH-treated milk by twenty-five to seventy percent.[81]

Research published in *The Lancet* in 1998 attributed a sevenfold increase in breast cancer risk among premenopausal women to IGF-1 content of milk. Blood from 32,826 nurses was collected and analyzed (in 1989) for IGF-1 levels; of these women, 397 eventually developed breast cancer. All of these 397 women had elevated IGF-1 levels when they were "healthy" and after they developed the cancer. The risk of breast cancer for women under fifty-one with the highest IGF-1 levels was seven times higher than women with lower levels. On this basis, the scientists stated there is "substantial indirect evidence of a relation" between IGF-1 levels and breast cancer.[82]

The Healthy Living Space Info Tip

For a source of copious information and public action/advocacy guidelines:
BioDemocracy and Organic Consumers Association,
6144 Highway 61,
Little Marais, MN 55614;
tel: 218-226-4164;
fax: 218-226-4157;
e-mail: campaign@organic-consumers.org;
website: www.purefood.org.

For another advocacy/public action source:
Genetically Engineered Food Alert,
1200 18th Street, NW,
5th Floor, Washington, D.C., 20036;
tel: 800-390-3373;
fax: 800-390-4751;
e-mail: gefoodalert@emediacy.org;
website: www.gefoodalert.org.

This organization is a coalition of seven other advocacy groups committed to the testing and labelling of GMOs. For more information about detecting the presence of GMOs in foods:
Genetic ID Inc.,
1760 Observatory Drive,
Fairfield, IA 52566;
tel: 515-472-9979;
fax: 515-472-9198;
e-mail: info@genetic-id.com;
website: www.genetic-id.com.

Another study, this one in *Science*, linked prostate cancer and IGF-1 in a study involving 152 men with prostate cancer. The researchers found "a strong positive association" between IGF-1 levels and prostate cancer risk. Specifically, they found that men with elevated but "normal" levels of IGF-1 levels were four times more likely to get prostate cancer. Among men sixty and older, if their IGF-1 levels were high, they were eight times more likely to get prostate cancer than men with the lowest levels of this hormone. The results were sufficiently vivid to "raise concern," the researchers stated, that sustained intake of IGF-1 through BGH-treated milk could increase the risk of prostate cancer. In fact, they suggested that elevated IGF-1 levels in the blood might well be used as an indicator of prostate and breast cancer risk, an early warning signal, if you like.[83]

The true extent of the health hazard of BGH-treated milk is not known. Yet. Consider it an experiment still in progress. "With the active complicity of the FDA," stated Dr. Epstein, "the entire nation is currently being subjected to an experiment involving large-scale adulteration of an age-old dietary staple by a poorly characterized and unlabeled biotechnology product." The experiment "poses major potential health risks for the entire U.S. population."

As with GMOs, a majority of consumers aware of the issue are demanding dairy products be clearly labeled if they contain BGH. Of 1,900 polled, ninety-four percent said BGH-milk should be labeled. Another study showed that already ten percent of consumers are taking evasive or preventive action by deliberately buying dairy products from nontreated cows, while seventy-four percent of consumers state they are concerned about the possible—eventual—discovery of negative long-term health consequences of consuming BGH-based dairy products.[84]

Until more is known about the long-term health impact of increased IGF-1 intake and blood levels in humans from consuming dairy products, it would be prudent for those wishing to minimize their intake of toxic substances to avoid consuming all dairy products not labeled organic (see figure 4-3). For the present, a label of organic on a dairy product is the only guarantee that the milk was not produced with BGH. Sheep or goat's milk products are exempt because BGH cannot be used on them; therefore, goat's and sheep milk products by definition (at present) are BGH-free. Also, certain imported cheeses are BGH-free, specifically from the countries that have banned BGH including Canada, France, Italy, Ireland, Great Britain, the Netherlands, Belgium, Luxembourg, Spain, Portugal, Germany, Austria, Switzerland, Norway, Sweden, Finland, Denmark, Greece, New Zealand, and Australia.

Good Reasons to Avoid
Irradiated Foods

The irradiation of agricultural produce and animal products poses another health threat for the toxic-substance-conscious consumer. As with GMOs and BGH, food irradiation represents another ill-founded toxic adulteration of our food supply.

The FDA began approving selective use of irradiation procedures on U.S. foods in the 1960s, starting with wheat, wheat flour, and potatoes; in the 1980s, pork, spices, herb teas, fruits, vegetables, and poultry were added to the list; and in 1997, meat started being irradiated before it reached the supermarket shelves. New foods likely to be approved for irradiation include deli meats, frozen foods, prepared fresh foods, fresh juices, seeds, and sprouts. Presently, thirty-five countries irradiate their foods.

The ostensible reason for food irradiation has been food safety, because it was believed that the radiation killed pathogenic organisms that might cause produce and meats to sicken consumers or spoil. However, the means to accomplish this goal are toxic. One of three energy sources is typically used: gamma rays from cobalt-60 or cesium-137 (which are radioactive waste products from the nuclear industry); X-rays; or high-energy electron beams.

When food irradiation received FDA support in 1987, the agency required all irradiated foods to be labeled as such, but in

 The Healthy Living Space Info Tip

For a list of organic and BGH-free dairy products, see:
"The Shopper's Campaign/Mothers' Milk List," at:
www.igc.apc.org/mothers/fieldwork/mo _field_milklist.html.
Prepared by: Mothers & Others for a Livable Planet,
40 West 20th Street,
New York, NY 10011;
tel: 212-242-0010;
e-mail: corevalues@mothers.org.

For more information and public advocacy action against BGH and other food contamination issues, see:
The Center for Food Safety,
666 Pennsylvania Avenue, SE, Suite 302, Washington, D.C. 20003;
tel: 202-547-9359;
fax: 202-547-9429;
e-mail: office@centerforfoodsafety.org;
website: www.centerforfoodsafety.org.

For information about organic standards (and complete document "International Certification Standards, March 2000") for agriculture:
Organic Crop Improvement Association (OCIA),
1001 Y Street, Suite B,
Lincoln, NE 68508;
tel: 402-477-2323;
fax: 402-477-4325;
e-mail: info@ocia.org;
website: www.ocia.org.

recent years, that requirement has been considerably relaxed. In 1997, Congress passed legislation allowing food packagers to reduce the label size (the words "treated with radiation" accompanied by a specific graphic design) and to exclude the identifying label if all the components of a food product had not been irradiated. In other words, if a product contains fifteen ingredients, and twelve have been irradiated, and three have not, the product does not have to say "treated with radiation." If the irradiated food will be used in a restaurant, deli, salad bar, hotel, airline, hospital, or school food service, labeling is not required.[85]

You must now be on guard, too, for semantic trickery in labels. The food industry is lobbying FDA to allow deceptive labeling such as "electronic pasteurization," "cold pasteurization," and "pasteurization with X rays" to disarm public disapproval (and awareness of) food irradiation.

What's wrong with radiation in foods? First, evidence suggests it reduces the nutritional content of foods. Vitamin C levels can be reduced by five to ten percent and vitamin E by twenty-five percent; thiamin, and vitamins A and K are especially susceptible to radiation damage. Some place the range of nutrient depletion between five percent and eighty percent, depending on how the produce is stored. Other research documents a ninety-five percent depletion of vitamin A in irradiated chicken, an eighty-six percent drop in vitamin B in irradiated oats, and a seventy percent depletion of vitamin C in irradiated fruit juices.

Even though irradiation destroys ninety-five percent of all bacteria (including beneficial ones), it also deactivates many essential digestive enzymes found in the produce, requiring the human system to work harder to process the foods.

Also, because radiation kills all bacteria, you can't smell a food to see if it's spoiled, even if it has, and botulinum, the toxic agent that produces botulism, is not affected by irradiation. This means your risk of unknowingly consuming tainted food is higher with irradiated foods. In addition, radiation is likely to have a mutagenic effect on bacteria and viruses present in the meat or produce, causing them to mutate into radiation-resistant strains. In fact, scientists have already developed a radiation-resistant strain of salmonella, one of the chief pathogens in animal products.

So you start off with your "fresh" vegetables being functionally and nutritionally already cooked. Insofar as most consumers cook their vegetables and thereby leach out further nutrients, nutrient loss due to irradiation adds to the nutritional depletion of our food supply and can contribute over time to selective or chronic nutrient deficiency or even subacute malnutrition.

Second, the so-called standard safe doses permitted for irradiation are shockingly high when compared to their equivalent in terms of X-ray exposures. For meat, the FDA permits the equivalent exposure of 22.5 million X-rays per piece; for poultry, 15 million X-rays; for spices, 150 million; fruits and vegetables, 5 million. That is an extraordinary number of X-rays.

Extensive research by nuclear radiation experts such as John W. Gofman, Ph.D., M.D., director of the Committee for Nuclear Responsibility, former professor of molecular biology at the University of California at Berkeley, and author of several important books on radiation exposure and cancer, indicates that far less exposure to X-rays can be carcinogenic. In fact, Dr. Gofman states that, over the course of a lifetime, X-ray exposure (including from mammograms) can account for seventy-five percent of all cases of breast cancer. Dr. Gofman found that the longer you are exposed to radiation, the weaker the dose it takes to produce damaging effects. When it comes to X-rays, less is very much more.[86]

An X-ray is a type of ionizing radiation, which means its high energy waves can rip electrons away from stable molecules. The principal means by which it is believed X-rays and thus all radiation produce biological damage is through the creation of free radicals, unstable molecules that destroy cells (see chapter 2). Overlooked in the FDA's "safety" standards is the fact that "food irradiation produces 'radiomimetic' foods—they *mimic* the effects of actual radiation when eaten."[87]

Third, even though, technically, irradiated foods are not radioactive as such, studies show that eating irradiated foods is still hazardous because they contain "radiolytic products," other toxic forms or byproducts of nuclear radiation. These byproducts have been associated with cancers, gene damage, birth defects, and other biological abnormalities. The radiolytic products also involve toxic chemicals found in foods, such as benzene, formaldehyde, formic acid, and quinines. In layperson's terms, the bombardment of the radiation shakes everything up in a food item, producing unstable molecules (free radicals) and new, bizarre, probably toxic products containing well-known toxic substances, such as benzene, formaldehyde, and the others.

Insofar as the "unique radiolytic products" are new to the food technology world, never seen before food irradiation, nobody can say for sure that they are harmless and that a diet of irradiated foods is safe. Like the long-term effects of GMO-based foods, it is entirely unknown to science what food irradiation will do to us. However, suspicions have been raised as to probable health effects, and they are distressing.

According to one estimate, for every 7.5 ounces of irradiated meat you consume, you are ingesting 2,560 potentially carcinogenic or mutagenic radiolytic product (RP) molecules that can affect liver cells. "Over a long period of time, the RP assault on the liver combined with fewer antioxidants in the diet [irradiation depletes antioxidant levels] will create a 'fertile field for the ultimate growth of cancer cells' and 'almost certainly evolve' to produce liver cancer."[88]

The ramifications of this calculation are that even at one-tenth the concentration of radiolytic products known by the FDA to be formed by food irradiation, "irradiation of foods in the human diet represents predictably unacceptable risks to the public's health." In other words, this one aspect of food irradiation may produce serious health consequences even if your exposure is only ten percent of the "safety" level established by the FDA.

Critics of food irradiation state that the technology has never been adequately tested for long-term safety and public health effects. In fact, the FDA approved food irradiation on the basis of only 5 out of 413 animal feeding trials under way at the time in 1982, and the key trial lasted only fifteen weeks. In the FDA's own review in 1982, it admitted that of these 413 studies, 344 were either inconclusive or inadequate and could not demonstrate or refute irradiation safety; 32 showed adverse effects; 37 appeared to support the procedure's safety; only 5 studies (1% of all studies reviewed) "appeared to support safety."[89]

There is strong evidence of health hazards from food irradiation. For example, in 1979, the Hungarian Academy of Sciences looked at all the available scientific studies on food irradiation. They found that the literature revealed food irradiation was responsible for 7,191 neutral effects, 185 beneficial effects, and 1,414 negative outcomes. The latter included tumor formation, damage to genes (including chromosomal polyploidy, or extra chromosomes in the genes), kidney and heart disease, and birth defects.[90]

Evidence linking gene damage to consuming irradiated foods was developed as early as 1973 in India. There scientists found that rats and mice fed irradiated wheat had increased levels of cells with abnormalities in their bone marrow chromosomes (called polyploid cells). Monkeys and undernourished children also developed abnormalities in their white blood cells after eating irradiated wheat. The cells became abnormal after only four weeks of the children's feeding program; it took twenty-six weeks for the abnormalities to dissipate after the program stopped. An increased number of polyploid cells is often associated with either rapidly regenerating tissues or rapidly growing malignant tumors, observed the researchers in presenting their data to the United States Congress in 1987.[91]

Opposition to food irradiation continues to mount as consumers become more aware of its potential health risks. The Center for Food Safety, a public advocacy group in Washington, D.C., states that "the use of food irradiation poses significant human and environmental impacts."[92] Another political advocacy group called Public Citizen, also in Washington, D.C., summarizes the negative health effects of food irradiation for which supporting research already exists:

• Increased chromosomal damage in animals and humans

• Formation of unique radiolytic products in the foods

• Increased frequency of cell mutations

• Formation of mutant bacteria

• Decreased nutritional content of foods

• Increased levels of carcinogens and other toxins in foods

The Healthy Living Space Info Tip

For more on the health hazards of X-rays and ionizing radiation and the work of Dr. John Gofman: The Committee for Nuclear Responsibility, P.O. Box 421993, San Francisco, CA 94142; tel & fax: 415-776-8299; website: http://radical.org/radiation/CNR.

For information and advocacy/action positions on food irradiation: Public Citizen, 1600 20th Street, NW, Washington, DC, 20009; tel: 202-588-1000; website: www.citizen.org. Public Citizen was founded by Ralph Nader in 1971 to represent consumers' interests.

• Increased frequency of tumors, reduced survival rate, and other health problems in animals

• Corrupted flavor and texture of foods.[93]

As with GMOs and BGH-treated dairy products, the U.S. public is overwhelmingly *not* behind food irradiation. A Louis Harris poll in 1986 reported that seventy-six percent of Americans considered irradiated foods to be a hazard. In 1997, a CBS News poll indicated that seventy-three percent of the public opposes food irradiation and that seventy-seven percent would not knowingly eat irradiated foods. An April 1999 survey found that eighty-eight percent of consumers support the labeling of irradiated foods.[94]

HEALTHY LIVING SPACE DETOXIFIER #12
Minimize Your Consumption of Foods Containing Trans-fatty Acids

In many respects, this next category of food adulteration is easier to pinpoint and to avoid than GMOs, BGH-dairy products, and irradiated foods. It pertains to the fats found in prepared foods, specifically, what are called saturated hydrogenated fats, or trans-fatty acids. Hydrogenated is a chemical term that refers to a fat in a semisolid state, such as margarine.

The recommendation here is simple: avoid consumption of all foods containing trans-fatty acids, or at least minimize your consumption. Trans-fatty acids are linked to heart disease, depression, and other long-term degenerative health conditions. You will have to read product labels carefully, looking for the words "hydrogenated fats" or "partially hydrogenated fats," and avoiding certain categories of prepared foods. But to understand why this is so important, we need to briefly review the chemical facts of fats.

Fats and oils are made of basic building blocks called fatty acids. A fatty acid is a chain of carbon atoms with a hydrogen atom at the end. The chains can have anywhere from two to thirty carbon atoms. When a fatty acid has all the hydrogen atoms it can hold in its configuration, it is saturated. Examples of this are animal fats and other fats that are solid at room temperature. If the fatty acid doesn't have all its hydrogen spots filled, it is unsaturated; examples of these are most vegetable oils, which are liquid at room temperature. Unsaturated fats are preferable in the diet and are called essential fatty acids; these include omega-6 oils, such as linoleic acid, and omega-3 oils, such as linolenic acid, all derived from natural plant sources.

A trans-fatty acid is an industrial alteration of the natural shape of oils. Although trans-fatty acids exist in small amounts in nature, that is nothing compared to the scale on which they have entered the food supply. The manufacturing process changes the way the hydrogen atoms bond to the carbon atoms in a fat. Hydrogenated fats or trans-fatty acids were originally synthesized and introduced into foods in 1910 (with a big push coming in the 1950s) to extend the shelf life of oil-based consumer foods. The oils were hardened or hydrogenated to prevent rancidity. This change in chemical configuration gives margarines a butter-like consistency and makes shortenings fluffy. However, from the viewpoint of some nutritionists, the introduction of trans-fatty acids into the food supply was not a good idea.

"The production of trans-fatty acids for human consumption is the most devastating, nutritional mistake ever made," claims Patricia Kane, Ph.D., a nutritional biochemist practicing in Millville, New Jersey.

"The production of trans-fatty acids for human consumption is the most devastating, nutritional *mistake* ever made," claims Patricia Kane, Ph.D., a nutritional biochemist practicing in Millville, New Jersey. It's a mistake because all traces of essential fatty acids are "obliterated" from processed foods, says Dr. Kane, and trans-fatty acids or hydrogenated oils take their place.[95]

The result of this substitution of hydrogenated oils for essential fatty acids is first a deficiency of the healthful oils in your body and a corresponding excess of unhealthful hydrogenated fats. This in turn has been identified as a contributing factor in obesity and heart disease. Fats are needed to produce cholesterol in the body, which in turn is needed to produce "a cascade of crucial hormones," explains Dr. Kane. All cholesterol is not "bad"; you actually need some to run your body properly.

Fatty acids have many key functions: they comprise sixty percent of the brain itself; they contribute to cell membrane fluidity, allowing biochemical "traffic" into and out of each cell; they help maintain the integrity of the gastrointestinal tract, enabling it to protect the body against pathogens. Disturbances in the energy activities associated with fatty acids, says Dr. Kane, "are reflected in every system of the body and can result in many physical and mental disorders, including depression." In fact, she states that in the difference between trans-fatty and essential fatty acids you have both the cause and the cure of depression. With a diet based on hydrogenated fats, "Prozac is only a few more wrong meals away."

Fatty acid chains are said to be like "tails": the tails of essential fatty acids vibrate fast and move quickly, a sign of molecular health, but trans-fatty acid tails are rigid and have no movement, says Dr. Kane. "A trans-fatty acid sits like a heavy blob inside you, shutting down the fatty acid metabolism within the immune, endocrine, and central nervous systems, and replacing the good, necessary fats (omega-3s and omega-6s) with something harmful to health."

Your body burns the trans-fatty acid for calories but can't absorb nutrients from it. The accumulation of trans-fatty acids in the body acts like a systemic poison and generates an abnormal biochemistry within you, Dr. Kane says. She recommends avoiding trans-fatty acids altogether to protect the integrity of your immune, endocrine (hormonal), and central nervous systems.

Research on trans-fatty acids has started to highlight their health hazards. As early as 1990, Dutch scientists showed that margarine consumption, thought to be healthy because it was not cholesterol-rich like dairy butter, actually increased the risk of coronary heart disease. Now new research links trans-fatty acids with elevated levels of LDL, the so-called "bad" cholesterol (HDL being the "good" kind). Scientists at Tufts University in Boston studied the effects on thirty-six men and women over the age of fifty of diets in which thirty percent of the calories came from fats. For the study, two-thirds of their fat came from soybean oil, semiliquid margarine, soft margarine, shortening, stick margarine, or butter.

The best results in terms of lowering LDL-cholesterol levels were obtained with soybean oil and semiliquid margarine (minimally hydrogenated) diets. It is interesting to note that for the most part the levels of trans-fatty acids used in the foods in this experiment were lower than what a typical American consumer is likely to get on a daily basis. For example, the soybean oil shortening contained 9.9 g of trans-fatty acids per 100 g of fat compared to 35-50 g of trans-fatty acids per 100 g of fat found in most commercially produced cakes, cookies, crackers, and doughnuts. The stick margarines used contained 20 g per 100 g of fat compared to 30 g typically found in popular stick margarines.

Those consuming only soybean oil had their LDL-cholesterol levels drop by twelve percent from pre-diet levels. They also found that trans-fatty acids raised the cholesterol levels more than saturated fats did. On the basis of their results, the researchers concluded that the general public and those with high blood cholesterol "should be encouraged to use vegetable oil in its natural state or after minimal hydrogenation." This is especially so since, as mentioned above, many people may consume trans-fatty acids at higher levels than those used as a basis in the study.[96]

Here is a summary of some of the research supporting the undesirability of consuming trans-fatty acids:

• Lowers levels of desirable HDL cholesterol, and raises levels of undesirable LDL cholesterol.

• Reduces the amount of "cream" or volume in the breast milk of nursing mothers.

• Increases blood levels of insulin, increasing the risk of diabetes.

• Decreases the response of red blood cells to insulin, potentially complicating the blood sugar balance in diabetics.

• Lowers immune response by affecting how the immune system's B cells respond.

• Causes unfavorable changes in the activities of enzymes that deal with carcinogens as part of the liver's detoxification process.

- Alters the functional properties of cell membranes such as transport and fluidity.

- Decreases levels of the male sex hormone testosterone, increases the level of abnormal sperm, and interferes with gestation in women.[97]

On a practical level, if you wish to minimize your intake of trans-fatty acids, you will need to avoid the following: fast-food burgers, french fries, and hash browns, as they will probably have been fried in hydrogenated fats; commercially baked cakes, cookies, muffins, doughnuts, corn chips, and pastries, as they probably contain hydrogenated fats; soft-tub and stick margarines and shortenings. French fries are the biggest offenders here, with four ounces containing 2.4 to 3.4 g of trans-fatty acids; doughnuts are close behind with a one ounce serving containing 3.19 g. As healthful alternatives, look for and consume products containing olive, canola, or other unsaturated vegetable oils.[98]

You will probably find that a great many foods you are accustomed to eating come under the trans-fatty acid ban. The average consumption of trans-fatty acids in grams per day for the United States is estimated to be between 11.4 and 12.1, comprising, respectively, 7.3% to 7.8% of total fat intake. However, for adults aged 20-65, that level is 14. 9 g/day or 8% of total daily fat intake, and for female teenagers, it is 30 g/day representing 28% of total fat intake. By comparison, Sweden is much lower at 5 g/day, Germany is 4.5 to 6.5, Canada is 9.1, England is 12, and the Netherlands is 17.[99]

Where does all this leave you in terms of what to eat? Essentially, if your sole guideline is to eat only organically produced food this in itself dictates a diet. By definition, an organic diet will eliminate a great deal of the nutritionally inferior, high-fat, sugar-based, additive-laden, preservative-rich, processed and prepared foods that are the carriers of many of the toxic substances you are trying to eliminate from your body. Beyond this, determining the most appropriate diet for an individual is one of the hardest tasks of medicine (and living) because everyone's physiology is specialized to some extent, unique to the individual, or at least uniquely idiosyncratic. You will need to give this matter considerable thought and further research to find the approach that works best to keep you nutritionally fit and minimally toxic.

HEALTHY LIVING SPACE DETOXIFIER #13
Do a 3-Day Water or Juice Fast to Rest and Regenerate Your Cells

By this time, you may be so dismayed with the state of the American food supply and the toxic burden it imposes on your body that the idea of fasting, that is, abstaining from solid foods for a limited period, may seem logical if not irresistible. The fact is, even if the food supply (and our air and water) were not so stunningly tainted, brief, recurrent abstention from foods is an old, well-proven remedy for improving one's health. Fasting has been practiced around the world in many traditions of medicine and spirituality.

Why fast? Think of it as a vacation for your digestive system and its "support staff," a break from business as usual for the gastrointestinal tract. Say you are a forty-year old man or woman and have never fasted. That means your digestive system has been running flat out for 14,600 days without stopping. It is almost impossible for your body to be entirely current with its digestive affairs; in most people, there will be a backlog of unfinished, incomplete, or even abandoned digestion.

As you will learn in chapter 5, the intestines, comprising about twenty-six feet of internal organ space, is a remarkably competent *storage* vessel for incompletely processed foods. Fasting for even a few days gives your intestines a chance to start getting caught up with its unending elimination demands. And it gives all the cells in your body, but especially those in the liver and kidneys, a chance for some rest and regeneration.

As a benefit of this respite from the ceaseless demands to process, assimilate, and eliminate foods, your body will have a chance to speed up its collection and excretion of toxins, from the colon, liver, kidneys, lymph nodes, bladder, lungs, even the skin. Your mind, too, will reap benefits from this brief abstention from food intake. It is quite likely you will emerge from a brief fast with enhanced clarity, focus, concentration, uplifted spirits, a general calmness, and a sense of heightened energy and vitality.

For the purposes of the detoxification recommendations offered in this book, the three-day water or juice fast can be undertaken as a preliminary to the more comprehensive intestinal, liver, kidney, and lymph cleansing regimens described in later chapters. You can do the three-day fast several times a year as a kind of routine internal housecleaning, if you wish.

There are a few precautions to observe regarding your limited fast:

First, do *not* do the fast if you have hypoglycemia (chronic low blood sugar), diabetes, weakened immunity, heart problems (such as low blood pressure), cancer, stomach ulcers, if you are pregnant, lactating, suffering from nutrient deficiencies or generally malnourished, excessively thin or anorexic, or under heavy medication for a serious illness. Or undertake it *only* under the supervision of a qualified health-care practitioner.

Second, don't start it tomorrow. Prepare your body for the drastic reduction in food intake it will experience. Over the course of a few days—a week perhaps—gradually reduce your food consumption to one light meal daily. Naturopathic physician Bruce Fife, N.D., author of *The Detox Book*, recommends following a natural foods diet for three to four weeks before starting the fast if you have been accustomed to a diet of fast, prepared, and convenience foods as that are notoriously deficient in nutrients. The preparatory health foods diet will fortify you nutritionally so that your system can function well during the fast. The natural foods diet Dr. Fife recommends includes only organically produced fruits, vegetables, and protein sources (in limited amounts), whole grains, and no prepared or packaged foods.[100]

Third, try the fast for one day to see how it feels. Then wait a week and, following the same preparation steps, try it for two or three days.

Fourth, expect a few transient symptoms to arise during the fast, such as headaches, mild muscle aches and pains, irritability, and old emotions or thoughts.

Fifth, after your three days of fasting, do not immediately return to a full-fledged solid foods diet. Build up to it gradually for three days, reversing your preparatory steps from before the fast. For example, you might continue with some of the juices, and add salads or steamed vegetables, followed the next day with well-cooked brown rice or millet.

Sixth, when you resume your regular diet, observe if any foods produce allergic reactions. Because your system has somewhat cleared itself of old debris and digestive backlog, hidden food allergies may now become apparent and you may find that wheat, eggs, chocolate, or corn, for example, produce allergic symptoms. If so, reduce or discontinue your intake of the specific food for a few weeks, then reintroduce at perhaps twenty-five percent of the previous intake rate.

During the fast you stop consuming solid foods and increase your intake of pure liquids, either in the form of water or juices. These liquids should not include stimulants such as coffee, tea, or alcohol; or milks, such as cow, goat, sheep, soy, rice, almond, or any other. Basically, consume small amounts of the selected beverage frequently throughout the day, perhaps hourly. Don't overtax your kidneys by drinking too much at one time, such as more than eight ounces. There are many options to choose from regarding what your liquid intake will consist of, and we'll review a few of these below.

Some detoxification experts, such as Elson Haas, M.D., director of the Preventive Medical Center of Marin in San Rafael, California, recommends a twice yearly fast, corresponding with the changes in season from winter to spring and summer to autumn. For example, as a general protocol, Dr. Haas advises consuming two to three quarts of liquids daily on the limited fast; these liquids can be fresh, pure water or specially blended vegetable juices.

Juices for Seasonal Cleanses

For the spring cleanse, Dr. Haas suggests drinking eight to twelve glasses daily of a blend of fresh lemon or lime juice (two tablespoons), maple syrup (one tablespoon), cayenne pepper (one-tenth of a teaspoon), and eight ounces of pure water. This can be supplemented with peppermint or chamomile tea, consumed at different times. For the autumn cleanse, the blend includes pure water (three cups), chopped, blended ginger root (one tablespoon), soybean miso (one to two tablespoons), chopped, blended green onion (one to two stalks), cilantro (a few pinches), cayenne pepper (a few pinches), olive oil (two teaspoons), and lemon juice (from one-half a lemon). Simmer the ginger root for ten minutes in water, stir in the miso, turn off the burner, and add the remaining ingredients; steep for ten minutes, then consume.[101]

Cleansing Juices from Fruits and Vegetables

Among the fruit juices that can be helpful during the three-day fast are watermelon, grape, papaya, pineapple, lemon, apple, pear, black cherry, and citrus. You can experiment with finding the blend that is most pleasing, but it is prudent to mix no more than three at one time. According to Dr. Haas, you can also make a juice of any of a number of vegetables that are beneficial for cleansing during a fast, including potatoes, radish, dark leafy greens, spinach, parsley, wheat grass, cabbage, beet greens, watercress, comfrey, carrots, beets, celery, cucumber, Jerusalem artichokes, garlic, or radish. Again, don't mix more than three or four vegetables together at one time.

Unless you have a juice bar in your neighborhood (which is possible if you live near a good natural foods store and it has a fresh juice bar), you will have to blend the fruits and vegetables yourself in a juicer. Remember to cleanse them of pesticides and bacteria, as described above in Healthy Living Space Detoxifier #10. Don't use canned, frozen, or bottled juices, as their enzymes will probably be weakened if not destroyed, and you need the living enzymes to spark digestion during the fast. Even though bottled juices from a natural foods company are still wholesome, they may be not fresh enough to best serve your detoxifying purposes.

Vegetable Juices, Herb Teas, and Potato Broth

Here is a tested variation provided by health journalist Lewis Harrison, author of *30-Day Body Purification*. During the three to four days before the fast, reduce your food intake to fresh fruits and vegetables and eight ounces of plain yogurt or buttermilk. Then during the fast, drink freshly pressed vegetable juices, especially those from beets and green leafy vegetables at the rate of one quart daily. Supplement this with an herbal cleansing tea, such as red clover or ginger, at the rate of twenty-four ounces daily and with sixteen ounces of an alkaline potassium broth. This broth can be prepared from potatoes, green beans, celery, and zucchini, says Harrison. Cook them in pure or distilled water, then blend the mixture. Other beneficial herbal teas to consume during the fast are peppermint, chamomile, or rose hips.[102]

Detoxifying Green Drink

Part of your daily liquids intake might include a few glasses of this detoxifying blend of herbs and vegetables, says Jacquelin Krohn, M.D., a practitioner in environmental medicine based in Los Alamos, New Mexico. Dr. Krohn suggests adding any of the following to a liquid base of fresh pineapple juice in a blender: celery, radish tops, comfrey leaves, burdock root, parsley, Swiss chard, plantain, dandelion, sprouts, carrot tops, wheat grass, or raspberry leaves.

Dr. Krohn also describes a "basic vegetable broth fasting drink" consisting of red potatoes (two large ones with skins intact), celery (three stalks), beets (three), carrots (four), plus small amounts of cabbage, turnip, onions, or beet tops. Chop up the vegetables, boil, simmer for forty-five minutes, then blend into a puree; consume in small amounts throughout the fast.[103]

Special Lemonade for a Water Fast

If you choose to undertake the water fast for three days, abstaining even from fruit and vegetable juices, here is a recommendation from Dr. Fife. "Fasting is the primary mechanism nature has given us for cleansing and detoxification," he comments. If you are fasting for longer than three days or if you are planning to consume only water during your three day fast, this dilute form of lemonade can be beneficial, advises Dr. Fife. Mix fresh lemon or lime juice (two tablespoons), raw honey or unprocessed maple syrup (one tablespoon), and filtered or distilled water (eight ounces).

Consume this lemonade regularly during your fast as part of your overall liquid intake, which Dr. Fife advises should be at least six glasses daily, or forty-eight ounces. The lemon is "a good cleanser and astringent that rids tissues of toxins," he says, and it stimulates liver detoxification. The honey or maple syrup provides minimal simple carbohydrates to provide energy to the body.[104]

HEALTHY LIVING SPACE DETOXIFIER #14
Do a Media/Image Fast to
Cleanse Your Mind and Energy Field

A character in John Updike's novel *Rabbit Redux* comments on the oppressive clutter in her mind: "The things I have in my mind, Hassy, it reminds me of when they clean out a drain.

All that hair and sludge mixed up with a rubber comb somebody went and dropped down years ago. Sixty years ago in my case."[105]

This is an excellent description of the mental sludge that builds up in our mind and energy fields over the months and years of being continuously subjected to a barrage of images, words, slogans, and sounds. Thus is our lot as participants in a media-intensive, highly literate, advertising-based society. Consider the sources of daily input: magazines, radio, television, Internet, billboards, books, newspapers, conversations, movies, commercials, advertisements, slogans, and signs, among others.

The nervous system, mind, and the body itself are bombarded by this array of insistent images and words. If the source is commercial in nature, be assured it is structured to influence you, to persuade you to do something, think something, get something. If the source is intellectual in nature, it is still designed, though at a more subtle level, to have a particular effect on you, such as giving you a certain slant on history or current affairs. Your consciousness, even your sense of self, are perpetually assaulted by a myriad of influences, each vying for your attention and their chance to produce a shift in allegiance in its favor in your thinking and way of being.

Some forms of media, such as television and movies seen in a theater, have an energetic effect on you, even to the extent that sensitives, or psychics, can observe energy residues in the aura surrounding the body of a person who has just watched television or sat through a movie. Like swirling reflections in a soap bubble, images from the television show or movie are still observable in your aura for at least an hour, sometimes longer, following your immersion in the energy field of that media. Everyone is familiar, too, with the queer sensation of lyrics and melodies repeating themselves, unbidden, in our minds, like a radio that cannot be easily shut off. Or perhaps you catch yourself about to automatically repeat something someone else said, perhaps a news commentator, or a salesman for a product advertised on television.

All of these sensory inputs have an impact on your mind and energy body. Like undigested (or hard to digest) food in the intestines, these media inputs can, if left unprocessed, act like toxins in your system and eventually contribute to an illness process. But we can take this further. What if the inputs are deliberate distortions of the truth, or prejudiced spins on the facts, or mean-spirited commentaries, or lies cast to protect special interests?

Untruths can be toxic substances, too. Our parents, grandparents, siblings, and friends tell us who we are, and this telling can become a mask we wear over our true identities. If we never strip off the mask—*their* mask imposed on us— we never know who we are. There are some who say what we take for history is a lie, a fabrication, a fantasy; others point out that what we take as our family history or the nature of our family interactions may be a tissue of untruths; indeed, perhaps much of what we tell ourselves in our interior mental monologues is similarly misleading. From a certain angle of observation, we could say that the total of media/image input acts as a straitjacket on human consciousness, forcing it into a groove (a rut) in which only one-way movement is possible. Put more simply, we live in a trance state induced by someone else when we weren't looking.

Consensus reality, like untruth, is unnatural and can be a toxic substance.

Some call this consensus reality, and some say consensus reality is a toxic substance for consciousness. It has guidelines for behavior, perception, self-definition, for how reality works, including what produces illness (germs) and what accomplishes healing (drugs and doctors). As children, we become entranced by the prevailing mode of cultural consensus reality. We develop what Charles Tart, Ph.D., calls "'consensus consciousness' to reflect the fact that our so-called ordinary state of consciousness, or 'normal consciousness' (which is a culturally relative term of course) means we have actually constructed the habits of our thinking and feeling and perceiving to reflect the consensus of what our culture thinks is important and good." Consensus reality is not what consciousness is really like; it is "a semi-arbitrary construction."[106]

Consensus reality, like untruth, is unnatural and can be a toxic substance.

Recommendation: Devote a week, perhaps in conjunction with the food fast and/or with the relaxation baths as described in the next section, and abstain entirely from media/image inputs. Don't read anything: books, newspapers, product labels, billboards, signs. Listen to as little as possible: radio, music with words, television, other people's gossip or conversations, your own interior monologue. Stop absorbing other people's view of the world, your family's definitions of roles and identities, even your own constantly reiterated identity statements. Allow your mind to cohere, to collect itself, to facilitate self-awareness, self-observation: *who are you*? Even if you think you know, even if you have spent years unpeeling the family and societal masks, you may be surprised by what emerges when you turn off the cultural tap.

Let your mind and energy body relax deeply, divesting themselves of a lifetime of media/image sludge. Consider meditating once daily, just sitting quietly in a comfortable position for a period of time, paying attention only to your breathing, and not chasing after any thoughts that come to mind. Perhaps you would like to go off for a week to a meditation retreat to make this withdrawal from input easier to sustain.

Or imagine that before you, a few feet away from your body, stands a very large red rose with absorbent petals; in fact, it has hundreds of petals, capable of surrounding you. This rose has a root system so deep it goes straight to the center of the Earth. Instruct the rose to absorb from you the energy residues of all the media/image input you have had in your lifetime. When the rose seems to have absorbed all it can, pluck it from the imaginary ground in which it grows and throw it away. You may need to imagine another rose—and probably many more—and do the same thing when it gets clogged with your energy effluent.

Alternatively, you could picture a large pipe connecting your body to the center of the Earth; it is a drainage pipe perhaps three feet in diameter, specifically suited to your body and energy field. Instruct your body to release the energy residues of all the images, words, songs, ideas, pictures, and other media/image input you have received in your lifetime. You may experience this as a kind of dark water or mucus flowing out of your body into the drainage pipe; or you may simply feel lighter, calmer, clearer, and see nothing.

You may wish to perform the meditation, rose, or drainage pipe exercises several times daily during your weeklong media/image fast. Just as your physical body can start to catch up on unfinished digestive business during the food fast, so can your mind and energy body catch up on processing a lifetime of energized media/image inputs. The process will free up a lot of your energy that was trapped or held hostage in the gravitational field of these inputs.

One of the benefits of this media/image fast is that you may find yourself opening up to new possibilities, to taste, perhaps, an infusion of what is often called the new paradigm, planetary transformation, or evolutionary global change under way. "Perhaps the most significant event in our lifetimes is the one that is taking place in our consciousness: Our collective view of reality, rooted in millennia of historical experience, is being shattered completely," stated the editors of *Cogenesis Journal*, an online magazine. "Our foundation of consensus reality is simply being swept away . . . *everything is changing.*"[107]

Our human understanding of how the world works, where we fit in the scheme of creation, our historical framework, our traditional cosmology—"all are being blown apart," add the editors. So the voluntary media/image fast could put you in synchrony with vaster changes in progress.

HEALTHY LIVING SPACE DETOXIFIER #15
Make a Lifestyle Out of Nonstop Stress Reduction with Healing Hot Water Soaks

It is important to appreciate that stress is a global—that is, completely body-wide—experience. If your cells are stressed with toxins, it is likely your mind and emotions are stressed as well. If you are not relaxed, it is difficult for your tissues, muscles, and cells to be at ease. Remember, stress is a toxic substance, too. Let's take another tack to make the same point: when was the last time you felt so relaxed you felt you were melting into your chair or bed?

If you can achieve that delicious state of meltingness, you are well on your way to relieving your system of stress. Once you have the sense of how to melt, on cue, as it were, you can make stress reduction a continuous part of your general detoxification

If you can achieve that delicious state of meltingness, you are well on your way to relieving your system of stress. Once you have the sense of how to melt, on cue, as it were, you can make stress reduction a continuous part of your general detoxification program.

program. For the present, here are several practical approaches that may ease you into meltingness.

Epsom Salt-Aromatherapy Relaxing Baths

Epsom salt[108] is a 100% dissolvable salt that when added to warm bath water can relax your muscles, helping them to release accumulated stress, tension, aches, or discomforts. At the same time, your nearly full-body immersion (up to the chin, ideally) in an Epsom-salt-saturated bath can be excellently relaxing for your mind and emotions as well. Epsom salt, which is primarily magnesium sulphate ($MgSO_4$), is widely available in supermarkets and pharmacies; it is inexpensive (less than three dollars for a four-pound container of dry salts) and entirely safe. Pour two to four pounds of dry Epsom salt mixture into a tub of hot water and stir until it is fully dissolved.

Aromatherapy is a term that refers to essential oils prepared from herbs and plants that are used topically (diluted, applied on the skin as a massage oil), mixed with water in baths, or diffused in the air via special burners. For the most part, the effective therapeutic action of the oil comes from your inhaling its aroma. There are aromatherapy oils, or blends (available in most natural foods stores), for almost any minor physical or mental condition, including anxiety and stress. Add these after the Epsom salt to your hot water bath.

Relieving Anxiety

The following essential oils can help relieve general anxiety: clary sage, rose otto, frankincense, bergamot, mandarin, sandalwood, lavender, juniper, patchouli, vetiver, cedarwood, melissa, and Roman chamomile. However, you don't want to use all of these at once; generally, it's preferable to use no more than three different essential oils at one time.

Let's say you have muscle pain, your body feels tense, with aches and soreness. The essential oils helpful for this condition are sandalwood, lavender, clary sage, Roman chamomile, and patchouli. Or perhaps you are feeling a restless anxiety; you have been overactive, you're sweating, perhaps dizzy, and your stomach is upset. Here vetiver, cedarwood, juniper, Roman chamomile, or frankincense might help you. Suppose you are feeling on edge, are irritable, cannot concentrate or sleep well, and you feel exhausted most of the time. The oils to address this type of anxiety include bergamot, melissa, neroli, cedarwood, sandalwood, and rose otto. Or finally, your anxiety is marked by a feeling of apprehension; you're worrying, filled with unease, a sense of foreboding, even paranoia. Try some of these oils: bergamot, lavender, neroli, rose otto, melissa, or geranium.[109]

For each type of anxiety, choose one to three oils, then use a total of thirty drops of all oils, dividing them into ten drops each, or one at five drops, one at ten, one at fifteen. Don't use any more than thirty drops at first; these oils are strong, both topically and in terms of the emotional response they can provoke. (For some people, thirty drops may be too rich a mixture; start lower, at ten drops total, then gradually increase drops over a few weeks as you get used to their effects.) Dribble the drops into an empty plastic container (such as a quart yogurt container), fill with hot bath water coming out of the tap, then slowly dribble the water plus oils into the down-flowing stream of hot bath water from the tap. This helps disperse the oil droplets into the general bath water.

Relieving Stress

If your primary sense of discomfort is better labelled "stress," then any of the following ten essential plant oils can help relieve some of it: mandarin, geranium, clary sage, ormenis flower, eucalyptus citriodora, Roman chamomile, sandalwood, ylang ylang, petitgrain, or lavender.

As with anxiety, there are different types of stress, each requiring a different blend of aromatherapy oils. In *The Fragrant Mind*, aromatherapy educator and practitioner Valerie Ann Worwood states that there are three basic types of stress. In type one, you feel tired, irritable, achy, and sometimes depressed. To get some relief from this kind of stress, Worwood recommends eucalyptus citriodora, geranium, and lavender, or mandarin, ylang ylang, and petitgrain, a total of thirty drops for all three oils in either formula.

The second type of stress is characterized by anxiety or depression, food allergies, persistent infections, or chronic background discomfort. Here Worwood advises clary sage, Roman chamomile, lavender, and geranium, or ormenis flower, ylang ylang, petitgrain, and sandalwood. Again, use no more than thirty drops total for all four oils in either formula. If your stress is considerable, marked by stomach pain, suicidal tendencies, fear, despair, or a general retreat from social interactions, Worwood suggests Roman chamomile, clary sage, and ormenis flower, or geranium, eucalyptus citriodora, and mandarin.[110]

Progressive Body Relaxation

While immersed in your Epsom salt-aromatherapy-infused tub, why not practice a simple relaxation exercise borrowed (and somewhat adapted) from hatha yoga. Start with your toes, and visualize (or imagine) that all the stress is being released from all the tissues, bones, cells, molecules, and atoms of your ten toes, and that the stress (or toxins) is flowing like effluent into the bath water from your toes. Next do your ankles, then legs, knees, thighs, hips, pelvis, and on, progressively, up to your head, continually releasing tension from each body area.

Improve the Ambience

Why not infuse the air of your bathroom with some pleasing aromatherapy scents that will contribute to the growing mood of relaxation? British aromatherapist Chrissie Wildwood recommends using one of the four following mixtures in an aromatherapy burner or diffuser (usually sold where aromatherapy oils are found) or water-based electric vaporizer. Dribble three drops of neroli, eight drops mandarin, and three of ylang ylang into a small amount of water; or Roman chamomile (three drops), rose otto (two), and bergamot (ten); or frankincense (three), lemon (six), and juniper (four); or galbanum (one), lavender (six), and petitgrain (six).[111] Within ten minutes or so, the bathroom, and adjacent rooms to an extent, will be suffused with the relaxation-inducing scents of these essential oils.

Use only one blend of aromatherapy oils per bath. Stay in the tub at least twenty minutes, and forty-five minutes if you can. Immerse yourself to your chin, if that's comfortable. When you leave the tub, don't towel off, but lie down immediately on your bed (on a dry towel) and air dry for at least thirty minutes. A fair measure of the relaxation effect of the Epsom salt-aromatherapy oils bath occurs during this critical air-drying time. You may even fall asleep during this time. Arrange beforehand not to be disturbed during this time. As a general stress-relieving technique, you might wish to do this bath once a week, at least; if you have a high stress life, then consider doing it two to three times every week. If you have the time, there is no reason not to do it every day.

HEALTHY LIVING SPACE DETOXIFIER #16
Enhance Your Relaxation by Floating in 800 Pounds of Epsom Salt

If you enjoy the Epsom soak in your bathtub, you may relish this next suggestion. For a profound introduction to relaxation, try an hour in a float tank. Flotation REST (Restricted Environmental Stimulation Therapy), originally developed in the 1950s,[112] has you floating in very high salt concentration water inside an enclosed chamber (like a spa-sized fiberglass bathtub with a canopy) so that all your sensory input is minimized and your relaxation is optimized.

Approximately 700-800 pounds of Epsom salt are added to 170 gallons of water, which are kept heated to 93.5° F, or skin temperature. Your body experiences (no doubt unique in its experience) a gravity-free condition because the huge amount of salt keeps you effortlessly suspended on top of about ten inches of water. So you float and relax on a "bed" of salt water and in a darkened atmosphere of calm and warmth, free of outside stimulation or distraction.

The flotation tank shields the body and mind from external environmental stimulation, thereby reducing the body's workload by an estimated ninety percent. This in turn conserves a great deal of energy, both mental and physiological, which can be constructively directed inwards. The result is what medical science recognizes as the "relaxation response," or more technically, the parasympathetic response,[113] one pole of the central nervous system easing into relaxation. "Tension and stress wear down our bodies, lower our resistance to illness and injury, upset our emotional balance, reduce our ability to think clearly, and even make us more accident prone," states a floatation tank manufacturer. "Flotation releases deep muscular tension (often unconsciously 'locked' into the body) starting a chain-reaction that spreads throughout the body to every organ, tissue, and cell."[114]

Psychologists Roderick A. Borrie and Thomas H. Fine (director of the International REST Investigators Society in Toledo, Ohio) concluded that flotation REST "serves as a powerful relaxation inducer and has clinical potential in working with patients who have stress-related disorders." Borrie and Fine measured the changes in key stress-indicating biochemicals in the blood of subjects using the salt flotation tanks. Subjects spent thirty to forty minutes in the tank every third day for a total number of four to twenty sessions. Levels of hormones associated with stress, such as cortisol, ACTH, and epinephrine, decreased during REST sessions, as did hormones associated with the adrenal glands (the "stress" organs), such as aldosterone and renin.

Further, they found that the lower levels of cortisol (a key stress-associated hormone) as well as blood pressure did not immediately reset to normal when the REST session was over, but that there was a significant carry-over effect of the benefits obtained during the immersion in the flotation tank. The researchers also studied the "subjective" responses of over 1,000 REST experiencers and found that by their own reports, ninety percent of the subjects found the immersion "deeply relaxing," and that they had experienced an increase in positive emotions (joy, elation, happiness, contentedness) and a corresponding decrease in negative emotions.

On the basis of this data and that developed by other researchers, Borrie and Fine report that REST has merit as a medical treatment for high blood pressure, muscle tension, headache, anxiety disorders, chronic pain, insomnia, PMS, and rheumatoid arthritis. It can also work as a "mood elevator" for cases of depression. "Uniquely, Flotation REST provides an effortless introduction to deep mental and physical relaxation."[115]

The therapeutic benefits of floating are numerous, and include an increased release of endorphins, the pain-killing brain chemicals that make you feel good. According to research, floatation lowers blood pressure and heart rate, reduces oxygen consumption (an index of cell metabolism); increases concentration, motivation, and energy levels; improves skin quality; helps the body remove harmful stress-related biochemicals such as cortisol from the bloodstream; stimulates an increase in T-cells (key immune cells); and allows every muscle in the body to relax, surely an experience hard to come by under any other circumstances.

As the mind drifts into a deep state of relaxation, its two hemispheres start to balance out and synchronize, research suggests; creativity and problem-solving abilities can be enhanced. In the words of one manufacturer, floating users report "a tranquil, carefree, super-relaxed feeling, a light, happy exuberance, attended by deep calmness and a sense of wholeness."[116]

Other benefits include fatigue reduction, alleviation of mental and physical stress, improvement in mental clarity, intensification of acuteness of all the senses; further, floating diminishes fear, depression, and anxiety; it speeds up rehabilitation and recovery from illness; it accentuates any attempt at self-hypnosis or auto-suggestion; and generally rejuvenates and revitalizes.

According to another manufacturer, the flotation tank is designed to keep outside stimulation away, so that you can float in an enclosed, darkened environment with as little sensory input as possible. "Sight, sound, temperature, gravity, and the presence of other people are minimized. This is the environment to examine your own responses, free of external input."[117]

Why is there so much Epsom salt involved, and why Epsom in the first place? The quantity used is to ensure maximum, effortless buoyancy. The concentration of Epsom salt in the water is so dense it makes the user's body comparatively light, so it floats on top like a cork. Epsom salt (pharmaceutical grade magnesium sulphate) has a strong affinity for carbon and carbon compounds, and can absorb and nullify carbon in the form of harmful bodily waste products. The magnesium in the Epsom salt has the power to draw out various carbon-based wastes (toxic substances) from bodily tissues where they are stored, thereby enabling the body to excrete them through the skin.

Flotation tanks are often available in gyms, spas, health resorts, fitness and sports centers, and can be purchased from several different manufacturers for around $5000. The salt is not changed after every use, but it can be regularly sanitized by hydrogen

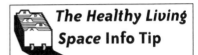

The Healthy Living Space Info Tip

For more information about flotation tanks:
Oasis Relaxation System, Biofeedback Instrument Corporation,
255 W. 98th Street,
New York, NY 10025;
tel: 212-222-5665;
fax: 212-222-5667;
e-mail: ac@inx.net;
website: www.biof.com/oasis;

Samadhi Tank Company,
P.O. Box 2119,
Nevada City, CA 95959;
tel: 530-477-1319;
fax: 530-477-1953;
e-mail: float@samadhitank.com;
website: www.samadhitank.com.

Also see: PathFinder, by ThinkTank International (Singapore) at www.thinktank.com.sg; and Floatworks (London, England) at www.floatworks.com.

For a partial list of flotation spas and places where you can float, see: www.floatation.com.

peroxide, ultraviolet light, or ozone with the result that there can be fewer bacteria remaining in the salt water than in the typical tap water.

HEALTHY LIVING SPACE DETOXIFIER #17
Use Music Therapy to Deepen
Your Sense of Melting Relaxation

All music has an effect on us, on our emotions, nervous system, and state of mind, but some music has been deliberately composed to heighten certain effects, specifically the beneficial effect of relaxation. The focused use of music to produce beneficial physiological and psychological effects is called music therapy, and while it is a large and well-researched discipline, it offers us a practical application in terms of producing deep, effortless relaxation.

One of the prime innovators in the use of specially composed music for heightening relaxation is Steven Halpern. One day in 1969, while meditating in a redwood grove in Santa Cruz, California, Halpern heard music in his head, fully realized, floating, ethereal, nonrhythmic music with sustained harmonies, overtones, and long pauses between phrases. "It was the most beautiful, soothing, and comforting music I had ever heard," he commented afterward.

This "aural vision" answered all of Halpern's questions about what healing music might sound like. "It was as if I had tapped into an ongoing concert, a wavelength that was broadcasting 'Music of the Spheres.' That was my quantum leap, a peak experience that changed my life." It also launched a very successful career as a composer of a genre of music Halpern variously calls Inner Peace Music, Inner Directed, Anti-Frantic, and Music Rx.

As a composer with a Ph.D. in music, Halpern deliberately keeps elements out of his music that will provoke a listener into thinking, anticipating, or looking ahead. These activities obstruct the relaxation response. Halpern's compositional strategy is to induce relaxation and inner harmony as fast as possible, "to go right to the desired outcome without going through the angst and tension build-up" that characterizes Western music. His "music of being, not doing" hovers around a steady tonal center so that the listener feels "always at home" and in the present moment, without the need to go somewhere, following a melodic theme to its future unfoldment.

"People in general not only do not know how it feels to be relaxed, but mistake bodily stimulus and intellectual entertainment as relaxing," says Halpern. "At its most basic, relaxation involves slowing down the heartbeat and breathing rate, as well as shifting from the everyday beta brainwave activity to the more tranquil alpha brainwaves. When practiced regularly, relaxation can help prevent many stress-related diseases such as heart attack, insomnia, migraine, and hypertension."

Most music, from Bach to rock, was not composed with the intent to relax its listeners, Halpern comments, but music can be composed that produces "predictable, positive results" of relaxation, or what he variously calls "push button serenity—as close as your CD player" or "stress relief at the speed of sound." The music creates a "background ambience" that in effect surrounds your body, envelops the nervous system and brain, and entrains them to a more relaxed mode of operation.[118]

Halpern composes music that produces "push button serenity—as close as your CD player" or "stress relief at the speed of sound." The music creates a "background ambience" that surrounds your body, envelops the nervous system and brain, and entrains them to a more relaxed mode of operation.

For example, in *Higher Ground*, Halpern creates a "sonic entrainment matrix" that quickly induces brain waves into states of relaxation, ease, euphoria, even harmonic resonance with the 7.83 hz electromagnetic field of the Earth itself. As a first-time listener to Halpern, I confess this CD was so richly relaxing, so luxuriously calming, that I felt as if my bones melted, as if my entire skeletal system sighed and dissolved. The mind-body, after all, has an inherent self-healing mechanism; it just needs a little boost. Halpern's intention is to bring a listener into a state of deep relaxation as a foundation for psychological insight, healing, meditative states, and spiritual illumination. "The body heals itself most effectively in a state of deep relaxation."

"My sense of the true function of art is to bring us back in touch with the divine, with our true Self," states Halpern. When we relax, we start hearing with our whole body; one of the reasons we feel so good is that we are tapping into the wholeness of our being, linking up "with a greater pattern of perfection that has been there all along," Halpern says. Halpern's music will relax a listener even if it's played as background, but focused listening is recommended. Then it becomes entrainment, not entertainment. More recent CDs by Halpern continue this focus on deliberately-induced relaxation, such as *Comfort Zone, Sleep Soundly, Serenity Suite*, and *Music for Sound Healing.*

Bear in mind that while Halpern may be one of the pioneers in this field, many other musicians have recorded music designed to heighten the relaxation response such that you will have a rich variety to choose from. You can easily get oriented to what is available by doing a web search under "relaxation CDs."

Recommendation: Listen to a relaxation CD while in the Epsom salt-aromatherapy bath, or while air-drying afterwards; or listen to it while lying down in a comfortable place in an environment free from distraction or interruption. Do not listen to music of this type while driving a car or doing anything requiring focused, linear concentration. Remember, the reason you are using music in your detoxification program is to help you deeply relax. Tension and stress impede the detoxification process; in fact, they are toxins in their own right. So as you "melt" to the music and Epsom salt, know that your cells are being freed of the energy grip of stress and tension, and are now a little more free to do their detoxifying jobs.

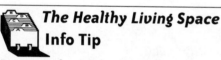

The Healthy Living Space Info Tip

For more information, contact:
Steven Halpern's Inner Peace Music,
P.O. Box 2644,
San Anselmo, CA 94979;
tel: 800-909-0707 or 415-485-0511;
e-mail:
innerpeacemusic@innerpeacemusic.com;
website: www.stevenhalpern.com.

This completes our groundwork for detoxification. Now that you have a sense of the role of dietary change and stress reduction in the detoxification process, we can move on to more focused strategies for helping the body purge itself of a lifetime of toxins, starting with the liver and intestines.

CHAPTER 5

Safe and Effective Cleansing Programs for the Liver and Intestines

You are now in a position to start a deliberate, planned, and supervised detoxification program, focusing on the liver and intestines. These three qualifiers are carefully chosen to emphasize the key elements in a detoxification program.

You can make the changes in food and water suggested in chapter 4 without any complications and with almost guaranteed benefit. But when it comes to relieving the liver and intestines of their toxic burden, it is well advised by detoxification authorities to do so prudently, with good advice, and in a sequential way. While there are many helpful components to a detoxification program, discussed below, they should be used in the context of a medically grounded internal cleansing program. That is, one that has solid clinical and evidential support, and one that you undertake with the supervision of, or at least consultation with, a qualified health-care practitioner.

The Healthy Living Space Expert Interview:
Jacob Farin, N.D., Naturopathic Physician

When it comes to finding a medically authoritative internal cleansing program, there is perhaps no better source than naturopathy.[1] In this well-established natural medicine discipline, relieving the body of its store of toxins is paramount, and developing ever more effective natural means to do so has occupied the medical attention of naturopathic practitioners and researchers for well over a century. One such practitioner is Jacob Farin, N.D., associate physician at the Center for Traditional Medicine in Lake Oswego, Oregon.

When Dr. Farin recommends a one- or two-week detoxification program to a client, he emphasizes that it must be centered around helping the liver, the body's prime detoxification organ. "You must talk about the liver because the liver is the main organ that detoxifies toxic substances in the body. There are other organs that support the detoxification process, such as the intestines, kidneys, skin, and lungs, and they all help expel toxins, but everything that enters the body needs to pass through the liver, so that is the main organ to support."

There are several conditions under which a person is likely to ask Dr. Farin for recommendations on detoxification. A person may want to feel better, to optimize their physiological functions. A person may be ill and suspect (or is told by a health-care practitioner) that detoxification may help. Or, more commonly, "they get stuck."

There are several conditions under which a person is likely to ask Dr. Farin for recommendations on a detoxification program, he explains. A person may want to feel better, to optimize their physiological functions. A person may be ill and suspect (or is told by a health-care practitioner) that detoxification may help. Or, more commonly, "they get stuck."

Something doesn't work for them anymore, or a well-recommended health-care regimen fails to produce the expected results. "A lot of times with certain protocols we get stuck, and the treatment plan goes nowhere. So I use the detoxification process as a way either to jump-start my protocols or as a way to help patients make necessary lifestyle changes." Dr. Farin mentions that detoxification can be particularly helpful to someone who is trying to make lifestyle changes and can't. "I've noticed that those who initiated a detoxification program had better results and had an increased ability to *sustain* the lifestyle changes I recommended."

What kind of lifestyle changes? Mainly food issues, says Dr. Farin. People eat too much, or are too dependent on sugar-based foods, coffee and other sources of caffeine, stimulants, or cigarettes. A detoxification program helps them see what their food issues are and how they use food cravings, dependencies, and indulgences to cover up emotional issues needing attention, says Dr. Farin. "During the detoxification program, I restrict the types of foods a person eats for a week or two," he explains. "When you restrict a person's foods, you take away their comfort foods, which is to say, their means of coping with stress. And when you take away that coping mechanism, they have to deal with those emotional issues head on. They discover they have been using food as a way to palliate their emotions." Thus an effective detoxification program has both physiological and psychoemotional benefits and, in either case, cleansing and supporting the liver holds the key to health.

"I think everyone has some degree of toxicity in their liver today," states Dr. Farin. Given the excessive degree of environmental and bodily pollution documented in the earlier chapters of this book, perhaps Dr. Farin's bold declaration will not strike readers as without foundation. A great number of our contemporary illnesses are the result of toxic overload, Dr. Farin explains, and central to toxic overload is a liver that is so burdened with the demands of detoxification that it becomes unable to keep up.

Like clogged plumbing, the liver develops a backlog of undetoxified substances. An unwholesome feedback loop develops between the liver and intestines, like a sink drain backing up into the sink itself. For example, in most people today you can find colon-derived bacteria in the portal vein, which is a large vein that leads to the liver, Dr. Farin notes. Somehow bacteria leak through the intestinal walls and get picked up by mesenteric veins, then are passed on to the larger portal vein and transported to the liver. This isn't the way toxic substances are supposed to move in the body. But what is more abnormal, he says, is that often the liver's key immune defense agents, called Kupffer cells, are unable to engulf the incoming pathogenic bacteria and keep up with detoxifying the backflow. The condition of colonic backflow, medically referred to as intestinal permeability, "plays a big role in liver toxic overload," says Dr. Farin.

Why does the liver get backlogged? Nutritional deficiencies account for some of it, and these in turn derive from malabsorption of nutrients, faulty diet (lacking the correct nutrients in their proper amounts and ratios), or from unsatisfied increased nutritional demands, as happens during a chronic illness or sustained athletic exertion. Emotional and psychological stress can also deplete the body of liver-focused nutrients, adds Dr. Farin. These stresses initiate hormonal changes in the body, requiring the body to adapt to the new, unhealthy, or unbalanced conditions. "If you don't have the nutritional support to produce these hormones to process them, then you put considerable additional strain on the liver."

As a general recommendation, Dr. Farin advises doing the following one-week liver and intestinal cleansing program once a year as a kind of preventive internal housecleaning. On the other hand, if you are pregnant or suffering from an acute or serious illness, the program is not recommended. He further advises doing a detoxification program under the medical attention of a trained health-care practitioner, at least to the extent that you have someone expert on hand to call if problems or uncertainties arise. "I would definitely consult a physician before initiating a detoxification program to rule out any conditions that would not warrant detoxifying," Dr. Farin notes.

While cleansing programs that specifically focus on the intestines have merit (and are discussed in detail later in this chapter), Dr. Farin emphasizes the importance of dealing with the liver first. An intestinal cleanse without liver support, or undertaken before the liver has been cleansed and supported, can further flood the liver with toxins and potentially be counterproductive.

The benefits of a liver cleanse are impressive and easily quantified, Dr. Farin states. "People have more energy. They feel better. They are happier. They can do more things without getting tired. They are not so fatigued in the afternoon. They find they can live without sugar and coffee, and they have a sense of empowerment that they can quit using these foods." Often a person emerges from the one- or two-week detoxification program with the sense of having clarified emotional issues, such as issues to do with anger, jealousy, and sadness, and having touched on uplifting ones such as happiness, radiance, and joy.

HEALTHY LIVING SPACE DETOXIFIER #18
Do a One-Week Elimination Diet
and Liver Cleansing Program

Dr. Farin's one-week liver cleansing program has three components. There is a dietary, a supplemental, and a self-care introspective element. Here are the procedural steps for each component.

Dietary Restrictions

Start by eliminating from your diet for a week the five top food allergens: glutinous grains, corn, potatoes, eggs, and dairy products. These may comprise your favorite "comfort" foods, but they are also well-documented allergenic foods, capable of regularly producing food allergy reactions and symptoms. These allergic reactions in turn burden your liver and intestines with additional toxic substances or incompletely digested food components.

For the week, you should also curtail your consumption of all members of the nightshade family (eggplants, tomatoes, peppers) because they can, for many people, quietly but persistently aggravate the digestive system. Other foods eliminated during the detoxification program include oranges, strawberries, sugars, red meats, coffee, caffeinated teas, and peanuts.

There is a sound reason for curtailing allergenic foods for a week. "Long-term allergies, to foods and substances, can be addressed through a detoxification program," explains Dr. Farin. "These allergies will invariably set someone up or predispose them for illness later. A detoxification program is a great way to clear those allergens from the body." To determine if a patient has unsuspected food allergies, Dr. Farin typically submits a patient's blood sample to an immunoglobulin analysis, specifically for IgG and IgE, which are indicators of allergic reactions to foods (see chapter 3 for more on this).

Thus the positive term for a diet that eliminates allergenic foods is "hypoallergenic diet"—that is, a diet comprising foods known to produce no allergic reactions. Once you stop the ingestion of irritating foods, then you add liver-supporting ones. These might include vegetables medically known to help liver function, such as the cruciferous vegetables—beets, broccoli, bok choy, Brussels sprouts, cabbage, cauliflower, swiss chard, and collard greens.[2] Dr. Farin recommends eating four cups of fresh vegetables daily.

Ironically, for many people, these vegetables are guaranteed producers of intestinal gas and bloating. However, if these symptoms arise, it means the person would benefit from digestive enzymes and perhaps supplementary hydrochloric acid (HCl, the stomach's main digestive "juice"), says Dr. Farin. A gaseous reaction to eating cruciferous vegetables generally means the body cannot digest the sulfur found in these vegetables, so enzyme support for the digestive process is indicated.

As another part of this one-week program, Dr. Farin limits carbohydrate intake although he makes sure his patients get a sufficient intake of protein. In the modified elimination diet, he allows or recommends some meat products such as lamb, chicken, turkey, and fish, but in the vegan hypoallergenic diet (a stricter variation on this approach), he disallows all animal products during the detoxification program. Instead, soybean tofu is relied upon for a protein source.

Nutritional and Dietary Supplements

The second component of the one-week program calls for specific nutritional support in the form of supplements and specialized nutrient formulas to provide support for the liver. Here Dr. Farin relies on two commercially prepared products: UltraClear and Phyto-Pro, both requiring a health-care practitioner's prescription. They are not drugs or medicines as such; rather, they are powerful formulas precisely designed for use in a detoxification program supervised by a health-care practitioner. Dr. Farin notes that both are free of cascara sagrada, a powerful herb often found in other liver and/or intestinal cleansing programs. This herb is widely recommended for detoxification, but its irritating effect on the intestines can sometimes be too unpleasant for users.

UltraClear is a "low-allergy potential nutritionally fortified food-based beverage mix" designed for use by patients who have food allergies or are environmentally sensitive, according to its manufacturer, Metagenics of Gig Harbor, Washington. "It can be used as part of a comprehensive elimination or rotation diet program as well as nutritional support for patients undergoing metabolic clearing or detoxification programs," says the company.

A blend of rice syrup solids and rice protein concentrates provides forty-four percent of its calories from carbohydrates. It is low calorie, containing only 170 calories per 44g serving. It also offers high levels of various antioxidants needed to help the body reduce its toxic load (oxidative stress) and nutrients to support the liver's two phases of detoxification. Remember that during Phase I, the liver converts toxic compounds into intermediate toxins. In Phase II, the liver converts these intermediate toxins into substances that can be eliminated from the body, delivering them to the colon (through the gallbladder) or bladder for excretion. (For more on the liver's detoxification process, see chapter 2.)

Specifically, among the liver-supportive nutrients is L-glutathione. This amino acid is a crucial detoxifier of foreign substances and is found naturally in the liver, but it may be deficient in a condition of toxic overload. Other liver-supportive nutrients found in UltraClear include N-acetylcysteine (an amino acid that helps make L-glutathione), L-cysteine (an amino acid), molybdenum and selenium (both trace minerals, which with cysteine help support the liver's Phase I activities), and vitamins A, C, E, and beta-carotene (all antioxidants). The product also contains numerous other vitamins, minerals, and amino acids needed for detoxification.

Phyto-Pro is a natural vegetarian herb-based ("phytonutrient") protein powder complex that contains organic grasses, chlorella, spirulina, beneficial microflora, amino acids, adaptogens (specialized herbs that exert a nonspecific effect on the entire body by increasing resistance to stress and toxins and promoting a balancing or normalizing condition), antioxidants, and "cleansing botanicals," according to NF Formulas, its manufacturer.

Due to its high content of organic grasses and blue-green algae components (chlorella and spirulina), NF Formulas calls this a "green drink," noting it is high in vitamin B12 and protein, and is suitable for providing nutritional support "for those stressed by toxins in the environment and food." They also make a variant in capsule form called Phyto-Pro II; this contains soy sprouts and lecithin, green tea polyphenols, and the other ingredients from Phyto-Pro. Neither version contains gluten, yeast, refined sugar, or eggs.

Whether you use UltraClear or Phyto-Pro, Dr. Farin typically recommends two to three doses per day for the one-week elimination diet program.

If the patient declines using UltraClear or Phyto-Pro, then Dr. Farin urges them to try an old naturopathic recipe called Bieler's Broth. You can also drink this to ensure an adequate intake of detoxifying vegetables. Bieler's Broth is a special vegetable broth made at home to increase one's nutritional status. "It's a way to get nutrients into the body in a gentle way and so they are not so hard to digest," he comments. Use any or all of these vegetables: celery, zucchini, broccoli, parsley, beets, and cabbage. Chop up two cups of them and steam in two cups of filtered, pure water until they get soft. Then puree vegetables and broth in a blender. This is like a vegetable juice, but even better because you get the juice and the fiber, says Dr. Farin, who advises drinking one batch of this daily.

As an additional support for the liver during its intensified period of detoxification, Dr. Farin advises a lemon-based liver cleanse. Take the juice of half a lemon and mix with eight ounces of pure water; add, if desired, one teaspoon of flaxseed oil or olive oil, and one clove of crushed garlic (optional). Drink the beverage once daily, preferably first thing in the morning during the days of the detoxification program. The lemon supports the Phase I aspects of the liver's detoxification activities; the oils provide essential fatty acids to the body; and the garlic kills bacteria. Further, Dr. Farin encourages detoxifiers to drink at least thirty-two ounces of pure water daily, and preferably more.

Self-Care/Introspective Activities

In this third component of the detoxification program, Dr. Farin recommends journal writing, hatha yoga, regular walks, meditation, prayer, letter writing, and a media fast. "I ask people to refrain from television, radio, magazines, newspapers, and if possible, to avoid toxic people and toxic relationships." (See Healthy Living Space Detoxifier #14 in chapter 4.) "This phase helps bring a person's awareness to their emotions and to find appropriate ways to manage their emotional stress."

Variation: Two-Week Modified Fast and Liver Cleanse

This is a more intensive detoxification program, best undertaken after you have first gone through the one-week program and allowed a few months to elapse. For the first week, you follow the same procedures as described in the one-week program.

In the second week, you begin a modified fast and take UltraClear or Phyto-Pro five times daily, says Dr. Farin. For three days, your entire intake is only the five doses of either formula, so that during the three days you take a total of fifteen doses, he says.

"This way, you give the liver all the support it needs. You really get the liver cleansing going by restricting the amount of toxins entering the body." In other words, no foods ingested equals no toxins ingested. "You do not get the same effect from the dietary changes alone unless you are ultra-careful about the foods you consume. Even with organic foods, they can still come in contact with environmental pollutants."

This is different from a juice or water fast, comments Dr. Farin. "With a juice fast, you get the high carbohydrate intake, but there is no protein ingested to support the liver, and the liver relies heavily on enzymes, which are specialized proteins. With the water fast, you get neither the carbohydrates for energy production nor the protein."

Typical Results to Expect

During the two-week modified fast, about eighty percent of people experience a headache, ranging in discomfort from mild to severe, says Dr. Farin. There are usually three factors that contribute to the onset of these detoxification headaches: low blood sugar due to the limited calorie intake; caffeine withdrawal from going off coffee, teas, and sodas; and food allergy withdrawal symptoms, from going off allergenic foods such as wheat or corn.

As a palliative, Dr. Farin advises consuming small amounts of nuts or a piece of fruit to raise the blood sugar level, and a few cups of green tea, an herbal tea with a small caffeine content but additional antioxidants to help the liver. For coping with the symptoms of withdrawal from wheat and glutinous grains, Dr. Farin advises increasing your intake of pure water.

On the positive side, you can expect to move your bowels more often. If you have not been regular, expect to become regular during the program, Dr. Farin explains. "It's partly because I've increased the amount of vegetables in their diet to four cups daily. For many people, that is a significant increase. If they are experiencing constipation, they will start going more often due to this increased fiber intake. What also occurs due to the increased fiber consumption is that their system binds onto bile[3] more readily. The bile passes into the intestines from the liver and has a beneficial irritating effect. So a person, if they are constipated, will start going more because of the increased presence of bile in the intestines."

HEALTHY LIVING SPACE DETOXIFIER #19
Use Natural Foods and Herbs to Aid Your Liver in Cleansing Itself

Dr. Farin's detoxification programs call for a one- or two-week commitment, but there are dietary changes you can make that will provide detoxifying benefits all year round. Or you can use them as a follow-up to an intensive liver cleansing program. Here are a few recommendations culled from various health authorities and researchers. The idea here is simple: try to find ways to consume many or all of these foods and herbs on a regular basis to make detoxification and liver support a year-round activity.

Liver Cleansing Foods

Try to incorporate some or all of these liver-cleansing foods into your regular diet: dandelion greens, watercress, and mustard greens. These bitter greens are known to stimulate bile flow and therefore to aid digestion and liver cleansing. They are also high in chlorophyll, which nutritionists believe has a cleansing and revitalizing effect on the whole body, but especially for the intestines and liver.

Other whole foods with generalized liver-supporting benefits include carrots, beets, endive, grapefruit, lemons, limes, parsley, and romaine. A salad of bitter greens every day supplemented with a dose of herbal bitters formula (available in natural foods stores) is recommended by some nutritionists as a way to reduce indigestion.

Burdock (*Arciium lappa*) is an especially helpful vegetable for the liver, enjoyed as cooked fresh root or as an herbal tea or tincture. Besides its high nutrient content, burdock root "helps to cleanse the blood through its action on the liver, and its gentle diuretic properties promote the elimination of toxins through increased kidney function."[4] It also stimulates the immune system and the production of digestive juices. Burdock seeds contain volatile oils that aid in neutralizing and eliminating toxins from the liver and body. Herbalists regard this plant as nature's best blood purifier; herbalists traditionally used burdock concoctions to treat snakebite. Burdock also stimulates bile flow, is a gentle laxative, and helps cleanse the blood by stimulating the body as a whole to improve its efficiency in removing waste products. Herbalists generally recommend three to four cups of fresh burdock root tea per day.

Ginger root (*Zingiber officianale*) is also highly recommended as a liver-supporting vegetable. According to medical research, fresh ginger root can prevent the liver from destroying (metabolizing) other medicinal herbs, allowing them to remain in the bloodstream to complete their detoxifying activities. Ginger is also noted for its ability to aid the intestine in its absorption of herbs and to move their medicinal elements into the blood.[5] Ginger root can be enjoyed fresh, grated or sliced in salads or cooked vegetable dishes; as a component in a blended vegetable juice; or as an herbal tea. Ginger is regarded as a classic tonic and stimulant for the digestive system; it also keeps the intestinal muscles toned, which in turn makes the movement of substances through the intestinal tract easier and less prone to produce irritation of the intestine's mucosal lining.[6]

Burdock (Arciium lappa) *is an especially helpful vegetable for the liver, enjoyed as cooked fresh root or as an herbal tea or tincture. Besides its high nutrient content, burdock root "helps to cleanse the blood through its action on the liver, and its gentle diuretic properties promote the elimination of toxins through increased kidney function."*

The Detoxifying Benefits of Beets

Beets are an excellent fiber source and can thereby work as a natural laxative, helping to stimulate peristalsis and purge the intestines of old fecal matter. According to traditional Chinese medicine, beets can purify the blood, benefit the liver, and moisten the intestines; they can also treat liver stagnancy and liver problems in general and relieve constipation, especially the type that results from fluid dryness.[7] One way to enjoy beets is to mix fresh beet juice with equal amounts of carrot or apple juice; another way is to slice and sauté them in a wok. When they are fully cooked, you can season them with soy sauce, Dijon mustard, and nutritional yeast.

Hot Lemon Juice Cleanser

Many experts in natural healing extol the benefits of freshly squeezed lemon juice for helping the system detoxify. Rejuvenation and detoxification expert Helene Silver recommends drinking an eight-ounce glass of hot lemon juice first thing every morning during the detoxification program. Mix the juice of one-half of a squeezed lemon with eight ounces of pure *warm* water, and add a pinch of cayenne pepper (up to one-eighth of a teaspoon is permissible) or one drop of cayenne tincture, she suggests. "Lemon juice helps to break up and dislodge the sticky mucus deposits that tend to clog up the system," she states.[8]

Liver Cleansing Herbs

Herbalists recommend teas or herbal tinctures made from any of the following liver-cleansing herbs: gentian, barberry, yellow dock, Oregon grape, sarsaparilla, dandelion root, burdock, or milk thistle. As with the bitter greens, it is the bitterness itself that produces the beneficial effects. When the digestive system encounters the striking bitter taste of the greens or herbs, it stimulates digestive secretions throughout the gastrointestinal system, including bile flow in the liver. Anything that sparks increased bile flow benefits the liver.

Milk thistle (*Silybum marianum*) and its active constituent, silymarin, is considered by many herbalists "nature's offering for optimal liver protection." In fact, this herb is prominent among effective treatments for chronic liver disease produced by alcoholism and hepatitis. "It is also emerging as an important supplement for those desiring to optimize liver function and maximize the detoxifying potential of this important organ," explains naturopathic physician Donald J. Brown, N.D.

According to Dr. Brown, milk thistle extract protects liver cells and even helps regenerate them. Specifically, silymarin acts as an antioxidant (a fighter against free radical damage from toxic substances), helping liver cells produce glutathione (increasing its levels by up to fifty percent), a key agent in liver detoxification. Given milk thistle's multifaceted support for liver function, Dr. Brown states it benefits people exposed to toxins at work or who already have multiple chemical sensitivities. Milk thistle, Dr. Brown says, can provide "critical support" for the liver during a detoxification program. In general, he recommends an 8-week course of 420 mg of silymarin in three divided doses per day; after 8 weeks, reduce the dose to 280 mg daily for preventive purposes.[9]

Nutrition researcher Laurel Vukovic recommends a strong, dark herbal tea (called an herbal decoction) made of the roots of dandelion and Oregon grape. To two tablespoons each of fresh sliced dandelion and Oregon grape root, Vukovic adds one teaspoon each of ginger and licorice root, simmered in three cups of water for about fifteen minutes. As part of a gentle and generalized detoxification program lasting three to six weeks, Vukovic suggests consuming three cups daily of this "robust" tea in between meals.[10]

Numerous liver-cleansing herbs are now available as teabags. For example, you can get roasted dandelion root in convenient teabags at most natural foods stores. Simply steep the teabag for at least three minutes in freshly boiled water then enjoy the strong roasted-grain-like beverage. Try having at least three cups per week as a general liver-supporting activity. Dandelion (*Taraxacum officinale*) is specifically recommended for liver conditions. Herbalists regard it as an effective blood and liver purifier. Clinical research shows that it helps the body recover from liver disease including hepatitis, as well as liver congestion.

Even more impressive is the fact that it can increase bile secretion by fifty percent; liver conditions in which insufficient bile secretion is the hallmark are particularly benefited by dandelion. Further, inflammation of the bile duct and/or gallbladder, obstruction of the bile duct, and jaundice of the liver are all relieved by dandelion.[11] The herb can also alleviate indigestion, encourage the free flow of urine, and improve the functioning of the pancreas, spleen, liver, bladder, and kidneys. It is "completely free" of any toxic side effects.[12]

Herbal Liver Tonic

Master herbalist David Hoffmann recommends a general liver tonic, to be consumed as a tea after each meal. Mix dandelion root (two parts), meadowsweet (two parts), fringetree bark (one part), and goldenseal (one part). Hoffmann recommends using these herbs in their whole, fresh form. Boil the herbs in water, simmer, and then strain to make the tea. Hoffmann states that the liver and entire digestive system will benefit from the use of herbal bitters, especially gentian, goldenseal, and/or wormwood. These will have a decongestant action on the liver. While taking these bitter herbs (including dandelion root, "the simplest and most widely applicable one," Hoffmann says), take some meadowsweet tincture to help the stomach.[13]

Bile Lubricants

According to naturopathic physicians Peter Bennett, N.D., and Stephen Barrie, N.D., four herbs, one vegetable, and one naturally derived substance are excellent bile lubricants. This means they stimulate and enhance the flow of bile from the liver. The herbs include dandelion root, turmeric, milk thistle, and chelidonium; the vegetable is artichoke; and the naturally derived substance is lecithin from soybeans.

Regarding specific recommendations, Drs. Bennett and Barrie suggest dandelion root at the rate of 1 teaspoon of solid extract three times daily or 8 g taken as tea; 4 capsules of tumeric after each meal or 1 teaspoon of extract with water after each meal; and 500 mg of lecithin three times daily. They warn that taking too much lecithin at one time can overstimulate bile flow, producing headaches and pain in the gallbladder.[14]

Detoxification Support Nutrients

A carefully chosen short list of nutrients in supplement form is often recommended for a detoxification program. Bear in mind that during detoxification, your nutrient requirements are higher than usual. If you are deficient in essential nutrients, this can block key biochemical pathways and possibly make you more toxic since your body can't finish its cleanup of toxic substances. Below are a few critical nutrients with intake recommendations by Drs. Bennett and Barrie.[15]

- *Antioxidants.* These nutrients work against free radicals, the unstable molecules created by toxic substances that damage cells. Chief among the antioxidants is vitamin C, sometimes called a "universal antitoxin." Recommended general dosage: 4,000 to 20,000 mg daily (in divided doses) during detoxification. Ultimate dosage is determined by bowel tolerance; this is the dosage after which (usually within three hours) you spontaneously have one movement of diarrhea. This means your body cannot handle any more vitamin C for a while; wait about twelve hours then resume intake but at a reduced dosage.

  There are two other helpful detoxification support antioxidant nutrients. Vitamin E helps protect cell membranes from damage by lipid peroxides, free radicals sometimes produced by detoxification itself. Recommended general dosage: 200 to 1,200 IU daily. Alpha-lipoic acid is both an antioxidant and a rich source of B vitamins. It helps cells generate energy and it protects the body and liver against poisoning from toxic substances such as heavy metals. Recommended general dosage: 600 mg, twice daily.

- *Amino Acids.* These are protein building blocks, and they are capable of bonding with toxins in the system and removing them from circulation. N-acetyl-cysteine (NAC) is a precursor to glutathione, a critical liver detoxification nutrient. NAC helps to maintain adequate levels of glutathione, thereby enabling the liver to complete its two phases of detoxification. Taking NAC is considered more effective than taking glutathione. Recommended general dosage: 500 mg, three times daily. Even though glutathione is the major player, Drs. Bennett and Barrie do not recommend taking it as a supplement; rather they contend that ingesting it through foods is preferable, notably fresh fruits and vegetables.

  Glycine is another amino acid involved in the liver's detoxification pathways. Like NAC, it is a building block in the production of glutathione. Recommended general dosage: 1,500 to 3,000 mg daily, taken between meals.

  Methionine helps remove fat from the liver and contribute essential molecules to the detoxification pathway. Recommended general dosage: 1,000 mg two or three times daily.

• *Oxystat.* This is a commercially prepared formula (it requires a doctor's prescription) comprising twenty-two natural substances (including the ones listed above) needed to support both phases of the liver's detoxification.

HEALTHY LIVING SPACE DETOXIFIER #20
Do a Natural Liver Flush to
Improve Your Internal "Plumbing"

One protocol many naturopaths, herbalists, and acupuncturists often recommend as part of a detoxification program is a liver flush using natural substances to stimulate the liver to flush itself clean of its toxic overload. Generally, the flush takes a few days, and there are a number of variations on the basic theme, which we will review below. The goal is to help your liver unburden itself of excess toxins and thereby enhance its natural ability to detoxify the body. The strategy behind the flush is that when you ingest the substance on an empty stomach, your liver gets stimulated (without the obstruction of other foods) to release stored toxins into the bile so they can be excreted from the body.

The strategy behind the flush is that when you ingest the substance on an empty stomach, your liver gets stimulated (without the obstruction of other foods) to release stored toxins into the bile so they can be excreted from the body.

While several different liver flush protocols are reviewed below, it is prudent to select one and follow *only one* protocol during your detoxification program. At a future date, try another of the variations.

However, all natural health practitioners who recommend or describe liver flushes strongly advise undertaking a flush *only* under the supervision of a trained health-care expert. While it is a safe, self-care procedure, complications or physiological symptoms may arise, requiring qualified review. For example, the flush may inadvertently dislodge gallstones from the gallbladder; this is a good thing, but it can be painful for a short period as the stones pass through the common bile duct to the stomach. More likely is the possibility of experiencing some odd or transiently uncomfortable symptoms, so having a practitioner on call to explain them can be psychologically reassuring.

Garlic and Cayenne Pepper Flush

Noted author, herbalist, and expert in Chinese medicine Michael Tierra, L.Ac., O.M.D., A.H.G., suggests a four-day flush, optimally undertaken in the spring or summer. It is based on drinking eight ounces of distilled water with eight ounces of apple juice blended with one to four cloves of garlic, a small piece of fresh ginger, and one to four tablespoons of olive oil. This is to be consumed every morning on an empty stomach for four days. Dr. Tierra advises following this immediately with a cup of herbal tea made from dandelion root and fennel seed.

Dr. Tierra further recommends eating a generous amount of green vegetables or going on a warm apple juice fast during this four-day period; add a teaspoon of agar flakes to the juice. Take two capsules of cayenne pepper, or one-half teaspoon cayenne powder mixed in a small amount of water, three times daily, he adds. Cayenne pepper (its major component is called capsaicin) elevates the activities of at least two liver enzymes and stimulates the mobilization of lipids from fat tissue, a necessary step in detoxification.[16]

Finally, Dr. Tierra advises taking two liver-supporting commercially prepared supplements during the four-day flush: Bupleurum Liver Cleanse (containing thirteen herbs such as wild yam root, dandelion root extract, ginger root, and milk thistle) and Turmeric Extract Full Spectrum at a dose of two tablets of each formula three times daily. The liver flush, says Dr. Tierra, "is invaluable for dredging and removing stored toxins and fat accumulated from a sluggish liver and stored throughout the body."[17]

Organic Apple Liver Flush

Herbalist and rejuvenation expert Helene Silver recommends this liver-flushing beverage—based on the juice of organic apples—as part of a detoxification program. The malic acid in the apples helps to cleanse the intestines and heal inflammation of its mucus membranes, says Silver, while the other components stimulate the liver to dump toxins. Combine freshly squeezed organic apple juice (one cup), freshly squeezed lemon

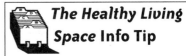

The Healthy Living Space Info Tip

For Oxystat, see:
NF Formulas,
9775 SW Commerce Circle, Suite C5,
Wilsonville, OR 97070;
tel: 800-547-4891 or 503-682-9755;
fax: 503-682-9529;
e-mail: info@nfformulas.com;
website: www.nfformulas.com.

For Bupleurum Liver Cleanse and Turmeric Extract Full Spectrum:
Planetary Formulas and Planetary Herbology,
P.O. Box 275,
Ben Lomond, CA 95005;
tel: 800-717-5010;
fax: 831-336-4548;
e-mail:
herbcourse@planetherbs.com;
website: www.planetherbs.com.

juice (from two lemons), grated fresh ginger root (one tea-spoon), crushed garlic cloves (one to three), cold-pressed saf-flower oil (one tablespoon), cold-pressed olive oil (one tablespoon), and cayenne pepper (a pinch) or cayenne tincture (one drop).

Once the ingredients are combined, consume the beverage in the morning, and do not eat any foods for two hours after-wards. However, Silver recommends drinking one or two cups of a specially prepared Herbal Purification Tea, consisting of fennel seeds (one-fourth cup), fenugreek seeds (one-fourth cup), licorice root (one-fourth cup), flaxseed (one-half cup), and pep-permint leaves (one-half cup). Mix four teaspoons of this dry blend in four cups of pure water, boil, simmer and steep for ten minutes each; strain out the herbs and drink.[18]

Citrus and Olive Oil Flush

Acupuncturist-herbalist Christopher Hobbs, L.Ac., offers this variation on the liver flush, noting, "I have taken liver flushes for many years now and can heartily recommend them." In gen-eral, Dr. Hobbs recommends doing this flush in the morning, pre-ceded by some gentle exercise, such as stretching and breathing exercises (hatha yoga, for example). It is best to eat nothing for an hour after taking the flush mixture, he says.

Produce one cup of fresh juice by squeezing fresh lemons or limes, then dilute the juice slightly with some distilled or pure spring water. Add to this the juice of garlic (one to two cloves, freshly pressed) and ginger (freshly grated and squeezed in a garlic press for the juice). Then add one tablespoon of extra vir-gin olive oil to the citrus, ginger, and garlic juice. Blend or shake the ingredients until all are mixed together, then drink the mix-ture, says Dr. Hobbs. An hour later, drink two cups of Polari Tea, an herbal blend containing dry portions of fennel (one part), flax (one part), burdock (one-fourth part), licorice (one-fourth part), fenugreek (one part), and peppermint (one part). Simmer all the herbs except the peppermint for twenty minutes, then add the peppermint and steep the entire mixture for ten min-utes; then consume, says Dr. Hobbs.

Continue with the liver flush for ten days, taking the flush mixture once every morning, followed, an hour later, by the herb tea, he says. He recommends taking a three-day break, then resuming the flush for another ten days. He further advises doing the flush twice a year, preferably in the spring and fall, two cycles each time.[19]

Castor Oil Compress

Many natural medicine practitioners recommend the use of a compress of castor oil (also known as ricinus oil) applied to the liver during the liver cleansing program. The therapeutic benefits of castor oil compresses were first introduced to Western medicine by Virginia psychic Edgar Cayce in the 1930s, and the practice has been taken up by many people ever since, often for relief of menstrual cramps or pain in the joints.

To prepare a castor oil pack, lightly heat enough castor oil to thoroughly wet, but not soak, a ten-by-twelve-inch flannel cloth. Immerse the flannel in the hot oil, then fold to make three to four layers and place against the skin over the liver (at the bottom of the rib cage on the right side). The oil helps to draw out toxins, release tension, and improve blood circulation, especially in the lower abdomen. Wrap a heating pad or hot water bottle in a towel and place this over the pack, then cover pack and bottle with another towel to retain heat. Keep in place for one to two hours. After you remove the compress, spend five to ten minutes gently rubbing small amounts of extra virgin olive oil into the skin over the liver. Following the treatment, you can wrap the oil-soaked flannel in plastic and store it in the refrigerator for later use. After the flannel has been used twenty times, discard it.

It is generally recommended that you apply the castor oil pack three times per week for about three months, but for women, not during menstruation. The therapeutic action behind the castor oil pack is that the oil is absorbed through the skin and stimulates blood flow and thereby produces improvements in sluggish liver (even cirrhosis), gallbladder inflammation, constipation, and numerous other conditions. Cayce stated that the technique would also stimulate lymph circulation, facilitating the drainage of toxic substances collected by the lymph system.

Intestinal Cleansing: Emptying Out a Storage Space the Size of a Tennis Court

Our intestines are not something we routinely, or perhaps ever, think about, yet when it comes to detoxification, they are crucially important. Here is a fact that may help spark a different attitude about your small intestine. If you were to stretch out smooth and flat the inner convoluted surface of the small intestine, which is about twenty-one feet long in an adult, it would cover the size of a tennis court. Think about your small intestine in this way for a moment: think about a lifetime of food choices, of digestion, assimilation, and elimination, or of indigestion, constipation, gas, cramps, or infrequent elimination. What have you put into your tennis court? Is what you put in still there?

The small intestine, one inch in diameter and stuffed in coils into a small space in your abdomen, absorbs about ninety-five percent of your dietary fats and ninety percent of the amino acids from your foods. Its inner surface, due to a remarkable design concept, is expanded about 600 times by being folded into millions of villi. These are finger-shaped projections and creases, little corners and in-tuckings, called crypts. Each villus has special cells for nutrient absorption and a minute lymph vessel called a lacteal. Each villus is made of thousands of smaller units, called microvilli. These act like a microscopic brush border, facilitating absorption at the molecular level. The purpose of all this intricate design is to multiply the area available for nutrient absorption. Food typically remains in the small intestines from two to six hours in a healthy individual (see figure 5-1).

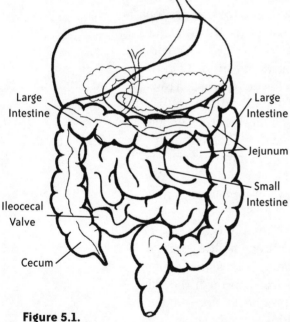

**Figure 5.1.
Large and
Small Intestines**

The large intestine, or colon, is five feet long and two and one-half inches in diameter. There is less of it and it is more ponderous, forming a kind of fence or border around the small intestine. The large intestine is responsible for reabsorbing water from digested foods, that is, foods processed and moved on by the small intestine. The large intestine organizes the various undigestible cellulose fibers as well as some of the "friendly" bacteria (resident in the colon and responsible for maintaining intestinal health) for eventual elimination as feces.

Average transit time in the colon is about twelve hours. This means the amount of time it takes for food—say yesterday's lunch—to pass through the entire gastrointestinal tract, from the mouth though the twenty-six feet of the small and large intestines, and be excreted as feces. Slow transit time is the same as constipation, a problem that concerns many today, especially the elderly. A normal, or healthy, transit time is less than twenty-four hours, although due to the low-grade toxic condition of many people today, this norm is not widely found any more. Slow transit time means that toxic substances present in the feces—for example, growth hormones and pesticides from animal products—remain longer in the intestines where they can begin working as carcinogens. Fast transit time means they don't have the chance to do any harm. Remember, in a constipated person, the transit time for both intestines can be more like thirty to fifty-five hours, according to medical studies.

Slow transit time means more than constipation, even unnoticed or uncomfortable. It means immune system stagnation. That is because both the large and small intestines are functional parts of the body's immune system. In fact, "the intestinal mucosa and some of its sub-mucosal structures constitute the largest immunological system of the body," explains Serafina Corsello, M.D., an expert in intestinal detoxification and director of the Corsello Centers for Nutritional-Complementary Medicine in Huntington, New York. The mucus layers of the intestines collect cellular debris and pathogenic material as the active, defense front of the immune system.

Aside from the skin, the intestines constitute the body's largest organ, thereby being an excellent place to mount a major immune system initiative. According to medical estimates, the intestines account for some eighty percent of the body's immune and lymphatic resources. They are one of the body's first "screening systems" against the daily intake of toxic substances, such as bacteria, viruses, and parasites (discussed later in the chapter), that if not dealt with, would move deeper into the body's blood and tissues, creating illness.

"A healthy intestine is immunologically *vigilant* against undesirable pathogens and toxins," says Dr. Corsello, but one that is "overburdened and compromised" cannot be an immune defensive front. Toxic intestines can thereby contribute seeds of illness to the body. When the intestine's immune vigilance falters or is dysfunctional, then our health is in trouble.[20]

The crucial relationship between intestinal health and overall physical well-being has been recognized for a long time. Almost a century ago, a prominent natural healer named John Harvey Kellogg, M.D., founder of the Battle Creek Sanitarium in Michigan (and the cereal empire named after him), declared that ninety percent of the diseases of civilization are the result of "improper functioning of the colon." In a sense, it's all due to transit time.

About one century ago, most Americans had a short intestinal transit time, of about fifteen to twenty hours, but today, it is much more likely to be fifty to seventy hours. That means that today's lunch will sit inside your body, unprocessed, or being *slowly* processed, for the next three days, or longer. This means there is more time for the stool to putrefy, to spoil inside you, and thereby for harmful intestinal bacteria to flourish and for toxins to develop and enter the bloodstream, taxing the liver. It is a bit like having meat going bad inside your small intestine; in fact, if you are a meat eater and have slow transit time, that is essentially what happens. If you eat low-fiber, high-fat, high-calorie, processed, prepared, or fast foods, especially ones high in mucus (dairy and flour), your transit time is slowed down even more.[21]

Slow transit time and colonic stagnation are the foundation for what physicians call a toxic bowel, and this is the seedbed for numerous illnesses. These can include chronic headaches, allergies, skin blemishes and acne, infections, various autoimmune disorders, in which a confused immune system starts attacking the body's own tissues, and cancer, among many others.

The colon-cancer connection is scientifically well established, ever since a key study of 88,751 women was published in 1990. Women, aged thirty-four to fifty-nine, without a history of cancer or intestinal pathology, were interviewed in 1980. In 1986, they were interviewed again, and this time, 150 cases of colon cancer were noted. The researchers were able to "positively" associate the intake of animal fat and the heightened risk and incidence of colon cancer. In fact, the risk of getting colon cancer was 2.5 times higher among women who ate beef, pork, or lamb as a main protein dish every day. Consumption of processed meats and liver was also "significantly associated" with increased colon cancer risk. In contrast, skinless chicken and fish were related to a decreased risk.

The scientists further noted a correlation between low fiber intake from fruits and vegetables and the risk of colon cancer. "These prospective data provide evidence for the hypothesis that a high intake of animal fat increases the risk of colon cancer," the researchers concluded.[22]

The essential point for our purposes here is not only the conclusion that animal products in themselves may act as carcinogens (based on their injurious chemical content of hormones, pesticides, and other contaminants), but that they take longer to digest (due to their low fiber content), may be incompletely digested, and are more likely to contribute to delayed transit time.

In 1990 researchers provided proof that high-fiber diets may help prevent colon cancer. Researchers at the Fox Chase Cancer Center in Philadelphia, Pennsylvania, studied the evidence from thirty-seven studies on the relationship of diet, fiber, and cancer. They reported that the majority of the cases "gave support for a protective effect associated with fiber-rich diets."[23] A related study in Majorca, Spain, of 286 cases of colorectal cancer (compared to 295 cancer-free subjects) showed that not only was an increased risk of colon cancer associated with the consumption of fresh meats, but a high intake of cruciferous vegetables "afforded protection" against the onset of cancer.[24]

Once slowly or incompletely digesting foods, such as animal fats and protein, start to spoil in the intestines, free radicals are produced. These unstable toxic substances are created by the body's metabolism or brought into the body from toxic materials in the environment, including foods. Once produced and distributed, free radicals start to damage and destroy cells; they are also regarded to be carcinogenic.

Researchers at the Biomedical Engineering Center at Purdue University in West Lafayette, Indiana, studied the production of free radicals from bacterial metabolism inside the colon and were amazed to find it corresponded to that which would be produced by over 10,000 rads of gamma radiation per day. They noted a connection between the high free radical levels and high iron concentrations in the feces; the iron interacts with bile pigments to support free radical generation from resident bacteria.

"Such free radical generation in feces could provide a missing link in our understanding of the etiology of colon cancer," the scientists concluded. It also helps explain why most gastrointestinal tract cancer occurs in the rectum and colon, and why a higher incidence of colon cancer is observed in red meat eaters. It is because red meat increases the iron content of the feces, and the excessive animal fat increases the fecal content of bile pigments and "procarcinogens." These are substances (in this case, bacteria) that, once oxidized (by free radicals), can become full-fledged carcinogens. The presence of animal fats in the colon provides the ideal conditions for this.[25]

Remember the basic equation: high fiber means faster transit time, which means less chance of fecal stagnation and toxicity, which means less chance of free radical production, which, in turn, means less chance of toxicity-related diseases (such as cancer) developing.

Remember the basic equation: high fiber means faster transit time, which means less chance of fecal stagnation and toxicity, which means less chance of free radical production, which, in turn, means less chance of toxicity-related diseases (such as cancer) developing.

A toxic bowel almost always means a body-wide state of toxicity exists, in which toxins "leak" out of the dysfunctional intestines into the bloodstream, the liver, lymph, and other body tissues. Your body now exists in a state of "intestinal toxemia and autointoxication." Your body is absorbing its own toxic waste products, like a drain or garbage disposal backing up into the sink. "It is the root cause of many of today's disorders and illnesses," explains Bernard Jensen, N.D., a naturopathic educator, author, and detoxification expert. Death begins in the colon, he states.

The bowel holds on to waste material much longer than people suspect, says Dr. Jensen. He cites the case of an autopsy that revealed a stagnant colon weighing forty pounds; in other words, that body had accumulated nearly forty pounds of uneliminated fecal matter over a lifetime. Dr. Jensen also describes a distended colon that was nine inches in diameter but had only a pencil-width open passage for the movement of feces. The rest of the nine inches was taken up with multiple layers of encrusted mucus and rubber-like feces.

Figure 5-2. Typical Symptoms and Results of Intestinal Stagnation and Toxicity

fatigue	pain in the lower back
nervousness	sciatica
problems in the gastrointestinal tract	allergies
nutrient malabsorption	asthma
skin problems	illnesses of the eye, ear, nose, and throat
endocrine disturbances	heart problems and abnormalities
irregularities in blood flow and circulation in the brain and nervous system	pathological changes in the breasts (fibrocystic breasts)
headaches	
arthritis	

Source: Dr. Bernard Jensen, *Dr. Jensen's Guide to Better Bowel Care*, Avery Publishing Group, Garden City Park, New York, 1999, 38.

Health-care practitioners at the Angel Healing Center, a colonics and detoxification center in Las Vegas, Nevada, amplify Dr. Jensen's observation. "The average American male colon today carries within it about five pounds of putrid, half-digested red meat, plus another five to ten pounds of foul toxic waste impacted for years in the folds of the colon with mucus." They also cite Dr. Kellogg as having made this remark: "Of the 22,000 operations I have personally performed, I have never found a single normal colon."[26] What would Dr. Kellogg say one hundred years later about the state of the North American colon?

Following Dr. Kellogg's original research, Dr. Jensen claims that if you have only one bowel movement per day, the large intestine will hold the residue of six previous meals; if it holds nine or more meals, you have chronic constipation. Your intestines are healthy, he says, if you eliminate the residue of a given meal fifteen to eighteen hours after consuming it (see figure 5-1).

Constipation is only one of many signs of intestinal toxemia, states Dr. Jensen. According to his research, at least seventy-four different medical conditions can be attributed to improperly functioning intestines, including depression, drowsiness, concentration difficulties, indecision, dry eyes, nausea, bad breath, body odor, insomnia, arthritis, high blood pressure, ovarian cysts, boils, clammy skin, muscle twitches and inflammations, and bladder infections. Intestinal toxemia generally shows up in any of sixteen major symptom categories (see figure 5-2), says Dr.

Jensen, who adds, "All of these conditions have responded to therapy for intestinal toxemia."[27]

There are many effective therapies for purging the intestines of its possibly lifelong backlog of uneliminated fecal matter. Many natural medicine practitioners recommend some form of colon hydrotherapy, more popularly known as colonics. These procedures involve flushing the large intestines with filtered and temperature-regulated pure water to soften the hard, impacted feces; the water is introduced through the rectum with a sanitary plastic tube. The intestines are stimulated to pass a fair amount of the stored waste matter. Sometimes herbs, ozone, and other natural substances are used in the colonics program as well. Colonics require a trained practitioner, which means you will need to visit a facility to have the procedure. It is painless and almost always effective.

While colonics is a viable option for intestinal cleansing, it does not necessarily provide a thorough cleanse of the full twenty-six feet of both small and large intestines, and it is not something you can do on your own. The next section reviews six substances you can take on your own as part of a gentle, home-based, self-care detoxification program with modest cost and no risk.

HEALTHY LIVING SPACE DETOXIFIER #21
Use Six Natural Substances
to Help Cleanse Your Intestines

Just as herbs, nutrients, and natural substances can be used to stimulate and support liver decongestion, so are there natural substances perfectly suited to get your intestines into a cleansing mode. In large measure, cleansing has a laxative effect. When you stimulate your intestines to cleanse, they will increase their evacuation of old fecal matter. So from an experiential viewpoint, using any of the substances described below will seem as if you have taken a remarkably effective laxative.

However, do not use all six substances at the same time. You may wish to try a few at one time, but it is probably most prudent to use *only one* at a time, depending on the desired effect you wish; there are exceptions to this, which are reviewed at the end of this section. Some can be used for an extended period of time (such as bentonite clay, which might be used productively for a month), but others are meant only for a short time (charcoal and psyllium husks, which shouldn't be used much more than seven to ten days).

Activated Charcoal

Activated charcoal, a reliable and very effective poison absorber, is a traditional remedy with a long history of use in many cultures. The charcoal is prepared by carbonizing organic matter such as wood or peat in a kiln, then activating it with oxidizing gases (steam or air) at high temperatures. One typical source of the carbon matter is coconut shells heated in the absence of air; then the partially burned shells are granulated to a size that maximizes their optimal absorption capacity. The high steam (applied at 800° C for 12-24 hours) opens up and enlarges the pores of the charcoal, thereby creating an enormous internal surface area, estimated to be 800 square meters per one gram of charcoal.[28]

If you suspect food poisoning from tainted restaurant food, taking two to four charcoal tablets (easily obtained at drugstores and natural foods outlets) can help reduce the toxic effect on your intestines and hasten the removal of these toxins from your body. The charcoal absorbs the poisons in the small intestines along with chemicals secreted in the bile, thereby preventing their re-uptake into the liver and blood circulation. It is even more effective when combined with two to four drops of oil of oregano.[29] Charcoal is also effective against flatulence and excessive intestinal gas.

As a general aid for detoxification, activated charcoal is often recommended to help in the systemic clearance of drugs and intoxicants and is regarded as a "universal antidote" to the ingestion of poisonous substances. Activated charcoal helps detoxify the body in several ways: it purifies the six to eight liters of various digestive fluids secreted daily in the body; it absorbs noxious chemicals (both the poisons and their breakdown products, called metabolites) from the bile duct; it absorbs ingested drugs that would otherwise diffuse back into the stomach and small intestine; and it reduces the liver's detoxification burden. Further, charcoal can absorb a fair amount of the toxins produced by a systemic yeast overgrowth of *Candida albicans*, preventing these toxins from being reabsorbed into the bloodstream.

Charcoal is also said to counteract decomposition products from ingested foods (such as beans) that would otherwise produce flatulence, diarrhea, or odorous stools.

In fact, according to one authority, "activated charcoal is the best single supplement for enhancing detoxification . . . [understood to be] an ongoing biological process that prevents toxins (from infectious agents, food, air, water, and substances that contact the skin) from destroying health." Richard C. Kaufman, Ph.D., recommends twenty to thirty-five grams of activated charcoal as a daily detoxification protocol, divided into two or three doses (morning, midday, and before bed—on an empty stomach in all cases), taken on two consecutive days for one week. For intestinal complaints, he recommends 4-10 g taken twice daily; for *Candida albicans*, 20-35 g daily until the problem is cleared.[30]

However, charcoal also removes nutrients from the intestines, so it should not be used routinely, or if employed during the detoxification program, it should not be used regularly afterwards. Charcoal can produce short-term constipation and, of course, black-gray stools.

Bentonite, or Liquid Clay

The term bentonite refers to a natural clay deposit found in cretaceous rocks, notably in Fort Benton, Wyoming, and throughout the Great Plains region of the United States, but also in France. In France, the active mineral in bentonite is called montmorillonite and is found in weathered volcanic ash that has become clay over time. A third term, smectite, is sometimes used to describe this same therapeutically active natural substance. Essentially, all three terms are interchangeable.

For our purposes, the key information is that bentonite or liquid clay—the clay is hydrated with water into the consistency of a very thick milkshake or tasteless pale grey gel—contains minerals that can absorb toxins from and deliver nutrients to the gastrointestinal tract. Since liquid clay is inert (not biologically active), its effects are physical, not chemical, and it passes undigested through the system, bearing its toxic load out of the body through the stool.

Like charcoal, bentonite has an extensive adsorptive surface area. So vast is this area, that one manufacturer claims a quart bottle represents 960 square yards of surface area, or about the size of twelve American football fields. Once inside the body, bentonite adsorbs toxins such as heavy metals, pesticides, and free radicals by attracting them to its generous surface area; then it gathers the poisons up for excretion in a way that has been compared to how a magnet draws filings to it.

The research supporting the beneficial detoxifying claims for bentonite is solid and impressive. Bentonite expands like a super-absorbent sponge and can adsorb selected pathogenic viruses (reovirus type 3 and a bacteria, coliphage T1, both common to sewage, aquatic, and land environments), according to a study involving soils and sediments. The study showed that bentonite has a "specificity" to adsorbing "mixed populations" of these microorganisms.[31] Another study suggested that bentonite clay solids had some ability to collect poliovirus microorganisms from tap water.[32] A Russian study showed that bentonite can effectively adsorb selected species of poliomyelitis type II viruses, monkey disease rotavirus, Coxsackie B1 and B6, and Picornaviridae and Reoviridae.[33]

It also has been observed to specifically bind up the herbicides Paraquat and Roundup as well as aflatoxin (a toxic mold that infests grains and nuts).[34] A poultry study involving 528 chickens showed that bentonite "partially neutralizes" the toxic effects of aflatoxin, a potent developmental poison for animals.[35] Comparable results were shown in a rat study; rats were fed an aflatoxin-infected diet, then given bentonite and another binding substance. None showed any developmental defects, indicating the bentonite and second substance had adsorbed or neutralized the aflatoxin.[36] A pig study showed bentonite added to aflatoxin-contaminated corn feed led to the partial restoration of liver performance and function, again indicating the clay's ability to collect and deactivate the toxins.[37] A cow study showed that bentonite could remove a toxin (lantana, a dairy poison) as effectively (but not as quickly) as activated charcoal, thereby showing "promise as a cheap alternative" to activated charcoal for lantana poisoning.[38]

According to Ran Knishinsky, a bentonite enthusiast and author of *The Clay Cure*, the benefits of using bentonite for only two to four weeks are numerous and impressive. They include improved regularity in intestinal evacuation; relief from chronic constipation, diarrhea, indigestion, and ulcers; an increase in physical energy; improved complexion; greater mental alertness; uplifted emotional mood; and increased resistance to infection. In other words, with liquid clay you get a lot of the general benefits expected from detoxification.[39]

Knishinsky contends that taking one to three tablespoons of liquid clay daily, in divided doses, can help eliminate intestinal parasites, provide relief from allergies and hay fever, clear up acne, and turn around anemia (because of its high iron content). Liquid clay manufacturers state that the substance shines as a general internal cleansing agent, because it scrapes and cleans the lining of the intestines at the same time as feeding it with essential and trace nutrients.

One liquid clay product (Mineral-Rich by Earth Essentials/White Rock) offers seventy-one trace and ultra-trace minerals, which the body needs to be able to absorb the bigger nutrients like vitamins. It works as both a mineral supplement and an internal body cleanser. According to this manufacturer, the bentonite begins adsorbing toxic substances as soon as it reaches the stomach (in this case, excess stomach bile); then it moves into the small intestine where its large surface area adsorbs toxins and releases minerals. Users of this product report that a variety of symptoms have abated, including hair loss, acne, insomnia, brittle nails, allergies, joint problems, spastic colon, digestive problems, and low energy.

Several brands of liquid clay are available in natural foods stores. A general usage recommendation is to start with one tablespoon daily mixed with juice or water and observe the results for a week. Gradually increase your intake to up to four tablespoons daily, in two divided doses, morning and evening. As part of an intensive detoxification program, manufacturers suggest a *short-term* dose of one tablespoon per hour through the day. You will probably notice a gentle laxative effect in the range of about a twenty-five percent increase in daily intestinal elimination. Use the bentonite for up to a month, then take a month off, and repeat, if you wish. It is important that you drink extra amounts (at least double your normal intake) of pure water during the time you take liquid clay.

Chlorella

This single-celled freshwater green algae (*Chlorella pyrenoidosa*) is noted for its ability to eliminate toxins from the body through the feces. Chlorella binds to toxic metals and chemicals, thereby facilitating their removal. The substance also has antibacterial and antiviral properties and is believed to stimulate the immune system. According to Earthrise, a chlorella manufacturer in Petaluma, California, the hard cellulose cell wall of chlorella helps to remove impurities from the body, and it may be involved in absorbing toxins from the intestines. Earthrise further states that chlorella "may have the ability to improve bowel function and stimulate the growth of beneficial [intestinal] bacteria."[40]

Chlorella, with a higher chlorophyll content per gram than any other plant and a complete array of essential amino acids, is known as the "unpoisoner" because it can detoxify the body of cadmium, lead, and the effects of uranium radiation. One way chlorella might do this is through its antioxidant effects on albumin.

Albumin, a substance continuously secreted by the liver and the most abundant protein found in human blood, is a major antioxidant. It appears both to transport vital nutrients and remove toxins from cells in the body's connective tissue. Perhaps because of albumin's detoxifying effect, high blood levels of albumin have been linked with longevity, which is to say, low levels of albumin are associated with increased states of toxicity. One estimate has it that chlorella supplementation can raise albumin levels by sixteen percent to twenty-one percent.[41]

A Japanese study demonstrated that chlorella is a first-rate detoxifying agent, capable of removing alcohol from the liver. The study showed that taking four to six grams of chlorella before consuming alcohol prevented hangovers in ninety-six

---

The Healthy Living Space Info Tip

For Mineral-Rich:
Earth Essentials,
P.O. Box 910,
Springville, UT 84663;
tel: 888-328-2529;
fax: 801-489-3175;
e-mail: support@earthessentials.net;
website: www.earthessentials.net.

For Great Plains Bentonite:
Yerba Prima, Inc.,
740 Jefferson Avenue,
Ashland, OR 97520;
tel: 800-488-4339 or 541-488-2228;
fax: 541-488-2443;
e-mail: yerba@yerba.com;
website: www.yerbaprima.com.

For Chlorella:
Earthrise Nutritionals, Inc.,
424 Payran Street,
Petaluma, CA 94952;
tel: 800-949-7473;
fax: 707-778-9028;
e-mail: info@earthrise.com;
website: www.earthrise.com.

For Triphala Internal Cleanser:
Planetary Formulas/Planet Herbs,
P.O. Box 275,
Ben Lomond, CA 95005;
tel: 800-717-5010;
fax: 831-336-4548;
e-mail: herbcourse@planetherbs.com;
website: www.planetherbs.com.

For Ultimate Cleanse:
Omni Nutraceuticals,
5310 Beethoven Street,
Los Angeles, CA 90066;
tel: 800-841-8448; fax: 310-306-1790;
product information: 888-297-3273;
website: www.naturessecret.com.

percent of cases, even following a night of heavy drinking.[42] Numerous studies demonstrate that chlorella is effective in use against tumors and in reducing the negative effects of chemotherapy and radiation treatments (and against gamma rays in particular). Another chlorella manufacturer states, "Numerous research projects in the United States and Europe have indicated chlorella can also aid the body in the breakdown of persistent hydrocarbon and metallic toxins such as DDT, PCB, mercury, cadmium, and lead, as well as strengthening the immune system response."[43]

Randal Merchant, M.D., of the Department of Neurosurgery at the Medical College of Virginia provides support for this last claim. Dr. Merchant is conducting clinical trials on chlorella and has summarized much of the key research on chlorella's health and detoxification benefits on a health-related website. Dr. Merchant states that a physician at Kitakyushu City Institute for Environmental Pollution Research in Japan gave thirty patients with PCB exposure daily chlorella doses of 4-6 g for one year, after which time, the key symptoms of PCB toxicity—exhaustion, poor digestion, abnormal bowel movements—had all improved.[44] From his own research he reports that twenty patients with brain tumors took chlorella (20 g in tablet form, and 150 ml in liquid form) during their cancer treatment and experienced fewer than expected respiratory infections and flu-like illnesses. They stated the chlorella helped them maintain their strength and resist common colds and infections prevalent among cancer patients.[45]

Chlorella seems to be effective in reducing symptoms in many conditions that involve toxicity. A study at the School of Medicine of West Virginia University showed that chlorella, given to rats, increases the rate of detoxification of a harmful pesticide called chlordecone. Chlorella was shown to remove the toxin from the

> *A Japanese study demonstrated that chlorella is a first-rate detoxifying agent, capable of removing alcohol from the liver. The study showed that taking four to six grams of chlorella before consuming alcohol prevented hangovers in ninety-six percent of cases, even following a night of heavy drinking.*

body twice as fast as the control substance; it reduced the half-life of the toxin from forty to nineteen days.[46] Chlorella is also competent at enhancing the excretion of the heavy metal cadmium in people suffering from cadmium poisoning.[47] Once chlorella binds with cadmium, it does not re-release it to the body while still in the intestinal tract, but removes it definitively from the body.[48]

Chlorella given daily to patients with fibromyalgia (chronic, often body-wide, muscle pain) for two months (at a dosage of 10 g of a dry powder and 100 ml of liquid form) produced a twenty-two percent reduction in pain intensity.[49] In a similar study (conducted by Dr. Merchant), 34 fibromyalgia patients took 50 tablets of chlorella and 100 ml of liquid chlorella every day for three months, after which they reported a fourfold decrease in pain and a 25% reduction in anxiety.

According to Dr. Merchant, chlorella achieves its detoxifying effects through at least three mechanisms (in addition to the albumin explanation above). First, it stimulates the body's immune system to produce more macrophages, immune cells that "eat" toxic substances. Macrophages "actively clean the blood, body fluids, and cavities of harmful substances," explains Dr. Merchant. Second, in the intestines, chlorella stimulates the growth of beneficial microflora, specifically the "good" intestinal bacteria called Lactobacillus; this family of bacteria help to destroy foreign and toxic substances and keep the ecology of the numerous microorganisms present in balance. Third, chlorella's thick cell wall adsorbs toxins in the intestine, and in so doing, reduces stool odor.[50]

Unlike activated charcoal, bentonite, and psyllium (discussed below), chlorella can be taken both during the intensive phase of a detoxification program and regularly as a supplement. During the detoxification program, you might wish to take more chlorella than during routine times, due to the increased mobilization of toxins in the body as a result of the various herbs and fibers you are taking to stimulate cleansing and evacuation.

Triphala, an Ayurvedic Herbal Cleanser

Triphala, an Ayurvedic herbal medicine, is the most popular herbal formula in India. Ayurveda,[51] which is India's classical and ancient medical system—still practiced today there and around the world, including to a limited extent in the United States—holds that Triphala is an effective but gentle laxative, capable of supporting the body's strength.

The name means "three fruits," and refers to the three Indian herbs used in it: *Haritaki* (*Terminalia chebula*), *Amalaki* (*Emblica officinalis*), and *Bhibhitaki* (*Terminalia belerica*). Each of these herbs is said to rejuvenate one of the three constitutional categories (called *doshas*) described in Ayurveda, namely, *vata, pitta*, and *kapha*. Haritaki balances the air element (vata) and the large intestine; Amalaki balances the fire element (pitta) and the liver; and Bhibitaki balances the water element (kapha) and reduces mucus and fats in the circulatory system. "Triphala uniquely cleanses and detoxifies at the deepest organic levels without depleting the body's reserves," explains Michael Tierra, L.Ac., O.M.D. "This makes it one of the most valuable herbal preparations in the world."[52]

Dr. Tierra makes an interesting observation about intestinal cleansing herbs and formulas that work as laxatives, explaining that there are two basic types. One type is called purgative; strong bitter herbs, such as senna, cascara, and others stimulate the intestine's peristaltic action by promoting bile secretion by the liver. Triphala is primarily a purgative. The other type is a lubricating bulk laxative, typified by herbs such as psyllium and flaxseed; this approach does not directly affect the liver or bile secretion, but works as an "intestinal broom" or sponge, absorbing fluids, says Dr. Tierra. He notes that people who require purgatives have a bowel irregularity caused by congestion in the liver and gallbladder along with some blood toxicity. People who need lubricating bulk laxatives tend to have intestinal dryness caused by metabolic imbalances (including nutritional deficiency).

Notwithstanding these distinctions, Triphala is effective for all types of constipation except those caused by a lack of vital energy, Dr. Tierra states. While Triphala will gently help move the bowels, it will also effectively purify the blood, stimulate bile secretion, promote liver detoxification, clear up stagnation, enhance digestion and nutrient assimilation, and significantly reduce blood levels of cholesterol and fats throughout the body. Indians believe that Triphala is "able to care for the internal organs of the body as a mother cares for her children," says Dr. Tierra.

He notes that one of his patients who was forty pounds overweight was able to lose twenty pounds in only a month by taking Triphala, without making any major dietary changes. Dr. Tierra also relates the arresting story about a yogic master he once met in California. The man was in his late eighties but could outwalk anyone in terms of speed or distance. His secret: regular meditation, kicharee (mung beans, rice, ghee, and spices), and a daily dose of Triphala.

Triphala is now available in prepared pill form from several manufacturers, although Ayurvedic physicians recommend preparing it from scratch, using the dry herbs. One practitioner suggests pouring boiling water into a cup in which you have put one teaspoonful of Triphala herbs; let it stand overnight; in the morning, strain it, then drink. The taste is "bitter, sour, pungent, astringent, and, at the end, thankfully, slightly sweet."[53] As with chlorella, you can take Triphala routinely to promote regularity and detoxification without causing any weakness or deficiency during your detoxification program. Planetary Formulas, one of the makers of Triphala, recommends taking it once weekly on the same day on a continuing basis, or one to three times daily for "balanced detoxification."

Psyllium Husks and Seeds

Not only do we need to remove intestinal toxins, we need to evacuate the bowels more often and more thoroughly. One of the easiest ways to do this is through increasing our intake of fiber or roughage. Of course this can be accomplished routinely by increasing the vegetable and whole grain content of our diet, but during a deliberate detoxification program, one method frequently recommended by natural health practitioners is the temporary use of psyllium husks (*Plantago ovata*).

Think of it as a natural laxative. But it is actually more than that. As a bulking agent, psyllium husks and seeds (taken in powder form) help "eliminate toxins and xenobiotics [foreign substances] by binding them in the feces so they are not absorbed back into the bloodstream," explains one detoxification expert.[54] Psyllium consists of about seventy-five percent to eighty percent dietary fiber, of which sixty-five percent is water soluble and ten percent to fifteen percent is insoluble (meaning it is not digested or absorbed, but passes through the system intact).

One of the main benefits of taking psyllium is that it speeds up intestinal transit time. A study involving men and women, age sixty-five and older, all of whom suffered from chronic constipation, showed that by taking psyllium daily for one month (at the rate of 24 g per day), transit time was nearly cut in half, from 53.9 hours to 30 hours. The patients also experienced an increase in bowel movements, from 0.8 per day to 1.3, again almost double. "Fiber supplementation appeared to benefit constipated older patients clinically, and it improved colonic transit time," the researchers concluded.[55]

A similar study looked at the effects of giving twelve subjects various daily fiber supplements containing wheat bran, psyllium gum, and/or a combination of both for two weeks. Fiber supplementation reduced transit time and increased the frequency of bowel movements. While wheat bran reduced transit time the most, psyllium had a greater effect on the amount of water in the stools, which means they were less hard and compacted, and therefore less painful or difficult to pass. One of the causes of constipation is dryness in the stools; they get tight, dense, and compacted, and thus hard for the intestine's innate rhythmic pulsing to move; it's like trying to push a boulder with a whisk broom. In this study, patients who had no fiber supplement said fifty percent of their stools were "hard," whereas those taking fiber said only ten percent of their stools were hard.[56]

A third study further supported these conclusions. This study involved twenty patients, all of whom suffered from chronic constipation and half of whom also had irritable bowel syndrome (which is a kind of spasticity of the colon, leading to frequent, unpleasant bursts of evacuation of irregular consistency and accompanied by abdominal pain). Patients took psyllium daily for one month, after which their weekly rate of bowel motions had increased from an average of two to eight, a fourfold increase, and their transit time was reduced from forty-eight to eighteen hours. Even better, no "side effects" or adverse effects such as flatulence were observed.[57]

A fourth study involving twenty-two subjects with chronic constipation reported pronounced improvement after the subjects took psyllium daily for two months. Their stool frequency increased from 2.9 to 3.8 stools per week, stool consistency improved (meaning higher water content and thus easier movement), pain on defecation decreased, and the weight of the average stool increased from 405 to 665 g per motion, which means they had a more thorough elimination.[58]

Lest all this sound unpleasantly clinical or too biologically intimate, it's important to see in these numbers and medical reports the nature of chronic constipation. Ideally, the healthy human is meant to have a bowel motion two to three times daily, based on food intake; in the study just summarized, the people had barely three bowel movements a week, and with pain. The mere addition of psyllium was able, over a few weeks, to almost double the output.

Psyllium has another beneficial effect, namely, an ability to reduce cholesterol levels and thereby help regulate a condition called hypercholesterolemia, which means, excess cholesterol.[59] This benefit was demonstrated in a study involving forty-four men and women with this medical condition. They took a psyllium-enriched cereal daily for seven weeks; at the end of this time, they all showed "significantly lower" levels of blood cholesterol and low-density lipoprotein (LDL) cholesterol. LDL is regarded as the undesirable form of cholesterol, in contrast to the "good" kind, called high-density lipoprotein (HDL)[60] When study subjects took a blend of psyllium husks, pectin, guar, and locust bean gums (various sources of water-soluble dietary fiber) for only four weeks, they had an 8.3% reduction in total cholesterol and a 12.4% decrease in LDL cholesterol.[61]

Again, you can clearly see the vital importance of intestinal cleansing and purging for health. Merely by increasing the intestine's ability to eliminate fecal matter, you reduce your chances of heart disease from high cholesterol. On the other hand, living with a stagnant colon in which excess dietary cholesterol is not regularly or effectively removed can lead to various life-threatening medical conditions. Either way, you are improving your health by reducing your body's toxic load.

There are now numerous commercial intestinal cleansing formulas containing psyllium available at natural foods stores or websites. Psyllium is available on its own in a dry powder, or in blends with other detoxifying herbs. In some people, psyllium can produce flatulence, abdominal distension (bloating), and/or pain. These symptoms are generally transient, but if they persist, it is advisable to use a different bulking agent. While taking psyllium, it is essential to drink generous amounts of pure water.

Dosages will vary with the product, but the following is a general recommendation. According to Yerba Prima, a provider of psyllium based in Ashland, Oregon, adults and children over twelve should take one rounded teaspoon of dry psyllium husks one to three times daily. Children between six and twelve should take one-half to one level teaspoon, one to three times a day. Take the psyllium a half-hour before or one hour after eating.

Plan on taking the psyllium once or twice daily—no more than three times in one day—for ten to fourteen days. There is a buildup phase of perhaps four to six days depending on your state of long-term constipation and intestinal stagnation. To an extent, most adults in Western industrialized countries have stagnation in the intestines, so don't worry that you are an exception to the healthy norm. The healthy norm is rarely observed anymore. For perhaps the first two days, you may actually not move your bowels at all, and you may feel bloated, even uncomfortably so. The psyllium is building up a head of steam, so to speak, moving slowly through the intestines, seeping into all the cracks and fissures. Around the third or fourth day, you will start evacuating much more than usual.

You will probably feel transient symptoms of discomfort, such as headaches, flu-like symptoms, congestion, a sore throat, aches and pains, or a slight fever. These will last for perhaps two days and are called the Herxheimer reaction.[62] When you mobilize toxins in the body—that is, identify and collect them—there is a short-term heightening of toxicity in the system. This is sometimes call the "die-off" phase of detoxification; toxic substances are neutralized but temporarily remain, like corpses, within the system, making it feel deeply poisoned. It's like sweeping a very dusty floor; at first, there is dust everywhere, and the place seems far messier than before you contemplated cleaning it. Ultimately, the floor will be much cleaner, as will your intestines. The arrival of Herxheimer symptoms is your body telling you that the intestinal cleanse is working. After a few days, your Herxheimer reaction will dissipate.

One way to palliate feelings of extreme toxicity—you may feel dreadful for an hour now and then—is to take a high dose of vitamin C, something on the order of 3000-6000 mg, perhaps in two divided doses, over a two-hour period. Vitamin C used this way acts the way aspirin does for a headache. Be sure to drink at least sixteen ounces of fresh water with the vitamin C intake any time you feel the Herxheimer effect.

By the peak of the cleanse, perhaps days six to nine, you may be passing three to four times your normal amount; six or seven evacuations per day for a few days is not unusual if this is the first time you have done an intestinal cleanse. This may not appeal to you, but you will notice (if you look) that around the time of the peak elimination, the bowel movements are strangely shaped, like twisted, moldy old rope. This is the "old stuff," finally being dredged up out of the immense storage space of your intestines for elimination. To a large measure, this is why you are taking psyllium in the first place: to get this old stuff moving and out of your body.

One way to palliate feelings of extreme toxicity—you may feel dreadful for an hour now and then—is to take a high dose of vitamin C, something on the order of 3000-6000 mg, perhaps in two divided doses, over a two-hour period. Vitamin C used this way acts the way aspirin does for a headache.

Bear in mind that taking psyllium should not be a lifestyle, a way of coping with the high-fat, high-sugar, low-fiber fast foods diet that many rely on; rather, it should be a component in an occasional (as in twice yearly) detoxification program. In other words, it is not advisable to take psyllium (or any other high-fiber supplement) routinely and continuously; it will make your intestines lazy and may irritate their mucosal linings as well. A high-fiber, whole-food diet consisting of fresh, organic, living foods is the preferred way to keep a steady intake of roughage. That is all your intestines need to do their nature-appointed task of frequent and thorough elimination of unwanted, toxic matter.

Cascara Sagrada

In the same family as buckthorn, this herb was once known to Native Americans as "sacred bark," as reflected in the Spanish name given to it by European explorers (botanical name: *Rhamnus purshianus*). Used in its dry bark form, it has been, on its own or in combination with other herbs, a popular and successful natural laxative for many years. Its chemical components are effective in stimulating intestinal peristalsis. A particular component (an anthracene derivative) gives cascara its distinctive laxative effect by increasing the motility of the colon. That means it stimulates it to move—to enhance its peristaltic motions. Thus, the feces move faster through the colon and absorb less water.[63]

Cascara is perhaps "the best researched" of the laxative herbs, notes Daniel B. Mowrey, Ph.D., in *Herbal Tonic Therapies*. Its mildness and nonhabituating qualities are widely noted. In other words, your intestines will not become dependent on its presence for continued bowel motions once you stop taking the herb. It does not lose its effectiveness with use, and you do not have to take increasingly larger doses to get the same laxative results. Cascara is an intestinal tonic, which means it can "nurture, soothe, stimulate, and condition" the intestines, says Dr. Mowrey. Cascara can be used in small doses to "restore and maintain tone" in the colon and it can be used daily in small doses "to enhance the health of the liver and other organs."[64] However, long-term use can lead to a loss of electrolytes (key minerals).

Although cascara sagrada can be taken on its own at the rate of 50-100 mg per dose, depending on the degree of constipation, it is more common to use it in prepared herbal detoxification formulas where it is combined with other detoxifying herbs. It is often the major player in detoxification formulas.

There are many such detoxification-laxative formulas, but one that has received considerable attention and garnered favorable public and medical opinion is called Ultimate Cleanse, originally designed by a naturopath-nutritionist and produced by Nature's Secret, now a subsidiary of Omni Nutraceuticals of Los Angeles, California. This formula consists of twenty-nine cleansing herbs and thirteen sources of fiber and is designed to cleanse and tone all channels of elimination, including the bowel, kidneys, lungs, skin, and lymphatic system, according to its manufacturer. This formula also includes Siberian ginseng, included for "extra energy and support against stress while cleansing." The program is meant for daily use, in the morning and evening, for about two weeks.

In closing this section, here are some general usage recommendations for the six substances just reviewed.

• Activated charcoal: use on its own

• Bentonite: use with chlorella, triphala, and psyllium or cascara sagrada (not both)

• Chlorella: use with bentonite, triphala, psyllium or cascara sagrada (not both)

• Triphala: use with chlorella or bentonite

• Psyllium: use with chlorella or bentonite; take at different times

• Cascara sagrada: use with chlorella or bentonite; take at different times

In many respects, it is better to use each substance on its own to gauge its effects. Later, you might consider using several at the same time.

HEALTHY LIVING SPACE DETOXIFIER #22
Remove the 50+ Feet of False
Mucoid Lining from Your Intestines

The use of any of the above-described natural substances will definitely stimulate your intestines to purge a fair amount of their stored waste matter. But there is a more biologically arcane level of old intestinal matter that these herbs will not address. It is called mucoid plaque or false mucoid lining. It "bizarrely resembles hardened blackish-green truck tire rubber or an old piece of dried rawhide," observes naturopathic practitioner and detoxification expert, Richard Anderson, N.D., N.M.D., of Mount Shasta, California.

In 1986, Dr. Anderson developed (and started to market) a four-phase, four-week, all natural colon cleansing program (called Arise & Shine and the Cleanse Thyself program) that dredges out this mucoid plaque. When the mucoid plaque comes out in an intensive intestinal cleansing program, it is characterized by "ropelike twists, striations, overlaps, folds, creases—the shape and texture of the intestinal wall," says Dr. Anderson.

It can be hard and brittle; firm and thick; tough, wet, and rubbery; soft, thick, and mucoid; or soft, transparent, and thin; and its color can range from light brown, black, or greenish-black to yellow or grey, and it usually stinks. Even more stunning is the fact that it is not unusual to pass thirty-five to forty-five feet of mucoid plaque during a four-week intestinal cleanse program; some pass more than sixty feet, and at least one of Dr. Anderson's clients passed a record single length that was fifteen feet long.

So what is mucoid plaque? The term is one of Dr. Anderson's devising. He uses it to indicate a film of mucus, different from the intestine's natural mucosal lining, which is the result of the unhealthy accumulation over time of abnormal mucus matter on the intestinal walls. Medicine knows this plaque as a natural layering of mucin or glycoproteins (comprising twenty amino acids and fifty percent carbohydrates); it is natural in that the intestines secrete it as a protection against acids, salt, heavy metals, parasites, and numerous other toxic substances. In fact, mucoid plaque starts out as mucin, or a layering of glycoproteins, then just about everything else in the intestines gets added: water, electrolytes, epithelial cells (that line the intestinal walls), bacteria, bacterial metabolities and toxins, digested food, blood proteins, bile salts, enzymes from the pancreas, drug residues, antigen-antibody complexes (from allergies), and toxins produced by bacteria, yeasts, and parasites.

Mucoid plaque appears to develop in the presence of acids, or in acid pH conditions in the intestines; a large measure of this requisite acidity is provided by the standard American diet, which is acid-producing, says Dr. Anderson. So this "gel-like, viscous and slimy mucus" gets deposited in successive layers over the inner lining of the intestines.

When the diet is unbalanced and biochemically toxic to the intestines, additional amounts of mucoid plaque are formed, says Dr. Anderson. Even though it is a natural protective mechanism, if you were healthy, your intestine wouldn't need to protect itself with mucoid plaque in the first place, comments Dr. Anderson.

Mucoid plaque does not routinely get excreted. Rather, it collects in the folds and crevices of the large intestine, and can remain there in storage for years, even for a lifetime. "Over time, the mucoid plaque grows thicker, firmer, and more widespread—colonizing, as it were, the tennis court-sized interior of the small intestine," says Dr. Anderson. Newly created feces adhere to it and the plaque grows, slowing down peristalsis and harboring intestinal pathogens; it thereby adds to bowel toxicity, emitting toxins continuously into the bloodstream and creating a favorable atmosphere for disease.

The plaque accumulation weakens overall intestinal function, interferes with nerve meridians, acts as a barrier to nutrient absorption, and may cause protein and carbohydrate intolerance (food allergies). Further, Dr. Anderson explains that prescription antibiotics and an unhealthy or unbalanced diet, comprising sugar, soft drinks, wheat products (allergenic for many people), rancid or spoiled foods, salt, and animal products containing hormones and antibiotics, can help negatively alter and transform the mucoid plaque into a toxic substance and the seedbed for "various disease states." "The hundreds of testimonies I have received clearly indicate that mucoid plaque contributes towards a high percentage of pathological problems, as well as premature death," says Dr. Anderson.[65]

At the other end of the spectrum, completion of Dr. Anderson's four-week self-care cleansing program yields impressive results, an undoing of numerous latent and full-blown pathological problems. A woman, age fifty-five, had suffered from a skin rash for thirty-five years. No medical treatment had been able to reverse this condition. After the four-week program, ninety-five percent of her rash had disappeared. Another woman, age forty-two, had chronic bronchitis and could not exercise or climb stairs without wheezing. All these problems cleared up after the cleanse. Yet another woman, forty-seven, had suffered with hip pain for seven years and needed a cane for walking. X-rays showed that her hip nerves were pinched and the cartilage of the femur (the tip of the thigh bone that connects to the hip bone) was actually worn off. On the second day of the four-week program, fifty percent of her pain disappeared; on the third day, she could stretch and exercise gently; and over the next several months, her pain continued to diminish.

Other benefits reported by users, says Dr. Anderson, include emotional release and cessation of problems such as menstrual pain, migraines, joint pain, skin problems, colds, sinus congestion, fibrocystic breasts, overweight, and poor concentration. Dr. Anderson explains that often old, unprocessed, negative emotions, states of consciousness, and thinking patterns are held in the body-mind system in association with old fecal matter. As you purge the intestines, you inadvertently purge the emotions. "I estimate that about 70% of those doing the intensive colon cleanse will experience long-forgotten memories and buried emotions," says Dr. Anderson.

In fact, often emotions surface "with all their original charge" and this is followed by a discharge of a section of mucoid plaque, he says. It's as if somehow the old fecal matter held—bound up—the old emotions in place. Dr. Anderson further proposes that, at an energy level, a negative state of consciousness born of these held emotions and thoughts is often at the root of the particular physical problem we have.[66] (See chapter 8 for more on emotional detoxification.)

The Arise & Shine Cleanse Thyself program consists of a series of herbal preparations and natural substances taken in specific order over a period of four weeks. The program provides herbal laxatives (including cascara sagrada), herbal nutrition, bentonite, psyllium, probiotics ("friendly" bacteria, discussed below), electrolytes, and antioxidants. As you take the various preparations, you alter your diet, and during the intense phase, you severely restrict it to enable the natural substances to produce the maximum benefit.

Each successive stage of the program calls for stricter dietary controls, offers a higher degree of nutrient supplements, and produces a deeper level of cleansing. Usually, it takes three to four weeks to complete the Pre-Cleanse phase of the program. This is followed by the Cleanse phase, which lasts one week. Typically, the mucoid lining comes out in the Cleanse phase, although some may start being eliminated a little sooner.

Because the last week of the program can be intense—involving the frequent intake of program substances, mostly in the form of "shakes," and no food intake—it might be prudent to schedule this as a vacation period unless you work at home where it is easier to handle the requirements of the Cleanse.

The mucoid plaque removal program is best undertaken after you have tried some of the gentler intestinal cleansing steps outlined in Healthy Living Space Detoxifier #21. This is especially true if this is the first time you have ever done anything to detoxify your intestines. The steps in #21 will *ease* you into the practice and experience of detoxification. Although the mucoid plaque removal phase, as presented by Arise & Shine, is a complete program requiring no previous experience or preparation, it can be intense, which is why I recommend some preparatory detoxification before trying it. After completing some of the steps in #21, wait a month or two, then start the mucoid plaque removal program.

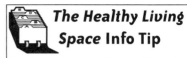

The Healthy Living Space Info Tip

For Arise & Shine Cleanse Thyself: Arise & Shine Herbal Products, P.O. Box 1439, Mt. Shasta, CA 96067; tel: 800-688-2444; fax (orders): 530-926-8866 or (main office) 530-926-0891; user support: 530-926-8867; website: www.ariseandshine.com.

HEALTHY LIVING SPACE DETOXIFIER #23
Purge the Parasites from Your Intestines

Mucoid plaque is not the only unsuspected and undesirable resident in the twenty-six feet of your intestines. Increasingly, Westerners have been beset by a variety of unwholesome intestinal parasites. Parasites are microorganisms that do not belong in the human intestines, but once there, disrupt the delicate balance of microflora, deplete the body nutritionally, and help to generate numerous symptoms and illnesses.

It was once thought that a Westerner needed to travel in exotic lands and be subjected to unsanitary conditions, notably food and water, before parasites became a worry. This is no longer the case. In 1993, for example, hundreds of thousands of residents of Milwaukee, Wisconsin, were parasitized by an outbreak of *Cryptosporidium parvum* through their muncipal tap water. The parasite produced diarrhea in many of those who drank the water. Also, it used to be the case that when someone mentioned the word "parasite," people would think of a tapeworm. This is a gross example of the problem, but it is now no longer the sole or even typical expression of intestinal parasitosis, as parasitic infection is clinically known.

Parasitic infestation does not have to be biologically dramatic, producing terrible symptoms and scores of deaths. In most cases, once inside the body, parasites act as silent invaders and relentless sickeners. Because conventional Western physicians still discount the growing prevalence of intestinal parasites in otherwise seemingly healthy individuals who have no record of travel to countries where parasitic infestation is likely, the problem tends to get overlooked. Fortunately, alternative medicine practitioners are starting to become aware of the problem and to develop effective protocols against parasites. To many laypersons, the idea of parasites in the intestines is bizarre, troubling, or unbelievable, but once you understand *how* they can get in, it begins to make more sense.

Parasitic infestation does not have to be biologically dramatic, producing terrible symptoms and scores of deaths. In most cases, once inside the body, parasites act as silent invaders and relentless sickeners.

The key idea that makes sense of parasitic infestation in the human intestines is a medical term called intestinal dysbiosis. This term refers to an imbalance in the microflora that populate the intestines. Here the community of living microorganisms—the natural ecology, the *bios*—is abnormal, disrupted, disturbed, or unfavorable (*dys*). Microscopic life in the intestines has become disordered— hence, disordered intestinal life. When a condition of intestinal dysbiosis exists, the healthy ratio between friendly and unfriendly, benign and pathogenic, microorganisms has shifted.

Bear in mind that the human body contains an estimated several trillion beneficial bacteria comprising over 400 species; all of these are necessary for health, nutrient assimilation, waste processing, and numerous other essential biological functions. In a healthy person, these friendly microorganisms (such as *Lactobacillus acidophilus* and *Bifidobacterium bifidum*) and unfriendly microorganisms (*Escherichia coli* and *Clostridium perfringens*) exist in an ecological balance in which the friendly ones predominate.

However, a number of factors arising from the typical Western lifestyle are shifting the balance the other way. Among these are overly acidic body conditions, chronic constipation or diarrhea, insufficient stomach acid, diminished output of pancreatic digestive enzymes, dietary/nutrient imbalances, the excessive use of antibiotics or consumption of animal products containing antibiotics and hormones, poor digestive function, and suboptimal immune function. In a sense, it is a two-way situation biologically: intestinal dysbiosis creates conditions favorable for parasites, and parasitic infestation (such as from contaminated tap water) can create intestinal dysbiosis.

In dysbiosis, the unfriendly or pathogenic bacteria dominate the intestine's beneficial microflora population. In the United States, the most common parasites, apart from head lice, are microscopic protozoans. These include *Giardia lambia,* a virulent form found in the contaminated waters of lakes, streams, and oceans, and a common cause of traveler's diarrhea; *Entamoeba histolytica*, which can cause dysentery and injure the liver and lungs; *Blastocystis hominus*, which is increasingly linked to acute and chronic illnesses; *Dientamoeba fragilis*, associated with diarrhea, abdominal pain, anal itching, and loose stools; and *Cryptosporidia*, which is particularly dangerous to those with compromised immune function.

Arthropod parasites include mites, fleas, and ticks. These in turn can carry smaller parasites that are also infectious to humans including, for example, the microorganism responsible for Lyme disease. Larger parasites, often referred to as "worms," include pinworms, tapeworms, roundworms, hookworms, filaria (thread-like worms that inhabit the blood and tissue), and flukes (which invade the liver). It is estimated that more than 300 kinds of parasites can live in the human body, where often they reside as what microbiologists call the "great masqueraders."

Parasites live off the life and nutrients of another living organism, usually to the host's detriment. Certain types can cause malabsorption of certain nutrients, such as iron, and vitamins A, B12, and beta-carotene. They begin a fermentation process, producing toxic byproducts, such as ammonia, amines, nitrosamines, phenols, cresols, indole, and skatole, which interfere with the normal elimination cycle. While they tend to stay in the intestines, parasites can also migrate elsewhere in the body—the blood, lymph, heart, liver, gallbladder, pancreas, spleen, eyes, and brain. They begin to eat us from the inside out, robbing our systems of nutrients and energy.

They generate numerous symptoms that are usually, and mistakenly, associated with other illnesses and never with a parasitic infestation. For example, if you have parasites, you may have headaches, back pain, energy loss, spaciness, vomiting, weight loss, colitis, gas, uncontrolled appetite, acne, bloating, diarrhea, constipation, irritable bowel syndrome, aches in the muscles and joints, anemia, allergies, depression, yeast infestations (*Candida albicans*), skin problems, sleep disturbances, chronic fatigue, and a weakening of the immune system response.

Dysbiosis is also considered a primary cause or major cofactor in the development of many health problems, such as PMS, rheumatoid arthritis, and cancer. You could easily be set to wandering through a labyrinth of unsuccessful treatments for each of the symptoms because the attending physicians never suspect—and therefore never treat—a parasite infestation. On the other hand, those practitioners aware of the principles and practices of natural medicine often report impressive clinical results when they accord the possibility of parasitic infestation some reality. "Over the years, I have seen a multitude of patients with symptoms of chronic fatigue, hypoglycemia, food allergy, spastic colon, and respiratory disorders get well when parasites were eradicated from their systems," states nutritionist Ann Louise Gittleman.[67]

How can you tell if you have parasites somewhere in your body and if they are slowly but steadily compromising your health? If you suspect contamination, a Comprehensive Digestive Stool Analysis and parasitology profile (explained in chapter 3) can be very helpful in confirming (or refuting) intestinal parasitosis and in identifying the species. However, sometimes a consideration of one's symptoms helps to clarify the situation.

In the course of presenting six case studies involving parasites, naturopathic physicians Silena Heron, N.D., and Eric Yarnell, N.D., both based in Sedona, Arizona, highlight some of the key presenting symptoms reported by their patients. One woman said she had a heavy feeling at the top of her stomach (where the esophagus empties into it), occasional aching there, and fatigue; a man had sporadic lightheadedness, vertigo, and hemorrhoidal irritation and pain that was worse for poor food choices; a woman had chronic constipation; a man had low energy, nausea, bloating, pain in his stomach and upper abdomen, and night sweats; a woman had lethargy, heat and light sensitivity, diarrhea, and occasional nausea; and a man had allergic rhinitis that was worse during certain seasons, flatulence, bloating, and abdominal pain. Only two of these individuals had been to an "exotic" land (India) where parasite infestation might have been expected.

Among the parasites identified in the preceding case histories were *Cryptosporidium* species, *Giardia lamblia*, *B. hominis*, *D. fragilis*, and *E. nana*. Also of interest was the discovery that in several of the patients there were low levels of secretory IgA. This is an immunoglobulin, one of the immune system's five such defensive and protective substances.[68] "In our experience, decreased gut IgA levels are common in patients who are infected with *Cryptosporidium* and may allow the organism to survive in such patients—this can happen despite normal systemic immune function," state Drs. Heron and Yarnell. They further state that low levels of this substance, which is supposed to protect the body against parasites, "have been shown to predispose people to contacting giardial [*Giardia lamblia*] infection."[69]

How common is the problem of parasite infection? Shockingly common, according to medical research. One New York physician found that out of 197 consecutively seen patients who complained of gastrointestinal symptoms, 95 of them (almost fifty percent) had giardiasis (an infestation of the parasite *Giardia lamblia*), and ninety-eight percent of these reported improvement of their complaints after completing a parasite elimination program.[70] This same physician discovered giardiasis in 61 of 218 patients who sought treatment for chronic fatigue; 42 of these patients experienced partial to complete recovery from their symptoms when treated for parasites.[71] Further, parasites were detected in 20% of 200,000 stool samples analyzed; most notable among the invaders were *Giardia lamblia* (in 7.2% of samples), *Entamoeba coli* and *Endolimax nana* (each 4.2%), *Blastocystis hominis* (2.6%), hookworm (1.5%), *Trichuris trichura* (1.2%), *Entamoeba histolytica* (0.9%), *Ascaris lumbricoides* (0.8%), and lesser amounts of other parasites.[72]

Additional evidence supports the conclusion that parasite infestation is a problem that affects all age groups and is both prevalent in but not limited to people living in Third World or developing countries. For example, stool samples were analyzed from 112 physically handicapped residents at a medical institution in Korea. In forty-two percent of the samples, evidence of at least two different parasites was found; three cases of *Trichuris trichiura* and one case of *Enterobius vermicularis* infection were found. Further, researchers found that 25% of the adults tested had an infection with *Entameoba coli*, 21% with *Endolimax nana*, 1.8% with either *E. histolytica* or *Iodameoba butschlii*, and 0.9% with *Giardia lamblia*. It's important to note that these men and women were institutionalized due to their physical handicap, not because of a reported or inexplicable gastrointestinal complaint; the discovery of the various parasites resident in their colons was a surprise to the doctors.[73]

How parasitized is the Third World? Korean researchers analyzed stool samples from sixty-four children and adolescents in Legaspi City in the Philippines. The overall parasitic infection rate among these children was seventy-eight percent; for those of this group living in rural areas it was ninety-two percent and for those living in cities, fifty-six percent. The most prevalent protozoan cysts were *Trichuris trichiura* (51%), *Ascaris lumbricoides* (40%), hookworm (23%), *Iodamoeba butschlii* (15%), *Endolimax nana* (14%), *Entamoeba coli* (9.4%), and *Giardia lamblia* (7.8%). Among the children, more than half (thirty-three) had multiple parasitic infections, and fifteen children had evidence of three or more parasites.[74]

Researchers at Yarmouk University in Irbid, Jordan, analyzed stool samples from 265 children under age five suffering from acute diarrhea. They found parasites in sixty-six percent of the children, one of which was common to fifty percent of the cases; fifteen percent of the children had multiple pathogens. Most notable among the pathogens (bacteria, viruses, and parasites) found were rotavirus (in 32% of cases), three types of *Escherichia coli* (5.7% to 12.8%), *Shigella spp.* and *Entamoeba histolytica* (4.9%), and Salmonella (4.5%).[75] In three provinces of Morocco, stool samples were studied from 1682 individuals representative of the urban and rural population. About sixty-six percent of samples from those living in rural areas and fifty percent of those from urban areas had parasites.[76] Further examples such as these can be found by the dozens.

Naturopathic physician Joseph Pizzorno, N.D., emphasizes that often parasitic infestations can be asymptomatic—you will not necessarily notice any overt or obvious symptoms of their presence. Such an infestation is most easily confirmed by seeing an actual worm of some kind on the stool or when "chronic inexplicable symptoms" develop after visiting a Third World country or being in close contact with someone who has, he says.

Dr. Pizzorno cites the case of a man who every month for ten years had a two- to three-day bout of an unexplained fever combined with a worsening of his existing symptoms of chronic fatigue and intestinal upset. He had spent over $10,000, fruitlessly, in consulting various specialists for an effective diagnosis and treatment. It turned out he had two kinds of parasites, and the periodicity of his symptoms was due to the reproductive cycle of these parasites, explains Dr. Pizzorno. When they reproduced—once every month during a two- to three-day period, the patient's symptoms were at their worst, exacerbated by the parasitic activities.[77]

In a related way, a person infested with parasites may seem to be asymptomatic only because the parasites are producing symptoms in an unexpected and therefore unexamined area, namely, personality changes. Researchers at Charles University in Prague in the Czech Republic found that among 230 women who had been diagnosed with acute toxoplasmosis (from the parasite *Toxoplasma gondii*) during the preceding 14 years, noticeable and quantifiable personality changes could be documented according to standard personality profile tests. In a related review of fifty-five younger women with latent toxoplasmosis, the scientists correlated various psychological factors with the length of the infection. "We suggest that the parasite induced the changes in personality profiles of the women because of our observation of an increasingly different personality profile over time between women with latent infection and controls."[78]

Berberine

Dr. Pizzorno stresses that generally parasites should not be self-treated and their removal requires expert medical care; however, in mild cases or as a preventative, he recommends goldenseal (1,500 mg, three times daily), whose constituent, berberine, can stop the growth of several types of common parasites.[79] There are a few other berberine-containing plants that are helpful against parasites: barberry, Oregon grape, and goldthread. When using these herbs, the dosage should be based on the berberine content at the recommended level of 25-50 mg, three times daily for adults, and for children, 5-10 mg of berberine per kilogram of body weight.[80]

Berberine has been shown to be effective in treating seven different types of parasites in children. In one study, 65 children (younger than 5) were given berberine tannate (25 mg every six hours) for relief of acute diarrhea caused by five different parasites; they responded better than children given conventional antibiotics.[81] In another study with 40 children (ages one to 10) infested with *Giardia*, the children received either berberine (5 mg per kilogram of body weight each day), the standard drug metronidazole (called Flagyl commercially, at the rate of 10 mg per kilogram of body weight each day), or a placebo of vitamin B.

Six days later, forty-eight percent of the children who took berberine were free of parasitic symptoms, and sixty-eight percent of these were free of all signs of *Giardia*, based on their stool samples. Thirty-three percent of the children who took the standard drug were free of symptoms, and the stools of all were free of *Giardia*. Berberine was more effective in relieving symptoms at half the dose of metronidazole, but was less effective than it in removing the parasites from the body, the scientists concluded.[82] In a third study involving 200 adults with acute diarrhea, those who had berberine with antibiotics recovered more quickly than those who had the antibiotic treatment alone.[83]

Parasite Purge Formula

Based on their extensive review of the scientific data supporting the herbal constituents involved, Drs. Heron and Yarnell recommend this liquid herbal blend for treatment of parasites. (While their protocol can be done on one's own, it is prudent to do it under the supervision of a qualified health-care practitioner.) Drs. Heron and Yarnell suggest mixing two parts each of wormseed (Epazote), Jamaican guassia, and Sweet Annie with one and one-half parts of gentian; one part each of garlic, black walnut, Oregon grape, ginger, male fern, tansy, and wormwood; and one-half parts each of greater celandine, anise, and Turkey rhubarb.

They recommend taking one teaspoonful of the mixture three times daily until the problem has cleared up. In addition, they advise taking grapefruit seed extract (ten drops three times daily, mixed in water); the commercially prepared antiparasite herbal tannate formulas Tanalbit (six capsules, three times daily) or Viracin (two capsules, three times daily), and garlic (four fresh cloves, two to three times daily, or extract at the rate of 5,000 mcg of allicin per capsule and eight capsules, two to three times daily).

The active ingredients of Tanalbit are plant tannins, astringent natural substances that attach themselves to the cells of fungi, yeasts, and bacteria and prevent them from metabolizing and colonizing, and ultimately cause them to die. Viracin is similar but a different strength, and contains extracts of Norwegian maple fruit, Babul bark, and wild rhubarb. Grapefruit Seed Extract (commercially available as Citricidal and made from the bioflavonoids [vitamin C helpers] found in grapefruit seed and pulp) is regarded to be effective against a broad spectrum of pathogenic microorganisms. It is also regaled as a general purpose disinfectant, dental rinse, and skin cleanser.

Over the course of two to four weeks, slowly build the daily dose of these substances to the amount above, Drs. Heron and Yarnell recommend. Then continue with these doses (regarded as the maximum) for about two months, they say. The substances should not be taken with food, and if diarrhea develops or the Herxheimer reaction sets in (due to parasitic die-off inside the body), take one level teaspoon of bentonite once daily. Drs. Heron and Yarnell also suggest that during and after the program you should take some form of probiotics, or "friendly" bacteria, such as *Lactobacillus acidophilus*, discussed below, as a way of replenishing beneficial bacteria in the intestines.

Bitter Melon

This is a bitter-tasting cucumber-like green vegetable (*Momordica charantia*) common to Asian cooking and Ayurvedic and Chinese medicine that can be used as a gentle food-based vermifuge, or agent against intestinal parasites. The fruit is best described as an oblong warty-looking gourd, although it tastes better than it looks. Traditionally, the food is used as, among many other things, a treatment for worms and parasites; in Western herbal medicine, bitter melon is increasingly used in the treatment of diabetes, hypoglycemia, colds, flus, HIV and other viruses, and psoriasis.

Scientific research is beginning to substantiate the folk claims for the antihelmintic (worm-killing) actions of this fruit. An herbal preparation made from bitter melon was more effective in treating infestations of *Ascaridia galli* worms in birds than the conventional drug.[84] Bitter melon is also effective against infectious diseases transmitted by microorganisms. Bolivian researchers reported that extracts of bitter melon were "moderately active" against an antibiotic-resistant strain of malaria.[85] Puerto Rican scientists found that out of fifty plants tested for activity against tuberculosis-producing microorganisms (*Mycobacterium smegmatis*), bitter melon was one of six that possessed "inhibitory capacity."[86]

Bitter melon has also been shown to improve factors necessary for liver detoxification, namely, significantly increasing the levels of glutathione and acid-soluble sulfhydryl, two substances crucial to the liver's two-phase detoxification pathways (see chapter 2).[87] Finally, Italian researchers have determined that bitter melon, in addition to other herbs used in Ayurveda, contains "antioxidant principles that can explain and justify their use in traditional medicine in the past as well as the present."[88] This would suggest bitter melon is effective against free radicals, such as the metabolites or toxic byproducts of parasites or the intestines' action against them.

One general antiparasite recommendation is to eat two bitter melons (cooked) daily for about ten days. Bitter melon is available in Asian food stores and in dry form as an herbal capsule.

Pumpkin Seeds

Another vermifuge folk remedy that is gaining scientific acceptance is the ingestion of pumpkin seeds, derived from autumn and crookneck squash and the Canada pumpkin. This treatment is believed to rid the body of intestinal parasites, especially roundworms and tapeworms. A typical regimen is three doses of 20-150 grams of seeds; other research shows that

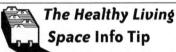

The Healthy Living Space Info Tip

For Tanalbit and Viracin, contact:
Scientific Consulting Service,
1972 Republic,
San Leandro, CA 94577;
tel: 800-333-7414 or 510-632-2370;
fax: 510-632-8561;
e-mail: intensivenutrition@pacbell.net;
website: www.intensivenutrition.com.

For Citricidal:
Nutriteam,
P.O. Box 71,
Ripton, VT 05766;
tel: 800-785-9791 or 802-388-0661;
fax: 815-377-2198;
e-mail: support@gfex.com;
website: www.nutriteam.com.

chewing twelve pumpkin seeds (sometimes in combination with Rangoon creeper fruit seeds, *Quisqualis indicae*) in the morning on an empty stomach for two weeks can help the intestines purge themselves of parasites. The treatment is believed to paralyze the parasites, causing them to loosen their grasp within the intestines and enabling their elimination from the body. An amino acid called cucurbitin, found in pumpkin seeds, is believed responsible for the worm-expelling effects.[89]

HEALTHY LIVING SPACE DETOXIFIER #24
Get Proactive with Probiotics—
Plant Food for the Intestines

Probiotics is a term used earlier in this chapter to denote the friendly, beneficial bacteria, or microflora, that inhabit—or ought to inhabit—your intestines. They are *pro*biotics in that they support and enhance the natural life functions performed by the intestines on behalf of the life of the body.

Among the two most prominent (and researched) probiotics are *Lactobacillus acidophilus* and *Bifidobacterium bifidum*. Others include *B. longum*, a primary resident of the large intestine, where it protects this organ from invading yeasts and bacteria, detoxifies the bile, and helps make B vitamins; *B. infantis*, the most prevalent probiotic in the intestines of infants; and *Streptococcus thermophilus* and *L. bulgaricus*, which are commonly found in yogurt and, although only transiently present in the intestines, produce lactic acid—encouraging the growth of other probiotics—and bacteriocins, natural antibiotic-like substances that kill pathogens. Other probiotics include *L. casei*, *L. plantarum*, *L. sporogenes*, *L. brevis*, and *Saccharomyces boulardii*.

Overly acidic bodily conditions, chronic constipation or diarrhea, dietary imbalances, consumption of highly processed foods, and the excessive use of antibiotics and hormonal drugs can interfere with probiotic function and even reduce the number of these microbes, setting up conditions for illness. One of the factors contributing to slow transit time is a deficiency of friendly bacteria which otherwise stimulate peristalsis.

At the same time, if you do a deliberate intestinal cleansing program, you must replenish your intestines' supply of friendly bacteria. Some inadvertently get flushed out of the system;

others get used up in the struggle to restore proper intestinal microfloral balance; and some you may have been deficient in for a long time due to untreated toxicity.

Recolonizing your intestines with a new population of probiotics is a bit like giving your lawn plant food to make the grass grow better. Introducing probiotics into the intestines enables them to perform their functions better, to counteract long-term antibiotic damage, and retune their immune activities. Think of recolonizing the intestines as a preventive measure against possible future illness. The body of scientific evidence supporting the benefits of *L. acidophilus* is large and irrefutable, as this brief overview will show.

If you do a deliberate intestinal cleansing program, you must replenish your intestines' supply of friendly bacteria. Some inadvertently get flushed out of the system; others get used up in the struggle to restore proper intestinal microfloral balance; and some you may have been deficient in for a long time due to untreated toxicity.

L. acidophilus is effective in inhibiting the growth of *Helicobacter pylori*, a pathogen believed to be the cause of acid-peptic disease of the stomach. In fact, it stopped the growth of seven different strains of *C. pylori* recovered from human gastrointestinal tracts.[90] Several strains of acidophilus had a "bacteriostatic" (bacteria-killing or suppressing) effect against the spoilage pathogen *Listeria monocytogenes* in dairy milk.[91]

Related to this benefit is the proven ability of *L. acidophilus* to act as a powerful antioxidant. It can inhibit the peroxidation of linoleic acid (the process by which this essential fatty acid is made into a damaging free radical) by twenty-eight percent to forty-eight percent; it can scavenge between twenty-one percent and fifty-two percent of three dangerous free radicals present in cells; and it has a "high inhibitory effect" against a particular cell-killing chemical, reducing its activities by fifty percent. Even better, *Bifidobacterium longum* demonstrated all these abilities, but was able to curtail ninety percent of the activity of the cell-killing chemical.[92]

L. acidophilus can also inhibit the growth of coliform bacteria (such as *Escherichia coli*, the food-borne pathogen) and reduce their existing populations, which makes it highly serviceable clinically for people suffering from gastrointestinal distress caused by coliforms.[93] A review of forty-nine studies on probiotics showed consistently that *L. acidophilus* intake can shorten the duration of diarrhea produced by rotavirus infection by one day.[94] *Lactobacillus* also exerts a protective effect against induced colon tumors (in rats), reducing the incidence by ten percent to twenty-five percent (depending on the strain of *Lactobacillus*), and reducing the tumor mass (or general size of the cancer that emerged).[95]

Giving infants pure cultures of *L. acidophilus* prevents "dysbacteriosis" (intestinal dysbiosis, or the state of being overrun by pathogenic bacteria, notably *Staphylococcus aureus*), thereby reducing the incidence of disease in very young children (in their first year) and improving the overall health and immune vitality of the gastrointestinal tract; acidophilus supplementation may contribute to resistance to potential food allergens in later life.[96] In a trial, *L. acidophilus* given to sixty infants (orally and dabbed in the nose), resulted in sixty percent of the infants leaving the maternity home with "normally formed intestinal microflora"; additionally, eighty percent had normally formed nasal microflora and seventy percent normal skin microflora, attesting to the bacteria's ability to reduce opportunistic pathogens in the three areas.[97] Dietary supplementation with three strains of *Lactobacillus* (in a mice study) also led to an enhancement of several key elements of natural and acquired immunity, such as the activity of white blood cells and the generation of immune cells by the spleen.[98]

It is also impressive to note that many of the friendly bacteria produce viable natural antibiotics in the colon, all of which have been studied by scientists. For example, *Bifidobacterium bifidum* produces bifidin; *L. acidophilus* produces acidolin, acidophilin, lactobacillin, and lactocidin; *L. brevis* makes lactobrevin; *L. bulgaricus* produces bulgarican; and *Streptococcus lactis* makes nisin. Once produced, these natural antibiotics do not so much destroy harmful bacteria, but make it impossible for them to flourish in the colon. Inhibition is better than destruction because the latter would leave toxic debris in the colon, thereby contributing to toxicity. Bulgarican and acidophilin are "exceedingly active against a wide variety of organisms," including pathogens, researchers have reported.[99]

So the case for taking *L. acidophilus* and related strains of friendly bacteria is strong, but how best to ingest it? You would think fresh unsugared yogurt would be ideal, but it actually is not because in most instances it primarily contains *L. bulgaricus* and *S. thermophilus*, friendly bacteria that only *temporarily* inhabit the intestines. This means their populations will die off after a short time in the colon. Another problem to overcome is the stomach. You need to get the friendly bacteria alive, active, and intact into your intestines, past the stomach's powerful digestive apparatus. The best way to ensure this is to use enteric-coated *L. acidophilus* capsules, which means they will not be digested until they reach the intestines.[100]

It's advisable to take a probiotic supplement during the active detoxification program, as a complement to the liver and intestinal cleansing. But it is better to take it *after* the intestinal cleansing substances—that is, when you have finished that phase of the detoxification program. The regular intake of friendly bacteria after the program is also a good idea, at least for a month or so, because it offers broad-spectrum protection and disease prevention in the same way as vitamin C.

In times of illness or medical treatment, taking *L. acidophilus* can be beneficial, especially if you are taking antibiotics or have recently done so. It can also be beneficial if you use birth control pills or steroids (as these deplete intestinal probiotics); if you have chronic constipation, a yeast infection, or bacterial vaginitis; if you have a gastrointestinal infection or inflammation; or if you are lactose intolerant (cannot digest milk sugar). As a regular dosage, 3 to 7 billion organisms (primarily *L. acidophilus* and *B. bifidus*) daily—most brands of probiotics specify their estimated organism count—is advised.[101]

There are many brands and formulations of friendly bacteria now on the market, giving consumers many choices. To give you an idea of what is out there, here are two offerings that exhibit interesting features. First, Culturelle, according to its manufacturer, contains 20 billion live and active cells (*L. acidophilus*) per capsule, and it's the same strain as appears in the human intestines, making it the "ideal probiotic." It is capable of surviving stomach and small intestine digestion to arrive in the colon where it implants itself on the cell walls and starts colonizing. Second, Jarro-Dophilus combines six species of friendly bacteria, including four species of *Lactobacillus* and two of *Bifidobacteria*. According to the manufacturer, each of the species colonizes its "own separate regional niche" in the colon, based on appropriate biochemical factors. Each capsule contains an estimated 3.36 billion organisms of the six species specified.

HEALTHY LIVING SPACE DETOXIFIER #25
Fertilize Your Bifidobacteria with Prebiotics

The idea of prebiotics was developed in Japan in the 1980s around the concept of introducing nutrients that directly feed the friendly bacteria already in place in the intestines, mostly *Bifidobacteria* and *Lactobacilli*. In effect, prebiotics supply the essential building blocks—the nutrient foreground, if you will—for beneficial intestinal bacteria.

Foremost among the prebiotics are natural carbohydrates called fructo-oligosaccharides, or FOS for short. FOS occurs naturally in foods such as garlic, honey, Jerusalem artichokes, soybeans, burdock, chicory root, asparagus, banana, rye, barley, tomato, onions, and triticale, but in minute amounts, too minimal to be of much use therapeutically. In fact, you would have to eat an estimated 429 garlic cloves to derive the same FOS as you get from FOS in supplement form. Made by fermenting sucrose with a fungus called *Aspergillus niger*, FOS (called neosugar) is now found in over 500 commercial foods in Japan as a beneficial, slightly sweet nutritional additive.

It's interesting to note that in the infant gastrointestinal tract, *Bifidobacteria* represent an estimated ninety-five percent to ninety-nine percent of all friendly bacteria, but this amount declines with age. Once introduced into the intestines, FOS, available as a white powder, acts as a kind of fertilizer that selectively feeds and nurtures the friendly bacteria so that their numbers will increase. FOS also helps lower the intestinal pH (the ratio of acidity and alkalinity) to a slightly more acidic condition so that the friendly bacteria will thrive, and the pathogenic bacteria will not.

According to information provided by the primary manufacturer, GTC Nutrition Company, FOS has been shown to increase the total count of beneficial bacteria by five to ten times after supplementation for two to four weeks. Other benefits attributed to FOS include relief from diarrhea and constipation, the promotion of bowel regularity, lowering of cholesterol and blood pressure, control of blood sugar levels, enhancement of immune function, improved B-vitamin synthesis and calcium absorption, better digestion of dairy milk proteins, and an easing of the liver's toxic burden.[102]

GTC Nutrition puts forward at least fifteen scientific studies supporting the major claims that FOS (and friendly bacteria in general) assists and protects the immune system, protects the body against the encroachment of pathogenic and putrefactive bacteria such as *E. coli* and *Clostridium* that would otherwise produce diarrhea and other intestinal disturbances, and promotes better health. A University of Illinois study showed that fermentable fiber—the study used NutraFlora as a food source—promotes the growth of beneficial intestinal organisms that retard the colonization by the pathogen *Clostridium difficile*. In fact, the scientists could find "no culturable counts" of *C. difficile* after the intestines had been "modified" by the introduction of FOS.[103] Another study examined the effect on twelve healthy adults of supplementing the diet for 42 days with 4 g of FOS daily. They found that the FOS altered the fecal microflora in a beneficial way by decreasing the (undesirable) activities of certain enzymes by seventy-five percent to ninety percent, thereby protecting the colon.[104]

FOS is not without its critics, however. It is not digestible in the mouth or small intestine, but only in the colon, where it could alter that organ's metabolic function; it can stimulate the growth of a few unfriendly microorganisms, such as *Klebsiella*; it is specific to probiotic strain and species, not to all beneficial bacteria; and if you have a yeast infection (*Candida albicans*), as a sugar, it will undesirably feed the yeast.[105]

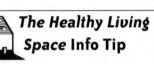

CHAPTER 6

Whole-Body Cleansing Routines:

Extending the Detoxification into Everyday Activities

Cleansing the liver and intestines represents the intensive phase of self-care detoxification. It is something you need do only once or twice yearly. But during the rest of the year, there are gentler but equally beneficial detoxification activities you can pursue to reinforce, and even deepen, the positive effects you obtained from the liver and intestinal cleansing.

These additional, regular cleansing routines tend to provide detoxification benefits for the entire body. It's not that liver and intestinal cleanses only benefit those organs; of course their effect is body-wide, but their application is organ specific. In the exercises outlined in this chapter, the application itself encompasses the entire body. For example, in this chapter we'll review the whole-body benefits of stimulating the lymphatic system by bouncing on a trampoline, dry skin brushing, getting regular exercise, taking a sauna, or enjoying an herbal detoxification bath. You may easily engage in any or all of these activities throughout the year as part of a continuing detoxification program—as new components of an evolving healthy lifestyle.

HEALTHY LIVING SPACE DETOXIFIER #26
Bounce on a Trampoline to
Improve Your Lymphatic Drainage

The human body has another detoxification system of equal importance to the liver and intestines in effecting removal of toxic substances. It's called the lymphatic system, but it doesn't get the attention it deserves from conventional medicine, and even in some areas of alternative medicine, it is a whole-body cleansing system that is underemphasized.

The lymphatic system consists of lymph fluid and the structures such as vessels, ducts, and nodes involved in transporting it from tissues to the bloodstream. Lymph fluid occupies the space between the body's cells and contains plasma proteins, foreign particles, and cellular waste. Lymph nodes are clusters of immune tissue that work as filters or "inspection stations" for detecting and removing foreign and potentially harmful substances in the lymph fluid (see figure 6-1).

While the body has hundreds of lymph nodes (more than 500), they are mostly clustered in the neck, armpits, chest, groin, and abdomen. The lymph nodes contain different types of scavenger cells that destroy toxic substances. The tonsils, for example, are part of the lymphatic system; so are the adenoids, the thymus gland (behind the sternum in the chest), the spleen (at the bottom of the left rib cage), the appendix, and Peyer's patches in the small intestine. The familiar sensation of having "swollen glands" in the throat refers to congested lymph nodes in that area of the body. Regrettably, conventional medicine regards the tonsils, adenoids, and appendix as largely expendable (surgically removable without physiological consequence), not understanding that these structures are key players in the body's lymphatic drainage system.

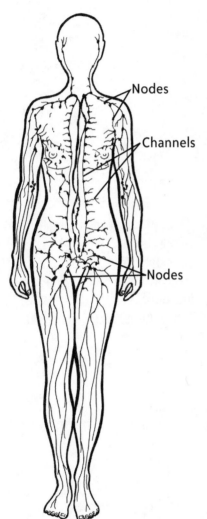

Figure 6-1. The Lymphatic System

Nodes

Channels

Nodes

The essential function of the lymphatic system (see figure 6-1) is twofold: to provide immune defense, and to maintain the fluid balance in the intracellular environment. For example, if the system didn't collect this interstitial fluid (the fluid between cells which leaks out of capillaries), the body's tissues would swell up dangerously. The lymphatic system is the body's master drain, collecting and filtering the lymph fluid and conveying it to the bloodstream, thereby clearing waste products and cellular debris from the tissues. But it also delivers food nutrients and oxygen to the cells, fulfilling its unique role as a connecting medium between the body's cells and tissues and the arteries, veins, and capillaries of the cardiovascular system.

As a fluid, lymph consists of water, inorganic mineral salts, and white blood cells (lymphocytes). Among its many cleansing, immunological, and defense activities, the lymph removes excess proteins resulting from a number of sources (such as dead cells and complexes of antigens and antibodies that form in an allergic reaction); collects protein wastes from the fluids in the regions between cells; removes foreign material and environmental toxins from the tissues; and maintains the fluid balance in body's web of connective tissue.

As with the intestines, if the lymphatic system does not work optimally, not only does it help create a condition of vulnerability to disease, it impedes your body's ability to heal itself from the disease.

Lymph system activity increases during illness (such as the flu) when the nodes (particularly at the throat) visibly swell with collected waste products. Some doctors have likened the lymphatic system to the "metabolic garbage can" of the body. The nodes and fluid collect the body's dead cells, metabolic wastes, pathogenic bacteria, toxins, and other foreign or injurious substances and remove them from circulation. It is a parallel and complementary detoxification track to the liver-intestines.

On the other hand, the lymphatic system, if it is clogged, dysfunctional, or sluggish, can be a health problem, participating in and slowly contributing to a condition of body-wide toxicity. As with the intestines, if the lymphatic system does not work optimally, not only does it help create a condition of vulnerability to disease, it impedes your body's ability to heal itself from the disease. Inadequate lymph flow, or a generally stagnated lymphatic system, has been correlated with numerous health problems, such as bursitis in the shoulders, joint stiffness, bunions, spasms in the soft tissues, bad breath, body odor, skin that is dry and flaky, lethargy, depression, and cancer. When the lymphatic system is egregiously blocked, you get the disfiguring disability called lymphedema, in which certain lymph nodes and channels get blocked and filled with water and literally balloon out to grotesque proportions.

In effect, the lymphatic system is the beginning and end of all disease, of aging, and *premature* aging, and of general toxicity or toxemia. Typically, as people age, they exercise less; one of the results is that lymph circulation slows down. Proteins and debris do not get flushed out by regular exercise and tend to accumulate in the nodes. The lymph, which should be clear, becomes cloudy and thick, changing its consistency from that of milk to yogurt then cottage cheese, and it begins to stagnate.

Thickened, stagnant lymph saturated with toxic wastes is an ideal setup for many illnesses, including cancer. "When the collecting terminals [lymph nodes] become blocked, it's like a bottleneck: lymph starts backing up in the system creating a toxic, oxygen-deprived environment conducive to degeneration."[1] The lymphatic system can store stagnant, toxic lymph fluid just as the intestines store old fecal matter; but just because storage is possible does not mean it's physiologically desirable. It's not.

To fulfill its function as a detoxification system, the lymphatic system needs a little help from the "user." It does not have a pump—like the heart in the circulating system or peristalsis in the intestines—to move the fluid. The fluid does flow on its own, at the average slow rate of 125 ml/hour, but this is mostly uphill, that is, against gravity. The natural slow movement of lymph is facilitated by breathing and skeletal muscle contractions.

There are three manual ways to get the lymph moving faster from the tissues into the blood: muscular contraction from movement and exercise; gravitational pressure; and internal massage of the lymph ducts. Lymph fluid movement is dependent on the body as a whole moving; in practical terms, that means when we exercise—run, walk, jump, swim, or move about with some degree of vigor—then the lymphatic system is primed and starts moving. One of the best ways (and one that is well-researched medically) to decongest the lymph nodes and move the lymph is to jump, and one of the easiest ways to jump is on a trampoline.

You don't need a gymnasium-grade trampoline to move the lymph. Smaller versions called mini-trampolines or rebounders are available and deliver the same results with less danger of injury from falling off. Typically, a rebounder is about three feet in diameter and about six to eight inches off the floor. Rebounding changes the gravitational forces affecting the body—at the height of the bounce you are for a moment free of gravity; when you land, you hit the trampoline with twice the force of gravity—thereby facilitating greater blood flow.

In fact, researchers have found that this twice-gravity bounce affects every muscle and cell in the body. It delivers gravitational pressure and an internal massage to the valves of the lymph ducts, enhancing their function. Rebounding also provides a gentle massage of the spinal column through its low-impact bouncing. This in turn enhances the amount of waste products flushed out of cells into the lymph and the movement of the lymph itself to its penultimate destination in the intestines and final excretion. Somehow exercise makes the lymph nodes expand and the flow of lymph becomes active; when you are not exercising, or remain physically inactive for a long time, the lymph flow becomes sluggish.

Rebounding is quintessentially a lymphatic exercise, and it satisfies all three physical requirements cited above needed to move the lymph. "The bouncing motion effectively moves and recycles the lymph and the entire blood supply through the circulatory system many times during the course of the rebounding session."[2]

Medical research suggests that during vigorous exercise, such as rebounding, lymph flow rate can increase by as much as fourteen times the resting state.[3] Further, if a 150-pound man exercised for one hour on a rebounder, he would burn 410 calories compared to only 355 calories if he spent that hour running approximately five miles. In fact, for similar levels of oxygen intake and heart rate, the "magnitude of the biomechanical stimulation is greater with jumping on a trampoline than with running," researchers concluded in 1980 based on a study of eight exercising males.[4] The key point is that by increasing your lymph flow, you are moving toxins out of your body that much faster.

Medical research shows that rebounding has numerous health benefits, extending beyond the biomechanical stimulation of lymphatic flow. Rebounding benefits the heart and blood circulation, it can slow the effects of aging, revitalize vision, reduce stress, and help children with cystic fibrosis and learning disabilities. One medical authority has cited thirty health benefits. Rebounding increases the capacity for respiration (oxygen intake); reduces arterial pressure during exertion; reduces the time blood pressure remains abnormal after extreme exertion; strengthens the red bone marrow's ability to produce red blood cells; promotes body growth and repair; stimulates metabolism; enhances digestion and the elimination processes; affords deeper relaxation and easier sleep; and produces better mental performance and keener learning abilities.[5]

If a practice has therapeutic benefits in helping to reduce or reverse a health problem, it is logical to assume it may produce positive gains in people who don't have those problems. In other words, if rebounding helps those with cognitive deficits, it may enhance the brain function of those who are more or less healthy and normal. For example, researchers writing in the medical journal *Rehabilitation* reported that trampoline therapy "is a useful part" in rehabilitating brain-injured children and adolescents (especially with partial brain paralysis, or hemiparesis) and that it improves standing balance and movement coordination.[6]

A Norwegian study showed that exercising on a rebounder for almost two hours weekly for two months produced positive improvements for children with cystic fibrosis. In this disease, the ducts in the pancreas, sweat glands, and lungs get clogged with thick mucus and cannot work properly. Two children in this study with the most serious lung congestion were able to significantly increase their oxygen intake as a result of rebounding.[7]

The recommendation for rebounding is simple: *bounce often*. How long? The American Institute of Reboundology in Orem, Utah, recommends a forty-minute moderate workout at least three times weekly. Rebounders for home use are available in the price range of $200 to $300.

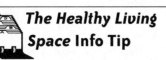

The Healthy Living Space Info Tip

For more information about rebounding and information about the ReboundAIR rebounder, contact: American Institute of Reboundology, 1240 East 800 North, Orem, UT 84097; tel: 888-464-5867 or 801-377-0570; fax: 801-377-0655; website: www.healthbounce.com.

For Needak Soft-Bounce rebounder: Needak Manufacturing, P.O. Box 776, O'Neill, NE 68763; tel: 800-232-5762 or 402-336-4083; fax: 402-336-4941; e-mail: needak@inetnebr.com; website: www.needakmfg.com.

HEALTHY LIVING SPACE DETOXIFIER #27
Dry Skin Brushing —Tone Up Your
Body's Largest Elimination Organ

It sounds a bit peculiar, but brushing your skin with a dry brush can help move the lymph and aid the body in detoxifying through the skin. Don't overlook the benefits of perspiration, or heavy sweating. Throughout a day the skin can eliminate an estimated pound of wastes and toxic products in the form of perspiration through the skin, the body's largest eliminative organ, sometimes dubbed the third kidney. As discussed in chapter 2, the skin can also absorb substances from the environment— helpful substances such as vitamin D, and toxic ones such as chlorine.

Dry skin brushing appears to work partly through gently massaging many of acupuncture's treatment nodes across the body's surface. These nodes are little areas of heightened vital energy (or qi) along the numerous energy channels, or meridians. These nodes are believed to correspond, by way of subtle energy connections, with various organs and organ systems throughout the body.

So by applying friction to these points (with a brush against the skin), energy is stimulated to move from the node to the organ in question, be it the liver, intestines, or lymphatic system. In its most elementary sense, dry skin brushing opens the skin's many pores, allowing it to "breathe," but it also increases blood flow. This helps to draw out stored wastes and toxic substances that otherwise result in a buildup of cellulite (fat deposits close to the skin surface, especially prevalent in the legs, thighs, and buttocks).

Dry skin brushing also encourages lymph fluid to move through the channels to the central place in the chest where it dumps into the blood circulation system, thereby dumping its collected toxins and waste products. Other benefits include the following: nerve endings are stimulated, thereby rejuvenating the entire nervous system; the skin is better toned so it can more efficiently purge itself of toxins; blood circulation improves, facilitating better toxic substance collection and removal; stress is reduced; tissue metabolism is improved, reducing fatigue; the amount of cellulite (toxic material stored in the body's fat cells) is reduced; dead layers of the skin are removed, opening pores.

Recommendation: Use a soft natural vegetable fiber bristle brush with a wooden handle and *gently* brush all the surfaces of your body for about five to ten minutes daily, until the skin appears rosy. Some doctors suggest brushing the skin daily for three months then cutting back to twice weekly as a standard ongoing detoxification routine. Make sure your skin is dry, which means, do the exercise before your morning shower, not after. Begin at your feet and brush vigorously in a circular fashion, moving slowly up the front of your body to the lower neck, then proceed down the back side to the feet again. Try to brush *toward* the sternum throughout the exercise. Brush from the hands up the arms to the shoulders. Wash and sanitize the brush every several weeks, because it will accumulate dead material from the skin. You might do the dry skin brushing immediately before a hot shower or a bath.

Scrubbing with Sea Salt

This complementary, whole-body cleansing scrub is recommended by detoxification expert Helene Silver. Silver says to put four to five handfuls of 100% sea salt in a plastic container; into another container, pour a quart of very hot water. Stand or sit in an empty bathtub and, using a sponge in one hand, daub parts of your body, such as your arm, your leg, and your abdomen with the hot water. Then use your other hand to apply the dry sea salt to those lightly moistened areas, rubbing it in with circular motions.

The goal is cover your entire body with the salt (avoid the genitals, as the salt will sting and irritate the urethra). Then take the dry skin brush and gently massage the salt into the skin. Relax for ten minutes with the salt in place until your skin begins to tingle. "As the salt dries, it is drawing the toxins out of your skin," says Silver. Finally, rinse off all the salt under the shower, using first hot then cold water.[8]

Epsom Salt and Cider Vinegar Scrub

This variation is part dry skin brushing and part detoxification bath, as suggested by iridologist-physician Farida Sharan, M.D. Add one tablespoon of an organic vegetable oil to one cup of dry Epsom salts in a plastic container. Rub the salt-oil mixture all over your skin while you stand in the bathtub. In this instance, the tub should already be filled with hot bath water, to which you've added one cup of apple cider vinegar.

The salt-oil rubbing helps the skin shed its old dead cells and the toxins they carry, leaving the skin smooth and soft, says Dr. Sharan. As you scrub, the salt will fall off your body into the tub. When you have finished the rub, lie down in the hot water and soak for thirty minutes; apply cold washcloths to your forehead if you get too hot. Complete the detoxification routine with a three-minute cold shower. Dr. Sharan adds that it is useful to drink herbal teas that encourage perspiration, such as yarrow, sage, catnip, pleurisy root, peppermint, or spearmint—ideally about thirty minutes before your bath.[9]

HEALTHY LIVING SPACE DETOXIFIER #28
Exercise Regularly to Enhance Blood Circulation and Toxin Removal

Seemingly all health authorities are constantly urging us to move, to be physically active, to exercise. Usually the reason given is better heart performance, longevity, prevention of muscular stagnation, even the joy of movement. All of these reasons are medically valid, yet there is an additional benefit to regular exercise. It is one of the easiest but most comprehensive forms of body-wide detoxification you can perform. The means are simple: walk, run, swim, play tennis, climb, ski, paddle, roller blade, ice skate, jump rope, bicycle, row, dance, bounce on a trampoline, stride on a treadmill.

Personally, I like to walk. Writers tend to sit around a lot, and sometimes, when the ideas and words are flowing well, it is easy to convince yourself not to move at all. So I walk two miles a day perhaps five to six days a week. Nothing too athletic, just a brisk, comfortable pace in which I feel muscles get stretched and the lungs work a little harder. In the summer, I supplement this with swimming in a nearby lake; again, nothing too fancy or professionally athletic here, just some informal laps with whatever swimming stroke I feel like or remember. What is important is not so much the vigor with which you exercise or even the duration (although research suggests that you need a minimum of twenty minutes), but the *regularity* with which you provide this benefit to your body.

When exercising, you breathe more oxygen, expand your lungs, stretch and work your muscles, and get your blood moving and your heart rate elevated, and here is the detoxification key. When you move your body during exercise, it stimulates the blood and lymph circulation to flow better, more vigorously, to catch up on unfinished or postponed business, to finally dump those protein wastes or collect the byproducts of those toxins you ingested last week, or last year, or deliver more life-supporting oxygen to the cells so they can continue detoxifying themselves.

When you move your body during exercise, it stimulates the blood and lymph circulation to flow better, more vigorously, to catch up on unfinished or postponed business, to finally dump those protein wastes or collect the byproducts of those toxins you ingested last week, or last year, or deliver more life-supporting oxygen to the cells so they can continue detoxifying themselves.

Exercising enhances your body's circulation of vital nutrients and the flushing out and elimination of stored toxins from the cells. It also stimulates the peristaltic rhythm in your intestines, encouraging this organ to move its contents along more quickly, thereby reducing bowel transit time and potential constipation. Further, some pathogenic organisms are anaerobic, which means they don't use oxygen to survive and can't exist in an oxygen-rich environment. Breathing more means oxygenating your cells, which in turn means suffocating the non-oxygen-breathing microorganisms. And don't overlook the obvious here: when you exercise you are likely to perspire, and the sweat itself carries toxins out with it through the skin.

These considerations are of vital importance during the intensive detoxification phase outlined in chapter 5, when your cells are dumping, collecting, and eliminating toxins at a rate far beyond normal. Exercise and physical movement will greatly facilitate toxin removal at a time when your body most needs it. Also, the exercise helps clear your head; during detoxification, old emotions and stray, scattered, or simply weird thoughts arise like vapors in your mind, and physical movement, even as simple as walking, helps blow the obnoxious mists out of your head.

The other obvious benefit to regular exercise is weight reduction or ideal weight maintenance. The exercise stimulates the removal or utilization of excess body fat stored in the fatty tissues. Remember that the body's fat reserves are its primary storage site for toxins, so if you start reducing body fat, you are also dumping toxins. If you are in your forties, you may have noticed that your weight is now much more sensitive to excesses or deficiencies in your diet or to the proportion of time during which you are luxuriously sedentary. In other words, if you are of this age, or older, you can't get away with overeating, indulging, or lounging about the way you used to. You will probably start putting on weight and your metabolic, digestive, and eliminative processes may start slowing down noticeably.

Scientific studies have shown that even though strenuous aerobic exercise in a person new to this kind of exertion can produce free radical activity and possible muscle injury as a result of this oxidative damage, the same exercise strengthens your body's ability to withstand free radical activity. Exercise fortifies your body's antioxidant defense system; you can gain even more benefits from this natural positive activity by taking vitamins C and E as daily supplements. These are both antioxidants (free radical fighters). Studies show that both these vitamins counteract whatever free radicals are produced during exercise, and that they have other specific benefits for the immune system and its specialized defense cells.[10]

The good news about the "exercise paradox," as fitness experts call it, is that when your body reaches the plateau of being used to the exercise you are doing, you will be able to exercise even more, or perform more strenuous work, without a corresponding rise in oxidative damage. Once you reach this plateau, you can actually get ahead on the paradox, and generate more antioxidants than free radicals. This is why scientists at the West Los Angeles Veterans Administration Medical Center in Los Angeles, California, concluded, after studying the effects of exercise on twenty patients, that "physical exercise training can reduce potential chronic health effects associated with daily activities by contributing to an overall reduction in exercise-induced free radical production."[11]

If you are among the "elderly"—let's say seventy and older—the relationship between the free radicals generated by exercise and the antioxidant strengthening that exercise also produces is more of a crucial factor, and there is a greater risk that too much exercise can tip the scale towards a predominance of oxidative damage. However, all that this means, in practical terms, is that it is essential to keep your antioxidant nutrient intake at an optimal level, and the easiest way to do this is through vitamin and mineral supplements. With this balance in place, the benefits to the elderly of regular exercise are numerous. It reduces age-related lean body mass loss and the concomitant risk for various chronic diseases such as coronary artery disease, high blood pressure, diabetes (non insulin dependent), anxiety, depression, functional decline, and frailty.[12]

Once you see what the game is and are aware of its stakes, you will probably be inclined to get moving. "Motion is life. Stagnation is death," comments naturopathic physician Bruce Fife, N.D. "Without movement we deteriorate and head toward disease and death. Physical activity is the closest thing we have to the fountain of youth."[13]

Recommendation: Most health experts advise exercising for twenty to thirty minutes per session, preferably every day. If you sweat a lot or sweat easily when you exercise, be sure to replenish your electrolytes[14]—these are essential minerals that are sweated out of your body—by drinking some form of electrolyte-enriched water immediately after exercising. However, try to avoid the sugar-loaded kinds (such as fructose-sweetened drinks and/or those containing artificial colors and flavors), because these will bring yet *more* toxins into your system.

HEALTHY LIVING SPACE DETOXIFIER #29
Sauna Detox: How Heat Therapy Can Help Your Body Release Toxins

A logical activity to take up after your exercise is basking in a dry heat sauna. First, you tax your muscles and cardiovascular system and work up a healthy sweat, then you relax in a hot, dry space. This sequence is logical from the viewpoint of the detoxification process, too.

Sitting in a dry or radiant heat sauna[15] produces hyperthermia, or "heat stress," which is an effective way of getting your cells to release fat-stored toxins; it also induces profuse sweating which, as we understood above, is an excellent, natural way for your body to excrete toxins through the skin. Saunas are no longer exotic, "something Scandinavians do," or even hard to find. Many fitness facilities, public gyms, health clubs, and upscale hotels now offer saunas, and relatively inexpensive home sauna units are available as well (see below).

The therapeutic function underlying heat stress is temporarily to raise the body's internal temperature to 101-103°F, in effect, to produce a transient fever. Heat stress is actually a fundamental premise of natural medicine, harking back some two thousand years to Hippocrates, the reputed progenitor of Western medicine, who said, in effect: Give me the power to create a fever and I shall cure any disease.

Once this internal heat has been generated, the cleansing process can begin. The artificial fever, or hyperthermia, works as an immune system stimulant by accelerating the output of white blood cells. There is some discussion among fitness experts and researchers whether you get the most efficient internal heating through a dry or wet sauna approach. Exponents of the wet or moist heat approach (we'll consider an example called aromaSpa below) say the high ambient humidity keeps the perspiration coming out on your skin from evaporating; further, ambient moisture condenses on the skin and acts as a heat insulator, making your body hotter. In dry heat conditions, your perspiration evaporates and you lose body heat and you may have to spend longer in the sauna until you reach the desired internal temperature.

Sitting in a dry or radiant heat sauna produces hyperthermia, or "heat stress," which is an effective way of getting your cells to release fat-stored toxins; it also induces profuse sweating, which is an excellent, natural way for your body to excrete toxins through the skin.

Scandinavian researchers were able to measure the actual changes in various physiological aspects in people taking regular saunas for a week. The researchers studied the changes in heart function and metabolism in ten healthy males who were exposed to the dry heat (80°C and higher) of a Finnish sauna for one hour twice daily for seven days. They found that after each session in the sauna the body temperature of the men rose by almost one degree and the body weight dropped by almost one kilogram.

While one aspect of the blood pressure[16] (systolic, when the heart contracts) did not change, the other (diastolic) decreased noticeably; the pulse rate rose from an average of 75-80 to 106-116 beats per minute, indicating increased heart rate, although this change was less noticeable after the third day; and metabolic rate increased by twenty-five percent to thirty-three percent after the first day. The researchers noted that the men tended to have lower levels of certain minerals such as potassium, sodium, and iron after the third day, indicating the need to supplement sauna use with electrolyte intake.[17]

Generally, sauna use is well tolerated and safe for people of all ages, from infancy to old age, and it does not pose any undue risk for people with heart problems such as a history of heart attacks or high blood pressure. As a rule of thumb, many doctors recommend that if you can walk into the sauna, you can walk out of it, and you will derive a measure of its cardiovascular benefits. "The normal sauna bath, with moderate cool-off phases, increases the cardiac workload about as much as a brisk walk."[18] Even patients who have recovered from acute heart attacks (myocardial infarctions) "can enjoy the sauna without incurring any harmful cardiovascular effects."[19]

Anything that enhances cardiac output facilitates detoxification, but even more specific research establishes the sauna's role in chemical detoxification. Scientists in the Ukraine found good reason for advocating the use of a sauna as a means of detoxifying chemical industry workers. "[The] sauna increased excretion with sweat of toxic substances (lead, thiuram, captax, sulphenamide C) that penetrated the body during work."[20] Researchers at the Institute of Physiology in Moscow, Russia, concluded that the sauna is effective for alleviating psycho-emotional stress due to its relaxation effect; this is produced by the alternation of heating and cooling phases and its regulatory effect on the body's autonomic nervous system.[21]

Health Mate® Sauna

This is a prefabricated, portable dry heat sauna made of cedar ready to plug into an electrical socket wherever you situate it in your house. According to the manufacturer, PLH Products of City of Industry, California, this unit uses infrared thermal heat, which is felt by the body to be similar to direct sunlight and its heat. Its source in this case is radiant energy, which works directly on the body's tissues rather than having to heat the air around the body (an approach called convection).

The air temperature in the unit is thus much lower than in a conventional sauna, typically 110°-130°F compared to 180°-235°F, and as a radiant heat, it tends to penetrate the body by an inch or more, producing two to three times more perspiration than other types of saunas.

One of the intriguing benefits put forward for this sauna is that spending thirty minutes in its dry heat envelope is an equivalent cardiovascular workout to running six to nine miles. According to medical research, a moderately conditioned person can sweat off 500 g in the sauna, burning 300 calories. Regular use of the sauna "may be as effective" as the cardiovascular conditioning and calorie burn-off expected from running or other forms of vigorous exercise.[22] Here's how it works: the body absorbs heat from the sauna then strives to cool itself by sending blood to the skin (the body's periphery); this action raises cardiovascular activity and speeds up metabolism.

According to the manufacturer, you will burn about 300 calories if you run 1.5 to 3 miles, but you will burn 900 calories if you spend thirty minutes in the sauna. The unit costs about $4000 for a two-seater. It is not recommended for people with adrenal suppression, lupus, multiple sclerosis, or hemophiliacs, for people prone to hemorrhage, or for women during pregnancy.[23]

Finlandia Sauna

According to folk wisdom, the Finnish use of the sauna, which means "bathhouse," goes back about two thousand years to when the Finns invented it. There is an amusing Finnish bromide extolling the benefits of the sauna: "If the sauna, vodka, or pine tar can't cure your ills, nothing will." In the various sauna models made to order per customer specification by Finlandia Sauna in Portland, Oregon, the inside temperature is typically 180°F (with a range of 175° to 195°F) and the humidity a low twenty-five percent. The Finlandia has rocks placed around and over the heater so as to filter the heat (the sauna user dribbles water over the stones to produce some steam to induce sweating), and the walls are made of soft wood (cedar, redwood, or hemlock) so as to absorb the humidity produced and to keep the interior atmosphere relatively dry.

According to Finlandia, the soft heat and low humidity soothe and relax tired muscles, relieve stress, and promote a generally "wonderful" feeling of satisfaction. One way the sauna may do this is by stimulating the brain to release additional levels of its own natural pain-killing biochemicals, such as beta-endorphins and norepinephrine. Further benefits to spending a half-hour in the sauna include increasing the rates of blood circulation, respiration (the inhale-exhale cycle), and pulse rate (indicating the cardiovascular system is working a little harder, in this case, usefully so).

As the skin pores open up under the influence of the hot steam, the body accelerates its excretion of cellular waste products through the skin. In fact, it has been observed that heavy smokers will excrete tobacco toxins through the skin, often leaving a visible yellow stain on white towels used to pat dry the skin.

Aromatherapy Spa

This home unit, called the aromaSpa, is a free-standing, plug-in steam heat therapy unit (alternatively called an Aromatic Steam Capsule by its manufacturer) for one user. The unit weighs about seventy pounds, stands sixty-six inches tall, and has one chair inside. It has transparent walls of polycarbonate, the same window substance used in airplanes. It is portable and costs about $1500. The aromaSpa has a steam generator (which circulates one quart of distilled water during a forty-minute session) and an aromatherapy diffuser designed to infuse the aromas of hundreds of essential plant oils (the basis of aromatherapy) into the misty enclosed air.

This way you get both the heat therapy benefit and an olfactory one by breathing aromatherapy oils chosen for their focused therapeutic benefits, such as relaxation, invigoration, detoxification, mental clarity, and other purposes.

Independent scientific studies on the unit have shown that it can increase vascular flow (which enhances oxygen, nutrient, and lymph exchange at the cellular level), increase muscle flexibility, decrease the risk of everyday and athletic injuries, improve blood flow and oxygen delivery to the cells, and heighten immune response by stimulating white blood cell production. Moist heat therapy in the aromaSpa can also relieve the symptoms of allergies, hay fever, and sinusitis, according to the product's manufacturer. Research also suggests that the steam bath or moist heat chamber can remove toxic chemicals such as DDE (a byproduct of the pesticide DDT), PCBs, and dioxin (a pesticide breakdown product) from fat cells.[24]

Sitting in the aromaSpa for twenty to forty minutes can reduce lactic acid buildup in the muscles following exercise and thereby prevent post-exercise muscle soreness; it may also be able to reduce cellulite deposits (lumpy fat areas in the skin), especially if you use the following aromatherapy oils during the session: rosemary, sandalwood, juniper, geranium, and/or lemon essential oils. The manufacturer states that these oils, diffused into the enclosed chamber, can produce detoxifying and water-draining effects in only ten minutes.[25]

According to the manufacturer, Variel Health International, the unit can help induce muscle relaxation and detoxification, stimulate the immune system, ease fatigue, revitalize the skin, and generally rejuvenate your system.

As the skin pores open up under the influence of the hot steam, the body accelerates its excretion of cellular waste products through the skin. In fact, it has been observed that heavy smokers will excrete tobacco toxins through the skin, often leaving a visible yellow stain on white towels used to pat dry the skin. During a forty-minute session (the manufacturer's recommended standard length), the inside temperature of the unit can reach 115°-120°F, and temporarily elevate the body temperature from 101°-103°F.

Recommendation: Exercise for twenty minutes then spend thirty minutes (or less, if the heat is too intense for you) in a sauna or steam bath. Thoroughly wash yourself in a hot shower afterward to remove toxins that may have come out through the skin. If you can get someone to give you a good rubdown or

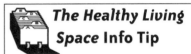

The Healthy Living Space Info Tip

For Health Mate Sauna:
PLH products, 16000 Phoenix Drive, City of Industry, CA 91745;
tel: 800-946-6001;
fax: 626-968-0444;
website:
www.healthmatesauna.com.

For Finlandia Sauna:
Finlandia Sauna,
14010-B.S.W. 72nd Avenue,
Portland, OR 97224;
tel: 800-354-3342 or 503-684-8289;
fax: 503-684-1120;
e-mail:
finlandiasauna@worldnet.att.net;
website: www. finlandiasauna.com.

For aromaSpa:
Variel Health International,
618 Variel Avenue,
Chatsworth, CA 91311;
tel: 800-800-7222;
fax: 818-407-0738;
e-mail: info@aromaspa.com;
website: www.aromaspa.com.

professional massage following the shower, this is another excellent complement to sauna therapy. If no massage or rubdown is forthcoming, try to rest for twenty minutes after showering, so your body can assimilate the relaxation benefits of the sauna.

HEALTHY LIVING SPACE DETOXIFIER #30
A Purifying Bath: Whole-Body Detoxifying Soaks in Herbs, Salts, Oils, and Other Natural Substances

One of the easiest and surely among the most inexpensive ways to detoxify through the skin is through whole-body soaks in special natural substances known for their cleansing effects, such as Epsom salt, seaweed, essential plant oils, apple cider vinegar, and mustard. This section will highlight several whole-body purifying soaks out of the range of possibilities.

Seaweed and Eucalyptus

For this bath, you need Epsom salts (one cup), baking soda (one cup), powdered kelp (one-half cup; you may have to pulverize it in your blender), eucalyptus essential oil (five to ten drops), and witch hazel (one teaspoon). According to herbalist Laurel Vukovic, eucalyptus oil has an antiseptic effect, and is also a capable respiratory system tonic and stimulant if you suspect a cold or flu coming. Vukovic suggests mixing the eucalyptus oil with the witch hazel and adding it to your bath after the tub is full to prevent it from evaporating under the hot running water. You can add the other ingredients earlier. It's important to stay in the bath at least twenty minutes, and you might try visualizing toxins seeping out of your body as you soak and perspire.[26]

Specialized Detoxification Baths

Noted naturopathic physician and educator Hazel Parcells, N.D., who took her own health advice to live to be 109, recommended using any of four therapeutic bathing formulas, depending on one's suspected toxicity.

For all four baths, Dr. Parcells recommended not showering or washing off for four hours after the soak; she also suggested doing the soaks just before going to bed at night.[27]

For exposure to X-rays or environmental radiation: sea salt (one pound) and baking soda (one pound) dissolved in a tub of hot water; drink a mixture of rock salt (one-half teaspoon), baking soda (one-half teaspoon), and warm water while you are having this soak.

For exposure to heavy metals, carbon monoxide, or pesticides: regular-brand Clorox bleach (one cup) to a tub of very hot water.

For exposure to low grade radioactive materials in the food or in irradiated foods: baking soda (two pounds) dissolved in a tub of hot water; drink a mixture of baking soda (one-half teaspoon) and warm water while soaking.

Dr. Parcells also described a general detoxifier, especially useful for building immunity when you feel you're getting sick, or if you have fatigue, muscle aches and pains, or emotional and mental stress: pure apple cider vinegar (two cups) mixed into the hot water in the bathtub.

Bentonite Bath

In chapter 5, we learned about the detoxifying benefits of bentonite clay. Bentonite can also be used as a bath ingredient. Put two to four pounds of bentonite in the water and allow it to sit overnight to mix with the water. Then add another two pounds of bentonite to your bath water and soak in it for one hour, or add four pounds and soak for thirty minutes. The more bentonite you use, the faster the detoxifying effect. Don't use a commercially prepared bentonite because it will be too dilute and you will have to use a great deal (at considerable cost) to get the same effect.

Pore-Opening Ginger

Add one cup of Epsom salts (or more, as you like, up to four pounds if you're feeling extravagant) and two tablespoons of fresh grated ginger to your bath water. Stay in the tub up to thirty minutes, but no longer. The ginger should make you sweat fairly vigorously after a while, thereby facilitating the release of toxins through the skin. The combination of Epsom salts and ginger helps open skin pores to excrete toxins, and it also helps eliminate pain throughout the body.

Mustard Bath

This is a traditional detoxifying soak in many parts of the world. Mustard is believed to increase blood circulation, open skin pores, stimulate the sweat glands, and generally draw out impurities and toxins through the skin. Mustard powder (about two large tablespoons per bath) may be supplemented with essential oils of wintergreen, eucalyptus, rosemary, and thyme (three drops each), for their antiseptic, cooling, skin toning, or stimulant effects. Stay in the bath at least twenty minutes.

Liquid Needle Soak

This bath, based on a commercial product called Liquid Needle® Rebalancer acts as a kind of liquid acupuncture needle on the body and provides the system with an energy rebalancing, according to its manufacturer, BioPhotanicals. The product is based on a blending of light (photons) and plant energies (botanicals).

BioPhotanicals claims that while you are soaking in a Liquid Needle Body Soak, "every pore and every acupoint on the skin is stimulated with the highly charged light-activated molecules." The pores and some 1,300 acupoints are stimulated simultaneously by "charged light signals" in the Liquid Needle mixture to collect and release toxic substances from inside the body. According to BioPhotanicals, reduced energy and energy blockages (addressed by Liquid Needle) are almost always the result of long-term toxic buildup as well as the presence of external or internal scar tissue. The company also states that each of their Body Soaks carries a photonic charge of 170-250 millivolts, which gives them considerable traction in addressing energy blockages or imbalances.

The company offers five types of Liquid Needle Body Soaks: Clear (to maintain vital energy balance affected by emotional stress); Gold (for maximum detoxifying effects); Blue (to gain a sense of increased energy and vitality); Amber (for those severely out of balance due to pain, inflammation, and stress); and Foot Soak (for those who can't use a bathtub).

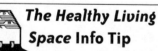

The Healthy Living Space Info Tip

For Liquid Needle Body Soaks: DNR (Developmental Natural Resources), 4193 Englewood Drive, Indianapolis, IN 46226; tel: 800-886-6222 or 317-543-4886; fax: 317-543-4880; e-mail: main@dnrinc.com; website: www.dnrinc.com.

CHAPTER 7

The Poisons in Your Mouth:

Specialized Dental Detoxification Programs

The subject of this chapter takes up relatively little space in your body, yet it can make your entire body sick, even seriously so, if left unattended. I am referring to your teeth and gums. In recent years, increasing attention has been accorded the teeth in the field of alternative and natural medicine. Physicians from various disciplines are starting to realize that the condition of a patient's teeth—more specifically, the nature of the dental materials used in dental work and how they interact with the body's physiology—have a great deal to do with many health conditions.

Evidence continues to mount in support of contention that many so-called standard dental procedures and substances—using mercury-based fillings, root canals, placing crowns, extracting teeth improperly—have toxic consequences, affecting the entire body. This chapter identifies the major toxic factors in modern dentistry and indicates effective ways to eliminate this toxicity from your system.

This is a crucial element of the detoxification picture. You may faithfully and successfully do all the other detoxifying steps described in this book, and not progress very much *if* your teeth are toxic themselves. It is by no means a sure thing that they are; the teeth of many people are in satisfactory condition and are not a major source of toxicity for the body. Either your immune system is strong enough to handle whatever toxins are released by the materials or conditions in your mouth, or, providentially, not too many are released. It is probably prudent to assume that some dental toxins are being released all the time, but they may or may not be seriously contributing to body-wide toxicity. One possible indication that your teeth are interfering with your body's ability to purge itself of its toxic burden is if you do not feel healthier and less toxic after performing the detoxifying steps in this book.

Unlike most of the other Healthy Living Space Detoxifier recommendations in this book, the action outlined below requires the services of a qualified biological dentist,[1] namely, one who is trained in the natural medicine protocols of what one dentist has termed "whole-body dentistry." This term refers to the many ways in which events and conditions in your mouth can affect any or all systems elsewhere in your body. Your action input is to *choose* to do something health promoting about the possible (some experts would say probable) dental poisons in your mouth. But how will you know if a dental matter is the cause of a seemingly remote, unconnected medical problem?

One way is to examine your symptoms and consider whether they seem to be treatment-resistant. In other words, despite well-indicated treatment, either conventional or alternative, your health problem has not improved. The reason might be your teeth. In 1996, a group called the Toxic Element Research Foundation in Colorado Springs, Colorado, interviewed 1,320 dental patients to seek correlations between dental procedures and substances and reported health symptoms. The subjects had received all kinds of standard dental work, such as root canals, dental restorations, dental implants, mercury fillings, orthodonture, and periodonture.

The researchers found that the people showed symptoms associated with thirty different diseases across a range of physical, mental, and emotional difficulties. For example, seventy-three percent reported unexplained irritability; seventy-two percent constant or frequent periods of depression; sixty-seven percent numbness and tingling in their extremities; sixty-four percent frequent urination; sixty-three percent unexplained chronic fatigue; sixty-two percent cold hands and feet even under conditions of external warmth; sixty percent constant bloating; fifty-eight percent memory deficits; fifty-five percent sudden, inexplicable anger; fifty-four percent regular constipation. Other frequently occurring symptoms in this group of 1,320 patients were tremors, twitches, leg cramps, shortness of breath, recurrent heartburn, itching, skin irritations, jitteriness, metallic taste in the mouth, suicidal tendencies, insomnia, chest pains, joint pain, irregular heart beat, headaches after eating, and more.[2]

Health-care practitioners who are aware of the dental link realize now that in most cases the connections are not obvious, direct, or even validated by conventional Western medicine. After all, how can something happening in your mouth—say a minor gum infection, a broken mercury amalgam filling, a poorly done root canal—have any effect on other systems in the body?

A Gallery of Possible Toxic Consequences of Modern Dentistry

The question is certainly a valid one, but to respond that they can have no effect because conventional medicine has no way of accounting for such a physiological causal chain or any mode of interdependent interaction, is not valid. You just need a broader, more comprehensive model of the body and how it works. This is to say, you need a medical model based on energy relationships in the human organism, and you find such a system primarily in acupuncture, or traditional Chinese medicine.

In this empirical way of viewing the body, based on many centuries of trained clinical observation, various energy channels running down the body connect the teeth to various organs and organ systems, such as the liver and the digestive system, respectively. If you have toxins in your mouth clustered around an upper back molar, this state of toxicity (which is also an energy imbalance) can get translated (or transported, as it were) to somewhere else in your body and start producing a disease or pathology. Cancer is the most extreme example, but it certainly makes the case vividly.

Swiss physician Thomas Rau, M.D., medical director of the Paracelsus Clinic in Lustmuhle, Switzerland, reports that both breast and prostate cancer can be caused by unaddressed dental problems. The relationship is called a dental focus: as it were, the toxicity in the tooth focuses itself on another part of the body. In fact, Dr. Rau is on record stating that in about ninety percent of breast cancer cases he has treated there is a dental factor. The breast lies on the energy channel acupuncturists call the Stomach meridian. So if you have a dental problem, such as a faulty root canal or a jaw infection (called a cavitation) in a tooth on this meridian, the flow of vital energy (called *qi* by acupuncturists) through this meridian will be blocked and lead to degeneration further down the energy channel.

In a sense, brushing your teeth faithfully has very little to do with any of this. A German study showed that only five patients out of sixty examined had sterile, germ-free teeth; fifty-five of those examined had various species of aerobic and nonaerobic bacteria present in their mouth. Each of these fifty-five patients had at least one tooth with a dental focus, that is, so infected with bacteria that it was transmitting toxicity energy signals to other parts of the body. In this particular case, the sixty subjects were tested because they were not responding favorably (or at all) to well-indicated treatments. The conclusion was that the dental foci or energetic disturbances were blocking their bodies' receptivity to the therapeutic efforts.[3]

Dr. Rau treated a man, age fifty-five, with prostate cancer. Even though the man's prostate organ had been removed, he still had cancer. A dental X-ray revealed that the man had a half-formed tooth impacted in his upper jaw, above the incisor. This extra tooth was affecting the patient's kidney and bladder energy channels and disrupting its energy flow through the groin, including the prostate. This imbalance was involved in the inception of the man's prostate cancer, concluded Dr. Rau, who promptly extracted the half-formed tooth. After the patient received various alternative medical therapies for his cancer, he regained his health and was cancer free.

Dr. Rau also treated a woman, forty-five, who had recently had part of her breast removed due to breast cancer, and she was about to begin chemotherapy. Dr. Rau, in examining the woman's teeth, discovered that one of her upper jaw incisors, which had received a root canal fifteen years earlier, was situated with respect to her kidney and bladder energy channels. A neighboring tooth, also on this channel, was poorly developed. Dr. Rau learned that prior to developing breast cancer, the woman had sustained an ovarian cyst (a noncancerous fluid-filled sac that forms in the ovaries) and had had it surgically removed. It was likely, said Dr. Rau, that the dental problem had initially focused itself in the ovaries, creating the cyst, which appeared two years after the root canal was performed. Again, removal of the two offending teeth, in conjunction with other medical treatments, helped reverse her health problems.[4]

Not only can toxic energies be transmitted through the body, but physical toxins can move outwards from the mouth, too. Dental toxins that leach from the mouth and migrate to other parts of the body are now associated with numerous health problems, including immune dysfunction, coma, multiple sclerosis, and leukemia. In the United States, one of the pioneering dentists to promote this concept is Hal Huggins, D.D.S., M.S., who is based in Colorado Springs, Colorado.

Here's how a dental problem can precipitate leukemia, a potentially fatal cancer of the blood-forming cells in bone marrow. A healthy young man of eighteen received two mercury amalgam dental fillings. Two days later he developed a high fever of 105°F, and the next day he was hospitalized with a diagnosis of leukemia, says Dr. Huggins. Within twenty-four hours of having the two mercury fillings removed, all signs of the boy's disease disappeared. Since Dr. Huggins caught the problem very early, it was easily reversible because he understood the true causal connection.

The mercury, which is a lethal poison on its own and regarded by the Environmental Protection Agency as an environmental hazard, somehow leached from the man's fillings in sufficient levels to destabilize his immune system and white blood cell count and precipitate a catastrophic decline into leukemia. It is ironic—and shocking—that a toxic substance the EPA calls a waste disposal hazard, something a dentist cannot throw out, bury in the ground, or dump in a landfill, is okay to put in a person's mouth. It is even more unbelievable that dentists who decline to do this and instead discuss the dangers of mercury with their patients are subject to professional reprisals, harassment, and legal action by medical authorities.

Sometimes it is harder to completely undo dental-caused leukemia if the problem has been developing for some time, as in this next example. A dentist, age forty-two, came to Dr. Huggins, after having been exposed daily to mercury amalgam materials for many years in the course of his dental practice. One day the man was exposed to yet another dose of mercury: in helping his father, a farmer, clean out a grain silo, he came into contact with a puddle of liquid mercury on the floor of the grain silo where the toxic heavy metal was used to keep the rats out. Within a week, the man was seriously ill and received a leukemia diagnosis.

One of the first treatment steps he took was to have all his mercury amalgam fillings removed; otherwise they would continue to slowly but steadily contaminate his system with mercury vapors and emissions. However, he was resistant to discontinuing his dental use of mercury as fillings for his patients. As a result, his recovery from leukemia was not complete, although it was satisfactory and enabled him to resume his life.

Thinking about having your teeth cleaned? Of course it's good for your gums and may prevent periodontal disease, but there is also the risk that it can scratch free some mercury from old fillings and allow a toxic dose to migrate through your body, states Dr. Huggins, who saw it happen. A young woman of twenty-nine who was in good health had a routine teeth cleaning by her dentist. The next day she detected a metallic taste in her mouth; her gums, lips, and mouth started tingling, then went numb; and her ears were ringing. Then things got much worse. She started to have seizures, lost her ability to speak, and slid into a state of near coma, oblivious of her surroundings. Her doctors expected her to die in a few days, and they had no idea what her medical problem was.

According to Dr. Huggins, "As a result of having her teeth cleaned, Sabina now had a higher level of mercury leaching from her twelve mercury-based fillings because the protective corrosion had been cleaned off." Her immune system could not handle this extra load of toxic mercury, and collapsed. It was a tough and delicate operation, but Dr. Huggins and his team removed all of the woman's mercury fillings while she was almost comatose. After the first day, she showed signs of alertness and three days later she was able to speak again; after a week or so, she was back on her feet, well again. This is a startling example of acute mercury toxicity and while, one hopes, relatively rare in occurrence, it shows the awesome health-debilitating effect mercury can have when it manages to seep out of a dental filling and migrate through the body.[5]

Here are two more patient studies that make a compelling case for systemic toxicity caused by mercury dental fillings. The first comes from an acupuncturist named David J. Nickel,

O.M.D., L.Ac., of Santa Monica, California. A man, age thirty-two, came to him with a list of debilitating symptoms: fatigue, anger, low blood sugar, prematurely greying hair, back problems, ringing in his ears, nervousness, and problems with concentration. At twenty-eight, he had had a nervous breakdown, and at the age of fifteen, he had developed anxiety and severe fatigue immediately following a root canal procedure.

Dr. Nickel did a mercury vapor analysis on the patient's mouth. He discovered that the man's teeth were outgassing mercury vapor from six teeth at levels forty-two times higher than the maximum allowable limit set by the Environmental Protection Agency had ruled. Dr. Nickel did a hair analysis on the patient and found high levels of other heavy metals (aluminum and copper; he also got confirmation of the presence of systemic mercury) and a dangerously slow rate of metabolism. Dr. Nickel advised the patient to have the six mercury fillings and the root-canalled tooth removed, and he put him on a nutritional supplement program to address his low metabolism and blood sugar imbalance.

A month after the corrective dentistry, the man reported his energy levels had returned to the high levels he had enjoyed seventeen years earlier. All his other symptoms had gone away as well, and he said he felt himself now in excellent health. There was no clinical doubt, as far as Dr. Nickel was concerned, that the mercury fillings and root-canalled tooth had produced the multiplicity of symptoms.

"Of the 90% of my patients with amalgam dental fillings, most have a mercury-induced copper toxicity, high calcium levels, and reduced thyroid and adrenal function," he states, outlining some of the secondary problems mercury produces, such as the dangerous link with copper, another toxic heavy metal. Dr. Nickel adds that mercury is linked with 258 different medical symptoms, and copper with at least 100. "Almost all my patients who have had their mercury-based fillings removed show moderate to dramatic improvement in their heath in usually less than one month."[6]

Here is another case from an acupuncturist. This time, a male patient, age thirty-seven, had suffered from seven years of unremitting fatigue. He also complained of swelling in his lymph nodes, headaches, light-headedness, irritability, and pain in his chest and muscles. M.M. van Benschoten, O.M.D., a doctor of

Oriental medicine practicing in Reseda, California, found traces of viruses and bacteria in the patient's system at sufficient levels to contribute to the chronic fatigue; but he also detected mercury toxicity from dental fillings at such levels as to suggest it was the "fundamental underlying cause" of the health problems.

Dr. Benschoten explains that in acupuncture theory, a toxic metal such as mercury interferes with the circulation of vital energy, or *qi*, through the energy channels of the body (meridians). Dr. Benschoten gave the patient a series of Chinese herbs to help deal with the viral, bacterial, and heavy metal toxicity, and he advised the man to have all fourteen of his mercury amalgams removed, which he did three months later. However, the dentist this patient employed for the mercury removal did not perform the procedure correctly, and the patient's body-wide mercury levels actually increased. This of course is the risk of mercury filling removal. If it isn't done right, it can enable dental mercury to be released into the body, increasing the body's total mercury load. In this case, Dr. Benschoten gave the patient a second round of Chinese herbs to round up the free mercury in the body, and after a few months, the man was symptom free.[7]

Another potent source of hidden dental infection comes from an incompletely performed tooth extraction, often of a wisdom tooth or an abscessed tooth. This type of dental focus is called a cavitation. A cavitation is an area in the jaw where a tooth has been removed, and the resulting bone lesion or tissue wound becomes infected and inflamed. When the bone of the extraction site is unable to heal properly, it cavitates, or forms a mushy depression (cavity) subject to infection and the eventual death of bone tissue. The dead bone can produce nerve pain, usually in the head, face, neck, or shoulders, but can sometimes create problems elsewhere in the body, such as the lower back, legs, or intestines.

Christopher Hussar, D.D.S., D.O., a dentist-osteopath who practices in Reno, Nevada, relates the case of a woman, fifty-five, who had suffered from severe facial pain for fifteen years. Nobody could figure out what was causing it, and she had consulted an estimated fifty doctors prior to seeing Dr. Hussar. Her dental focus was a deep chronic infection in her lower jaw where the infection had wrapped itself around the major nerve trunk in that area of her mouth, explains Dr. Hussar.

The problem most likely originated years earlier following a faulty wisdom tooth extraction in which the dentist had failed to thoroughly debride (clean out) all the unhealthy tissue and dead bone from the extraction site. This set in motion the chronic infection and in turn the referred pain, that is, *facial* pain rather than strictly locatable *dental* pain. As a secondary dental focus, the woman had a localized, but festering, jaw infection around the site of a root-canalled tooth. Dr. Hussar cleaned out the site of infection in her mouth and irrigated the area with disinfectants; following the two-hour procedure, the woman had no post-operative pain and her facial pain did not return.

Dr. Hussar notes that the inside of these dental lesions or cavitations can be quite gross. "Inside these jawbone cavities you may also encounter viruses, bacteria, yeasts, and parasites, all of which contribute to the harmful dental focal disturbance. The mouth is the filthiest place in the body." Dr. Hussar has seen direct clinical evidence linking untreated cavitations with irregular heartbeat, orbital pseudo-tumor, or pain around the eyes, headaches, blindness, hearing disorders, arthritic pain, rheumatological problems, "and all manner of unexplained pain disorders." All of these conditions were reversed when the hidden dental infection was treated correctly, says Dr. Hussar.[8]

With these examples as a conceptual starting point, let's examine in greater detail the potential toxic contribution of mercury amalgam fillings, root canals, and cavitations, and consider grounds for undergoing corrective dentistry to eliminate these sources of toxicity from the body.

HEALTHY LIVING SPACE DETOXIFIER #31
Make Your Mouth a Mercury-Free Zone by Having Your Mercury Fillings Correctly Replaced

The matter of mercury amalgam fillings and their effect on the body is a controversial and politically charged one. Most dentists in the United States are still resistant to the concept that mercury fillings might be hazardous to the patient's health. Many dentists claim they are unfamiliar with the argument, or have never seen evidence supporting the claim, or that the evidence is unsubstantial.

However, as a health-care consumer, you must see through the ignorance and duplicity of modern dentistry and consider the facts and theories on your own. Other countries have actually banned the use of mercury amalgam fillings, regarding the substance as too toxic for human contact, while the United States remains highly resistant to not only taking this action or openly discussing the evidence, but even to informing dental patients that such evidence exists.

It certainly doesn't help matters that in many cases state licensing boards come after dentists and basically punish (legally and financially) those who break away from conventional attitudes about dental mercury and start informing their patients that mercury is a hazard and ought to be removed from their teeth at the earliest opportunity. Let's establish the basic facts first.

Mercury fillings, or amalgams, have been used in dentistry since the 1820s, and today an estimated ninety-two percent of dentists routinely place them in their patients' mouths. Today's amalgam typically contains an alloy of several metals including mercury (fifty percent), silver (thirty-five percent), tin (nine percent), copper (six percent), and a trace of zinc.[9] An estimated 150 million are placed in mouths every year, representing seventy-five tons of amalgam alloy. Dentists say they like mercury fillings because they are durable, easy to manipulate and install, and don't cost much. However, the disadvantages far outweigh the benefits. Mercury is a toxic heavy metal, a noted carcinogen, an immune system damager, and generally a heavy-duty poison best avoided or handled with extreme caution in all other circumstances other than in your mouth.

Mercury as a heavy metal is also a potent free radical, capable of destroying cells and ruining cell membrane integrity, and even affecting DNA processes and producing cell death. Further, mercury interferes with the energy producing function of the cells by causing the mitochondria, the cell's energy "factories," to become dysfunctional. Not only does it increase the number of free radicals in the system, but it reduces the body's defense system, the antioxidants.

As a free radical, mercury can block the body's detoxification pathways by blocking the action of key enzymes.[10] Specifically, it can have "devastating effects" on the glutathione content of the body, which in turn facilitates the increased retention by the body of other environmental toxins.

Glutathione is one of the liver's key detoxification substances, so if its levels are diminished, so is the liver's detoxification capability.[11]

It was not until 1988 that the routine use of mercury raised serious enough questions for the Environmental Protection Agency (EPA) to declare scrap dental amalgam a hazardous waste. Dentists have to dispose of dental mercury with the same care as they would extend for any other highly toxic, lethal hazardous waste. Yet they routinely keep putting it in the mouths of millions of patients. It takes only a modicum of intelligence to ask why if this substance is an EPA-designated hazardous waste it is ever considered safe to store in the human mouth in teeth? Is the mouth a strange new kind of unregulated hazardous waste site?

The traditional answer has been that once in the amalgam composite filling the mercury is fixed fast and will not leach out of the dental filling, and if it did, it would not go anywhere in the body and thereby create a health problem. Medical research is refuting both of these assumptions, showing them to be dangerously incorrect. Mercury does leach and it does migrate through the body.

Mercury vapors from the fillings are continuously being outgassed in the mouth, entering the body through the blood or inhaled mouth air. Chewing or grinding your teeth contribute to this steady release of minute amounts of mercury vapor in the form of what chemists call elemental mercury. You don't have to be chewing or grinding your teeth to still be absorbing outgassed mercury vapors; in fact, sometimes just drinking a hot beverage such as coffee can increase the vapor release from the fillings. Scientists estimate that eighty percent of mercury vapor absorption from the teeth happens in the lungs, after which the mercury vapor rapidly enters the bloodstream; once in the body's tissues, it has a preference for lodging in the central nervous system and the kidneys.[12]

Potentially, your dental fillings can outgas mercury twenty-four hours a day, every day of your life. How much gets released in a single day? A Norwegian study involving 147 patients (measuring mercury release in the blood, urine, and exhaled air) found that people with more than 36 restored dental surfaces (36 mercury fillings, even if some were on the same tooth) absorb 10-12 mcg/l of mercury every day.[13] In 1985, the World Health Organization reported that a single mercury filling can release 3-17 mcg of mercury every day.[14]

Other studies estimate the daily release to be from 20-150 mcg per filling, although the ultramodern high-copper amalgams can release fifty times more mercury vapor than conventional mercury amalgams. The key point here is that the exact amount of mercury emission is not yet known, though the observed range has been documented, and this alone should concern us—that it is leaking from teeth continuously. A Swiss study showed that the greatest volume of mercury released into the body was during the first 24 hours after the filling was installed, ranging from 17.4 mcg/l to 34.5 mcg/l. After the fillings "annealed"(hardened and solidified over time) for two years, the daily mercury emission rate (for eight fillings, as used in the study) was 1.5 mcg.[15]

So while the amounts said to be absorbed vary according to the study, there seems to be agreement that some mercury is definitely absorbed.

A Danish dentist, H. Lichtenberg, D.D.S., undertook his own research to find out how bad the mercury emissions were from teeth. He studied oral mercury vapor emissions from the teeth of 103 patients, whose average age was 47. He noted that each of his patients in this study already had at least fourteen symptoms representative of mercury toxicity; each patient also had an average of twenty-two mercury fillings. The mercury emissions from a single mouth varied from 3 mcg to 329 mcg per cubic meter of air, with an average of 54 mcg, Dr. Lichtenberg reported. He found that people who had twenty-six or more mercury fillings tended to have emissions above fifty, and those who had less than twenty mercury fillings had levels below fifty.

The number fifty is important here because in Denmark levels above 50 mcg in a workplace are judged unsafe by the government. This means many of Dr. Lichtenberg's patients had oral mercury levels exceeding the legal safe limit for industrial workplaces. Put differently, they had a mercury exposure equivalent to a workplace exposure of 168 hours a week (twenty-four hours a day) *indefinitely*. How do Denmark's mercury exposure standards stack up compared to other countries? In Russia, only 10 mcg are allowed; in the United States, 100 mcg; in Canada, 1 mcg for a person weighing 150 pounds was recently judged a

Tolerable Daily Intake. Dr. Lichtenberg's patients were getting a daily mercury exposure fifty times higher than this safety norm.[16]

So mercury is being released from fillings—is this a lot? According to one study, it takes only one microgram (mcg) of mercury to damage nerve tissue. Further, "the bad thing about mercury release is that it is cumulative," explains Hal Huggins, D.D.S., M.S., an outspoken opponent of mercury amalgams and author of *Uninformed Consent*.

"In the fastest elimination mode, if one microgram is absorbed, it will take 70 days to several months to eliminate half of it." The next day you absorb another microgram, then perhaps you get another mercury-based filling, and still another one cracks, doubling the outgassing volume. The math suggests that unless you take major action to detoxify yourself of mercury, you will never get it all out of your body on your own by depending on natural internal detoxification processes. "You will still increase your total body burden of mercury daily."[17]

Inhalation of mercury vapor from the teeth and its absorption by the lungs is only one of three possible routes by which mercury can pass from your fillings into your body. Once in the intestines, soluble mercury compounds break down into mercuric ions that are easily absorbed and transported from the intestines throughout the body along with nourishing fluids. A third route is through the mouth itself. Mercury outgassed from the fillings can be absorbed by the nerves and tissues beneath the fillings and possibly also in root canals.

Once in the bloodstream, bacteria convert mercury to methylmercury, the organic form of mercury that is one hundred times more toxic than the form of mercury that starts out in your dental filling. The methylmercury form of the heavy metal is capable of crossing the blood-brain barrier, usually a physiologically sacrosanct threshold that keeps toxic substances out of the brain. Methylmercury is also distributed throughout the body. The blood readily absorbs it because it mixes easily with fat molecules; it can potentially be distributed to every cell in the body.

Croatian scientists studied the migration of mercury from amalgams in rats over a two-month period. Rats were exposed to either four mercury amalgams or were fed powdered amalgam in their diet. After two months, the kidneys and brains had "significantly higher" concentrations of mercury than other organs for both groups compared to the controls, which had no mercury exposure. Rats with actual amalgams had mercury levels eight times higher than controls and two times higher than those fed the amalgam powder, and they had kidney concentrations of mercury five times that of the control group.[18]

Evidence now shows that mercury amalgams are the major source of mercury exposure for the general public, six times higher than mercury exposure from fish and seafood. A study of the effect of abrasion (chewing) on amalgam surfaces (using real teeth with mercury amalgam fillings but in an artificial mouth to simulate chewing) showed that the "steady-state" release of mercury every day from a *single* filling is 0.03 mcg.[19] Again, you can see the range of estimated levels of emission.

A Danish study of a random sample of 100 men and 100 women showed that increased blood mercury levels were related to the presence of more than four amalgam fillings in the teeth. As Dr. Morton Walker concludes in *Elements of Danger*, an indictment of the toxic practices of modern dentistry, "In my opinion, anyone who allows dental amalgam fillings to remain as part of his or her oral cavity has elected to commit slow but steady suicide by mercury poisoning."[20]

Mercury toxicity has been shown to have destructive contributory effects on kidney and immunologic function and in cardiovascular disease, neuropsychological dysfunction, reproductive disorders, and birth defects, to name a few. Symptoms of or diseases resulting from mercury toxicity make a very long list: anorexia, depression, fatigue, insomnia, arthritis, Alzheimer's, moodiness, Parkinson's, Lou Gehrig's disease, periodontal disease, irritability, memory loss, nausea, diarrhea, gum disease, swollen glands, headaches, multiple sclerosis, antibiotic resistance, and many more.[21]

Researchers have found that hair analysis of multiple sclerosis (MS) patients reveals significantly higher mercury levels than those found in non-MS patients. They also found that MS patients with mercury amalgams have thirty-three percent more MS exacerbations (flare-ups of debilitating symptoms) in a twelve-month period than MS patients without mercury fillings.[22]

Researchers have also established that MS patients with mercury fillings tend to have a poorer mental health status than those patients with no mercury fillings. When forty-seven MS patients with mercury fillings were polled using standard psychological questionnaires, scientists found that they had higher rates of depression, anger, hostility, psychosis, and symptoms of obsessive-compulsive disorder compared to MS patients with no mercury fillings. Further, MS patients with mercury amalgams had forty-three percent more MS symptoms over a twelve-month period. The researchers concluded that the lowered psychological health profile of MS patients may be due to mercury toxicity from dental fillings.[23]

A 1993 study of 1,569 patients drawn from the United States, Denmark, Sweden, and Canada tabulated the correlation of numerous health problems with mercury amalgams. They found that 705 patients reported fatigue, 531 headaches, 347 depression, 343 dizziness, 270 concentration problems, 265 memory loss, 260 metallic taste in the mouth, 231 intestinal problems, 221 allergies, and the list continued.

The study also correlated improvement in reported symptoms with mercury amalgam removal: eighty-six percent with fatigue reported a cure or improvement in this problem after amalgam removal; eighty-seven percent of those with headaches, ninety-one percent with depression, eighty-eight percent with dizziness, eighty percent with concentration deficits, seventy-three percent with memory loss, ninety-five percent with metallic taste, eighty-three percent with intestinal problems, and eighty-nine percent with allergies. In other words, the causal connection between systemic mercury poisoning produced by mercury amalgams and numerous minor to serious health conditions was well established in this study. The report further showed the dramatic improvement in health conditions with the removal of the mercury fillings.[24]

In 1991, a large group of dentists submitted themselves to a study on the effects of systemic mercury toxicity resulting from their prolonged professional contact with the heavy metal. At the annual meeting of the American Dental Association, 1,502 dentists had their urine analyzed for mercury levels. Of this group, 2%, or 29 dentists, had levels of 29 µg/l (micrograms/liter) and were classified as "exposed." Their mercury levels exceeded the safety level of 19 µg/l, and it was seven times higher than the mean level measured in dentists. The "exposed" dentists placed 50% more mercury fillings per week than nonexposed dentists; they had worked an average of 19 years in the same office, and averaged 2.3 mercury spills in their offices compared to only 0.1 for nonexposed dentists. This data suggested clearly that mercury toxicity is related both to duration of exposure and degree of regular contact.

Next, the dentists volunteered to take a behavior test based on sixty-five different mood descriptors to register mental and emotional function. The results were "very significantly linked" to urine mercury levels, the researchers found. The strongest associations between mood and mercury were found in the areas of tension, fatigue, and confusion, as well as reduction in vitality and increased depression. Correlations were also noted between mercury exposure and poor mental concentration, emotional lability (mood fluctuation), and nervous system irritation. The study found "some evidence of adverse preclinical effects at mercury doses averaging 36 µg/l in urine." The report suggested the World Health Organization safety standard of 50 µg/l should be critically reevaluated, and observed that "this is the first U.S. dental study to detect potential behavioral deficits at such a low level of exposure."[25]

Another study demonstrated the mood-altering effects of mercury toxicity. Researchers interviewed twenty-five women with mercury amalgams and twenty-five without, using various standard psychological inventories employed by psychologists to gauge and quantify emotional states. They found that women with mercury fillings had higher scores overall (higher meant they were more reactive), with more symptoms of fatigue and insomnia. They had a greater tendency to express anger without provocation; to experience more intense angry feelings and a greater level of general anxiety; to feel less pleasant, satisfied, happy, secure, or steady; and to have a harder time making decisions. Women without mercury in their mouths had an easier time controlling their anger. On this basis, the researchers concluded that mercury toxicity may be a causative factor in states of depression, excessive anger, and anxiety.[26]

A study of the teeth of military personnel showed that the more fillings in the mouth, the greater the body load of leached mercury. Researchers at the National Institute of Dental Research examined the teeth of 1,127 adult male military personnel, average age 52, with an average of 19.9 mercury amalgam fillings (surfaces of the teeth exposed to mercury fillings, meaning one tooth might have multiple fillings). The total and inorganic mercury concentrations in the urine were 3.09 mcg/l and 2.88 mcg/l, respectively, while the average blood level for both were 2.55 mcg/l and 0.54 mcg/l.

Not only did this study show conclusively that mercury from amalgams leaches and migrates into the body, but the researchers concluded that "on average, each ten surface increase in amalgam exposure is associated with an increase of 1 mcg/l of mercury in urine concentration." In other words, for every new filling you can count on there being *at least* one more microgram of toxic mercury released into your system. One microgram of mercury may be excreted in the urine, but how many micrograms remain in the body?[27] "Mercury is more effective as a killer of cells (cytotoxicity) than many cancer chemotherapies," comments Dr. Walker. "There is *no* harmless level of mercury vapor exposure."[28]

For prospective parents, there is yet another cause for concern for mercury fillings. Research shows that women can pass on mercury to their fetuses in the womb, as mercury can cross the placenta from mother to fetus. Studies have shown that the fetus can store eight times more mercury than the mother's own tissues, where it tends to store in the breasts and get passed on to infants through breast milk.[29]

Summarizing the scientific research and clinical evidence, Dr. Huggins says mercury "can express its toxicity" in ten ways (see figure 7-1). It can:

1) Alter cell membrane permeability. Mercury binds to the cell membranes, affecting how the cell discriminates between "good" and "bad" substances to let cross its border.

2) Change the shape of molecules, affecting their ability to bond with other molecules.

3) Alter enzyme function. Mercury binds to sites on enzymes, slowing down their reaction time and ability to react.

4) Interfere with nerve impulses. Mercury blocks the synaptic gap between nerve cells, hindering transmission.

5) Affect the genetic code. Mercury cleaves DNA, producing genetic defects in fetuses.

6) Inhibit DNA repair mechanisms.

7) Disrupt endocrine gland activity. One atom of mercury can deactivate an entire hormone molecule.

8) Contribute to autoimmune illnesses. Mercury, attached to cells, distorts their shape and confuses the immune system, which judges it to be a foreign and not a host cell.

9) Change digestion and absorption functions.

10) Contribute to antibiotic resistance. Mercury causes some bacteria to alter their shape, inadvertently enabling them to resist conventional antibiotics.[30]

On this last point, researchers at the University of Georgia at Athens reported that mercury exposure through dental fillings can produce antibiotic resistant bacteria in the intestinal flora of otherwise healthy and nonmedicated subjects. They studied 640 people, of whom 356 had not had a recent exposure to antibiotics, and found that those with a high prevalence of mercury resistance in their intestinal flora (the "friendly" bacteria resident in the intestines) were also likely to resist the action of at least two standard antibiotics. In other words, the mercury changed

Figure 7-1. 10 Ways Mercury Can Interfere with Vital Body Systems

1. Alter cell membrane potential, affecting what it absorbs
2. Change the shape of molecules, affecting their ability to bond with other molecules
3. Alter enzyme function, slowing down important chemical reactions
4. Interfere with nerve function
5. Affect the genetic code, producing genetic defects in fetuses.
6. Inhibit DNA repair mechanisms
7. Disrupt endocrine gland activity
8. Contribute to autoimmune disease
9. Change digestion and absorption functions
10. Contribute to antibiotic resistance by altering bacteria

the internal bacteria (mostly oral *Streptococcus* organisms) in such a way that they became resistant to the effect of antibiotics designed to kill them.[31]

"Mercury amalgams are as close as you can get to the center of the illness universe," comments Bruce Shelton, M.D., M.D. (H), Di.Hom., a physician specializing in homeopathy and natural medicine based in Phoenix, Arizona, where he runs The Allergy Center. "Their use in dentistry has set us up for most of the health problems we see today."

For example, there is a "domino effect" that starts with mercury toxicity, explains Dr. Shelton. The overwhelming majority (ninety percent) of the patients he sees who report allergies have an overgrowth of the yeast *Candida albicans*, and they often have this yeast infestation because of heavy metal toxicity in the body, notably of mercury.[32] Candida is an effective, natural absorber of mercury, so in a perverse but logical move, the body attracts the yeast to it so it will absorb the toxic mercury. The logic is that of a tradeoff: the yeast overgrowth will be less toxic overall than unguarded free mercury, so the body opts for a *Candida albicans* infestation to contain the mercury—chronic allergies instead of multiple sclerosis, as it were.

However, it's really a bad trade-off, because the yeast overgrowth sets the stage for intestinal permeability, or what's popularly known as leaky gut syndrome. This is a kind of backwash into the blood from clogged, dysfunctional intestines. Food allergies develop and soon the person is allergic to everything; the next step from here is multiple chemical sensitivity, environmental illness, or chronic fatigue syndrome, says Dr. Shelton. "Environmental illness is then the end-product of a string of health problems that stem from mercury and build, one upon the other."[33]

Candida albicans is not the only thing in the body that has an affinity for mercury. Research now shows that nerve endings in the peripheral nervous system[34] voluntarily absorb mercury (that has leached from teeth and migrated into the body at large) even though it is a neurotoxin—toxic to nerve cells. According to Dietrich Klinghardt, M.D., Ph.D., an innovative physician who practices in Seattle, Washington, these nerve cells absorb mercury "out of curiosity," transporting it up the spinal column. It is their natural function to scan their environment

continuously and inspect all foreign substances for their threat potential.

The trouble is that when mercury moves up the spinal column, it destroys a crucial substance called tubulin, which is necessary for moving substances in the nerves. In effect, the mere presence of mercury destroys the nerves and their transport mechanisms, so it is a one-way and deadly "visit." The intent of the peripheral nervous system in examining the mercury, explains Dr. Klinghardt, is to make an antineurotoxin against it to neutralize and eliminate it from the body. But the mercury is too deadly and overpowers the nerve cells.

Dr. Klinghardt states that scientific studies establish that within twenty-four hours after injecting a tiny dose of mercury into a muscle anywhere in the body (in this study, it was monkeys), it is detectable in the spinal cord and brain, as well as kidneys, lungs, blood, connective tissue, and adrenal and other endocrine glands.[35] It is also now known that mercury prefers the brain's hypothalamus gland (which regulates the sympathetic nervous system[36]) and the brain's limbic system (which is believed to be the organic seat of the emotions).

These affinities help explain the range of physical and emotional symptoms attributed to mercury toxicity. "As soon as anybody has any type of medical illness or symptom, whether medical or emotional, the amalgam fillings should be removed and the mercury residues should be eliminated from the body, especially the brain," states Dr. Klinghardt.[37]

But let's say you don't have an overt or manifest illness at the moment. Should you have your mercury fillings removed? How can you tell if you have mercury in your system at levels beyond what your immune system can handle? In chapter 3, we reviewed five different laboratory tests that can give you an answer about your body's mercury load. These tests include hair analysis for heavy metals, a urine elements profile, a fecal metals stool analysis, an oral toxicity test called ALT, and the DMSA mercury provocation test.

The recommendation here is before you have your mercury fillings replaced, find out if you have too much mercury in your body, and do this by employing one or more of the tests just cited and described in detail in chapter 3. As a complement, get a reading on the vitality of your immune system and your general nutrient status; find out if you are nutritionally and immunologically equipped to handle whatever toxic load your teeth may be putting on your body. Intelligent, focused nutrient fortification may enable your system to handle the mercury load for a while longer until you decide what permanent course of action to take, or if you elect to have a few fillings replaced at a time over a two-year period, for example.

The reason for the conservative approach here is that not only is mercury amalgam replacement expensive and not necessarily reimbursed (if at all) by dental insurance plans, it is potentially dangerous if not done correctly. Minute mercury particles can be swallowed and minute amounts of mercury vapor inhaled during the procedure, and you can end up with more mercury in your system than before. If your immune system is already on the edge, at its limit of being able to handle your body's toxic load, this additional toxic input may be too much, and you may get sick as a result, even *very* sick.

At a minimum, for safe mercury amalgam removal, your dentist must use a rubber dam (a rubber latex sheet or dental dam) in your mouth to prevent you from swallowing mercury. Your dentist should also use strong air suction to collect vapors, and frequent water suctioning and washing out of the mouth. The patient must be draped so no mercury chips get carried home; ideally, the patient breathes oxygen through a nosepiece during the procedure rather than through the mouth or nose to avoid any possible inhalation of mercury vapors.

Perhaps the following data will help clarify your thinking. A researcher polled sixty patients who had undergone replacement of their mercury fillings, followed up with a nutritional program and heavy metal detoxification using DMPS (see below). Of these people, seventy-eight percent said they were either satisfied or very satisfied with the results. In terms of the patient's own assessment of their medical problems before having the fillings replaced, the most common complaints were memory and concentration deficits; pain in the muscles and joints; anxiety; insomnia; problems in the stomach, intestines, and bladder; depression; food or chemical sensitivities; numbness; tingling; or eye problems, in that order. Of the symptoms that bothered them the most, the patients cited headaches, backaches, fatigue, and memory and concentration problems.[38]

Evidence exists that even with these precautions, "significant" new deposits of mercury in the body (lungs, kidneys, endocrine organs, liver, and heart) can occur. This means you need an effective way to bind up (chelate) existing mercury in the body so as to effectively escort it out of the body.

Cilantro

Research conducted by Chinese acupuncturists found that cilantro (*Coriandum sativum*) can effectively collect and bind up mercury and other heavy metals in the brain and central nervous system. Another mobilization agent, such as chlorella, is then needed to facilitate the excretion of these toxic substances from the body.

For patients who were having their dental amalgams replaced, the acupuncturists prescribed cilantro, also known as Chinese parsley, at the oral dose of 100 mg four times daily (in conjunction with other "drug-uptake enhancement methods," e.g., the essential fatty acids EPA and DHA) to collect and remove the mercury from the body, including the new deposits that resulted from the amalgam removal. They recommended taking cilantro before the amalgam removal, and then for another two to three weeks afterwards.[39]

The Chinese researchers also found that cilantro worked synergistically with antibiotics and natural antiviral agents (EPA and DHA) against several otherwise intractable infectious organisms that had been unresponsive to the antibiotics alone. When cilantro was given in tandem with these other treatments, it "rapidly reduced the generalized symptom and infection." Cilantro "accelerates" the excretion of mercury and lead from the body through the urine, they reported. They postulated that the infectious microorganisms used the heavy metals in the body (lead and mercury) to protect themselves from the antibiotics.[40]

Cilantro of course is available without a prescription, and you can also take it as a cooked herb (stalks), at the rate of one to two teaspoons daily.[41] Dragon River Herbals offers a blend of cilantro and yellow dock to be taken at the rate of 5-15 drops 2 times daily for the first 5 days; stop for 2 days, then resume at this dosage for 30-120 days.

DMSA

This substance—dimercaptosuccinic acid—was mentioned above (and in chapter 3) as a provocative agent to reveal mercury load in the body as measured in the urine. A nontoxic, water-soluble substance, DMSA chelates mercury and excretes it out of the body, giving the physician an indication of the body's mercury burden. But it can also be used as the official chelation agent to remove mercury following mercury amalgam replacement.

DMSA, administered orally, has been used since the 1950s as an antidote to heavy metal toxicity such that today, according to some experts in the field of alternative medicine, it is considered "the premier metal chelation compound."[42] As an example of its "premier" abilities, nine children were exposed to vapors of metallic mercury from an external source (not teeth). Their initial urinary mercury levels ranged from 61 to 1,213 mcg/g, with an average of 214 mcg. Immediately after DMSA treatment, the urinary mercury average soared by 268% to 573 mcg/g, then after six weeks, leveled out to an average of 102 mcg/g, or only fifty percent of the average level originally detected after the exposure. None of the children experienced any adverse side effects.[43]

Swedish researchers found that when they gave oral DMSA to twenty dental patients (suspected to have mercury toxicity from their fillings) for 14 days at the rate of 20 mg/kg of body weight, it resulted in an average increase in urinary mercury excretion of 65%. The DMSA also reduced blood mercury levels by 0.04 mcg/l/day. The mercury kept coming out of their bodies for three months even though the DMSA was only given for two weeks. The patients also experienced a decrease in their levels of reported fatigue and inertia.[44]

Researchers at Odensk University in Denmark gave fifty patients with environmental-illness-type medical complaints a program of DMSA (30 mg/kg body weight) for five days. These patients had elevated levels of overall distress, obsessive-compulsive tendencies, depression, anxiety, reduced extroversion, and greater emotional volatility, according to standard psychological profiling. Six weeks later, when they were queried again, the patients said most of their distress symptoms had "improved considerably." The tests showed they had excreted a great deal of mercury and lead in their urine during that time.[45]

DMPS

2,3-dimercaptopropane-1-sulfonic acid is another favored chelating agent for increasing the removal of elemental mercury from the human body. It can be given orally, intravenously, or intramuscularly, and is useful for people who have been exposed to mercury amalgam through their dental fillings, or for those who show evidence or suspicion of heavy metal toxicity from other sources. DMPS has been used with a good safety record for many years in Russia (since the 1960s) and Germany (since 1978) and is used by some progressive physicians in the United States as part of a post-mercury-amalgam-removal protocol.

Like DMSA, it can also be given as a challenge to see how much mercury the body is carrying. For example, twenty-eight dental personnel (dentists, dental technicians, and office staff) were given DMPS, after which their urinary excretion of mercury was eighty-eight times higher (for the technicians who formulate amalgams), forty-nine times higher (dentists), and thirty-five times greater (office staff).[46]

American researchers found that giving dental patients an oral DMPS dose of 300 mg increased their excretion of mercury through the urine from 0.70 to 17.2 mcg among patients with mercury amalgams and from 0.27 to 5.1 mcg for those without mercury amalgams in only nine hours. The scientists gauged that two-thirds of the excreted urinary mercury in the patients with amalgams came from vapor released by those fillings, the rest from environmental sources of mercury contamination, such as air pollution and fish.[47]

In Mexico, scientists monitored the urinary excretion of mercury from dental technicians, dentists, and office personnel who had taken DMPS. They compared the rate before DMPS was given and six hours afterwards. For the technicians, before DMPS, they excreted 4.84 mcg of mercury, but after, 424 mcg; for dentists, 3.28 mcg before, and 162 after; and for office staff, 0.7 mcg before and 27 mcg after. The researchers concluded that it is more meaningful to determine how much mercury the kidney is burdened with based on the excretion rate after DMPS is given.[48]

DMPS may be somewhat more effective than DMSA in removing mercury from the kidneys. Researchers at the Mercer University School of Medicine in Macon, Georgia, used both chelating substances to monitor mercury removal from the kidneys of rats. Both substances increased the rate of mercury elimination from the body during the first twenty-four hours after administration, but DMPS was more effective at reducing the "renal burden" (the amount of mercury stored in the kidneys).[49]

At the National Institute of Public Health in Prague in the Czech Republic, researchers studied the effect of DMPS on three groups of subjects: industrial workers exposed to workplace mercury, dentists, and rats injected with mercury. Two doses of DMPS were given, spaced one day apart. After two days, the urinary mercury excretion rate in the workers was 1513 mcg; in the dentists, 132 mcg; and in human controls, 3.78 mcg. Two doses of DMPS decreased the kidney content of mercury in the rats by thirty percent when given orally and fifty percent when injected into the muscles. The scientists found that in the human subjects, two doses of DMPS reduced their kidney mercury content by seventeen to twenty percent (oral dose) and twenty-five to thirty percent (injection) in only forty-eight hours.[50]

Alginate

This substance derives from the Fucales seaweed, *Ascophyllum nodosum,* and is accumulating a good track record for its ability to bind up heavy metals and radioactive solutions in the body. The body is not able to break down or digest alginate, so the substance passes through intact, bearing its heavy metal burden. Alginate is commercially available without a prescription under the brand name ProAlgen (from Nordic Naturals), which is comprised of *Ascophyllum nodosum* and Fucus and Laminaria algae (containing 40 minerals and trace elements) in 600 mg capsules. You can use alginate following mercury amalgam removal, or even after every meal, to collect any mercury

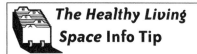

The Healthy Living Space Info Tip

For cilantro:
Dragon River Herbals,
P.O. Box 74,
Ojo Caliente, NM 87549;
tel: 505-583-2348 or 800-813-2118;
fax: 505-583-2339;
website: www.dragonriverherbals.com.

For ProAlgen, Alginate Detox Supplement:
Nordic Naturals,
3040 Valencia Ave., #2,
Aptos, CA 95003;
tel: 800-662-2544 or 831-662-2852;
fax: 831-662-0382;
website: www.nordicnaturals.com.

For information about
biological dentistry:
Hal Huggins, D.D.S., M.S.,
P.O. Box 49145,
Colorado Springs, CO 80949;
tel: 888-843-5832 or 719-522-0566;
fax: 719-548-8220;
website: www.hugnet.com.

For nutritional and homeopathic protocols for mercury detoxification:
Daniel F. Royal, D.O.,
The Royal Center of Advanced Medicine,
2501 N. Green Valley Parkway, Suite D-132,
Henderson, NV 89014;
tel: 888-DANROYAL or 702-433-8800;
fax: 702-433-8823;
e-mail: royal@drroyal.com;
website: www.drroyal.com.

🏠 *The Healthy Living Space* Info Tip

For information for dentists contemplating biological dentistry (protocols and standards):
International Academy of Oral Medicine and Toxicology,
Michael E. Ziff, Executive Director,
P.O. Box 628531,
Orlando, FL 32860;
tel: 407-298-2450;
e-mail: mziff@iaomt.org;
website: www.iaomt.org.

For patients to get referrals for biological dentists:
Holistic Dental Association,
P.O. Box 5007,
Durango, CO 81301;
tel: 970-259-1091;
e-mail: had@frontier.net;
website: www.holisticdental.org.

For more information about biological dentistry, conferences, and research:
American Academy of Biological Dentistry,
P.O. Box 856,
Carmel Valley, CA 93924;
tel: 831-659-5385;
fax: 831-659-2417.

For information about healthy treatment options for periodontal disease:
International Dental Health Foundation,
2414 Black Cap Lane, Suite L-1,
Reston, VA 20191;
tel: 703-860-9244 or 800-368-3396;
fax: 703-860-9245;
website: http://members.aol.com/idhf.

that might have been released into your system through chewing.

Timing Your Amalgam Removals

If you decide to have your mercury fillings removed, Dr. Huggins has a tip about finding the best time to do so. Apparently your immune system has a cycle in which it replenishes its supplies of white blood cells or lymphocytes. You don't want to hit that low time with a big challenge to the immune system generated by removing your mercury fillings.

Dr. Huggins reports that about seven days after an immune challenge—mercury exposure during amalgam replacement, having an immunization shot, a bad case of the flu, serious emotional trauma from death or accidents—your body's defenses are weakened. The lymphocytes are in the process of being replaced, so there are several hours on day seven when your immune defenses are down and vulnerable. On day fourteen, the lymphocytes are again regrouping, regenerating, and you are immunologically vulnerable. So "if there is an additional [immune] challenge on day 7, 14, or especially 21, then your genetic weak link is apt to be stretched, and you may become ill," says Dr. Huggins.

In other words, don't have any mercury amalgam work done on days seven, fourteen, or twenty-one. He advises not having dental appointments on the same day of the week during a two-month period, and don't have dental work two days in a row, or procedures that last longer than two hours. In practical terms, he suggests having dental appointments on Monday, Wednesday, and Friday of one week, then Tuesday, Thursday, and Saturday the next week. It is immunologically preferable to have all the amalgams removed in a thirty-day period, if possible.[51]

Nutritional Support for Amalgam Removal

In conjunction with having your amalgams replaced, and especially as an immediate follow-up, many alternative medicine physicians recommend a targeted nutritional program to help your body cope with the mobilization and removal of mercury.

Daniel F. Royal, D.O., an osteopath who practices in Henderson, Nevada, recommends the following: chlorella (1-3 capsules daily); L-glutathione (150 mg daily); kyolic garlic (1 capsule with meals, three times daily); silymarin (1 capsule, twice daily); vitamin C (2,000-8,000 mg daily, depending on tolerance, in divided doses); vitamin B complex (25-100 mg daily); DHEA (an adrenal hormone precursor, 5 mg for men, 2.5 mg for women, daily); pregnenolone (a steroid building block made from cholesterol; 10 mg for men, 30 mg for women, once daily*); Mercurius solubilis* 30C (a homeopathic remedy; thirty drops, 2-3 times weekly, for a few weeks); selenium (50 mcg, three times daily); and *Lactobacillus acidophilus* (one teaspoon daily). Dr. Royal also recommends time in a sauna to sweat out mercury and other toxins through the skin (see chapter 6).[52]

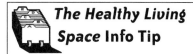

The Healthy Living Space Info Tip

For detailed information on mercury hazards and mercury-free dentistry:
DAMS (Dental Amalgam Mercury Syndrome),
P.O. Box 64397,
Virginia Beach, VA 23467;
tel: 800-311-6265;
website: www.amalgam.org.

HEALTHY LIVING SPACE DETOXIFIER #32
Have Your Cavitations Cleaned Out and Reduce Possible Jawbone Infections

As explained above, a cavitation is a formal term from dentistry to describe a hole in the upper or lower jawbone following a tooth extraction in which an infectious process is occurring, usually unbeknownst to the person. The cavitation typically is the same size as the tooth that was removed from that site. It is a problem because it is a site of incomplete healing.

When a tooth is root-canalled and then later removed, often a little bit is left behind, called the periodontal ligament, half of whose fibers come from the jaw, the other half from the tooth. When the tooth is removed but the ligament is left in place, it starts to release neurotoxic chemicals that slowly seep into the body; these chemicals were originally produced by the harmful bacteria in the root of the decayed, dying tooth.

Now if the root-canalled tooth is extracted and the ligament left there, a small cap of bone forms over the socket "leaving a cesspool of these chemicals lining the hole, and sealed within the bone," explains Dr. Huggins. The cavitation then serves as a breeding ground for bacteria and the toxic substances they excrete. It also creates osteonecrosis, or bone death, through the progressive impairment of blood circulation through that part of the jawbone. Biological dentists also postulate that the toxic cavitations can block the flow of *qi* through the acupuncture meridians that pass through the mouth and also transmit the energy signal of toxicity to other organs and organ systems in the body through this same network of energy channels. There is some evidence that cavitations can act as reservoirs for leeched amalgam mercury.

Unfortunately, this setup is not easily detectable with X-rays, so many dentists can overlook it. On close examination of the X-ray, the cavitation may appear like the shadow of a tooth, or a phantom tooth. "Almost always, this is indicative of a cavitation," states Mark A. Breiner, D.D.S., in *Whole-Body Dentistry*. Dr. Breiner notes that the most common site for a cavitation to form is at the extraction site of a wisdom tooth, and the second most common site is a root-canalled tooth extraction site.

Dr. Huggins reports that cavitation in dental patients is "an *extremely* common finding." The third molars, or wisdom teeth, are the most prevalent site, such that out of 354 extraction sites examined, 88% had cavitations. The second molars had a seventy percent incidence of cavitations, and in the first molars, eighty-two percent had cavitations. For all molars examined, eighty-five percent had cavitations (441 sites out of 517 examined). In nonmolar sites, the incidence of cavitations was much lower, at fifty-five percent.[53] This is a shockingly high incidence of a dental condition (and source of dental toxicity) still largely unrecognized by most dentists.

Insofar as the wisdom teeth have energy correlations through the acupuncture meridians with many of the body's important organs, including the heart, a cavitation at this point—also known as a focal infection, as mentioned earlier—is highly undesirable and a potentially serious health threat. Dr. Breiner recounts how his own episode of an irregular heartbeat was traced to a cavitation in the wisdom tooth area of his jaw. Surgical debridement (cleaning toxins and dead bone material out of the cavitation) resolved the arrhythmia in a few days, he reports. Cavitations can also produce chronic facial pain (trigeminal neuralgia), as well as some headaches and phantom toothaches. Dr. Breiner calls cavitations SICO, for Sickness Inducing Cavitational Osteonecrosis (dead bone material) to highlight their ability to negatively affect many aspects of a person's health.[54]

In support of Dr. Breiner's sweeping indictment of cavitations is evidence developed by Boyd Hailey, Ph.D., a prominent dental researcher at the University of Kentucky. His research shows that all cavitation tissue samples tested contain toxins that are able to significantly block the activity of one or more of five critical body enzymes involved in the production of energy. The toxins produce health problems both localized (in the jawbone) and systemic (throughout the body).[55]

There also is a succession of bacterial species in the cavitation. Swiss dentists reported that in advanced root caries ninety percent of the microflora found were bacteria, and of these, in the early stage of tooth infection, *Actinomyces naeslundii* was significantly higher than other species. In the advanced stage of decay, the predominant bacteria was *Streptococcus mutans*. In other words, there was a succession of bacterial populations observed during the "destruction process" of a single tooth.[56]

As noted earlier in this chapter, Dr. Christopher Hussar has remarked that the mouth is a dirty place. He was not exaggerating. Over 300 different species of bacteria exist in the mouth, creating a population estimated to be several hundred billion. In an insufficiently cleaned mouth, that number can be a thousand billion. These billions of bacteria create their own ecological niches inside the human mouth, reproduce, metabolize, and thereby threaten oral and systemic health.

Scientists know the action of these bacteria is associated with the incidence of rheumatoid arthritis, dermatitis, nephritis (bacteria-induced kidney inflammation), bacterial pneumonia, pregnancy troubles, blood circulation problems, and coronary heart disease.[57] Periodontal disease can also lead to bacteremia (bacteria in the blood), diabetes, respiratory disease, prosthetic device infection, and atherosclerosis.[58] Periodontal disease is seven times more likely to be linked with a preterm delivery of a low birth weight infant than other factors, including the mother's age and tobacco and alcohol use.[59]

Infections in the gum and jawbone have been linked to 150-350 different anaerobic bacterial species, depending on the type of periodontitis; dental treatment and tooth extraction can cause these toxic microorganisms to move into the bloodstream where they are free to circulate around the body. If a person has a pre-existing heart problem (such as an ineffective heart valve or a vascular disease), the circulation of these bacterial species can lead to serious problems, including heart attacks.[60]

In an odd way, brushing your teeth is potentially bad for your heart. English researchers studied the effect on 150 children of tooth brushing, professional cleaning, and scaling on the release of bacteria into the body. They found that all three methods of cleaning the teeth released at least three species of bacteria implicated in the development of bacterial endocarditis (inflammation of the membrane lining the heart). In other words, the average mouth has these toxic bacteria in residence, and cleaning the teeth mobilizes them and gets them moving through the body.[61]

The connection between oral focal infections and/or periodontitis (inflammation and degeneration of the supporting structures of the teeth) and the heart is well established in scientific research. Finnish researchers examined the microbial population in the mouths of fifty patients (average age sixty-five) about to have abdominal aortic surgery. They found that eighty-two percent had evidence of oral infection. On average, most of the patients had only nine teeth, and twenty-one percent of these were potential focal infection sites; further, twenty-six percent of the patients had oral candidiasis (an infection caused by *Candida albicans*). "Oral infectious foci occur frequently in patients needing aortic surgery," said the researchers, adding that untreated focal infections may contribute to heart infection.[62]

When 261 patients with suspected focal-infection-produced diseases were examined for chronic inflammatory problems in their mouths, researchers found that 83% had periodontal problems, such as dead tissue and inflammation. These oral problems are frequently detected as factors in chronic cardiac disorders, eye problems (uveitis), and skin diseases, the researchers said.[63]

It is also possible for oral bacteria to first start a systemic infection, like endocarditis, then indirectly stimulate a brain abscess.[64] Various oral bacteria (including Streptococci species) can cause sinusitis, either acute or chronic.[65]

These are examples of how an oral focal infection—the human mouth as a focus of infection—can produce a range of specific and systemic diseases throughout the body. This is a medical insight at least one hundred years old, but largely ignored until recently. The term focal infection can encompass many problems in the mouth: cavitations, cavities, extraction sites, infected teeth and pulps. While periodontitis is not the same as a cavitation, it is a potent source of oral focal infection that can exist alongside or in conjunction with a cavitation, adding to the total toxicity present in the mouth.

The crucial point to keep in mind is that bacterial and viral microorganisms or their toxic products can enter the body tissues through the mouth and thereby produce health problems. Arthritis is a good example. In one study, an antigen (foreign protein) was injected to the mouth and soon after produced a knee inflammation, leading scientists to postulate that a dental focal infection may be involved in arthritis of the knee and arthritis in general.[66]

Should you, if you have extraction sites in your mouth, automatically have your cavitations debrided? Not necessarily, says Dr. Huggins. If you feel well, enjoy good health, and have normal laboratory profiles for nutrient and antioxidant defense status, it probably means the toxins are stable, staying in place in the jawbone, and that your immune system is coping. But if you get sick or develop a chronic problem, then you should consider investigating the possibility that you have cavitations acting as focal infections, and get them treated.

"Cavitations can progress over time, with more and more adjacent jawbone dying," says Dr. Huggins. You may not have a problem this year, but perhaps in five or ten years, you might. As J.H. Meurmann, a dental researcher at the Institute of Dentistry at the University of Helsinki in Finland remarks, "Chronic dental infections may worsen the conditions of medically compromised patients." Dr. Meurmann adds that if a person is acutely or chronically ill, frequent dental checkups to determine possible focal infections in the mouth are highly advised.[67]

When a biological dentist cleans the cavitation, the walls of the jawbone socket must be cut out with a dental burr, then the toxic material is scraped out. Since some of the toxic material then enters the lymphatic system as part of the body's natural (and now freed up) detoxification pathway, the patient may feel sick for a few days while the body processes the toxins, Dr. Huggins says.

HEALTHY LIVING SPACE DETOXIFIER #33
Think Twice before Digging Another Root Canal in Your Mouth

Having a root canal "dug" in one of your teeth is generally regarded as a highly unpleasant experience by most people. It may be a miserable experience, but in 1996, an estimated 25 million were installed in American mouths, and for 2000, the dental industry predicted 30 million.

Most dental patients and dentists regard it as preferable to having the tooth extracted because, depending on the location, this can destabilize the jaw and lead to other dental problems later. In the root canal procedure, the dental pulp, dying (or dead) and infected, is removed and replaced with a wax material called gutta percha. Technically the tooth is now dead, but as biological dentists have known for decades, dead does not mean inactive. In this case, the activity is bacterial, and it is not good for you.

You may think the dental infection is terminated once the gutta percha is laid into the tooth and the painful abscess goes away, but research suggests it isn't. In fact, serious health consequences may result from a hidden, deep-set infection beneath the root-canalled tooth. According to George Meinig, D.D.S., author of Root Canal Cover-up, "root canal treated teeth have side effects that cause many disorders."[68] He made this statement on the foundation of forty-seven years of clinical practice as a root canal clinician and dentist.

It is almost impossible for a dentist to clean out all the infection from a decayed root canal; so pockets of infection remain when the canal is sealed up. The result is that bacteria get trapped within the estimated three miles of microscopic dentin tubules inside a single root-canalled tooth. The cementum (the outermost hard surface of the tooth) prevents the bacteria from migrating from the tooth into the bloodstream, but not the toxins produced by these bacteria.

Over the years, these pockets of infection can start spreading their process throughout the body, without the person suspecting it, at least directly. As toxins leak from the root-canalled tooth, they chronically trigger the immune system to react, and eventually the immunological defense system gets weary of the engagement. Infections under root canals are focal infections, which means they continuously disseminate toxins into the body, contributing, undetected, to a myriad of problems throughout the body.

As early as 1925, the connection between bacterially contaminating root canals and systemic health problems was known to professionals who read the scientific literature. Weston A. Price, D.D.S., reported that many degenerative diseases result from root canals, including endocarditis and other heart ailments, disorders of the kidneys and bladder, rheumatism, arthritis, lung problems, complications of pregnancy, bacterial infections, and even mental illness. Dr. Price demonstrated his point vividly when he implanted actual root-canalled teeth (from human subjects suffering from various diseases) under the skin of rabbits. The rabbits developed the same diseases as the humans whose teeth they were.[69]

Dr. Price discovered many changes in blood chemistry as a result of root-canalled teeth. The white blood cell count (lymphocytes) goes up considerably; in rabbits, it increased fifty-eight percent following the implantation of the human teeth. But at the same time, another kind of white blood cell (polymorphonuclear leukocytes) decreased by thirty-three percent in rabbits. These changes indicated both a mobilization of the immune response and a diminution of one of its prime components.

How can you tell if a root-canalled tooth is acting as a focal infection in your body? Consider undergoing the oral toxicity test developed by Boyd Haley, Ph.D., of Affinity Labeling Technologies in Lexington, Kentucky, as discussed in chapter 3. In conjunction with this, have your immune vitality tested based on a blood and urine sample, again, as described in chapter 3.

Whether a root-canalled tooth is making you sick depends a great deal on the vitality of your immune system. "If your immune system is strong, your body may be able to quarantine the toxins by 'walling off' the area [around the tooth]," says Dr. Breiner. This area might appear as a "more radiolucent" area suggestive of an abscess on a dental X-ray, he adds. The radiolucent sign is a good one, indicating the successful immunological containment of toxins. Sometimes, Dr. Breiner adds, a "drain" will open up under the root canal tooth and the toxins will slowly, almost imperceptibly drain out into the mouth over time.

Gutta Percha Alternative: BioCalex

One of the problems with gutta percha, explains Dr. Breiner, is that it contracts over time, creating a gap between itself and the tooth's remaining dentin. This allows bacteria from the bloodstream to enter and exacerbate the infectious process already under way.[70]

An alternative substance from France, newly introduced among biological dentists (1994), is called BioCalex, made from calcium and zinc oxide. Used in France since 1979, BioCalex seals the root canals more effectively than gutta percha, creating a tight bond and preventing bacterial ingress; it has been shown to penetrate into the most inaccessible of the tiny canals and tubules inside the tooth.

It is also alkaline (nonacidic), which creates an unfavorable environment for bacteria. This was demonstrated by Australian researchers who studied the changes in root dentin pH (the ratio of acidity to alkalinity on a scale of 0.1-14, with 7 being neutral) over a four-week period after they had been treated with calcium hydroxide. In the inner part of the dentin, the pH peaked at a high alkaline reading of between 9.7 and 10.8; after 2-3 weeks, the outer dentin reached a pH of 9.0 to 9.3. Although the pH change took longer to obtain in the outer dentin of the root, the study showed that calcium hydroxide could diffuse throughout the tooth and change its chemical nature.

In fact, the calcium oxide composition of BioCalex is very effective at destroying anaerobic bacteria found in teeth, according to BioProbe, its U.S. marketer. Greek researchers tested calcium hydroxide alongside a standard disinfectant (paramonochlorophenol, PMCP) against anaerobic bacteria isolated from infected root canals, and observed results at time intervals of five, fifteen, thirty, and sixty minutes.

They found that calcium hydroxide was "significantly more effective" than PMCP against the total bacterial population. Further, it was "quickly and highly effective" against several microorganisms (B. melaninogenicus, P. gingivalis, and Actinomyces species) associated with severe clinical symptoms.71 Preliminary tests show a considerably reduced level of toxicity associated with BioCalex used in root-canalled teeth compared to those treated with gutta percha.

Further, when calcium oxide combines with water, it forms calcium hydroxide, and this is one of the most biocompatible dental materials available. Biocompatibility will be discussed below, but it means the substance is nonallergenic and nontoxic to the human body; it will not produce overt or hidden allergic or immunological reactions when it comes in contact with human tissue, such as in the mouth.

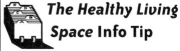

The Healthy Living Space Info Tip

For information about BioCalex, BioProbe Newsletter, and scientific documentation about mercury hazards, and for dentists wishing to obtain BioCalex:
BioProbe, Inc.,
P.O. Box 608010,
Orlando, FL 32860;
tel: 800-282-9670 or 407-290-9670;
fax: 407-299-4149;
website: www.bioprobe.com.

HEALTHY LIVING SPACE DETOXIFIER #34
Determine Your Biocompatibility with Dental Materials before Putting Any More in Your Mouth

Mention was made above about biocompatibility of dental materials. This is an important issue with regard to toxicity and allergic reactions to substances, yet it is not discussed enough in medical circles. Dentists routinely place many substances in our mouths—mercury, silver, and tin (in amalgams), gutta percha (in root canals), sealants, gold or chrome (in crowns), porcelain and plastic (bridges), nickel (orthodontic braces), titanium or ceramic (implants)—but who is to say a given dental patient is not allergic, or will not develop an allergy over time to these strange substances not meant by nature to be in the human body. Who is to say (who has tested them?) they are compatible with the immune system?

"Not too many dental materials are free from toxins," comments Dr. Huggins. "Unfortunately, the stronger materials are the most toxic," he adds. This is why he recommends compatibility testing for dental products to assess in advance the potential or likely allergenicity *to you* of any dental substance that might be placed in your mouth. Bear in mind that, to an extent, allergic reactions are individual, based on your total biochemistry and immune status; this means that if a given substance is said not to produce allergic reactions generally, it may still generate symptoms in you because of your biochemical specificity.

For example, scientists now know that toxic substances can be leaked from composite dental resins used instead of mercury amalgams and that these "exudations" into the mouth can be estrogenic—act like the hormone estrogen. Researchers at the University of Granada in Spain applied a dental sealant based on a substance called bisphenol-A diglycidylether methacrylate (found in dental resins) to the molars of eighteen dental patients. Saliva samples were tested one hour before this application and one hour after it.

Anywhere from 90 to 131 mcg of bisphenol-A were detected after the sealant had been applied. Further, the researchers found that certain biochemical changes typical of estrogenic activity were noted in these patients, and on that basis they made this conclusion: "The use of bis-GMA-based resins in dentistry, and particularly the use of sealants in children, appears to contribute to human exposure to xenoestrogens."[72] As you may recall from chapter 2, a xenoestrogen is a foreign estrogen; it is a synthetic chemical that acts *like* estrogen in the body, thereby upsetting the hormonal balance.

Another study showed that formaldehyde can be released by dental composites in your teeth. Researchers at the NIOM-Scandinavian Institute of Dental Materials in Haslum, Norway, found that nine different types of commercially used dental composites released formaldehyde into the mouth. "A continuous release of formaldehyde was evident during the first ten days [after placement]," they stated. Then it declined, but was still detectable after 115 days.[73]

These two examples of estrogenic dental factors are included here to give an introductory idea about biocompatibility. Obviously, estrogenic chemicals and formaldehyde from dental materials are not compatible with the human system and will contribute to body-wide toxicity and a heightening (and eventually a fatiguing) of the immune response.

A test called the Clifford Materials Reactivity Testing (CMRT) is now available to monitor dental biocompatibility. The purpose of the test, according to its provider, Clifford Consulting and Research of Colorado Springs, Colorado, is to screen a patient for sensitivities to chemical groups and compounds, to identify dental materials that can be used with that patient with the greatest degree of safety and least amount of risk, and to help the dentist put together a biocompatible treatment plan.

The test looks for specific antibody formation in response to various dental materials, and interprets this response as a gauge for biocompatibility. (When the body encounters a foreign or suspect substance in the bloodstream, it produces antibodies, or immune defense proteins, to tag and neutralize the intruding substance.) The test looks for antigens to various chemical groups such as acrylates, urethanes, toluenes, nickel, aluminum, and mercury. The testers take a small amount of blood and give it a "challenge" of the dental material (the antigen) to see whether antibodies are formed in response.

The test is recommended for people with existing sensitivity problems such as environmental illness or multiple chemical sensitivity, those who already have a compromised physiology (an illness or chronic condition), or those who have a prior history of reacting negatively to dental materials. It's also helpful if you are planning major dental restorative work, including dental implants, crowns, bridges, or mercury amalgam replacement. The results are cross-referenced with a list of over 1,900 dental and medical trade-named products so that the dentist can select materials of minimal reactivity for individual patients.

The test looks at how the patient will react not only to newly placed dental materials, but the corrosion byproducts of dental materials already in the patient's mouth. In other words, say you had a gold crown put on a molar five years ago; whatever trace amounts of metals or byproducts of the corrosion process have been generated and released by this crown will be accounted for in the test. For example, according to Clifford Consulting and Research, testing of more than 12,800 patients shows that 1% do not handle gold in the mouth well, and that twenty-five percent have problems with silver. In other words, "no single material is 100% suited to all patients."

Resolution of long-standing dental problems may turn around many chronic symptoms that you had previously never suspected were associated

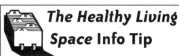

The Healthy Living Space Info Tip

For Clifford Materials Reactivity Testing:
Clifford Consulting and Research, Inc.,
P.O. Box 17597,
Colorado Springs, CO 80935;
tel: 719-550-0008;
fax: 719-550-0009;
e-mail: wjclifford@ccrlab.com;
website: www.ccrlab.com.

with events in your mouth. You may find that certain emotional states that came upon you now and then start to lift; you may have thought depression or anxiety were "just who you were," but now that your mercury amalgams are gone, so is your depression.

Now that you have removed a fair amount of physical toxicity from your system, from the protocols in chapters 4-7 encompassing your liver, intestines, kidneys, lymphatic system, and teeth, you have sufficient momentum to move a layer deeper into yourself—into the realm of emotions. Emotions, too, can be toxic; certain strongly held but unexpressed emotions can act like toxins if they are left to fester. So our next phase of detoxification in chapter 8 moves into the emotional life and offers ways to start resolving buried, repressed, or neglected emotional issues.

CHAPTER 8

Guidelines for Emotional Detoxification:

Unresolved Emotional Issues Can Become Toxic to the Body

In the course of following the detoxification suggestions in this book you have undoubtedly come up against some old, perhaps painful or intractable emotions. You may have been surprised by their existence, or by the energy with which they reminded you of their existence. It is highly common for people cleansing the colon to reexperience charged emotional material from many years back, as if they had unknowingly walked into some unsuspected personalized museum of hurts and trauma.

In many respects, physical detoxification makes it possible to get to the emotions, buried, as it were, under layers of physical toxins and dysfunctional physiological states. Internal organ cleansing often helps you identify this next level of toxicity.

Like the intestines, the body is a remarkable storage device for unprocessed thoughts and feelings. Most people spend a lifetime depositing unresolved emotional issues throughout the body; in fact, it is not only painful experiences that are stored; all sorts of memories get lodged in the body's tissues. In her book, *Being-in-Dreaming*, Florinda Donner, an anthropologist and compatriot of Carlos Castaneda in the mysteries of Toltec shamanism, explains how she uses a little wooden mallet to tap her body for memories. She systematically taps every inch of her body, noting that everyday events tend to get stored in the chest, back, and abdomen, while dream content tends to go into the legs and hips.

"All that concerns you now is that remembering dreams has to do with physical pressure on the specific spot where that vision is stored," she says, adding that events experienced in dreams are hard to remember "because the body stores them in different places."[1] I used to think this was a fascinating but unsubstantiated idea until in the course of giving a friend a backrub and probing the left shoulder blade, she suddenly remembered being chased by a large turtle in a dry riverbed when she was eight years old. She had stored the actual daytime experience—like a home movie, vivid with the fright, surprise, adrenaline rush—at the bottom of her left shoulder blade.

In many respects, physical detoxification makes it possible to get to the emotions, buried, as it were, under layers of physical toxins and dysfunctional physiological states. Internal organ cleansing often helps you identify this next level of toxicity.

While the body is almost endlessly accommodating in this coping strategy, eventually it runs out of space, or the load in one place is too big a burden. Then the price comes due for your long-term emotional storage: your unresolved, stored emotions become toxic to the body and will start to make you sick. In this chapter, then, we will explore the contribution of unresolved emotional issues to body-wide toxicity, and suggest a strategy for clarifying and dissolving this subtler level of toxicity. But first let's consider some more examples of the consequences of using the body as an emotional storage depot.

How Unresolved Emotions Can Contribute to Illness

Emotional issues carry a powerful charge capable of affecting your biology in profound and often undesirable ways. For example, unresolved emotional issues are often associated with gynecological problems, such as uterine fibroids, ovarian cysts, and excessive menstrual bleeding, because the body must express itself, explains John Diamond, M.D., a homeopathic physician who practices in Reno, Nevada.

Dr. Diamond, who was educated in South Africa, cites a saying in that country that "If you don't cry above, you'll cry below." The crying below refers to the uterus, whose "tears" are menstrual blood. Dr. Diamond explains that he frequently sees strong emotions, if left unaddressed, manifesting as body symptoms, such as excessive menstrual bleeding.

The body is always metaphorical, he says. "It always *listens* to the psyche of the individual and responds accordingly, in its own way, translating withheld tears into copious menstrual flow." The emotional issue is an energy that *has* to go somewhere, *has* to be expressed physiologically, says Dr. Diamond.

A uterine fibroid (a noncancerous fibrous mass that grows on the inside wall of the uterus) often is about emotional suppression relating to either sexuality or relationships with men; the heavy bleeding it occasions is often associated with prolonged internalized sadness and withheld emotions; and an ovarian cyst (a noncancerous fluid-filled sac on an ovary) can be correlated with a history of sexual abuse, according to Dr. Diamond.

He cites the case of Flora, a thirty-eight-year-old woman with heavy, painful menstrual bleeding occasioned by multiple uterine fibroids. The woman, a mother of four, related that her heavy menstruation started two years earlier when her husband talked about divorcing her. Even though the marriage remained "intact," Flora was anxious, unsettled, and fearful about the prospect of a divorce, and "stuffed" the emotions and sadness into her body, says Dr. Diamond. Why her uterus?

Here we see the role of individual constitutional weakness and genetic predisposition. Her mother at her age had had the identical uterine problem, and both had started menstruating at a late age (fifteen), which can be indicative of later reproductive system problems, says Dr. Diamond. Flora's uterus was the designated weak point in her body, so if she had strong emotional content to store (suppress) somewhere, it would go there, and when the body could no longer cope with the continuous toxic presence of these emotions, it would discharge them through this same weak point: the uterus. Metaphorically, the fibroid was saying to Flora that her "ugly secret" was out: she could no longer hide her emotional pain and the way she tried to bury it in a hard shell.

After a comprehensive treatment program involving homeopathic remedies and herbs, Flora regained her health and did not need a hysterectomy (surgical removal of the uterus). The homeopathic remedies helped bring her emotions to the surface for clarification and expression. Then she resolved her emotional problems with her husband and started having normal periods again.

A hysterectomy, which conventional medicine routinely recommends for fibroids and related uterine problems, would not have corrected the deep-set cause of the imbalance, says Dr. Diamond. It would not have addressed "the true pathology of the internalized emotional fear and anger she had harbored for so long." It could have driven these emotions even deeper into her body, producing a more serious health problem such as cancer or mental illness.[2]

Unexpressed, stuffed emotions can also contribute to the emergence of rheumatoid arthritis, according to board-certified rheumatologist Norman Levin, M.D., who practices in Aldie, Virginia. He cites the case of Tara, thirty-six, who came to him suffering from rheumatoid arthritis. In addition to addressing the physiological and biochemical aspects of her medical problem, Dr. Levin encouraged Tara to ask herself *why* she was having arthritis now. Nobody gets a serious illness out of the blue, as if you accidentally walk through an illness ray and emerge sick, he says. There are always emotional and psychological factors involved in the development of an illness, he says.

"Patients need to be encouraged to find the meaning in their health crisis," Dr. Levin notes. Echoing Dr. Diamond's observation, he adds: "The body speaks its own language, and often illnesses affecting different parts of the body are associated with certain emotional states." For example, Dr. Levin often finds that unexpressed anger or resentment underlie the emergence of arthritis; the arthritis is a physical manifestation or expression of those emotions, he says.

In Tara's case, she had been a successful realtor who was suddenly relocated to an unfamiliar territory, having to abandon the market area she knew very well. It *felt* to her like she was being fired. At the same time she was uprooted from the safe and familiar routines of her job and environment, a romantic relationship was breaking up. So the job change and termination of a relationship gave Tara a double hit of emotional trauma, acting as *precipitating* factors for her arthritis, which began soon afterwards, says Dr. Levin.

In the case of Michelle, thirty-nine, her fibromyalgia was emotionally linked to a feeling of carrying the weight of the world on her shoulders. Fibromyalgia is a highly painful and debilitating illness in which numerous muscles throughout the body are chronically inflamed and painful, severely limiting movement. Ironically, Michelle had been an aerobics instructor before her muscles refused to let her move without extreme pain, spasm, and fatigue. "She was the kind of person who tried to do and be everything for everybody," comments Dr. Levin. "As we discovered, this attitude was at the core of her muscle aches."

About four weeks into her treatment program (a comprehensive alternative medicine approach), Michelle had enough freedom from pain to start to examine her psychoemotional state to see why she had fibromyalgia. She saw that she was a superachiever, a woman who always sought to be the best in every situation, be it motherhood, teaching aerobics, being a wife. She cared so much for everyone else she forgot to care for herself. She saw how everybody in her life *leaned* on her for support, that she could never say no to *carrying* their burdens.

The words say it all: the burden she was carrying for others was too much for her muscles. She was like not the mythic Atlas, capable of carrying the entire world on his Titan shoulders; she was a human woman with limits. Following its own innate intelligence, her body manifested fibromyalgia—muscle gridlock, so to speak—to force her to realize her approach to life was toxic. Michelle realized she could say no, turn down another plea for help, and ask for help herself. This understanding was the final turn of the key in the lock of her recovery.

Not everyone with fibromyalgia has this exact state of mind, says Dr. Levin, but it is fairly representative of the broad strokes. "A person feels burdened and overwhelmed, as if everybody is *leaning* on their body, as if they are *carrying* the world's weight on their shoulders."[3] Eventually, the body translates this metaphorical self-assessment into biological reality, and the psychological weight gets shifted to the actual muscles, and they ache, spasm, and refuse to carry it.

The longer a condition like this persists without the person understanding—and undoing—the emotional etiology, the more entrenched the translation into biology becomes. In other words, the emotional state may be a prime precipitating factor, but because of its charge and power, it starts to rearrange the body's structure, physiology, and biochemistry—only the tip of the illness iceberg, the part that conventional medicine tends to focus on—in accordance with its view of reality. If I feel like I'm carrying the weight of the world on my shoulders, my shoulders will start to believe it, and hurt accordingly.

Think of it this way: the unexpressed or unresolved anger, fear, resentment, or whatever the emotionally charged issue might be, act as free radicals in the body, as toxic agents capable of destabilizing physiological structures and processes just as powerfully and effectively as mercury, an organochlorine, or any other toxic substance described in this book. This is no judgment on emotions; it is not saying some are good and some bad. Rather, the point here is that when they get *stuck*, emotions become a physiological problem for the body. When stuck, their powerful energy charge starts to work negatively on the body.

All emotions are healthy because they are what tie the mind and body together, explains Candace Pert, Ph.D., in *Molecules of Emotion*. But they need to be expressed and let go of so they don't fester, build, or escalate uncontrollably. When they are not expressed, and instead are repressed, this sets up a "disintegrity" within the body, causing it to act at cross-purposes with being a unified whole organism. This repression generates stress that leads to blockages and an insufficient flow of "peptide signals to maintain function at the cellular level." This blocked flow creates the conditions of weakened function and immunity that can precipitate disease, says Dr. Pert.

The peptide signals are modes of communication between the biochemicals of emotion, Dr. Pert explains. Emotional biochemistry consists of neuropeptides (key brain chemicals that translate thoughts and feelings into biochemical and physiological responses) and their receptors. Dr. Pert's research has established that emotions are equal players in the health or illness of the body, as considerable in their influence as chemicals, toxic substances, or other material biological substances. The neuropeptides are the "substrates of emotion," in continuous communication with the immune system and its cells. Emotions have a "cellular signal" that is involved in translating emotional and mental information into physical reality, "literally transforming mind into matter."

In fact, Dr. Pert says our brains are not really just in our skulls; they are *mobile* brains, with communication networks throughout the body. Intelligent information travels throughout the network, which includes the hormonal, gastrointestinal, immune, and central nervous systems. According to this model, as we think and feel, so do our molecules act. Emotions are part of our cellular consciousness, because every cell has receptors that are conduits for emotional energy. First the emotions happen, then the neuropeptides are released. The fact that information flows throughout the mobile brain network demonstrates that "the body is the actual outward manifestation, in physical space, of the mind."[4]

But what about the stuck emotions you are unaware of, the ones you have buried deep and cannot retrieve or even remember that they exist? Sometimes clinical hypnotherapy can be helpful in aiding your dive into the subconscious to retrieve them, according to Joseph Riccioli, M.D., N.D., a physician and naturopath practicing in Clifton, New Jersey, who uses clinical hypnosis to help patients get over depression, cancer, and other serious health problems.

Medical science has established that our thoughts and emotions "talk" to our cells. Ever since the 1970s, scientists (including Dr. Pert) have been building a case for this and calling it psychoneuroimmunology, or PNI. PNI says the mind and emotions (psyche) communicate with the nervous (neuro) and immune (immunology) systems, both to their detriment or advantage, depending on whether it is consciously or unconsciously directed, and depending on the content of that communication.

Unfortunately, most of the time this dialogue is unconscious, says Dr. Riccioli. We get the results (the health problem) without understanding the causes (the emotional content), or we may be aware of a part of the picture, but missing the other pieces to make it comprehensible. Below are a few vivid examples from Dr. Riccioli's clinical casebook that make the point.

Grace, thirty-six, had an embarrassing problem: she chronically pulled her hair out the way other people bite their fingernails. Her scalp was a mess of patchy, straggly hair and great gaps where she had ripped the hair out. In the course of working with Grace, Dr. Riccioli learned that she was using the hair-pulling as a way to discharge stress and tension associated with two traumatic events earlier in her life, in the thrall of which emotions she was still gripped. As a child, she had been publicly humiliated in school, and in early adulthood, her husband became an active alcoholic and deserted their marriage.

Psychoneuroimmunology says the mind and emotions (psyche) communicate with the nervous (neuro) and immune (immunology) systems, both to their detriment or advantage, depending on whether it is consciously or unconsciously directed, and depending on the content of that communication.

Grace thought these two events happened because of her and therefore she deserved to be punished for them, even though she couldn't figure out why. Her pent-up, conflicted anger was expressed through her hair-pulling; because she couldn't find rest or resolution with respect to these two intense experiences, she was transiting back and forth continuously from her present age and those earlier times. Once she understood the connection and remembered the earlier experiences clearly and in full, she was able to discharge the old emotions and stop pulling her hair, says Dr. Riccioli.

Vera, forty-two, was a woman with angry ovaries. She had a serious case of ovarian cancer and was about to undergo surgery. Dr. Riccioli learned Vera had endured a highly abusive marital relationship, such that she at times had to lock herself in a room to protect herself from her husband. She knew she had a lot of anger towards him, but had stuffed it away inside herself and never dealt with it. "Vera never dealt with her anger and it eventually turned into guilt," and she assumed she must have done something wrong to provoke her husband, notes Dr. Riccioli.

According to mind-body logic, if she had been wrong, guilty of bad behavior, she must be punished, and what better biological punishment than ovarian cancer, in one of the key organs of her femininity? "Just as her husband literally beat her up, so she symbolically transferred the beating to her ovaries," says Dr. Riccioli. "You might say Vera stored the energy of the abuse, and perhaps the unexpressed anger, too, in her ovaries." During the course of several hypnotherapy sessions, Vera understood the connections and interactions between her relationship with her husband, her emotions, and her bodily symptoms.[5]

The preceding examples illustrate the meaning of a useful term coined by noted women's doctor and health educator, Christiane Northrup, M.D. She calls them "toxic emotions." Toxic emotions are powerful, strongly held, and typically unconscious beliefs and emotions that act as precipitators, catalysts, or seeds for a variety of illnesses, from mild to mortal. Belief becomes biology when it remains unaddressed, undischarged, or even unidentified, says Dr. Northrup. When emotions are unexpressed, they stay *in* the body "like small ticking time bombs—they are illnesses in incubation." She relates a vivid case to make her point.

A forty-one-year-old business executive was suffering from hot flashes. This is early to have the first signs of menopause, but because she had had a hysterectomy with removal of both ovaries a few years earlier, the surgery probably speeded up the hormonal timetable a bit, edging her, if prematurely, into perimenopause. She was under stress at work, taking four times the normal dose of estrogen for women with hot flashes, and not getting any relief. Two years into her treatment with Dr. Northrup, the woman finally revealed she had been sexually molested at age six by an adult male. She had felt frozen, numb, unable to speak at the time. Later she felt ashamed and told nobody about the incident, thinking that somehow she must have done something wrong to warrant this kind of punishment.

The hysterectomy, which was done as a result of years of unremitting uterine pain, says Dr. Northrup, was actually a step in the right direction, not so much medically, as emotionally. It was her body's way of focusing the woman's attention on the "scene of the crime," in this case, literally. Even deeper, the woman felt oppressed by "the original sin of being female," and tried to compensate for this felt inferiority by overworking. She overworked to prove herself in the workplace and to avoid contact with the deep emotional pain she bore in her uterus and the shame that made her feel unworthy and bad, explains Dr. Northrup.

She adds that the "seeds" for the woman's physical problems were planted by the emotional trauma of sexual abuse. It did not necessarily create it in a linear chain of causality, but this early abuse "set a pattern of discomfort in her body-mind," and her body-mind expressed the pain continually at the place of the original trauma. Undoing the lifelong effects of this toxic seed meant going back in herself to experience and "expiate it, exorcise it" from her cellular memory bank.

Dr. Northrup calls this process of feeling, expressing, and releasing old repressed emotions "emotional incision and drainage." Buried emotions, festering and toxic, are like abscesses that a doctor needs to lance and drain. Similarly, emotions, walled off and generating pain, must be "lanced" and "drained" so healthy new tissues (metaphorically, self-attitudes and behaviors) can form.[6]

As Carolyn Myss, Ph.D., the highly popular advocate of the seamless mind-body model, remarks, the first principle of illness is that biography becomes biology. All our thoughts and feelings first enter our biological system as energy. "Every thought you have had has traveled through your biological system and activated a physiological response," she says. Some have dropped depth charges, causing physiological reactions throughout the body. "In this way our biographies are woven into our biological systems, gradually, slowly, every day."[7]

Most of us carry destructive beliefs and feelings around with us, and these steadily undermine our health, gradually converting our biology to be in accordance with our definition of reality. For example, if you are continuously "pissed off" at somebody or a situation, your body may translate this into chronic urinary tract infections in which your "piss" acidifies under the influence of this strongly held, undischarged emotion. Until you discharge the emotion, you may be subject to recurrent bouts of urinary tract infection.

Various emotions, such as low self-esteem or self-worth, have been associated with the development of cancer, and these toxic emotions can have a powerful influence on the course of the disease and the inability of well-indicated therapies to stop it. "Many cancer patients cannot recover from their cancer until these memories are discovered and treated."[8]

It sounds counter to common sense, but what you *don't* know can hurt you, "because the repressed memory of trauma is traumatic," explains Arthur Janov, M.D., in *Why You Get Sick and How You Get Well*. Dr. Janov is the well-known founder of the primal scream technique, which he introduced in the 1970s. It is our repressed memory of a painful or deprived or abusive childhood that is itself traumatic, exerting a continuous debilitating effect on our body, says Dr. Janov.

Neurosis, the state of carrying unresolved, conflicted emotion and states of mind, is the foundation of illness, he says. There is nothing more healing than to actually *feel* and fully experience the memories and emotions—our "internal reality"— from earlier in life that have been repressed or shunted out of our awareness. Childhood pain is like a psychological big bang that can set the course for the rest of our life, until we deal with it. We may spend a lifetime trying to repress the painful memory, but "all that energy and activation has to find its way into some kind of disease," says Dr. Janov.

Dr. Janov relates the case of a woman, twenty-nine, who had been bulimic for eleven years. After working with Dr. Janov and his primal therapy approach, she realized her bulimia was a coping mechanism traceable to her difficult birth. During her birthing, she got stuck in the birth canal and went into a frenzy— angry, afraid, and fighting for her life. She couldn't breathe and her body went into convulsions. In her adult life, during a crisis, she would stuff herself with food and then vomit. She realized her bulimia was mimicking the trauma of her birth. Throwing up was her way of disgorging the stress of not being able to breathe, and therefore of discharging the tension of the crisis.

"I seemed to have recreated the airlessness of my birth through the throwing up of my bulimia," she told Dr. Janov. When she had a crisis as an adult and felt her breathing start to constrict, she *had* to vomit; this was how her body learned to deal with crises. Once she understood this energy equation, she was able to free herself from the bulimia. "We have learned that what makes people sick is the key to making them well again," comments Dr. Janov. But to "fully respond to traumatic aspects of their childhood for the first time,"[9] people have to bring the content from out of unconscious storage back into consciousness.

The Healthy Living Space Expert Interview: Patricia Kaminski, Flower Essence Practitioner

There are many ways to access, express, and release buried emotions, but the one we will focus on in this chapter is called flower essence therapy. It is a gentle but deep practice originally developed in the 1930s by a British bacteriologist, Edward Bach, M.D. He found a way to use the subtle energies of plant blossoms to highlight, clarify, and resolve human emotions.

Dr. Bach created a series of thirty-eight formulas, now called the Bach Flower Remedies, in which an infusion of flower blossoms into distilled water—when taken orally as drops over a period of weeks—could produce profound clarifications in specific emotions such as grief, sadness, fear, anxiety, and others. His idea was to use these flower essences to address emotional, psychological, even spiritual issues underlying physical and medical problems.

In the late 1970s, Patricia Kaminski joined with Richard Katz to extend Dr. Bach's principles of emotional healing through flower essences to develop remedies based on plants grown in North America. Their assumption was that, it being fifty years later and another continent, the remedies might be more effectively produced from indigenous plants and encompass a broader range of emotional nuance. Humans are emotionally more complex today than in Dr. Bach's time, and the American psyche may need homegrown flower energies, botanical essences more in resonance with the landscape in which the end users live.

Today, their line of flower essences number more than 100 (based on the freshly harvested and infused blossoms of plants, bushes, and trees) and through their Flower Essence Society, based in Nevada City, California, they have an active network of colleagues, students, and practitioners throughout the world.[10]

Implicit in the model of flower essences, whether they come from Bach or Katz and Kaminski, is the startling idea that somehow the energy of plant blossoms has a relationship with the spectrum of human emotions. Flower essence practitioners suggest that the plant kingdom, through its blossoms, embodies in a pure, almost abstract form, the essence of human emotions. The purity of this expression enables the plant blossoms, when prepared in the right way, to have a clarifying effect on human emotions—clarifying in the sense of the impact an archetype (a pure emotion) can have on its manifestation (a pure emotion expressed, distorted, or blocked by a human psyche).

Flower essence practitioners also postulate that the human energy field, or aura (discussed in more detail in chapter 9), has a basic affinity with the plant kingdom. It is even suggested that in some manner the human energy field embodies the full spectrum of the plant kingdom and, analogically speaking, the myriad blossoms occurring in the plant world are like little stars, or points of pure consciousness, in the human energy field. Whatever the theoretical explanation, flower essence practitioners operate on the assumption—one backed by decades of empirical results and clinical observation of clients—that a flower essence can help a person experience, clarify, and resolve distorted emotions.

Flower essences "*encourage* rather than *compel* change, working by vibrational resonance rather than by biochemical intervention," explains Kaminski. They evoke and stimulate "an inner dialogue with hidden aspects of the Self, awakening profound psychological archetypes, and giving us access to their message." Through this kind of inner dialogue, Kaminski says, flower essences can catalyze "deep emotional and mental changes" powerful enough to in turn spark physiological alterations, reversals of symptoms, and often healings.[11]

As Kaminski sees it, flower essences "unite the human soul with the soul of nature" and "rekindle a vital connection" between these two expressions of soul. Flower essences "massage" the sensibilities of the soul, Kaminski explains. "They reinstill our capacity to receive living forces from nature, qualities that allow our souls to be permeable rather than hardened," as well as vital instead of mechanical.

In flower essence thinking, the term "soul" has a vital, real role, and would still have this quality even if matters of the soul were not now a nationally validated topic in publishing and teaching, ever since Thomas More's best-selling *Care of the Soul* was published in 1992. The soul is the substrate of our emotions and sense of self, the deep, pure feeling state within, the inner, permanent self. In her book *Flowers That Heal*,

How do we know if we're toxic, either physically or emotionally? "I think we should assume that we all are," says Kaminski. "The question is this: do we have ways of efficiently recycling that toxicity, processing it the way the liver handles toxins? What kind of soul apparatus do we have that helps us deal with toxicity?"

Kaminski says using flower essences dredges unpleasant emotions to the surface of our awareness. "As we witness these parts of ourselves, we have the opportunity to understand, to redeem and to cleanse these emotions."[12] With flower essences, we heal from the inside out.

How do we know if we're toxic, either physically or emotionally? "I think we should assume that we all are," says Kaminski. "The question is this: do we have ways of efficiently recycling that toxicity, processing it the way the liver handles toxins? What kind of soul apparatus do we have that helps us deal with toxicity? You can't medicate away the pain of the soul with psychiatric drugs. We need to be involved in creating in the soul those structures and processes analogous to the liver that enable us to process emotional toxicity. With flower essences, you actually flood the body with a positive 'medicine,' with positive emotional archetypes that shift the cellular structure in a different direction."

In other words, says Kaminski, toxicity is a condition we are bound to encounter on the emotional level, so we need to develop ways to *process* it. Even better, we need to process it in such a way that in the end we have gained in consciousness. We are more aware of ourselves, of our emotional totality. This way, Kaminski says, emotional detoxification through flower remedies can lead to more consciousness. She adds that flower essence therapy is "a cutting edge, vanguard 'medicine' that is trying to build a bridge between psyche and soma, or the body."

Here's an example from Kaminski's case files that illustrates these points. She consulted with a fifty-eight-year-old business executive who had sustained a heart attack. He had tremendous stress in his life and it seemed his primary way of relating to the world was through hostility. He was in advertising, a highly competitive industry, and his job description was virtually to walk all over everybody else, to triumph, win the client, do the best, make the most amount of money, and the usual ultra-Type A personality behaviors. Naturally, he had high blood pressure as well as a weakened heart after the "attack."

When he came to Kaminski, he had already started a nutritional therapy regimen and meditation. She started him on four flower essences specific to his condition of stress, hostility, and a rigidified heart, using Impatiens, Zinnia, Borage, and Holly.

In terms of its effect on human emotions, the flower Impatiens is aptly named: it dissolves impatience. This man was always snapping his fingers, tapping his fingers, expressing his impatience, says Kaminski. "The impatience was everywhere in him: the need to drive fast, to be somewhere in a hurry, to get things done in a hurry."

Individuals who need Impatiens "find it difficult to be within the flow of time; their tendency is to rush ahead of experience," comments Kaminski in her masterwork on flower essence prescribing, *Flower Essence Repertory* (cowritten with husband Richard Katz).[13] They have too much fiery force, and this flares up easily into irritation, impatience, intolerance, and anger. Impatiens as a flower essence actually imparts the opposite qualities: patience, acceptance, and the ability to flow with the pace of life and others, explains Kaminski.

Kaminski gave the man Zinnia flower essence because much of his joy of life was gone. He had lost his sense of humor and ability to easily laugh; he took himself too seriously. He had developed an overly somber sense of self, a dullness and over-seriousness, explains Kaminski. Zinnia would help reverse that by evoking "childlike humor and playfulness," a lightheartedness, an inner joyfulness, and a sense of detached perspective on oneself. It would help him appreciate the possibility that playfulness and laughter could have a role in a responsible life, says Kaminski.

The third flower essence prescribed was Borage. The emotional issues to do with Borage were to a large degree at the "heart" of the man's heart condition, says Kaminski. The patterns of imbalance that indicate the need for Borage are heavy-heartedness and a lack of confidence in facing difficult circumstances, Kaminski explains. Borage instills a sense of courage and buoyancy that helps one rise above difficulties. "Borage is often at the core of outer hostility because underneath this is grief and vulnerability that emotionally weigh down the heart and prevent the heart from expressing its own real emotion. Borage helps the heart to experience this ebullience and lightness, filling the soul with fresh forces of optimism and enthusiasm."

Finally, Holly was indicated to address this man's sense of feeling cut off from love, and of being filled with jealousy, suspicion, anger, and envy. On the positive side, Holly would help evoke the feeling of love and the ability to extend it to others, an open heart and a sense of compassion, says Kaminski. This remedy helps restore a person's "ability to feel unity and wholeness," she notes.

After a few weeks of taking the four remedies—he took them several times daily as drops—the man began to see changes in his emotional nature. Previously, when his young daughter walked into a room, he would be impatient for her to leave, talking to her briefly, feeling increasingly irritated. But now he found himself "fascinated" by what she had to say; he felt inclined to play with her as opposed to having to order himself to do so out of fatherly duty. He started to see he didn't have to "jump all the time into reality," but that he could sit back and allow it to unfold before him, says Kaminski. He didn't have to control everything any more.

"Learning to trust the world is the antidote for hostility," Kaminski notes. This man had not been trusting of the world, and eventually his body mimicked his core emotional stance and attacked him just as he was chronically attacking the world through his hostility. A key element in easing hostility is teaching a person to trust the world again, to let the heart relax its vigilance, she adds.

"Through the flower essences, he gained enough of an edge on himself that he could start to *witness* life rather than *react* to it all of the time. He has had remarkable changes in his heart condition since then. All of the physiological indicators for heart health are now very favorable for him." Through the flower essences and the way they worked to clarify his emotional knots and give him a position of detached awareness about them—what Kaminski calls the "witness" stance—he was able to dissolve much of his emotional toxicity and thereby relieve its steady, sickening pressure on his physical heart. He became able to have vulnerability and emotional space with himself in the context of his family, and this was intensely healing for him, says Kaminski. He no longer was "incredibly actively hostile" at work: he didn't *need* to exhibit that kind of behavior any more.

"For me, the question with emotional toxicity is not that we get the 'poison' out of the body, but that we learn how to handle the daily flow of it, that we learn how emotional toxicity originates. So the goal is not so much a cleansing of emotional toxicity but an active change in how we *deal* with it," Kaminski explains. Ideally, through flower essences, we can deal with it with more consciousness, more awareness of its true message.

HEALTHY LIVING SPACE DETOXIFIER #35
Remedying the Four Basic States of
Emotional Toxicity with Flower Essences

Based on more than twenty years of clinical consultation with hundreds of clients, Kaminski describes four basic states of emotional toxicity. Using these four categories, she says it is possible for a person to categorize oneself and thereby select appropriate remedies to start the process of emotional clarification. The four basic categories are hostility, depression, stress/tension, and anxiety/fear, all of which are presented in more detail below. The strategy is simple: a group of compatible remedies will undo the emotional knots that produce the overall style of reactivity, such as hostility or depression.

The idea is simple: examine your typical style of emotional reaction when you are pressed up against the wall. What is your usual response when "push comes to shove"? Do you get mad, depressed, stressed out, or afraid? From this small act of self-observation, you can see which of the four categories you fit into, says Kaminski. Then within the chosen category, decide again which of the nuances of that basic emotional state best describes your emotional style, and select one flower essence and use it for a month or two (see figure 8-1).

These are not absolute categories, by the way. They are meant only as provisional definitions of emotional experience, says Kaminski—general, perhaps broad, guideposts to help

Figure 8-1. The Four Basic States of Emotional Toxicity and Their Appropriate Flower Essences	
Hostility:	Holly, Oregon Grape, Willow, Beech, Zinnia, Borage, Bleeding Heart, Golden Ear Drops, Calendula
Depression:	St. John's Wort, California Wild Rose, Scotch Broom, Mustard, Gentian, Sweet Chestnut, Love-Lies-Bleeding
Stress/Tension:	Yarrow Special Formula, Five Flower Formula, Impatiens, Canyon Dudleya, Yarrow, Scleranthus, Indian Pink, Star Tulip
Anxiety/Fear:	Mimulus, Scarlet Monkeyflower, Sticky Monkeyflower, Buttercup, Sunflower, Penstemon, Mountain Pride, California Wild Rose, Blackberry.

orient you to your emotional reality. Further, the flower remedies are not first aid conveniences, like aspirin, producing a quick resolution of the problem. They work slowly, deeply, organically, from within you; generally you should allow a month or two for lasting results, she notes.

It is useful to compare the action of flower remedies to intestinal cleansers. A kind of dredging work is started by taking either. In the case of intestinal cleansers, odd, uncomfortable, but transient mental and physical states are experienced as the intestines get cleansed. Similarly, while taking flower remedies you can expect an upwelling of strange, unfamiliar, or deeply familiar emotions; the process may make you feel unsettled, but then, it's supposed to. You can't expect to clarify and resolve emotions without some confusion and seeming emotional chaos during the process. But remember: it is a *process*, and one with an eventual positive and beneficial conclusion. So it is worth it to stick out the ups and downs of the emotional process flower remedies can precipitate.

Hostility

This first category includes feelings of hostility and lack of trust. As we saw in the case study above, it especially afflicts the heart, both physically and as the center of our affective life. This affliction then gets projected aggressively outwards onto the world in overly assertive, aggressive, even potentially violent, behavior. It is about a loss of trust by the heart and a lack of open space for the heart, for a sense of vulnerability and emotional exposure. Borrowing a term from traditional Chinese medicine, Kaminski calls this state *yang*, meaning, fiery, intense, strong, hard, active, outward-tending. But it is a state of emotional imbalance.

Flower essences recommended for this emotional state to help curb the overly *yang* disposition of the heart:

Holly: Holly helps one develop an equanimity and sense of spaciousness in the soul, says Kaminski, freeing one up from the felt need to react hard against the world. It helps one be more inclusive and expansive, to feel less isolated from others, to experience love in connection with other people.

Oregon Grape: This is indicated if a person feels paranoid or self-protective or expects hostility from others even when this expectation is not warranted by the facts. The person tends to feel they are likely to be attacked, from anywhere. In contrast, taking the remedy will help generate a sense of loving inclusion of others, the expectation of good will coming from others, and the ability to trust in the goodness of other people.

Willow: This remedy is needed when one feels resentful, irritable, bitter, or that life is unfair and has cast one as a victim, or when one has too many hard edges to the personality. Willow will help produce a feeling of acceptance, forgiveness, a flowing-ness with life, the ability to yield and bend with circumstances, to stop rigidly holding on to negative emotions or some old, unnecessary part of oneself, and the willingness to take responsibility for one's life. Willow helps to decongest dammed up, internalized emotions that can lead to—as it were, congeal into—painful, stiff joints and muscles, even arthritis.

Beech: Beech is needed if you feel critical, judgmental, intolerant, and have perfectionist expectations of others; also if you have an oversensitivity to your social and physical environment. You project your inner sense of inferiority, imperfection, and insecurity onto others, and seek to feel safe by condemning others. Beech helps undo this by generating feelings of tolerance and acceptance of the differences and imperfections of others.

Zinnia: As described earlier, Zinnia helps evoke feelings of childlike playfulness, humor, amusement, and laughter as a counterbalance to the tendency to be heavy and hard-hearted.

Flower essences recommended to help heal the underlying lack of emotional vulnerability that accompanies hostility:

Borage: Borage also helps undo the heaviness of the heart and opens up the hidden areas of grief in the heart. Borage instills courage, upliftment, a sense of light-filled buoyancy, and "fresh forces of optimism and enthusiasm."

Bleeding Heart: This essence is indicated if you form relationships based on fear or possessiveness or emotional codependence, or if you have poured great amounts of love into a relationship that subsequently failed (or the person died or moved away), leaving you wounded and heartbroken. The remedy helps one rebuild heart forces from within, generating a capacity to love unconditionally with an open heart, and to forgive those who have hurt you.

Golden Ear Drops: You can benefit from this flower essence if there are suppressed toxic memories of childhood or feelings of pain and unexpiated trauma from earlier events that produce emotional instability. Look for evidence of emotional amnesia and the "unconscious residue of traumatic memories," says Kaminski. This remedy will help cleanse the heart and may literally produce tears as a form of emotional discharge, she adds. It helps you reconnect with your childhood and see it as a source of emotional well-being, not toxicity.

Calendula: A person can benefit from this remedy if one tends to use sharp, cutting, argumentative words as a psychological defense in communication with others. Calendula brings warmth to the spoken word, so that it generates good will and understanding and not division and hurt. It also helps to calm down the adrenal glands, which can be revved up in a state of chronic argumentativeness and verbal aggressiveness.

Depression

As the second category of emotional toxicity, depression is in many respects the opposite of hostility. It is a *yin* condition, a turning inward, a cold, damp, passive, soft, yielding, sinking quality. There is no fire here, and the person retreats from the world and, in effect, from active expressions of self and will. Cancer is typical of this state of emotional toxicity, says Kaminski. It would be mistaken to think of depression purely in biochemical terms, as only a brain-bound condition, she says.

It is also about whether our will has fire in it, and enthusiasm for life and taking action. A person with this condition is liable to develop alcohol dependency, but alcohol is poison for depressives, says Kaminski. "Alcohol has so much fire in it that it drowns out our own fire." Depression is often "a loss of connection (especially in the will) with the spiritual world and a loss of hope in that connection; one becomes submerged in the narrowness of the personality (the opposite of the hostile person who inflames their sense of self)."

Sometimes the person's sense of self is so uninflamed—so passive and watery, so to speak, so lacking in inner will—that one is easily overcome by foreign disease agents, such as cancerous cells, or even parasitic energy organisms, thoughts, and feelings from the outer world, Kaminski notes. "At its worst, one can become overcome and possessed by entities because one's ego is not strong enough to ward off these negative disease-producing influences." (For more on this subject, see chapter 9.)

Flower essences recommended to help heal the deep underlying wounds of depression include:

St. John's Wort: A need for this remedy is indicated by physical and psychic vulnerability, the lack of rootedness in the world leading to an overexposure to the light. Such people have a tendency to get sunburned and develop allergies as part of their oversensitivity, and they have a very active psychic life, but an ungrounded one, leading them to loose their connection to the physical body, says Kaminski. "This weak association to the body results in a propensity for invasion or attack from negative elemental forces or other entities, especially during sleep." This remedy helps a person *circulate* the light throughout the physical body and undo psychic blockages that drain off one's vital energy.

California Wild Rose: Here the condition is apathy, resignation, and the inability to organize and spark the forces of will through the heart so that one can take hold of one's responsibilities and life tasks. People needing this remedy find it hard to take emotional risks, need to insulate themselves against wounding, and may even be alienated from the social world. The remedy instills a feeling of love for the Earth and human life, and an enthusiasm to serve others. This flower gives one the courage to love, to love life, and even to wear the "crown of thorns" life inevitably gives you.

> *Sometimes the person's sense of self is so uninflamed—so passive and watery, so to speak, so lacking in inner will—that one is easily overcome by foreign disease agents, such as cancerous cells, or even parasitic energy organisms, thoughts, and feelings from the outer world.*

Scotch Broom: This remedy is indicated when a person feels weighed down and depressed, overcome with despair or pessimistic views, especially with regard to one's relationship to large social events. The soul feels burdened with negative scenarios of great social upheaval and travail, and this unrelieved weight leads to resignation, paralysis of the will, and depression. Scotch Broom sparks feelings of optimism about being able to affect the world positively; it imparts a sense of caring, encouragement, hope, and purposefulness.

Mustard: Feelings of melancholy, gloom, despair, and depression without obvious cause suggest this remedy. The soul

345

feels darkness and is overwhelmed by it, especially as its onset seems inexplicable. Mustard helps one gain emotional equanimity and joy, and identify forgotten or suppressed events that may have triggered or sustained the depression.

Gentian: If you feel doubt or discouragement after a setback, Gentian can help. Gentian helps build resilience in the face of impediments and obstacles, and it provides encouragement to see these setbacks as opportunities to learn more about oneself by shifting one's perspective on life and identity. Skepticism and doubt get transformed into faith and confidence.

Sweet Chestnut: This remedy is helpful when you feel strong despair and anguish and something akin to what is traditionally called "the Dark Night of the Soul." If you need this you are probably suffering acutely, seemingly being tested to the breaking point. You probably feel deeply alone, possibly suicidal. Sweet Chestnut helps instill a deep sense of courage and faith that comes from trusting the spiritual world to not let you down and to help you out of the "rock bottom" of your depression.

Love-Lies-Bleeding: In this case, a person feels an intensification of pain and suffering due to isolation. The suffering can be intense, either bodily or psychological in nature, and it pushes one's awareness deeply inward; such a person is "truly deep-pressed," comments Kaminski. This remedy does not so much provide immediate relief from this state as it helps the person move consciousness outward from the over-personal identification and isolation into something more transpersonal. It is a shift in perspective and meaning from the inside to the outside, from the personal to something beyond it; it provides a context that thereby eases the suffering because suffering now has a role and purpose.

Yerba Santa: This remedy is recommended when you feel emotionally constricted, especially in the chest; when you have internalized grief and melancholy; or have deeply repressed emotions stored away, as it were, in the deepest recesses of the heart. Typically, your breathing is disturbed and congested, and you are liable to respiratory diseases as the soul wastes away within, consumed by the intense energies of unrelieved sadness or grief. Yerba Santa helps free up the flow of emotions so that feeling and breathing may be harmonized.

Stress/Tension

These two conditions tend to go together. As a strong sense of pressure, stress/tension is "the younger brother of hostility and afflicts many," notes Kaminski. "Such persons are not as overtly hostile or aggressive, but they still are predominantly *yang* in their soul orientation. They need to develop more inner space, a quality of soul spaciousness. Such persons find it hard to be at rest; they always need to be doing something; they feel hurried and pressured; and they set up situations in their life in which they will be hurried and pressured."

Kaminski notes that in some respects, this condition is "a strong imprint or overlay from Western culture itself and may not be part of a person's true temperament. Many people are profoundly influenced by the overall speeded-up quality of the urban environment in which everything rushes by intensely; people end up unconsciously copying this energy pattern in their own life. Such persons could be called adrenaline junkies, because they thrive on tension, pressure, deadlines, and performance expectations, all of which tend to over-stimulate the adrenal glands. The faster something is, the more impatient they are to make it go even faster. They will switch TV channels constantly or upgrade their computer every year."

Two essences specifically deal with the overall quality of pressure, tension, and stress imparted by Western culture to all of us:

Yarrow Special Formula: This formula focuses on enhancing the integrity of our energy body, the flow of physical and subtle energies through our physical body and aura. It also helps undo the toxic influence of noxious environmental energies such as radiation, pollution, geopathic stress (harmful energies from the Earth itself—see chapter 12 for more details), and even computer stress. This remedy combines yarrow and sea salt to strengthen the human energy field with pure formative forces from the plant and mineral kingdoms so that we can withstand and resist the tension/pressure and noxious influences from the environment.

Five Flower Formula: This is an all-purpose first-aid remedy (also known as Rescue Remedy) combining five flower essences (Cherry Plum, Clematis, Impatiens, Rock Rose, and Star of Bethlehem). It is especially useful in cases of sudden, acute shock or trauma. "It is also a good overall balancer for tension, stress, emergencies, life in the fast lane, some cases of insomnia, subliminal levels of panic, and general *dis*-ease," comments Kaminski. It instills calmness and stability in the face of physical or emotional emergencies, high stress, sudden panic, disorientation, or loss of consciousness. It helps the soul stay connected with the body, and in cases of nonemergency, it can be used in the early stages of inner work as a way of stabilizing the self so that it can calmly contact the soul within.

Other essences helpful for easing the pattern of stress/tension:

Impatiens: As already mentioned, Impatiens can alleviate the sense of impatience, irritation, urgency, and tension, and allow instead a sense of patient acceptance of the flow of events and the movement of time.

Canyon Dudleya: This remedy is particularly indicated for people who have distorted psychic experiences, who are preoccupied with mediumism, or who need more order and less self-inflation in their soul lives. Canyon Dudleya will help catalyze a healthy, balanced, grounded spiritual opening.

Yarrow: People who experience extreme vulnerability to others and to their environment, who are easily depleted energetically, or who too easily absorb negative influences and psychic toxicity from around them will benefit from Yarrow. This flower essence instills a sense of inner radiance and auric strength, a sensitivity that is not vulnerable to constant permeation by outside influences. Persons who have allergies, environmental sensitivities, and psychosomatic diseases will benefit from Yarrow.

Scleranthus: Scleranthus deals with hesitation, confusion, indecision, and conditions of unresolved duality in the quest for inner wholeness. People for whom this remedy is indicated tend to vacillate when they need to make decisions; this chronic uncertainty can get translated into bodily symptoms, especially ones that continually shift, come and go, increase and decrease in intensity. Scleranthus can help produce inner resolve and decisiveness.

Indian Pink: The person requiring this flower essence tends to have their psychic forces easily shattered by overactivity and find it hard to remain centered and grounded during this intense activity. Indian Pink people tend to try to do too many things at once, and they spin out of control and out of focus. They can be emotionally volatile and appear haggard or depleted. Indian Pink helps such a person stay centered and focused even during times of stress.

Star Tulip: The Star Tulip person tends to feel hardened, cut off, unable to feel attuned to things or any sense of quiet inner presence as is needed to pray or meditate. The remedy helps one listen within, to become aware of the subtle influences perpetually at work within and around them; it enhances one's ability to pray, dream, meditate, or feel connected to the spiritual worlds.

Anxiety/Fear

This fourth basic state of emotional toxicity includes loss of confidence and low self-esteem in the context of low-grade chronic fear and anxiety. "This is the lesser sister of depression," says Kaminski. "It works predominantly in a *yin* way in the soul. These are persons who under-perform, who do not push or pressure themselves with respect to externals though they may carry a huge amount of pressure or anxiety that churns them up from within. Such persons hold in too much psychic force especially in the abdomen or solar plexus area of the body. They tend to cave in, give way to fear and limiting notions of self. They need courage and strength, more *yang* force."

These are the flower remedies recommended to help undo this condition of chronic anxiety and fear:

Mimulus: This essence is helpful for easing the effects of known, everyday fears, for people who are hypersensitive to small ordinary fears. The solar plexus churns with agitation and unease at all these unrelieved fears. Mimulus restores courage to the soul to face these fears and life challenges with confidence and inner light, and it helps highlight the deeper, more basic fear underlying the multitude of surface panics: "the fear of the physical body, or of physical life itself," sometimes traceable to the moment of birth, says Kaminski.

Scarlet Monkeyflower: The person needing this flower essence tends to fear intense feelings and represses all strong emotions, leaving them unable to resolve issues of anger and powerlessness. The person is afraid of their shadow-self emotions, the ones they believe originate from the unconscious.

Scarlet Monkeyflower helps instill emotional honesty and helps integrate the shadow feelings.

Sticky Monkeyflower: This one deals with repressed sexual feelings or acting out in inappropriate sexual behavior. It is also concerned with a person's inability to experience human warmth during sexual relations; in a sense, it is about a deep fear of sex and intimacy, says Kaminski, and even more, it is about a fear of exposure of one's essential self during moments of physical intimacy. Sticky Monkeyflower thereby helps a person integrate sexual urges with human warmth and intimacy.

Buttercup: Buttercup is indicated when one feels low self-worth and high self-doubt, and when one is unable to acknowledge one's own inner light and uniqueness especially when measured against conventional external standards. Buttercup, in keeping with its bright, almost glistening yellowness, helps one radiate an inner light so as to become free of the need for outer recognition. Buttercup helps you honor your own value from within and bring this quality out into the world.

Sunflower: The Sunflower person has a distorted sense of self, either tending to self-inflation or self-diminishment, to arrogance or low self-esteem. There is often an imbalance in their relationship to the masculine (or Father archetype), even if the person is a male. Sunflower evokes a balanced sense of ego or self-identity, neither too much nor too little, marked by light, warmth, and compassion.

"This is exactly what flower essence therapy is intended to achieve: not to mask outer symptoms but to help the soul find the right balance with regard to these basic soul dispositions." The toxicity comes when these soul aspects aren't being attended to in a conscious way.

Penstemon: Here one feels sorry for oneself and self-pity is the order of the day. One is also unable to bear the difficulties of one's circumstances (such as a handicap or disability from birth or an accident) and succumbs to a sense of persecution. Hence, Penstemon instills a feeling of inner fortitude, an ability to persevere despite the heavy challenges facing one.

Mountain Pride: The Mountain Pride person often vacillates and even withdraws in the face of a hard challenge, lacking assertiveness and the inner nerve to stand up for one's convictions. This is for people who confuse peace with passivity. Mountain Pride evokes a sense of "forthright masculine energy, a warrior-like spirituality that confronts and transforms," explains Kaminski.

California Wild Rose: See the Depression category for a description of this essence.

Blackberry: Here a person has a hard time translating goals and ideals into actual action in the world. It is as if the will cannot link itself with the world; there is a significant gap between aims and achievements. Appropriately, the person's metabolism is sluggish, mirroring the sluggishness of the will. Blackberry helps one develop a sense of "exuberant manifestation" in which one can clearly, directly channel one's will forces into concrete action.

As mentioned earlier, these categories and their subdivisions are not cast in stone. "As the emphasis here is emotional toxicity, I refer to the dysfunctional qualities we often see when these four temperaments are out of balance," comments Kaminski. "There is usually one we gravitate towards more than others, but certainly these are not mutually exclusive categories. In fact, we can switch into different basic responses as we go through different life cycles. Even the seasons can affect our responses." For example, there is a normal disposition to "depression" in the winter months when there is the least amount of sunlight.

Writers such as James Hillman, in *The Soul's Code*, wisely counsel us to cultivate this depression in the winter, to take time to go into our depths. If we did, he argues, we would see more depth in our culture, more ability to deal with grief and loss, and less need to medicate. "This is exactly what flower essence therapy is intended to achieve," notes Kaminski. "Not to mask outer symptoms, but to help the soul find the right balance with regard to these basic soul dispositions."

The toxicity comes when these soul aspects aren't being attended to in a conscious way, she explains. "I use the analogy of a river that flows harmoniously without being impeded, dammed, or otherwise regulated from without. This river (our emotional life) is able to cleanse itself of toxic waste effectively, even to regenerate itself from rather extreme states of toxicity if given the opportunity to come back into dynamic balance."

As Patricia Kaminski makes clear, flower essences can highlight, clarify, and help resolve emotional knots in the psyche. It can bring light into the dark regions of our emotional life and help us see where we have been tied up, repressed, or otherwise blocked by stuck or buried emotions. Flower essences, especially St. John's Wort, discussed above, can also make us aware of psychic blockages or even parasitic elements in our overall energy field. Sometimes these blockages or the presence of foreign energies in our aura can compromise us to a degree beyond which flower essence therapy can be therapeutic. That is because such blockages or presences operate beyond our emotional sphere, in the sphere of energy and psychic or spiritual influences, and require a different approach. This is the subject of the next chapter.

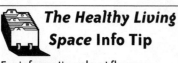

The Healthy Living Space Info Tip

For information about flower essences mentioned in this chapter:
Patricia Kaminski,
Flower Essence Society,
P.O. Box 459,
Nevada City, CA 95959;
tel: 800-736-9222 or 530-265-9163;
fax: 530-265-0584;
e-mail: mail@flowersociety.org ;
website: www.flowersociety.org.

CHAPTER 9

Guidelines for Spiritual Detoxification:

Cleansing the Space around the Body

Call to mind, if you will, the last time you walked into a room and felt accosted by the strange, unpleasant, possibly obnoxious energy in that space. It may not have been anything you heard, anyone in particular you observed, or even an odor you detected. But nonetheless you *felt* something, an almost baleful atmosphere emanating from the room—or movie theater, restaurant, store, basement, potentially any public or domestic space you find yourself in. Perhaps you felt a prickling at the back of your neck; maybe your skin went clammy, your breathing tightened, you felt panicked or anxious, or noticed anomalous aches or pains suddenly emerging in your body.

What's happened? Using senses common to humans, though ones not generally acknowledged, you have *sensed* the spiritual quality of a living space—"spiritual" in the literal sense of spirit, meaning not physically embodied but immaterial, an energy essence or influence, a vibration. The part of you that did the sensing is often called the aura, and this is the subtle energy field—a kind of sixth sense—said to envelop the body of every human being and to resemble a luminous egg, according to the reports of psychics. The aura can see where we can't with our ordinary eyes, and it can register subtle influences, both healthy and unwholesome, that can affect our minds and bodies. It is another aspect of our overall *living space* and like the other aspects, our physical body and our home, it can either support or hinder our well-being.

Poisons in Our Invisible Atmosphere

While the direct perception of the aura (and thus confirmation of its existence to skeptics) depends on one having psychic abilities, the inference that there is an invisible energy envelope around the human body is much easier to support. After all, you have just inferred its existence when you felt the unpleasant vibrations upon entering that room.

The matter of auric influences has been a topic of discussion for many centuries in both Western and Eastern cultures. The sixteenth century German philosopher Henry Cornelius Agrippa advised his readers against associating with people who were evil-minded because "their souls are filled with harmful radiations which will infect your surroundings in an unhealthy way." Agrippa recommended that his contemporaries interested in preserving their health associate with "good and fortunate people, for these can help us greatly by being near to us."[1]

More recently, in 1934, a German physician named Dr. Friedrich Markus Huebner noted that "one can be poisoned" not only by unwholesome foods, gases, and microbes, but by "unwholesome people." Dr. Huebner explained that "our invisible atmosphere" is the part of us that first senses the subtle poison, and it becomes "negatively charged by contact with harmful radiations." These radiations then exert unhealthy influences on the mind and body, eventually contributing to the emergence of symptoms of dysfunction and disease.

Dr. Heubner further noted that it was not uncommon for a person, upon coming in contact with a man or woman with a "malignant aura," to get sudden giddiness, stomach pains, perspiration, or a fit of nervous laughter. "Our organism is hard put to throw off an intoxication that menaces it or already seems to be active," he stated.[2] According to these experts, it is the energy field or aura around the body that registers, and holds, these influences, and it is from the aura, as if it were a staging ground, that these external energies work their way into the physical body.

So what does the aura look like? One way to conceptualize it is to think of it in terms of heat radiations seen over a flat landscape or over an empty tarred parking lot on a hot summer day. You can actually see the heat rising from the surface, even though normally "heat" is not visible. Another way is to think of an egg. The consensus among psychics describing the human aura is that it resembles a translucent white egg extending perhaps one to three feet away from the physical body on all sides. Others have called it a "radiant luminous cloud." Either way, every human has a "personal radiation field through which we touch our environment."[3] Clairvoyants report that in a state of vibrant health, a human standing in his aura resembles a figure inside a sun, as the brilliant aura radiates light in all directions.

However, the aura is a fragile energy field, subject to injury and compromise, according to psychic healer Ruth Berger. In her handbook on aura cleansing, *The Secret is in the Rainbow: Aura Interrelationships*, she notes that the aura can be ripped, torn, and penetrated. It can sustain cuts, slashes, gaps, slits, and openings, Berger reports. "Picture a piece of cloth or other material dotted with cuts, slits, tears, cigarette burns, and frayed edges, and you will be able to imagine what it would take to repair such an aura."

How does the aura get damaged? Powerful emotional events, focused insults, psychic and verbal abuse, accidents, violence, bad thoughts directed at you from other people, drunkenness, and substance abuse—there are numerous ways in which the delicate energy field around the human body can be polluted, soiled, or injured. All of us are subject to these auric influences, and the older we get, the more likely it is that our auric field matches Berger's description.

The cumulative effect of many energy insults to the aura is eventually tangible, physical symptoms, Berger explains. The aura develops splotches, dirty, murky, grayish areas like stains on blotting paper; it may also bear circles, checks, squares, lines, squares, or other strange unnatural-looking shapes, each of which is a kind of seed for an illness. In fact, psychic healers often report that observation of these abnormalities in the energy field is a valuable diagnostic tool, enabling them to see a health problem before it manifests physically.

For example, say somebody shouts at you and abuses you verbally and, in your view, quite unfairly. The abuse makes you feel bad, probably depressed, and it remains in your aura as a kind of repetitive thought, a harmful echo, a constant bruising influence, and thus a seed of illness. It weakens your aura and in turn makes your physical organism vulnerable, a little off balance. "This could result in colds, headaches, and general ill health," says Berger. "You must be aware of how negative thoughts can implant themselves in the body in order to take up the proper defense."[4]

According to psychic healers who work regularly with patients who have compromised auras, the energy field of the typical person bears hundreds of negative "seeds" of possible future illness left over from insults, abuses, traumas, strong emotional experiences, bad thoughts, and the rest.

According to psychic healers who work regularly with patients who have compromised auras, the energy field of the typical person bears hundreds of negative "seeds" of possible future illness left over from insults, abuses, traumas, strong emotional experiences, bad thoughts, and the rest. In fact, not only have "seeds" been observed, but numerous anomalous and frankly bizarre energy aberrations and "devices" have been noted. In fact, some have reported the presence of foreign sentient beings in the aura, even the spectral presence—auric ghosts, if you will—of deceased family members, relatives, or generational forebears.

As long as these "seeds" remain in the aura, they continue to exert an influence as "spiritual toxins." Metaphorically, they are another kind of free radical, less tangible than the molecular kind but equally capable of producing illness. Your aura is part of your overall living space and thereby is subject to toxic influences. Over time these spiritual toxins can contribute to a general weakening of the immune system and the body's physical integrity and to the emergence of numerous mental and physical symptoms, even degenerative disease—*unless* they are expunged. This chapter provides practical techniques to accomplish this.

The Outer and Inner Aura in Disease

The link between unseen influences in the energy field around the body and the emergence of mental and physical symptoms has occupied progressive researchers and physicians for the past one hundred years. Similarly, devising workable methods for auric detoxification has been the concern of psychic healers for a long time. Among scientific researchers, the effort of course has been to somehow quantify, even to make visible, the auric field and to use it as a diagnostic tool in assessing a patient's health and predisposition to illness.

While the aura and its "contents" have been discussed for millennia by healers, spiritual leaders, and psychics, in 1908, the scientific world took a major step forward in demonstrating the existence of the aura. Dr. Walter Kilner, a physician at London's St. Thomas' Hospital, developed a photographic process called the Kilner Screen that made the human aura relatively visible, thereby offering doctors a remarkable diagnostic potential.

The aura is triple-layered, transiently disfigured in infections but permanently distorted in pathological conditions, Dr. Kilner reported. With the Kilner Screen a physician could now see aspects of the human auric field, a perception that formerly had been available only to medical clairvoyants. In fact, Dr. Kilner devoted many pages to medical descriptions of the aura in disease, drawing correlations between observed energy anomalies in the aura and diagnosed medical conditions or pathologies in the physical bodies of patients. In Dr. Kilner's view, the connection between auric status and physical health was unassailable. "It is extremely difficult to imagine any departure from health that can occur without in some manner influencing one or more of the auric forces, and in consequence the aura itself."[5]

The human raiment of light received further clarification through the more recent work of John C. Pierrakos, M.D., a physician and practicing clairvoyant. Dr. Pierrakos described the "thrilling phenomenon" of the cloudlike auric envelope and its precise chromatic pulsations relative to body metabolism, breathing rate, emotional state, humidity, and air ionization. According to his own observations, the aura, which appears nearly perfectly oval, pulsates in a continual expansion-contraction rhythm at the rate of fifteen to twenty-five times per minute in a person who is in a wakeful state.

"The auric envelope viewed as a whole is blue-gray to sky blue, and it illuminates the periphery of the body in the way the rays of the rising sun light up the profile of dark mountains." Dr. Pierrakos postulates that the aura springs from a "longitudinal core of energy" in the physical body (possibly connected with the central nervous system) that radiates outward through the skin to activate the immediate atmosphere and form the aura. For those who can see the aura, it provides information about "the systemic implications of an illness, whether the primary symptoms surface in physical disabilities, emotional imbalances, or warped thinking."[6]

The practical, diagnostic correlations of the subtle human anatomy (energy features that work in complement with organic ones) with medicine were advanced in 1967 by neuropsychiatrist Shafica Karagulla, M.D., when she investigated the applications of clairvoyance for aura diagnosis. Dr. Karagulla worked with a team of psychics, matching their psychic perceptions of internal organs, auric colors, and the functional integrity of the chakras with known physical pathologies. For Dr. Karagulla's sensitives, the healthy energy field is a matrix of light frequencies penetrating the body like a "sparkling web of light beams."

This energy web can be tightly or loosely woven around the person; it can appear coarse or fine, dull or bright, she said. The auric web of unhealthy people, however, shows gaps, breaks in the pattern, holes, minute energy whirlpools that have separated from the normal energy stream, and a jumble of lines of force whose texture is like scar tissue. The essential point is that "the energy web or body showed the condition clearly many months before it became apparent in the physical body," commented Dr. Karagulla.

Dr. Karagulla described the case of "SA" in whose thyroid gland (in the throat) a nodule had been found and excised. The energy field of SA's throat was dull, ranging from gray and blue to a darker shade of gray. The energy level of the thyroid gland was "flabby, extremely low, as though dead," said Dr. Karagulla. Describing the overall impression made by SA's aura, she noted: "There was an unusual granular, sandlike appearance of the etheric energy distributed over the surface of the whole etheric field [another name for the auric energy field], which dipped deep into the physical body as well."[7] In other words, Dr. Karagulla saw confirmations of SA's poor health in the low energy state of and deformations in her aura.

Dr. Karagulla described the abdominal region of another patient. The solar plexus energy region of this person was "wilted" and "broken into fragments," especially around the belly button, while the energy outside that area, but still in the abdomen, moved at a faster rate and was brighter, all of which indicated an energy imbalance in the abdomen. The medical diagnosis was that this person had a blocked colon in the part near the spleen (on the left side).

Dr. Karagulla further reported that within the auric envelope are a series of whirling wheels of color, known anciently in both the East and West as chakras. These energy centers are arranged vertically with reference to the spinal column and in association with the endocrine glands. The chakras are "spiral cones of whirling energy," reported Dr. Karagulla in *Breakthrough to Creativity*. Breaks or disturbances in these spiral cones indicate an imbalance in the function of the physical body in that area, Dr. Karagulla explained. "If any of these major vortices show a dullness or irregularity or 'leak' in this central point or core, we look for some serious pathology in the physical body in the area."[8]

HEALTHY LIVING SPACE DETOXIFIER #36
Salting Your Energy Centers

Because the focus of this book is pragmatic rather than theoretical, it's time to try a technique that will both produce noticeable immediate benefits and demonstrate the reality of the aura and its influence on the mind and body.

You can use this technique as a once-weekly mind-body detoxifier, as an emergency auric detoxification method (for moments in which you feel "polluted"), as an occasional auric toner for improved well-being, or every morning (or evening) before your shower or bath. In this

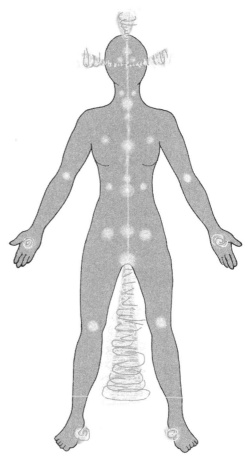

Figure 9-1. Locations of the Chakras.

exercise, you use a heavy saltwater solution to anoint different parts of your body to cleanse your energy centers, or chakras, thereby cleansing them of auric pollution. It is generally agreed that there are seven major centers along the spine from groin to head, but there are also numerous minor centers (some say as many as seventy-two) arrayed across the rest of the body; both major and minor energy centers are addressed in this detoxification technique (see figure 9-1).

Before you begin this exercise, notice your state of mind and body: How do you *feel*? What is your emotional state? Are you irritable or calm? Does your body feel comfortable or tense? Do you feel sluggish or alert? Do you have a headache? Is your breathing loose or tight? What kinds of thoughts are occupying your attention?

Directions: Fill a plastic quart container (such as a yogurt container) with one-half pound of food-grade salt, then add warm water to the top. Stir to mix the salt with the water. Take your clothes off and step into a shower stall; pull the shower curtain to keep the salt water from splattering your bathroom. Put your hand into the salt water (make sure the salt is thoroughly mixed in) so that a small amount of the thick salty water remains on your palm when you remove your hand. Daub the top of your head in a circular motion with this salt water in your hand.

You may wish to make a statement as you apply the salt water; one such statement is: "In the name of the Father, the Son, and the Holy Ghost, may these centers be clear and full of light." You can say anything you wish; the principle is that by making a statement it helps to focus the physical action. Make the statement each time you daub an energy center.

There are many energy centers on the head. After you daub the crown, daub your brow, then both sides of your nose, behind both ears, the temples, at the top back of the head, the back of the neck, the front of the neck. Next do your upper chest, then your solar plexus, pubic area, and groin. Be careful (especially men) not to get salt water directly on your genitals; it can irritate the urethra. With each energy center (chakra), take a fresh portion of salt water from the container. Finally, do the soles of your feet.

Now return to the top portion of your torso and do the armpits, insides of the elbows, the wrists, and the palms. Next, anoint your liver (lower front right side), spleen (lower front left side), both kidneys (same place, but in the back), the two shoulder blades, the inguinal lymph node area at the tops of the thighs (a few inches down from the groin on each leg), the front and back of the knees, the ankles, and the soles of the feet again.

If there is any salt water remaining, daub it any place where you sense it is needed and empty the rest over your head. One clue to where else may need salting is that during the anointing you may find you shiver or shake as you apply the salt to certain areas. Commonly, the back of the neck and the solar plexus (upper abdomen) reflect a great deal of auric pollution; the contact of the salt water with these sites can produce temporary physical sensations. Often the occurrence of shakes, shivers, sighs, groans, or even shouts as you apply the salt can be interpreted as a kind of feedback, confirming the appropriateness of the salt-based detoxification technique. In other words, getting a reaction of this type tells you there was in fact some auric pollution there; however, not reacting in these ways does not mean your aura was clear. People react differently to energy clearings.

Remain standing with the salt all over your body for about ten seconds, then shower off all the salt. Take another inventory of your state of mind and body. Do you notice any differences? I am certain you will feel better. The more you use this technique and the closer you observe your starting and finishing mind-body state, the more you will come to appreciate the cleansing effect of the salt water. Also, the more acute the sense of auric pollution—recall that contaminated room we imagined entering at the start of this chapter—the more immediate and unarguable the psychic and physical relief you will probably experience after salting your energy centers.

This technique is not curative, in the sense of permanently removing deeply embedded influences from your aura, but it is definitely palliative. You will feel better after doing it and can preempt the influence of unwholesome auric energies upon your thoughts, feelings, and actions. You will probably come to realize that sometimes that spike of irritation, that surge of anger, that flare-up of pique, is not *you*; it does not come authentically from you but from a transiently resident energy influence, in a sense, something you picked up at the mall.

Variations: Should you be so fortunate as to live near the ocean, a daily swim, float, or simple immersion in the salt water will accomplish the same effect as the anointing of your energy centers in the shower stall. If you own or have access to a flotation tank, thirty to sixty minutes in this salt-rich enclosed water environment will produce excellent results. Not only will your energy centers have a cleansing, but your whole body will feel astonishingly relaxed, rested, and clean.

Charting the Subconscious Mind in the Aura

The medical applications of auric diagnosis have taken a great leap forward with the innovative work of Shakuntala Modi, a board-certified psychiatrist based in Wheeling, West Virginia, who has successfully used hypnotherapy to help relieve patients of numerous physical and psychological symptoms due to spiritual toxins. Dr. Modi's approach is to hypnotize patients, then interview them while they are in a light trance state to ascertain the subconscious factors underlying their health problems, both physiological and psychological in nature.

Based on her research with hypnotized patients, conducted over more than fifteen years, Dr. Modi is confident in correlating numerous health conditions, such as stammering, panic disorder, headaches, weight gain, allergies, schizophrenia, uterine disorders, and others, with various types of unresolved energy field disturbances. What Dr. Modi refers to as a person's "soul history" is arrayed in the aura. She explains that this energy field can get "polluted" with unhealthy thoughts and influences just as the physical body gets overburdened with toxins.

Research conducted among her patient base showed that 77 out of 100 patients reported having foreign "beings" in their aura (they described them as "demons") who were responsible for the psychological and physical symptoms for which they were seeking help, reports Dr. Modi. These inimical energies were described as being black, red, or gray blobs in various shapes, "ranging from tiny dots to giant-sized creatures," as "black and gray pebbles all over the body," or a "piece of coal," but they could also assume shapes more like animals, gargoyles, devils, or monsters; while in hypnotic trance, some people said their bodies seemed to be infested with "freckles," which they understood to be the foreign energies; still others said they perceived these bizarre external energies to exist in many layers in the aura.

These toxic energies can make patients "convulse, shake, jerk, froth at the mouth, spit, hiss, growl," and to feel other strong, negative emotions, says Dr. Modi. Her research demonstrated that these foreign energy beings are "the most common cause for depression" and "the single leading cause for psychiatric problems in general, directly or indirectly." In one case, persistent shooting nerve pain in the heel was due to gray and dark foreign energies "packed in multiple layers" in the patient's heel; in another case, a man had chronic back pain due to a similar layering of toxic energies; while still other patients reported "black blobs" in their

Figure 9-2. Picture of Body Showing Energy Interferences.

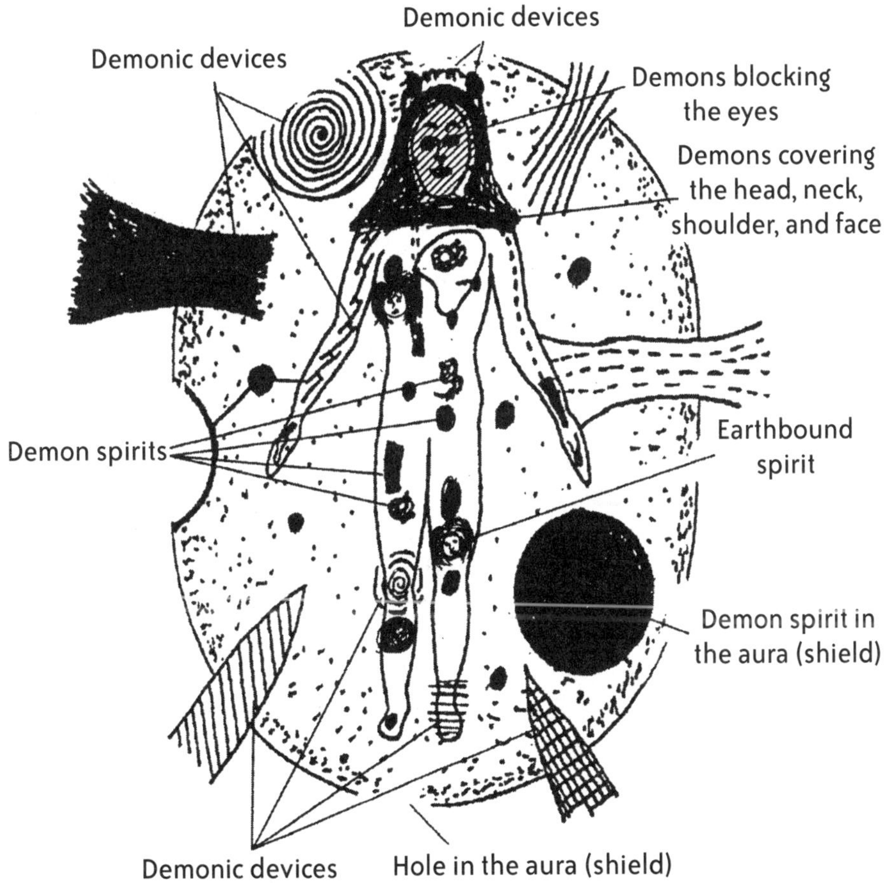

Demonic devices

Demonic devices

Demons blocking the eyes

Demons covering the head, neck, shoulder, and face

Demon spirits

Earthbound spirit

Demon spirit in the aura (shield)

Demonic devices   Hole in the aura (shield)

Reprinted with publisher's permission from *Remarkable Healings*, by Shakuntala Modi, M.D., Hampton Roads, 1999.

stomach, bladder, shoulders, jaw, eyes, hands, or head, producing chronic pain and discomfort in those areas (see figure 9-2).

Of equal strangeness is Dr. Modi's report that many patients, under hypnosis, discovered that various foreign "devices" were lodged in their auras. These devices act as spiritual toxins, draining the body of energy or inducing symptoms and the energy conditions for physical illness. For example, Dr. Modi found that some patients had "energy absorbers," which interfered with nerve impulses. Their effect is to absorb a person's energy, "making them chronically fatigued, sluggish, and sleepy," and they can interfere with memory and brain functions as well. One patient reported detecting a "yellow-green slime" in the digestive tract. This had the physical effect of interfering with digestion and nutrient absorption, and produced stomach pain, comments Dr. Modi.[9]

The crucial point is that once this realm of toxic influence is acknowledged—once you accept that it is possible such things can exist—the deep roots of a great deal of toxicity, illness, and disease have been identified.

There are a multitude of cases showing the deleterious effects of spiritual toxins in the aura from the casebooks of Dr. Modi and other "spirit releasement" practitioners, whether psychics or psychiatrists. The crucial point is that once this realm of toxic influence is acknowledged—once you accept that it is possible such things can exist—the deep roots of a great deal of toxicity, illness, and disease have been identified. Not to remove these bad energy influences is to ensure their continuing negative impact on our health and well-being and to relegate many people to *unnecessary* (because it is treatable) discomfort and suffering.

When these foreign presences and devices were removed from the patients' auras through a process called spirit releasement, says Dr. Modi, the acute symptoms "often cleared up immediately," relieving patients of their long-term discomfort.

It's not always spirit attachment per se that creates the problem, sometimes it is only a matter of proximity. According to the late British psychiatrist, Arthur Guirdham, M.D., many common illnesses can be attributed to the aura registering contact with evil entities or discarnate beings or with the onset of "far memory," otherwise known as recall of past lives. In this model, the body's reaction is to channel the mind's suppression of this information into certain illness categories, including migraines, epilepsy, asthma, childhood tics, intestinal distress, Meniere's disease, shingles, and later in life, obsessional neurosis, heart problems, and in some instances, cancer.

Dr. Guirdham, a psychic himself, recognized the psychic side of many illness conditions, both physical and mental. The illness results from the body recoiling from the inimical contact or from the force of the psyche's repression of the awareness of the contact, Dr. Guirdham says. He reminds us that epilepsy was once called the "sacred disease," and was associated with psychic abilities and contact with discarnate presences. It remains so today in most instances, even if it is not medically recognized as such. "In such cases, the individual is escaping in *petit mal* from what he is afraid to receive in full consciousness." Epilepsy is a defensive response, both crude and immediate, to the encroaching presence of "invading entities," and as the child grows older it is often succeeded by migraines and asthma. Asthma in a child, says Dr. Guirdham, is often "a straight response to night terrors," the semi-conscious perception of astral entities or discarnate beings, usually of an unwholesome valence.[10]

Increasingly, practitioners from diverse fields, such as psychology and medicine, are beginning to acknowledge this energy factor in disease. In fact, the matter of infestation by entities has a distinguished past, being one of the eight sections of classical Ayurveda, the traditional medical-mystical science of India. In Ayurveda, *bhuta-vidya* is the science of entities and considers the effect of bhutas, or entities, on human health and sanity, and the ways one can eliminate these noxious presences. One *bhuta-vidya* practitioner is Parisian-trained physician Samuel Sagan, M.D., who directs the Clairvision School in Sydney, Australia. A significant portion of his work involves clearing entities and "perverse energies" from the auras of clients.[11]

"Entity" is an all-purpose term denoting a nonphysical being or presence that gets attached to a human being and there acts as an energy parasite. Entities drain life force energy; they inspire perverse or inappropriate behavior; and they contribute to various types of ill health and disease, says Dr. Sagan. What do they look like? Patients have described them as blobs, clouds, amorphous black shapes, amoeba, octopus-like, spider-like, and other "monstrous" shapes.

In Dr. Sagan's view, for the most part, entities derive from human beings, specifically, from shattered fragments of the astral body after one has died. These float around like miniature persons, but with a singular, if not fixated, focus, usually upon a single desire for revenge, pleasure, or other strongly charged emotional condition. The entities get attached to humans in moments of stress, shock, or trauma; during electroshock therapy; during serious illness (involving fluid loss, hemorrhaging, or extreme energy depletion); under anesthesia or recreational drug use; *in utero* and during birth; and in other situations when the aura opens up or is vulnerable and when its natural defense system collapses.

In fact, Dr. Sagan advises having a "systematic entity checkup" with a qualified practitioner after undergoing high-risk situations, such as abortions, miscarriage, delivery, or the death of a close relative. Each of these is a condition in which one's natural defense system is vulnerable to entity penetration.

Entities are experts at camouflage, and are intent on not being detected by their hosts. Their goal is to decrease the person's mental acuity, to make the awareness blurry and confused, so as to enable them to elude detection. The last thing an entity wants is for the host to wake up to the fact they are being "tricked and manipulated by something foreign," says Dr. Sagan.

Entities in a human's energy field act like toxic substances, and are capable of producing numerous health problems, such as, for example, depression. Dr. Sagan relates a case in which a man, age twenty-six, a former heroin addict, was heavily depressed. During treatment (in which the patient is put into a kind of light trance enabling one to see the intruders in their energy body), he saw a black cloud around his heart. The primary emotion associated with this black cloud was fear of death. He understood it had entered his auric space when he began using heroin at age twelve, and been reawakened by a recent car accident.

The entity's purpose was to make the man suffer, to harm him, to make him take drugs. "It lives in people's minds like a headache," he told Dr. Sagan. "If you need a headache, it will come to you and give you one." The man further understood that the entity was creating his depression. "It secretes the depression like a dark cloud into my heart." Removal of the entity produced complete relief from depression in two days, says Dr. Sagan.

Here is another eye-opening case. In this one, a dead step-father returned to haunt his stepdaughter's womb and produce a fibroid, a noncancerous but medically dangerous fibrous growth in the uterus. In this woman, age forty-two, her fibroid had grown very large—uncomfortably so—and was producing increased menstrual bleeding. The stepfather had raped the woman when she was ten; when he died by suicide, the woman (as a girl) was unable to process her emotions and went through a "time of madness"; his despair and rage revisited the woman at this time of vulnerability and lodged in her uterus like a fetus. The fibroid started to shrink once the stepfather's presence was removed from it, says Dr. Sagan.

Here is a third case, this time involving entities and migraines. A woman, age forty-eight, had excruciating migraines that would take eight days to subside. She discovered that dug in around her skull was "a big insect," like a crayfish, with legs dug in around her occiput and eyebrows. The insect had a tube inserted into the woman's head and it was feeding off her brain's energy and her anger like a tick, she reported. Its purpose was to confuse her, to keep her from thinking clearly. "The migraine comes out of the tick like a poison," she said. It came out of its belly and was injected under her skin, producing terrible pain. Once Dr. Sagan removed the astral entity, the migraines stopped immediately.

Based on his clinical experience, Dr. Sagan concludes that "the work on entities has proved a remarkably quick and efficient way of improving the health and well-being of a number of clients." He adds that when you discover and clear the entity behind—that is to say, responsible for—a physical illness, the results can be "spectacular." The earlier you can do this, the better, before the body has translated a functional disorder, produced by an entity, into an entrenched, crystallized disease.

Entities do not necessarily produce all illnesses, and some-times they stop short at energy drainage or psychological inter-ference, such as producing emotional outbursts, sugar cravings, and alcohol or drug abuse. Their preferred "food" is strong human emotion, especially of a negative kind, such as anger, dismay, frustration, emotional pain, melancholy, sadness, or depression, as well as sensual enjoyment, says Dr. Sagan. The most common bodily locations for entities are the large intestine (especially the left iliac region), the vagina, uterus, and ovaries, mainly because, from their viewpoint, these are commodious, cavelike environments, suitable for staying resident and hidden.

Many—perhaps most—people still regard the concept of entities in the aura as something close to preposterous, yet Dr. Sagan reports that "hundreds" of clients who had never even heard of the possibility, much less dismissed it as being impossible, had, during a heightened state of perception, become aware of a foreign, parasitic presence attached to their energy body.

In most cases, a person doesn't have just one entity attached, but usually many, states William J. Baldwin, D.D.S., Ph.D., one of the country's preeminent educators and practitioners in the field of what he calls spirit releasement therapy. Dr. Baldwin is the author of *Spirit Releasement Therapy: A Technique Manual*, an accomplished remover of attached entities, and the director of the Center for Human Relations in Enterprise, Florida.

"A living person can have dozens, even hundreds, of attached spirits as they occupy no physical space," states Dr. Baldwin. Parts of the body that have a physical weakness tend to attract parasitic energy forms, especially discarnate but earthbound human spirits; the physical weakness matches an ailment or disability they had while alive. "The discarnate entity retains the psychic energy pattern of its own ailments following death and can produce in the host any mental aberration or emotional disturbance and any symptom of physical illness," explains Dr. Baldwin.

Similarly, any symptom, both mental and physical, or strong emotion (especially repressed strong feelings such as unexpressed grief or rage) can "act like a magnet" and attract a discarnate being or other energy form with similar emotions, conditions, needs, or feelings. He calls this situation in which a foreign energy is present in the aura and exerting a powerful but unsuspected influence on the host "spirit possession syndrome."[12]

For those initially skeptical of the possibility that essentially invisible and inimical energy entities reside in their auras, Dr. Baldwin suggests considering the following list of symptoms, odd sensations, and inexplicable feelings typically reported by people who later discovered such entities present around them: feelings of being blocked or sabotaged, especially when things seem favorable; hearing intrusive thoughts and voices; the sense that some of your behaviors or statements are inconsistent with your sense of yourself; recurrent dreams or nightmares; addictions; sexual or relationship problems; feelings of abandonment or of not being alone in your body; the sense of being followed or stalked; irrational fears, anger, sadness, guilt, or other negative emotional states; chronic unhappiness as if over everything and anything. Any, some, or all of these symptoms can indicate an attached negative—that is to say, toxic—entity in your energy space, says Dr. Baldwin.

There are also many empirical signs that are suggestive of entity attachment, says Dr. Baldwin. All it takes is a little extra measure of self-awareness and a comparison of present and earlier mental and emotional states, a kind of identity baseline, if you will. Dr. Baldwin explains that "a newly formed spirit attachment" can generate any of these symptoms: the sudden onset of drug dependency; speech or behavior that is out of character in terms of affect or content; unfamiliar, uncharacteristic reactions to otherwise familiar situations; bodily movements, especially repetitive ones, that seem out of your control; a sense of having lost one's normal sense of oneself; conspicuous but inexplicable personality changes; sudden change in beliefs, dietary preferences, or taste in clothing, or even subtle changes in facial features.

> ### The Healthy Living Space Info Tip
>
> Dr. Modi specializes in spirit releasement work using hypnotherapy in her clinical practice. To contact:
> Shakuntala Modi, M.D.,
> 1025 Main Street,
> 416 Holly Building,
> Wheeling, WV 26003;
> tel: 304-233-7246.
>
> Samuel Sagan, M.D., offers courses in training sensitivity to perceive foreign energies in the aura and techniques for removing them. Clairvision, P.O. Box 33, Roseville, 2069 Australia;
> tel: 61-2-9888-1999;
> e-mail: info@clairvision.org;
> website: www. clairvision.org.
>
> William J. Baldwin, D.D.D., Ph.D., Center for Human Relations, P.O. Box 4061,
> Enterprise, FL 32725;
> e-mail: doctorbill@aol.com;
> website: www.spiritreleasement.org .

HEALTHY LIVING SPACE DETOXIFIER #37
Request a Cleansing from Above

How does Dr. Modi remove these harmful energies? As with physical detoxification, a deep cleansing is involved, but this one has a twist. Here again, most of us need to make a leap of faith, but if we accept one end of the subtle world of invisible energies, namely, the role of negative auric entities, we may as well accept the other, positive pole; cleansers from above, so to speak.

"I routinely ask the angels to cleanse and heal the person by scrubbing every part and every organ of the patient's body, removing all the negative entities, energies, and devices, and any leftover residue," states Dr. Modi unabashedly. Next, Dr. Modi asks the angelic helpers to fill the person with light and to shield the body with light and "spiritual mirrors and rays of blinding hot white Light."[13] Dr. Modi also advises clients to visualize a bright violet flame burning around their bodies, incinerating impurities and infusing the energy field with a strong protective quality.

No special ability is required to request this kind of other-worldly cleansing, only the intent to be rid of the foreign energies and a belief that seemingly invisible help can accomplish this important task. Merely *asking* for assistance from above is a powerful technique in starting to clear the aura of pollutants. The power of asking is an open secret, and a paradoxical one. It works, but you have to believe in something you probably can't see. You will not necessarily be aware of anything during the subtle cleansing, but almost surely you will feel some easing of your symptoms shortly afterwards, probably within a day.

Directions: While sitting in a quiet place, request a cleansing from above. If you are comfortable with the concept of invisible benign helpers, then ask that beings of light, friendly spirits, angels, your higher self, inner self, guardian angel, a saint, or God—whatever form the numinous takes in your belief system— to remove any negative entities, energies, and devices from your aura. Ask that they then put a protective bubble or shield of spiritual light around your aura and reflective mirrors on the outside to keep away further contaminating energies. Visualize a column of brilliant pure white light coming from the highest divine source above you and entering your body through your head, filling all of your body down to your toes, cleansing every aspect of your physical body and surrounding aura. Finally, ask that you be protected from this point forward from any further inimical influence.[14]

The Healthy Living Space Expert Interview: Rev. Leon S. LeGant, Psychic Healer

To an extent, once we grant the possibility that the energy field surrounding our physical body can contain injurious energies and presences, it is possible to take steps on our own to rid ourselves of these intruders. At the same time, it is a good idea to arrange a consultation with a qualified psychic healer to do a thorough job of cleansing your aura. The combination of self-help steps and professional treatment is generally advisable. After all, as we discussed in earlier chapters, there is much we can do to effect a cleansing of our digestive system, including liver, kidney, and intestinal detoxification, but a few acupuncture treatments, for example, can help a great deal in balancing the overall energy flow within the body and through these organs.

Since 1994, Rev. Leon S. Legant, a self-described "clairvoyant reader and spiritual healer" practicing in San Rafael, California, has removed unsuspected spiritual toxins from the energy fields of some two thousand clients. Working with this world of subtle influence and effect every day for years has given LeGant an "insider's" view of the mechanics of spiritual toxicity.

The energy field is "basically a storage unit," LeGant explains, containing information packed in layers on "survival, our emotions, how the body runs its energy, how it drains it, our affinities, self-image, and much more." Foreign energy affects and tends to lodge in one of the layers of the aura, depending on its nature and the corresponding location it chooses in the aura. If it lodges in the auric storage area for survival issues, the foreign energy will stimulate thoughts, feelings, fears, even outer episodes to do with survival, explains LeGant. How does one know if there is something foreign in the aura? You will first notice the problem it is causing, says LeGant; you will not necessarily (unless you are trained in this kind of sensitivity) notice the energy itself.

"The first thing for people to realize as a step in their healing is to acknowledge that many of their problems are not produced by their own energy. What they are feeling isn't really who they are in many cases; there is something foreign causing these states of mind or feelings about themselves." Once the foreign energies are removed, you can then sense the difference in yourself made by their absence, LeGant adds. You will feel the change, and looking back to how you felt earlier, see the effect on you of the foreign energy and the degree to which you thought it was yourself.

Our auras, like the skin on our physical bodies, are subject to bruises and penetrations every day, says LeGant. The difference is that we usually are unaware of when our energy field has been breached, leaving us vulnerable to harmful energy influences. "When someone's aura is ripped or torn open, this is called a whack. A whack happens when someone or an experience contradicts a person and injures the aura." Harsh, insulting, demeaning words, or any kind of strong verbal abuse, can "whack" the aura, especially when they focus on the person's weak, sore, or painful spots. You may get over the words, but their effect still resonates in your aura; in a sense, the words are still lodged there.

LeGant explains that "sometimes the aura looks like someone fired buckshot at it, or there is a giant rip starting at the aura's outermost edge. Once there is a whack, the person's energy begins to drain out through that rip or opening in the aura, instead of flowing evenly through the aura." Once the aura's integrity has been violated, it increases our vulnerability to further pollution by inimical energies, says LeGant. The situation is similar to when your immune system is weakened by illness or an unbalanced lifestyle; this leaves your body open to the effect of opportunistic germs in your environment. In this case, the aura is your energetic immune system, and, once weakened by "whacks," it can allow unwholesome energies to enter and attach themselves to our vulnerable spots.

Those painful areas or points of vulnerability exist in the aura like pictures or condensed images of experiences, says LeGant. He calls these "core pictures," and he says they are central to an understanding of how spiritual toxins work.

Those painful areas or points of vulnerability exist in the aura like pictures or condensed images of experiences, says LeGant. He calls these "core pictures," and he says they are central to an understanding of how spiritual toxins work. "Because of the intense stimulation of an event, the body believes it is having an important experience, causing it to store all that information from the experience within the brain. From a clairvoyant perspective, that stored information looks like a mass of energy about the size of a softball, located in the limbic system but 'bleeding' into the brain's cortex."

Typically, a person has thousands of core pictures, says LeGant, accumulated (and unprocessed) from this and other lifetimes. Each is a condensed, crystallized picture or residue of an emotional intensity, be it trauma, injury, insult, abuse, or humiliation. When something happens in our outer world that is similar to the content of a core picture, the core picture gets lit up, emphasized, and reactivated, and we see our reality through it. If it involved illness or dysfunction, these conditions too start to manifest. In essence, each core picture is an "energetic block" that acts like a toxin and detracts from our mental clarity, emotional well-being, and physical health.

"When a core picture becomes stuck in the brain, its influence is extreme. It wraps around our flame of consciousness. Our essence shines through the core picture and projects that past time experience into our mental body [our thoughts and mental processes construed as if they are a body on their own] and thus into our reality." For example, say a young girl has an abusive, alcoholic father. The girl stores her memories of her father's abusiveness in a "solidified" form as a core picture. This core picture then becomes a filter throughout her life for how she sees her reality and relationships with men.

"Now as your consciousness projects that core picture into your reality, you are in your fifth relationship with an alcoholic and abusive man. With each new relationship, you attracted someone like your father. It only takes one core picture to produce such devastating effects." But it gets still more complex for two reasons. First, most of our core pictures are not derived from our current life, which means it is unlikely we would ever suspect they are in play; and second, it is the core pictures that attract the spiritual toxins described above by Dr. Modi. "Core pictures are like cheese on Ritz crackers for unwholesome energies and beings," says LeGant.

Core pictures are "anchor points" allowing "demons," discarnate earthbound entities, and other injurious energies to attach to the person's aura. LeGant uses the general term "spirit guides" to describe the range of beings that can occupy (or infest) our auric space—"beings without bodies, sources of influence." A spirit guide in this model is not necessarily a beneficial presence; in fact, it can be literally demonic.

The larger point is that spirit guides, whatever they are, claim "seniority" over the host's thoughts, feelings, actions, health—life. They are parasites that have claimed a person's body as their own. "Most people have many dozens, if not hundreds, of spirit guides in their auric space, and only a very small percentage of people have seniority to their spirit guides."

The combination of core pictures and attached entities often explains why people are not able to clear out the bad energy by themselves, notes LeGant. "I first ask why the spiritual consciousness of the client has not or is not healing those blocks on their own. I believe everyone knows how to heal himself. But if they are not doing so, that usually means their consciousness is sitting in a core picture that is stuck in the system."

One of the central points in this book is that toxicity affects every aspect of our being, from the physical body to the energy field surrounding it. The combination of core picture and attached entity is similar to a situation observed on the molecular level and known as circulating immune complexes (CIC), a key issue in physiological toxicity (see chapter 2, p. 74).

To review: foreign proteins "leak" into the blood system, usually from the intestines. The immune system tags these proteins as foreign invaders (antigens) and surrounds them with immune cells (antibodies); the antigen-antibody complex is known as a CIC.

In a healthy person, CICs are neutralized, but in someone with a compromised immune system, they tend to accumulate in the blood and burden the detoxification pathways or produce allergies. If too many CICs accumulate, the kidneys are usually unable to excrete them through the urine, and they get stored in the body's soft tissues where they produce inflammation and further stress on the immune system. The overload can lead to a variety of chronic health conditions.

Meanwhile, the entity complexes, left unresolved in the auric space, produce numerous symptoms, conditions, and illnesses, just as a glut of free radicals and CICs do in the physical body. A "spirit guide" may lodge itself in an organ and start depriving the person of the full use of this organ, explains LeGant. Say it is the lungs, and the person is a smoker. The tobacco smoke is the entry point for a type of being. "Once the beings get into the lungs, they start to lodge themselves in the cells and there becomes less room for the person's own energy in that organ and more of this foreign energy."

LeGant explains that sometimes "just the presence of that foreign energy in an organ for so long and not having your own healing energies running through the tissues can cause a health problem, even cancer." He further states that sometimes foreign energy beings can activate cancer genes and start a cancer process, or attract viruses to the host to produce serious illnesses, or provoke the host into taking self-destructive actions, such as neglecting their health or exposing themselves to infection.

"However, as a rule of thumb, the spiritual toxins come first and that attracts or produces the physical problems," says LeGant. "You can clairvoyantly 'read' someone who has a cancer being in their body *before* they have cancer, and you can remove that cancer being and enable the person to avoid developing cancer." This can be taken one step further, he adds. If you remove a fair amount of the spiritual toxins from a person's aura, that person tends to be less affected by or can better handle physical toxins they come across. "You can reverse whatever physical manifestations are present if you remove enough of the foreign energy and are very thorough about this. A cancer can go into remission, a disease can go away."

The practical conclusion from this information is that it is advisable to undertake a physical detoxification program in conjunction with work that removes spiritual toxins as well, advises LeGant. "It is prudent to deal with *both* poles of toxicity, the physical and the spiritual sides." If you do a physical cleanse program and overlook possible auric toxicity, you have not removed the seeds of the physical toxicity. At the same time, the body always needs a helping hand when it comes to handling an extra load of detoxification, so if you remove spiritual toxins, be sure to undertake a complementary physical detoxification program because the auric shifts will provoke corresponding physiological ones.

Typically, LeGant, using psychic methods, removes a layer of four or five core pictures and numerous attached entities, then watches his client's "subconscious or spiritual self release the remaining anchor points throughout their body, aura, and energy centers. If they are not healing themselves at that point, I will remove another layer of core pictures and then another until they are successfully able to clear themselves."

During a typical session, which may last from 30 to 120 minutes, LeGant "erases" core pictures and "removes" the attached beings according to what is most prominent in the client's aura. Current life experiences tend to "light up" specific core pictures, making them more noticeable and the client more uncomfortable under their influence, says LeGant, but it is the foreground core pictures to which he devotes his attention in a clearing session. If you schedule regular clearings at the rate of once monthly, the subconscious starts cooperating, shifting material towards the forefront of your awareness such that in the few days before a session, new core pictures and their attached beings become illuminated in the aura—"lit up," LeGant calls it. It is as if they start to queue for their forthcoming release.

How do you know if you have spiritual toxins in your aura? LeGant's estimation is that most people have them, but usually go about their lives oblivious of their presence, attributing their effects to other causes. One rule of thumb is that if you keep coming up against a brick wall in your life—an attitude that won't shift, a destructive or self-limiting self-definition, an obstacle, opponent, or seeming enemy that won't go away—then it is likely you have a foreign energy of some kind at work, invisible to you, in your space.

Another way to think of this is in a way parallel to how we view the intestines. Many people with regular eliminations would consider it ridiculous to suggest that nonetheless they might be chronically constipated and benefit from an intestinal cleansing. Yet many are, and many would. Similarly, it would surprise many Westerners to learn that they have intestinal dysbiosis and possibly some parasites, yet the trend in laboratory testing indicates that many do (see chapter 3). Pollution in the intestines, pollution in the aura—in essence they are the same.

We tend to become accustomed to our dysfunctions, and mask them or account for them in ways that enable us to keep living with a minimum of disruption. While this may seem pragmatic, it's not curative; we're still stuck with these invisible yet potent energies in our space that can often make our life a lot harder than it needs to be. The best confirmation that you need a psychic clearing of your aura comes afterwards, when you look back and wonder how you managed to function before all this negative energy was removed, just as, in the weeks after a colon cleanse, you wonder how your intestines ever functioned properly—because now you can *feel* the difference in yourself.

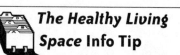

The Healthy Living Space Info Tip

Leon S. LeGant does most of his spirit releasement and psychic healing work over the telephone, and works with clients across the United States. To contact:
Rev. Leon S. LeGant,
27 Aquinas Drive,
San Rafael, CA 94901;
tel: 888-459-4585.

HEALTHY LIVING SPACE DETOXIFIER #38
Do a 30-Minute Spirit-Detoxifying Bath

While you are likely to feel immediate relief from some mental or physical symptoms during or immediately after a session (LeGant calls it a "reading"), in the following one to two weeks, the physical body starts to deal with the ramifications of this major energy shift in its auric field. Also, if LeGant removes five beings, your auric space, now freed from the magnetizing core pictures, can release perhaps thirty more beings on its own, and possibly shatter a few pictures as well.

The way you experience this is similar to what we defined earlier in the book as the Herxheimer effect in terms of physical detoxification. In the physical case, the body temporarily feels more toxic as toxins are mobilized, neutralized, and released from the body. Similarly, in the auric case, your state of mind, emotions, and thoughts, and to an extent, your body as well, feel more toxic for a short while as the aura purges beings and energies and your physical body makes the corresponding adjustments.

What experts in physical detoxification call the Herxheimer Effect, psychic healers like Leon LeGant call a "growth period." Removing foreign energies, pictures, and beings from your auric space generates a profound shift in your mind-body constitution, says LeGant. In a sense, you have disturbed a long-term ecology, although it is an unbalanced ecology in which your body has learned to accommodate "hostile demons, painful core pictures, and energy blocks" in much the same way your liver and intestines learn to accommodate environmental toxins. "As spirits, we can change our energy in the snap of a finger, but our bodies require a period of time to catch up and adjust to those changes."

In the weeks following a psychic clearing, you continue to heal yourself, bringing up and releasing physical, emotion, and mental pain, as well as more beings, says LeGant. "As that energy releases, you may experience its effects, which include an edgy and uncomfortable sensation. You may feel that your life is falling apart, that chaos has broken loose in your mind, that you have lost all sense of your self, among other transient mind states." These pass, just as the Herxheimer reaction to detoxification subsides. Typically, the intense phase of the growth period lasts only one week. "Once a person finishes releasing, they begin to recreate themselves and their environment. I have seen these kinds of transformations thousands of times; after removing demonic influences, a person has the freedom to change any and every element of their life they choose."

It is advisable to give your body some tangible support as it reorganizes itself now that it has been freed from the deleterious influence of negative energies. One practical way is to take specially formulated baths, and it is especially helpful to do this in the days *immediately* following a psychic clearing, says LeGant. "Epsom salts baths are very useful for clearing pain out of the body and for releasing beings, foreign energy, and stress," says LeGant.

Directions: You may have tried the Epsom salts bath following directions in chapter 4 for the purposes of general stress relief. Now the focus is more refined—to help your body release accumulated energetic toxins.

Fill a bathtub with very hot water, as hot as you are comfortable lying in. Add bubble bath and an aromatherapy essential oil to the water to provide bubbles, scent, and additional detoxifying agents. If you wish to relax deeply, use lavender or melissa essential oils; if you need to center, reintegrate, and reorganize yourself, use rosemary; if you need a cleansing, rejuvenating energy, use pine, juniper, or eucalyptus.

Here is a tip about adding bubbles and oils: Measure the bubble bath into a plastic quart container; dribble in the aromatherapy oils, anywhere from five to thirty drops, understanding that more equals stronger. Then fill the container with hot water and dribble its contents into the stream of water coming out of the faucet. This improves the miscibility and dispersion of the bubble bath material and oils into the hot water.

Add two to four pounds of Epsom salts (magnesium sulfate) to the water, stirring well. As with the aromatherapy oils, more Epsom salts equals a deeper relaxation, but don't use more than four pounds per bath. Epsom salts typically come in a four-pound milk-carton-like package, costing between two and three dollars.

As additional support for your post-spirit-releasement detoxification bath, consider bringing a CD-player into the bathroom and playing your favorite music while you soak. It is advisable, however, to use a calming music, something that might evoke a meditative, relaxed state of mind, such as Chopin's

Etudes, or Steven Halpern's *Spectrum Suite* (see chapter 4 for more on music therapy for stress reduction). Also supportive of the detox mood is dim lighting, such as candlelight or indirect lighting from another room, while the bathroom itself is dark.

Soak for at least twenty minutes, but thirty or longer is better. You may find yourself sighing, moaning, groaning, whimpering, shouting, or emitting other surprising vocal noises while you soak. You may also experience transient emotions, such as grief, anger, sadness, or despair—any of the gamut of feelings. Do not be alarmed, but be amused if you wish: your body is doing its releasing work. In a sense, you are only becoming aware of what was already there in your emotional field.

When you are finished soaking and climb out of the tub, do not towel dry. Lie on some dry towels on your bed and air dry over the next thirty to forty-five minutes. Your skin is still covered with a film of Epsom salts and aromatherapy oils, and these will continue working while you air dry. Often this phase of the detoxification bath is the most relaxing; don't be surprised if you fall asleep for a short time.

Variation: Try substituting Dead Sea mineral salts for the Epsom salts for a twenty- to thirty-minute growth-period soak. The mineral salts concentration of Dead Sea bath salts is 27-33% higher than the average ocean concentration of 3.4%. The specific salts include magnesium, potassium, sodium, and calcium chlorides. For presumably thousands of years, the Dead Sea has been the destination for millions seeking the therapeutic benefit of its mineral salts for muscle pain, muscle tension, arthritis, and other conditions.[15] You can also mix Dead Sea bath salts with aromatherapy oils (such as citrus, eucalyptus, lavender, rose) for extra detoxifying benefits.

Here is a general recommendation: add a full cup (250 g, or about 1/2 pound) of Dead Sea bath salts to a tub of hot water; stay in the water fifteen to twenty minutes, but do not use any soap, then rinse off and rest in or on your bed for thirty minutes.

According to one Dead Sea salts processor, the high mineral content of the salts "stimulates blood and lymph circulation, an effect that helps drain out the

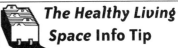

The Healthy Living Space Info Tip

For a source of Dead Sea mineral salts (unprocessed, in their natural form):
Masada Marketing Corp.,
P.O. Box 4118,
Chatsworth, CA 91313-4118;
tel: 800-368-8811 or 818-717-8300;
fax: 818-717-8400;
website:
www.secondwave.net/masada-marketing;
e-mail: sam@masada-spa.com.

Also: Ashtar Natural Dead Sea Products,
Amig Group,
P.O. Box 53, A.1.E.
Amman, Jordan 11512;
fax: 962-6-5534562;
website: www.fjcc.com/amig.

trapped fluid in the joints, which causes arthritic pain, thus improving joint movement." Further, the salts "exfoliate and revitalize the skin, eliminating toxins" and they help relieve aches and pains, relax the muscles, and relieve neck and back tension and stiffness.[16]

HEALTHY LIVING SPACE DETOXIFIER #39
Shake Yourself Free of Toxic Energies

Think of a dog just out of the rain or from swimming in a lake: it shakes itself vigorously, sending water droplets everywhere, perhaps on you. It's an effective drying technique, at least for the dog. In the same way, vigorously shaking your whole body is an effective way to scatter negative, heavy energies that have adhered to it, suggests psychic protection expert William Bloom. A leader of psychic protection workshops in Europe, author of several books on the subject, and a man especially "sensitive to atmospheres" since infancy, Bloom has developed a variety of practical techniques for clearing the energy field of obtrusive, foreign energies.

"Moving and shaking your body will free up your own frozen energy, as well as moving any that belongs to someone or something else," he explains. Energy, whether it comes from our own emotional reactions or the energy extrusions of others around us, can get stuck in the aura. It can get "blocked or glued into you," Bloom says. When the energy doesn't move, it can start to stagnate in your energy field and eventually create symptoms, such as pains and aches, heaviness or weariness, distress, and illness.

"The quickest way to unload it is to move your body." Bloom suggests shaking, stretching, skipping, bouncing—moving around vigorously, doing any kind of strong physical movement that gets your entire body moving and shaking. Make sure you move everything: elbows, hands, shoulders, head, torso, hips, legs, and feet. Wobble your body, even your cheeks and tongue. One simple way to produce the desired body-wide shaking is to use a rebounder or mini-trampoline, recommended in chapter 6 with reference to stimulating the lymphatic system.

It might help to pretend you are that wet dog scattering water droplets in all directions. Think of the water droplets as "molecules" of toxic energy. This moving will loosen and release the stuck energy, Bloom states. Feel free to make noises, too, such as screams, gasps, and moans.

Other activities of similar effectiveness include putting your hands under running water, taking a shower, standing in a windy place or before a fan, and changing your clothes and giving your worn ones a good shake and thumping to remove the energetic traces of the contaminants in question.[17]

HEALTHY LIVING SPACE DETOXIFIER #40
Scrub Your Aura Clean with a Golden Sponge

While it is hard to duplicate the masterful auric cleanse you get from a professional psychic healer, there are several practical steps you can take on your own to do a fair amount of auric scrubbing, says LeGant. The following is a self-help technique for removing energy imprints, influences, detritus, and residual after-effects of arguments, encounters, or excursions into unpleasant environments such as we pick up every day.

Directions: This is an exercise developed by LeGant, which you can do while soaking in an Epsom salts bath (Healthy Living Space Detoxifier #38), as you lie in bed waiting to fall asleep, or any time during the day when you feel aurically toxic. Visualize your aura as a big golden bubble extending a few feet out from your skin in all directions. Give it an electric blue fringe to help see where its edges are. Tell your aura, which might be extended further out, to retract to within two feet of your body.

Next, visualize a golden sponge and instruct the sponge to move around inside your aura and energy centers (chakras) to collect (sponge up) all the "pictures and energies that allow whacks in the aura to exist," says LeGant. Tell the golden sponge to absorb everything of this nature. If, for example, you have been obsessing about a topic—an insult, abuse, argument, money, sex, an embarrassment, an unexpressed grievance—specifically direct the sponge to absorb all the energy associated with it.

When you feel the sponge is full and has absorbed all it can, put it in an imaginary container, seal the lid, throw the container away from you, and explode a bomb under it. Sometimes you may need to do several sponges in succession to collect all the negative energy. Be sure to blow up every sponge you use for this purpose. "If you feel you want to keep clearing your aura, keep creating sponges, bringing them into your aura, sponging things up until you feel clear," says LeGant.

It's a good idea to consider the golden sponge technique a regular part of your detoxification routines, he adds. "People get whacked aurically very easily and frequently during the course of a day or week, and the older whacks get reactivated, too, so you need to be constantly clearing out the effect of these whacks."

HEALTHY LIVING SPACE DETOXIFIER #41
Turn Your Body into Transparent Glass

This exercise, which I have modified from instructions provided by Leon LeGant, is appropriately performed while in the tub or a flotation tank. For some people, water acts as a psychic enhancer, making it easier to visualize the steps in the exercise. The goal of this exercise is to make your body neutral and transparent, thereby highlighting all the foreign, undesirable energy, enabling you to remove it.

Directions: Immerse yourself in a bathtub full of hot water with all the additions specified in Healthy Living Space Detoxifier #38. Wait ten to fifteen minutes in the water before starting this exercise. When you feel relaxed and focused, begin. Starting at your feet, visualize that your body is turning to transparent, colorless glass. In other words, first see your feet and ankles as clear glass. You will probably have some obstacles or opposition to this, but this is the point of the exercise—to highlight the negative energies so you can remove them. As you try to see your body as transparent glass, all the foreign energies will become apparent; that's when you can remove them.

You may come up with a better way to do this, but try "pushing" the dark energies, when you see them, up through your body to drain out through the back of your neck. Why there? Because the back of the neck, a recognized energy center (chakra) is known as the psychic gate; it's like a swinging door for the entry and departure of psychic energies.[18]

Pretend that you can open a valve in the back of your neck, and as you push the energies up from the feet, they start draining out from your neck. Also, visualize a large, highly absorbent sponge situated on the outside of your neck, capable of absorbing all the toxic energy that will be draining out of your neck. You might focus on the neck drain, seeing more and more "liquid" or dark energy flowing out, thereby enabling dark liquids lower down in your body to move towards the drain. Or you may need to more aggressively push the dark energies to the drain, somewhat like using a squeegee to move water across a surface. Sometimes, when I perceive there is a great deal of energy rubbish present in my body, I visualize using a shovel or even a tiny bulldozer to push it all to the neck drain.

As the energy rubbish moves toward the drain, see the parts of the body from which this energy has just departed as being clear as glass. By the time everything has drained out of your neck (and don't forget to drain your head), you should be able to see your whole body as glassine, if only for a moment. You may have to repeat this exercise two or three times before you can feel confident you have become transparent as glass. When you have completed one pass through the body, blow up the sponge; if you are repeating the exercise, install a new sponge at the neck drain, and destroy it once you have drained the body. Don't be alarmed if during the drainage, you find yourself twitching, shaking, moaning, groaning, or even shouting. It is your body registering the energy transaction, and is a transient, though sometimes to others in the house a somewhat amusing, occurrence.

Your energy body, like your intestines once they get engaged in a detoxification program, has its own peristalsis, its own rhythm of pushing out foreign toxic energies. The more you can keep up with this natural energy rhythm, the better you will feel because you are always current with the latest batch of energy rubbish awaiting removal from your auric space.

In the week following a psychic clearing, it is highly beneficial to do this exercise every day, even twice daily. Your energy body, like your intestines once they get engaged in a detoxification program, has its own peristalsis, its own rhythm of pushing out foreign toxic energies. The more you can keep up with this natural energy rhythm, the better you will feel because you are always current with the latest batch of energy rubbish awaiting removal from your auric space.

You may experience the energy rubbish in many different ways. For example, I have seen it as thick green sludge, as dark blackish tar, as caked, dried, sandy-colored mud, and as a sickly pale green vapor. Sometimes you might experience a particular accumulation in one body area, such as the groin, solar plexus, or neck, although it can be anywhere in the body. You may find that the flow of energy rubbish up from the feet to the neck gets slowed down, perhaps halted, at one spot. Don't fight it. Visualize another sponge and use this to absorb the toxic sludge in this particular area; then blow up the sponge and resume your full body drain. Once the localized energy obstacle has been removed, the overall drainage may proceed rapidly and without obstruction.

The experience of purging your body and space of the foreign energies by doing the glass body exercise may feel intense for a few moments; it certainly requires some concentration. When you have completed your glass body exercise, get out of the tub, lie down on a towel on your bed for about twenty to thirty minutes, and don't do anything else. This gives your mind and body time to relax and reorganize after the intensity of the toxic cleanup.

HEALTHY LIVING SPACE DETOXIFIER #42
Cutting the Cords and Ties
That Bind—Psychic Plumbing

According to many psychic practitioners, one of the ways we receive a continuous stream of foreign and often toxic energy from other people, especially those emotionally close to us, is by way of psychic cords. These psychic cords, or energy connections, have also been described as "hooks, nets, cables, tree trunks, and many other variations linking us inextricably to the other person," explains Judy Hall, an expert in psychic protection and energy work.[19]

Energy cords are connections to people we have been close to (parents, siblings, relatives), are presently close to (spouses, partners, children, friends), or with whom we have some type of energetically charged relationship (employees, coworkers, neighbors, casual acquaintances, even strangers). Energy links are formed, connecting us to the person; perhaps we established the cord, perhaps they did—either way, it functions as a kind of umbilical cord through which thoughts, feelings, attitudes, and other charged emotional states or conditions of negativity can continuously flow. The effect, potentially, is to keep us constantly toxic from this source, receiving energy input that is not always in our best interests and may in fact be psychically injurious.

For example, you can count on having energy cords connecting you to your parents, regardless of their status, dead or alive, close or estranged. It is not always this way, but it is often the case that energy cords to your parents can exist all over your body; you may in fact discover dozens, even hundreds of cables from your mother and father hooked into your body. They may appear to you as an inch wide or five or six inches in diameter. You may detect a large trunk line surrounded by a dozen smaller input cables. They tend to be organized around the body's major and minor chakras, arrayed along the spinal column and all over the head.

Psychically attuned practitioners report that they can hear, sense, feel, or see emotional content flowing through these cables from their parents and other people. In some cases, these cables drain away our vital energy, as if a powerful suction device at the other end of the cable is steadily sucking our *qi* out of us. Sometimes people unconsciously establish cords into high-energy individuals to siphon off—some call it vampirize—energy, leaving us unaccountably depleted until we figure out what has happened and remove the drainage cord.

In infancy and early childhood, cables from our parents were useful, even necessary for our survival; but as adults, they can be toxic artifacts, riveting us to old, inappropriate, or regressive modes of being derived from our parents and our earliest relationships with them. You may feel you cannot sever your dependency on your mother or father, or that you keep hearing or feeling their personalities or attitudes; in both cases, the presence is inappropriate, even oppressive at times.

Cutting a tie or energy cord to a loved one does not mean you are severing all links with that person; it just means you are unencumbering yourself of inappropriate old energy links. Your relationship may actually improve because it has been clarified and updated—that is, brought into the present, out of the past where it had stagnated due to the energy cords. "If you feel you owe someone something, you probably need more than most to cut the ties," advises Hall. "Guilt is disempowering, and highly abusive on both sides."

The cords—whether they carry guilt, parental "shoulds" and "don'ts," or other forms of family invalidation—provide the energy antecedents for unhealthy emotional states (as discussed in chapter 8) and unbalanced physiological states (as discussed in chapter 5). Thus removing the cords can be a significant part of your detoxification program.

To cut energy cords, it first is necessary to see or at least sense them. Surprisingly, one doesn't have to be too psychic to accomplish this; the intent to discern these cords is often a sufficiently strong factor in making the existence of such cords apparent. One way that might be helpful is to look for the cords while you are having your detoxification bath. Name the person in question. You could say, for example: "I wish to become aware of energy cords from my mother." Or whichever individual you suspect of being corded into. It is quite likely that your mind will project some form of image in response to this request; you may see cords hooked into a certain part of your body, or you may sense some discomfort, tingling, heaviness, or other sensation in a particular area.

Once you see the cords, remove them from yourself and from the person to whom they are attached, Judy Hall says. How do you remove the cords? Hall recommends that you visualize cutting them with a pair of golden scissors, or slicing them with a sharp hoop of light. She also says it is effective to cut them with a visualized mental laser of light or to imagine yourself in a "mental bonfire" in which all energy ties named will be burned up, while leaving your own energies intact. You may wish to mentally tell the person to whom you are corded what you are doing and why. When you are finished with the exercise, pile the cords up like kindling for a bonfire and burn them so that no trace remains. You could also visualize tossing them into a swiftly flowing river. If you do not destroy the remains of the cords, Hall cautions, they can return to you or sprout and grow back again. She also advises

> *The cords—whether they carry guilt, parental "shoulds" and "don'ts," or other forms of family invalidation—provide the energy antecedents for unhealthy emotional states and unbalanced physiological states. Thus removing the cords can be a significant part of your detoxification program.*

sealing the part of the body from which the cords were removed with a healing light.

"In cutting the ties, the energy changes," Hall explains. Your life is likely to change for the better because cutting the ties that bind you to other people restores your autonomy and psychic energy. Hall recommends examining all your relationships to see if they are based on inappropriate cords. All relationships will benefit from cutting the energy cords, she notes. It makes good detoxification sense, she says, to "regularly clear our ties."

Leon LeGant also works with cord removals and offers a variant to Hall's approach. When you see the cords, unscrew them the way you open a tamper-proof bottle of pills, pushing down and turning; this frees the cords from your energy body. Then using the golden sponge image, instruct it to collect all the cords; then destroy the sponge by visualizing placing a bomb under it and blowing it up. Or put it in a large container and blow it up inside that. Somehow the psychic sponge handles the cord and collects its connections at the other end, says LeGant. It is advisable to work on one person at a time, allowing your body a few days to regroup to the new energy configuration, which is now free of a fair number of cords.

HEALTHY LIVING SPACE DETOXIFIER #43
Ground Yourself to the Center of the Earth

People often talk about "centering" themselves, and although the concept is sound and helpful, often the practice used does not accomplish the task. One method that ensures real centering is a technique called the "grounding cord," says LeGant. Not only does it provide deep centering—rooting yourself to the imagined core of the planet itself—but it acts as a kind of lightning rod, sending spiritual toxins straight through you (who remains unscathed) and into the Earth.

You can use this technique any time you find yourself in an unfriendly environment—remember the toxic room we mentioned at the start of the chapter?—or in a formal meeting, a charged situation among people, or every day as a regular part of your meditative or exercise routine.

Directions: Visualize a hollow energy tube extending from your waist to the center of the Earth. It might help to see yourself sitting on this tube as if it is a tree trunk (or a pillar) that comes out of the center of the planet. It is hollow like a chute, and you can throw things down it; it can be any color you choose, and it is about the width (plus a little) of your body. It starts around your waist and includes your groin (seat of the root chakra) and goes all the way down to the core of the Earth, in whatever way you can conceive this. Sometimes it helps to see the grounding cord anchored into a specific place, like a pylon in a rock face when climbing; you might for example see it as attached to a gold plate with your name on it on the subterranean rock.

By the way, don't worry about whether the center of the planet is molten lava or hollow, or that you don't feel you can even imagine what it might be. What is essential is that you purposefully connect yourself with the "center" of the planet and use this connection as a way of grounding foreign, hostile, or simply nonself energy, in the way a lightning rod functions on a house.

Foreign energy, which includes energy from those closest to you as well as from strangers and those who wish you (or everyone in sight) ill, now has a place to go upon hitting your aura. Without the grounding cord, hostile foreign energy lodges somewhere in your aura and works its way into your body; with the grounding cord, it can pass through you into the ground. You remain neutral to its influence. Generally, you will need to destroy your grounding cord every one to two weeks and generate a new one.

Once you become familiar with the workings of your grounding cord, you can extend its uses, says LeGant. "You can allow your grounding cord to release energy out of your body and aura, along with all of the pain in your body or from a particular place that is experiencing pain." If you have a headache, or stomachache, or menstrual cramps, try establishing a mini-grounding cord from that organ or body area to the center of the Earth and directing the cord to drain out the pain. Or perhaps you are feeling despair, apathy, or hopelessness; direct the cord to drain these negative states from your mind-body. Spend five to ten minutes focused on this draining.

If it helps your visualization of the grounding cord, imagine it has an on/off switch, suggests LeGant. When you are ready to "drain," flip the on switch; when you are finished, flip the off switch. Allow the natural gravity of the Earth to effortlessly suck out all the pain and negativity from your aura. You might view the pain as water circling a bathtub drain, flowing out of the tub (your body) down the pipe (grounding cord).

One final point on the grounding cord. Resistance is futile, says LeGant. If you come in contact with "unfriendly" energy or situations, resisting this undesired field of influence can be counterproductive, LeGant explains. It will actually draw the unwanted energy closer to you. "If you start resisting it, it's going to stick right to you." Further, you have to learn to be aware of when you're in resistance. "You have to learn to catch yourself doing it. The problem is if you go into resistance, you're actually going into fear. You're expecting it to attack or pollute you, and you are basically opening the door for that energy to slam into you and do exactly what you fear it will."

The best way to "repel" foreign, inimical energy is to go neutral to it; then you do not attract or repel it, but rather you act as if it didn't exist or that it had no ability to affect you. "You can have your own conversation with it. 'I see you, but I'm neutral to you and I'm senior to you and you don't have to effect me.'"

Then you send the energy down the grounding cord, or if it is a situation, put a grounding cord under it—the people, building, whatever the physical environment and its contents—and allow the hostile energy to funnel down the cord to the center of the Earth. One of LeGant's colleagues once defused an armed bank robbery in progress by putting a grounding cord under the robbery principals; after a few minutes, they got flustered, confused, even frightened, and ran out of the bank, abandoning the robbery.

As a further precaution, LeGant recommends generating a protection symbol around your aura, such as an outward facing red rose, a six-pointed star, a cross, "or whatever you're comfortable with." Place a clear mental image of this protection symbol on the electric blue edge of your aura, says LeGant. This is the energy equivalent of strengthening your immune system to protect your body against unwanted biological substances.

HEALTHY LIVING SPACE DETOXIFIER #44
Protect Your Space by Connecting to a Higher Source

At this level of detoxification and health maintenance, you need a kind of free-ranging spiritual antioxidant to protect your space against unwanted intruders and foreign energies, or in the language of Modi and LeGant, "beings." LeGant recommends going to the highest source possible, what he recognizes as the Supreme Being. Call this highest source God, divinity, the Creator, Source, Goddess, Allah, Brahman, Ain Sof—anything at all; the point is that you request spiritual assistance from the highest or most exalted or most evolved source you can conceive of and feel comfortable conceiving of, advises LeGant.

Directions: LeGant says to visualize a bright golden cord of light extending from the center of your head straight up to this highest source. You don't have to be a saint or mystic to do this; simply tell the golden cord to connect itself to this highest source, and it will do the right thing for you, says LeGant. "If your *intention* is to send the golden cord to the Supreme Being, that's where it will go. Hook yourself up and ask for healing, ask to have some of the foreign energy cleared out of your space."

You can also ask your higher source to guide you to information or experts to help you further detoxify your spiritual space. "You can also talk directly, have an interactive relationship with the Supreme Being. Just say hello and listen for responses. You will hear them in your mind, and you may think they are your own thoughts." LeGant recommends that after saying "hello" and requesting assistance, try to still your thoughts, then wait and listen, even if it runs to a few days, even months.

"You might hear that 'hello' come back." Naturally, we all will feel cognitively wobbly at this point, for how can we be certain it is the Supreme Being responding? It may sound preposterous, but LeGant suggests you "ask the Supreme Being to make itself real for you," however paradoxical, impossible, or wild that eventuality sounds. "Keep asking the questions, keep noticing the answers, keep seeing that back-and-forth relationship—then you will develop certainty about the dialog," says LeGant. This kind of connection surely is the ultimate immune defense.

Bear in mind that these approaches are palliative, not curative. In other words, they are effective short-term steps for spiritual detoxification and energy immune defense. Core pictures are deeply embedded in the auric space, however, and generally require a trained psychic practitioner to remove.

HEALTHY LIVING SPACE DETOXIFIER #45
Cleanse and Protect Your Aura with Pomanders and "Air Conditioners"

Wouldn't it be remarkably convenient if there was something natural but powerful you could spray into your aura that would help cleanse and protect it? It turns out there is, and it is known as a pomander. The term "pomander" is an old English word denoting a fragrant herbal bouquet once worn close to the body as an air freshener in a time when people didn't bathe very often or use deodorants. It might be comprised of small flower blossoms or small fruits flavored with spices. The pomander's intent was for protection, disinfection, or for clearing the local atmosphere (a few feet in radius) of psychic pollutants.

In recent years, British master color therapist Mike Booth has reintroduced and expanded the concept of pomanders. The fifteen Pomanders produced by his Aura-Soma Products company in Tetford, England, are capable of precise cleansing and protection of the aura. The application is simple: dribble three drops of the selected Pomander onto the left palm, rub the hands together, then drape the aura from head to foot with the delicious herbal scents, and gently inhale them through your cupped hands.

The Pomanders come in tiny crush-proof plastic bottles and in mister-sprayer dispensers, making them suitable for carrying with you during the day or while traveling. Each Pomander contains the essences of forty-nine herbs, essential oils, flowers, minerals, and crystals (preserved in a light alcohol base), in a special ratio enabling it to affect different aspects of one's emotional and psychic dimensions, explains Booth. Each is a different color as well. This makes sense because psychics describe the aura as a multicolored field surrounding the body, and that its colors and intensities change constantly in accordance with our moods and thoughts; so introducing the essences of colors to your aura is a way of reestablishing balance through resonance—like balancing like, color for color.

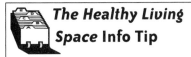

The Healthy Living Space Info Tip

For audio tapes, classes, and instruction including tips and techniques for psychic clearing and protection as well as psychic clearing practitioner referrals:
Berkeley Psychic Institute,
2018 Allston Way,
Berkeley, CA;
tel: 510-548-8020, 510-644-1600, or 800-433-5288;
website: www.berkeleypsychic.com;
e-mail: dejavu@dnai.com.

Another approach that clears auric energy blockages and balances the aura is called Noetic Field Therapy, based on original research by Dr. Robert D. Waterman (*Through the Eyes of Soul: Theory and Practice of Noetic Field Therapy*, 1999). For information and referrals:
John M. Browning,
tel: 800-251-3354 or 703-532-7796;
e-mail:
energytherapy@starpower.net;
website: energytherapy.net.

"The Pomanders are created mostly for the protection of persons who are in the process of [psychically] opening up," says Booth.[20] In practical terms, that would mean after (or during the time) you have tried some of the aura detoxifying exercises in this chapter. According to Booth, the Pomanders help balance the electromagnetic field of the user, providing protection against negative influences while allowing positive ones to enter the aura. "By placing these naturally fragranced colored essences into your hands and moving them through the aura, the electromagnetic field that surrounds your body, like a gentle breeze you create a delicate web around yourself," explains Booth. "This colored 'web' protects you from energies you do not want and allows the positive energies to enter. Kirlian photography [which photographs energy emissions from living organisms] has shown [that the Pomanders] create little valves within the electromagnetic field that allow the positive energies in and filter out energies that are less helpful."

The Pomanders can also change negative energy in rooms or houses. Here you apply the specific Pomander to your hand, as above, but then "wave" its fumes around the room in question, distributing the aromatic vapors to all corners. While doing this, it helps to visualize the fumes as sweeping away all negative energies in the room, says Booth. Especially helpful here are the mister-sprayer Pomander dispensers (suitable for spraying around the body) and the Air Conditioners, four-fluid-ounce spray bottles suitable for misting an indoor environment. "These enable you to clear and condition your space with the energies of color," says Booth.

With this in mind, we can move on to the actual Pomanders that will be helpful for detoxification.

White Pomander

The predominant essential oils in this blend include Kajeput, California laurel, and laurel. The crystal energies are morganite, quartz, and selenite. This Pomander is recommended for protecting and balancing all seven chakras of the body, for protecting the whole electromagnetic field, for mitigating the energetic effects of radiation, and which may help to alleviate allergies caused by outside toxic substances and energies. Of the fifteen Pomanders produced by Aura-Soma, the White

Pomander, the original one of the series, contains all forty-nine herbs in equal balance. "It is suitable for cleansing, purifying, and protecting, and may be used in any space to cleanse the atmosphere, bring the light in, and renew energies," says Booth. "It is also helpful during detoxification."

Deep Red Pomander

This one contains a predominance of cedar and laurel essential oils, as well as crystal energies of garnet, ruby, carnelite, strawberry-quartz, hematite, and neptunite. It is especially helpful in dealing with stress, and of the entire line of Pomanders "this is the one that grounds most intensively, energizes, and provides the most effective protection," says Booth. It is recommended for use after meditation and rituals. Further, "it protects against negative influences from Earth energies and on the other hand, it sensitizes for Earth energies." (See "geopathic stress" in chapter 12.)

For healers, the Deep Red Pomander is recommended for times when you feel your client is draining your energy. "This one provides the strongest protection for energy zapping, as it is energizing and may restore physical energies after tiredness and fatigue or depletion through drugs." It also supports the intuition and removes fears regarding survival issues surrounding, for example, money or health. "The Deep Red Pomander may help those in their teens who have poltergeist activity, and it may be used in house-clearing to neutralize the effects of psychic activity or when visiting sacred sites and power places that have very often been used in an incorrect manner," or whose energy aspects or water have become toxic, adds Booth. (Again, see chapter 12.)

Serapis Bey Master Quintessence

Serapis Bey is one of fifteen similar products made by Aura-Soma called Master Quintessences. In general, they deal with more refined energies and states of awareness than the Pomanders. As with the Pomanders, they are color-differentiated, and contain herbs, essential oils, and crystal energies. The Serapis Bey Quintessence is a clear formula suitable for cleansing, says Booth. It is recommended for healers and therapists to use to "clear" a treatment room of ambient energies and energy toxins following a session and to help the practitioner to cleanse and rebalance his aura.

It is believed that this spicy and flowery Quintessence "stretches" the electromagnetic field of the user, enabling one to integrate one's recent healing experience or insight. "Serapis Bey is good for detoxifying at all levels," Booth notes. As with the Pomanders, the Quintessence is available in a small plastic bottle or as a sprayer/mister dispenser.

Spiritual Detoxification Is a Lifelong Activity

Once you begin to purge spiritual toxins from your system, you have started a process that can, if you wish it, transform your life and give you a focus for meditation and inner work for the rest of your life. Once you enter the field of the aura, and the larger, even subtler energy fields beyond it (yet still connected to you), you find auric space is remarkably *larger* than you would have expected. In fact, some people, after doing spiritual detoxification work for a few years, are astonished at how vast is this auric space and how replete it is with beings and energies that can be purged.

It is not that we are phenomenally polluted, so contaminated that a life of constant detoxification is required to cleanse our space. Rather, the further you go with this level of detoxification, the more you enter the realm of basic spiritual growth and unfoldment. In so doing, you unavoidably enter the domain of the transpersonal—that is, the realm of parts of yourself you didn't know you had, and that are not necessarily even from this time, this life, this body. Let me put this in perspective by an example from an old religious tradition.

Jainism is an ancient religion of India, older than Buddhism and possibly Hinduism as well. One of its tenets is spiritual cleansing, but Jainists take a very broad view of what this entails. Jainism says that the condition and color status of the aura is an index to the soul condition of the individual. Originally, and in our pure condition, our essential "color" is a noncolor of stainless, crystalline, transparent clarity, but through our life actions, thoughts, feelings, and the rest of everyday living, other colors can appear in the aura. How we live and what kind of cumulative effect our actions have determine (and attract) what colors appear in the aura. Jainism calls these colors *lesyas*, and there are six of them: white, yellow (or rose), flaming red, dove-grey, dark blue, and black.

One of the chief goals of Jainist spiritual practice is to purify the aura and remove the colors (*lesyas*) so that only the original crystalline purity remains. As the noted scholar of Indian religions, Heinrich Zimmer, stated, "the advance of the individual toward perfection and emancipation is the result of an actual physical process of cleansing taking place in the sphere of subtle matter [our auric space]—literally a cleansing of the crystal-like life-monad."

Jainism proposes that when this life-monad (the original transparent clarity of our being) is purged of all the life-action colorings and contaminations, "it literally shines with a transparent lucidity" and that when it is completely cleansed, "it is immediately capable of mirroring the highest truth of man and the universe, reflecting reality as it really is."[21] Surely that's a benefit worth detoxifying for. But here is yet another way of framing the spiritual side of detoxification.

According to British psychic Mona Rolfe, Ph.D., in *The Sacred Vessel*, an essential element of the ancient tradition of initiation was preparation and purification. To understand more about one's deepest self and the cosmos, one had to purify the body and mind of all the aspects that weighted or darkened it. Candidates for initiation purified their bodies daily with fresh clean water and foods, what we would call "kosher" today.

The point of all this incessant detoxification was to enable the human form to contain more light, which is to say, more spiritual illumination. "Buddha is an immense force of light, the greatest force of light in the world," explained Dr. Rolfe, but equally powerful was the light of the Christ. For anyone desiring to be touched by these sources of immense light, they must first be purified and prepared. Toxic substances actually impede the entry of light—more consciousness, self-awareness, understanding, and insight—into the mind and body.

"Your soul is guiding your personality through certain experiences on Earth in order that you may become purified, body, soul, and spirit, sufficiently so that the Buddhic force may touch you and hold you for all time," explains Dr. Rolfe.[22] You needn't worry that spiritual detoxification will make a Buddhist of you; where Dr. Rolfe says "Buddhic," substitute whatever description of spiritual energy you prefer, or simply psychological insight. The essential point is that spiritual detoxification can make it easier for you to embody more spiritual light, insight, compassion, even wisdom, if you wish. And it might make it easier for you to extend this understanding to your living space, the subject of the next several chapters.

Part Three

Creating the Healthy
Home Living Space

CHAPTER 10

Cleaning Up the Home's Indoor Environment:

Overcoming the Effects of Sick Building Syndrome

When we consider the home as a living space that has something to do with our health, we find the same factors at play as we did with the body. Toxins. Certain factors about the modern house—specifically, its building materials, furnishings, and air quality and circulation—can be toxic factors and thus harmful to our health.

Just as we saw with toxicity at the physiological level of the body, it isn't always a question of a single poison negatively affecting our system. House-borne toxins often are multiple and together can produce a toxic, immune-system weakening effect. We may be able to tolerate one, or several, toxins in our home environment, but for each of us, there is a limit, a point at which our system can no longer accommodate the toxic load and we get sick. It may start as allergies, headaches, or irritability, but it may progress to a wide range of symptoms and baffling new health conditions including chronic fatigue syndrome, multiple chemical sensitivity, and environmental illness. Physicians are increasingly faced with a strange new kind of patient, the hypersensitive, one who is allergically reactive, seemingly to almost anything of modern manufacture.

The trouble is, with respect to toxins generated in our home living space, we are not yet sufficiently accustomed as a culture even to think of the home as a source of toxicity. Potentially, most of the structural elements of our inside living space, even many items we take for granted as part of everyday living, can be toxic: paints, lumber, carpets, sofas, furniture, household cleaning products, computers, overhead lights, appliances, the unfinished basement. It's a long list of potential suspects, potential toxic sources.

It's not that we should suddenly start to fear our living space as poisoned and out to hurt us, but the news that aspects of modern homes, schools, office buildings, and nearly all indoor living or work spaces may be hazardous to our health should counsel us to look carefully at the materials we surround ourselves with and to think about ways to neutralize their ill effects or replace them with nontoxic alternatives.

Sick building syndrome refers to the negative health effect of a building on its occupants. More formally, according to the EPA, it refers to "situations in which the building occupants experience acute health and comfort effects that appear to be linked to time spent in a building, but no specific illness or cause can be identified."

Since the majority of Americans probably spend about ninety percent of their time in indoor environments, the importance of that inside living space being health-promoting becomes strikingly evident. Since the 1980s, medical attention has started to focus on this previously unsuspected field of toxicity such that the negative health relationship between an interior living space and the health of its occupants is now often referred to as "sick building syndrome."

Sick Building Syndrome: The Disease of Modern Architecture

One of the dominant trends in late twentieth century Western architecture was to create increasingly self-sufficient internal environments, buildings whose inner space was almost completely sealed off from the outside world. To an extent, this trend gained emphasis in the wake of the 1973 oil embargo, which riveted attention on the need to conserve fuels and maximize their efficiency. The result was both office buildings and homes that were indeed more fuel efficient, but they achieved this savings at a hidden cost, one that is only now becoming clear. In effect, by saving heating fuel, we created a new illness, known as sick building syndrome (SBS).

Put as simply as possible, SBS refers to the negative health effect of a building on its occupants. More formally, according to a statement by the United States Environmental Protection Agency (EPA), sick building syndrome refers to "situations in which the building occupants experience acute health and comfort effects that appear to be linked to time spent in a building, but no specific illness or cause can be identified." EPA also describes a similar condition called "building-related illness" (BRI) for situations in which "symptoms of diagnosable illness are identified and can be attributed directly to airborne building contaminants."[1] SBS symptoms can be generated by almost any type of modern indoor environment, such as office building, school, hospital, public assembly hall, or home, in potentially any country.

From a layperson's viewpoint, there is not a great deal of difference between SBS and BRI: both describe how a building can make its occupants sick. Whether the exact individual causes can be identified, as in BRI, or cannot be pinpointed, as in SBS, is almost a moot point, because as we are instructed by alternative medicine, toxicity is a cumulative, additive influence. The body has a capacity to handle a certain amount of toxicity—the toxic load or total toxic burden—but when that capacity is reached, and exceeded, any additional toxic exposure will make us sick. So one specific factor in an interior environment may not sicken us, but when added to the toxic influence of several others, the end result may be illness.

SBS symptoms tend to fall into a familiar cluster that includes headache; eye, nose, or throat irritation; sinus infections; dry cough; dry or itchy skin; dizziness; nausea, concentration difficulties; reduced memory; fatigue; drowsiness; whole body weakness; hoarseness or changed voice; skin reddening; stinging or smarting of the skin; runny nose or eyes; and odor sensitivity, according to the EPA. BRI symptoms include cough, chest tightness, fever, chills, and muscle aches (see figure 10-1).

How widespread is the problem? According to the prestigious British medical journal, *The Lancet*, SBS is "an increasingly

Figure 10-1. Typical Health Symptoms of Sick Building Syndrome and Building-Related Illness	
headache	drowsiness
eye, nose, or throat irritation	whole body weakness
sinus infections	hoarseness or changed voice
dry cough	skin reddening
dry or itchy skin	stinging or smarting of the skin
allergies	runny nose or eyes
dizziness	odor sensitivity
nausea	chest tightness
concentration difficulties	fever
reduced memory	chills
fatigue	muscle aches

common problem." The symptoms of SBS, said *The Lancet*, can be "uncomfortable, even disabling, and whole workplaces can be rendered non-functional" as a result.[2]

According to a 1984 study by the World Health Organization, thirty percent of new and remodeled buildings worldwide may generate symptoms of SBS or BRI, mainly due to indoor air quality. The air circulation mechanics and quality of sealed in living spaces tend to be the prime carrier of a great deal of the sick building pollutants. A more recent estimate suggests that twenty percent of American office workers are affected by SBS.[3] A study by Honeywell Techanalysis of 600 of its own office workers found that 24% said they felt (based on symptoms experienced) there were air quality problems in their office environment. Also, between seven percent and eleven percent of these same employees reported having a tired feeling, stuffed up nose, eye irritations, headaches, or labored breathing.[4]

Researchers at Cornell University in Ithaca, New York, found that workers in poorly ventilated offices are twice as likely to complain of SBS symptoms as those in well-ventilated environments. The 1998 study looked at four multistory office buildings over a course of three consecutive days, measuring levels of thirty-six "potential worker irritants," such as temperature, carbon monoxide and carbon dioxide levels, dust mass, carpet dust, light levels, airborne particulate counts, and nicotine and formaldehyde levels. The researchers collected over 1,500 questionnaires from workers in the four buildings concerning SBS-type symptoms.

The study results were instructive and clearly supported the SBS thesis. "Both the workers with very few symptoms and those with more intense symptoms show a clear pattern of increased problems by the end of the day, suggesting that something is making the workers who are more sensitive feel sick," concluded head researcher Alan Hedge, director of the Human Factors Laboratory at Cornell's College of Human Ecology. The workers had a "clear pattern" of feeling worse at the end of each day.

While no single "culprit" was identified as the "cause" of SBS symptoms, Hedge noted that small accumulations of carbon dioxide from human breathing (due to inadequate ventilation) had been noted in these environments and are related to SBS. He further explained that workers were much more likely to report SBS symptoms when indoor carbon dioxide levels were higher than 650 parts per million (ppm). A typical outdoor concentration of carbon dioxide is 325 ppm. "This suggests that SBS symptoms may be associated with building ventilation performance." An earlier study (1993) by Hedge of 1,324 workers in nine buildings had linked SBS symptoms to "the amount of man-made mineral fibers in settle office dust," again pointing to poor air circulation as the main problem in SBS.[5]

Other studies have established the connection between carbon dioxide concentration and the incidence of SBS symptoms. Finnish researchers at the Helsinki University of Technology reviewed the results of 41 studies involving 60,000 subjects and found that almost all the studies showed that poor ventilation rates were clearly linked with a worsening of SBS conditions. They also reported that about fifty percent of the studies showed that as indoor carbon dioxide concentrations dropped below 800 ppm, the rate of SBS symptoms also dropped "significantly."[6]

Other studies, reported by Michael J. Hodgson, M.D., M.P.H., of the University of Pittsburgh School of Medicine, confirm and extend Hedge's conclusions. For example, Hodgson reported that in Germany, among 2,000 office workers with work-related symptoms, a fifty percent higher than average rate of upper respiratory tract infections was noted. These infections could be directly attributed to inadequate mechanically ventilated buildings—in other words, buildings where you couldn't open a window to get fresh air, but had to breath continually recirculated indoor air.

One study reported by Hodgson showed that seventy percent of buildings already classified as sources of SBS symptoms had poor circulation of fresh outdoor air. This study also showed that fifty percent to seventy percent of these buildings had poor internal air distribution (meaning the air didn't move much at all); sixty percent had poor filtration of pollutants derived from outside the building; sixty percent had indoor standing water (capable of supporting unfavorable biological growths); and twenty percent had humidifiers that functioned poorly. The result of this array of toxic indoor air pollutants—including toxic airborne compounds released from building materials, furniture, office machines, paints, glues, and other standard items found in the modern office or home—is "a complex mixture of very low levels of individual pollutants."[7]

A Danish study from 1987 examined the relationship of SBS-type symptoms and indoor air quality in 3,757 office workers and their environments in 14 different buildings. The researchers found that people working in the oldest buildings (and therefore not mechanically ventilated) had the least number of SBS symptoms; they also found the highest rates of certain symptoms (mucous membrane irritation, headache, fatigue, and lethargy) among workers who spent their time in buildings with mechanical ventilation, meaning, without the regular circulation of fresh outside air. The study also found that twenty-eight percent of the office workers said they had irritation in the mucous linings (nose, throat) and thirty-six percent had headache, unusual fatigue, or malaise (general poor feeling).[8]

A British study that same year examined the SBS incidence among 4,373 office workers in 42 different buildings and under 47 different ventilation conditions. The researchers found that eighty percent of the people had at least one work-related symptom and more than forty percent had SBS symptoms such as stuffy nose, dry throat, or headache. Women tended to have more SBS symptoms than men, and the typical range of symptoms per person in any of the forty-two different buildings was from one to five. In buildings in which the indoor air supply was cooled or humidified, the incidence of symptoms was much higher. The study further revealed that eighty percent had at least one work-related symptom, fifty-seven percent had lethargy, forty-seven percent a blocked nose, forty-six percent dry throat, forty-six percent headaches, nine percent chest tightness, and nine percent breathing difficulties.[9]

Another study in Denmark had fifty-four "air quality judges" assess the indoor air quality in twenty randomly selected offices and public assembly halls. They found that air quality deteriorated more from indoor pollution sources (from the outgassing of building and furnishings materials, tobacco smoke, and the ventilation system) than from the effects of the occupants (such as carbon dioxide exhalation). Specifically, twenty percent of the assessed indoor air pollution was due to the building materials, forty-two percent to the ventilation systems, twenty-five percent to tobacco smoke, and only thirteen percent to the people in those spaces.[10]

Government researchers at the Institute of Environmental Epidemiology in Singapore found that 19% of 2,856 office workers from 56 randomly selected public and private sector buildings reported SBS symptoms.[11] The same researchers, in studying a different group of 2,160 people in 67 offices in Singapore discovered that SBS symptoms are more prevalent among workers who report high levels of physical and mental stress; the study implied that stress makes one more susceptible to the toxic indoor influences that produce SBS symptoms.[12]

Not only can stress bring on susceptibility to SBS influences, but if you are already allergic, being in a "sick building" is likely to make your allergies worse, or produce SBS symptoms faster than in people who are not constantly allergic. Researchers at Kristianstad University in Sweden found that people with allergies (in this case, high school students) "note discomfort earlier" than people without allergies when exposed to sick building influences. A higher percentage of already allergic people suffered weekly symptoms than nonallergic people did, but even more interesting (or alarming) was the finding that only forty-five percent of the students in the Swedish high school studied were non-allergic, meaning fifty-five percent had regular allergies.[13]

Elsewhere in Sweden, researchers at the Department of Lung Medicine and Asthma Research Center at Uppsala

University found that 21% of a randomly selected group of 418 men and women, aged 20-45 years, reported experiencing one or more SBS symptoms on a weekly basis; these results led the researchers to conclude that "sick building symptoms are common in the general population."[14]

A study from New Zealand came up with similar results. Researchers at Massey University in Palmerston North found that 80% of 360 office workers studied experienced some SBS symptoms, with forty percent of these reporting lethargy, stuffy noses, dry throat, and headaches. These researchers used a British questionnaire from a study of an English population, the statistical results of which were the same. "Sick building syndrome was found to be sufficiently prevalent in both surveys to warrant concern."[15]

Often individuals suffering with SBS or BRI do not make the connection between their strange list of symptoms and where they spend the bulk of their time. Given the sealed-in nature of many modern homes and apartments, it is possible to be in a toxic living space twenty-four hours a day, on the job and at home. Similarly, most conventional physicians do not make the link between indoor environment and symptom picture, and often patients visit one doctor ten times or ten different doctors in search of a comprehensive diagnosis for their condition: not acutely sick, but not well either. You end up with what one SBS expert characterized as "a basket of symptoms with no clear cause."[16]

For some reason, women tend to have more SBS symptoms than men, according to a study at the University of Hamburg in Germany of 2,517 female employees. The women had a higher incidence than men in general bodily complaints and sensory irritations along with a "more negative evaluation of the indoor climate"—which may be scientific jargon for saying they were both more aware of and sensitive to the quality of their workspace.[17]

In especially sensitive individuals, typical SBS and BRI symptoms can progress to more long-term dysfunction and a constant state of allergic reaction, as in multiple chemical sensitivity, environmental illness, and chronic fatigue syndrome, which share overlapping symptoms. In these cases, one is hypersensitive to substances found in a typical indoor environment and is in effect unable to function in those environments.

Indoor Pollutants—A Matter of "Genuine Concern"

If one's reaction to SBS is caught early on, generally the symptoms can be reversed quickly, by removing yourself from the toxic space and/or neutralizing the toxic effect of various elements in that indoor living space. But if your exposure to SBS influences goes on unchecked for a longer period, it can start to produce deeper-set damage (to the liver and immune system, primarily), which though reversible, may take months to undo.

By way of illustration of the first situation—quick reversal of symptoms by leaving the toxic environment—here is a case history from Michael Hodgson, M.D., M.P.H. Dr. Hodgson describes a forty-year-old woman who started having headaches, dizziness, difficulty in concentrating, and runny nose soon after she started working in a "hermetically sealed" modern office building. Indoor carbon dioxide levels were 600-700 ppm, or about double, or more, than normal outdoor levels; there were also measurable amounts of formaldehyde and volatile organic compounds (outgasses of various equipment and building materials).

Various neuropsychological tests showed that this woman had symptoms of solvent neurotoxicity. This means the constant low-grade but poisonous gas emissions from various components of the office environment were affecting how her nervous system worked, to the extent that they were toxic to her neurons (nerve cells). When the woman stayed away from this unhealthy office for four weeks, working elsewhere, all of her test results returned to normal and the toxic effects went away. If she went back to the toxic office, her symptoms returned. According to Dr. Hodgson, when a formal study was made of the "toxic" building and its occupants, a definite relationship was shown between the level of "respirable suspended particulates" (airborne, breathable toxic substances) and the degree of symptoms in "a large proportion" of the people there.[18]

Here is a case that shows the long-term effects of not dealing with SBS symptoms when they first show up. Susan Lange, O.M.D., L.Ac., is a licensed acupuncturist, doctor of Oriental medicine, and cofounder of Meridian Center, an alternative medicine clinic in Santa Monica, California. It took her almost twelve years to figure out that the reason she had environmental illness was that she had endured exposure to numerous toxic substances much earlier in her life, and the effects were still active.

Specifically, Dr. Lange had sustained petrochemical toxicity, due to working in an office heated by kerosene gas stoves and with poor ventilation; later, she worked in a hospital whose building materials were contaminated with molds and fungus; then she worked in another "health" clinic in which the air conditioning filters were dirty such that they vented microbially contaminated air into the offices. Things got so bad for Dr. Lange that she even became allergic to her own house.

The combined effect of all the toxins she had been exposed to over the years made her "incredibly ill," with numerous SBS symptoms including heart palpitations, concentration difficulties, and allergies to seventy percent of the foods and substances in her environment. She nearly fainted when she inhaled perfume or gas fumes, and "when I walked into my own house, I felt like passing out." The story has a happy ending: Dr. Lange was able to undo the cumulative toxicity in her system through a carefully designed alternative medicine detoxification program.[19]

> *The liver, as the body's prime detoxification organ, gets overloaded and becomes unable to do its normal detoxification, so the body gets overwhelmed by toxins and moves into a state of constant dysfunction and, paradoxically, hypersensitivity to new toxic influences.*

That is the good news: despite the rising incidence of hypersensitive, highly reactive individuals, their condition is not permanent. With effective detoxification practices and alternative medicine-based restorative protocols, it can be reversed, enabling them to function once again in the modern world without getting sick every time they walk upon a new carpet or stand by a photocopier machine. As we learned in earlier chapters, in cases of hypersensitivity, often the liver is the key to both the problem and its solution. The liver, as the body's prime detoxification organ, gets overloaded and becomes unable to do its normal detoxification, so the body gets overwhelmed by toxins and moves into a state of constant dysfunction and, paradoxically, hypersensitivity to new toxic influences.

Even though its unhealthy results can be reversed, that doesn't change the fact that the problem of SBS is clearly widespread and probably increasing as buildings become ever more "modern" and thus sealed off from the outside environment. The main toxic sources, according to the EPA, fall into four categories.

First is inadequate ventilation. Before 1973, U.S. ventilation standards required that each building occupant have 15 cubic feet per minute (cfm) of outside air; after 1973, the amount was reduced by 66% to only 5 cfm.

Second are chemical contaminants from indoor sources, such as outgassing from carpets, adhesives, upholstery, manufactured wood products, photocopiers, pesticides, cleaning products, tobacco smoke, and unvented heating devices, all of which emit volatile organic compounds (VOCs).

Third are chemical contaminants from outdoor sources that enter the building through the ventilation system. These can include motor vehicle exhaust, and airborne toxins from plumbing vents, and building exhausts.

Fourth are biological contaminants, such as bacteria, molds, pollen, and viruses that may, for example, breed and spread in stagnant water present in ducts, humidifiers, air conditioners, ceiling tiles, carpets, or insulation. Toxic microorganisms such as *Staphylococcus*, *Streptococcus*, and *Aspergillus* can actually grow in a building's duct work and then get spread through the air through the building's ventilation system.

Managers of office buildings and large indoor spaces are beginning to get the idea that these spaces might be harmful to the health of the people who work inside them. A trade publication called *Today's Facility Manager* published a survey of an unspecified number of facility managers, which showed that 89% had heard of SBS and 100% considered it a "genuine concern," especially given the high incidence of allergies; 69% said their facility had already been tested for SBS and poor indoor air quality, and of these, 55% said the testing occurred because of employee complaints, 31% because of insufficient air circulation or filtration in their building, and 17% as part of a preventive maintenance program.[20]

The reader at this point might well ask: "What have SBS-conditions reported in office buildings, schools, and other large indoor spaces to do with my home or apartment?" The answer is that the data reported for SBS conditions in these larger modern indoor environments are highly relevant to the typical modern Western indoor living space. Many of the same toxic factors are

Figure 10-2. 8 Major Indoor Pollutants and the Symptoms They Produce

Here is a summary list of major building-related toxic substances, their sources, and the typical symptoms they produce:

TOXIC SUBSTANCE	SOURCES	SYMPTOMS
Benzene	paint, new upholstery, drapes, carpets	headaches, eye/skin irritation, fatigue, cancer
Ammonia	tobacco smoke, cleaning supplies	sinus problems, nosebleeds, eye/skin irritation, headaches
Chloroform	paint, new drapes and carpets, upholstery	headaches, eye/skin irritation, asthma attacks, dizziness
Formaldehyde	tobacco smoke, plywood, furniture, particle board, new drapes and carpets, office dividers, wallpaper, paneling	headaches, eye/skin irritation, gynecological problems, respiratory disorders, drowsiness, fatigue, memory loss, depression, cancer
Benzopyrene	tobacco smoke	respiratory irritation, asthma attacks, eye/skin irritation
Hydrocarbons	tobacco smoke, gas burners, furnace outgassing	headaches, fatigue, nausea, breathing constriction, vertigo
Trichloroethylene	wallpaper, furniture, glues and paints	respiratory, eye/skin irritation, headaches
Xylene	cleaning supplies, new carpets and drapes, paints	headaches, dizziness, fatigue

at play in the home (and will be discussed later in this chapter, along with their practical remedies), and while perhaps many homes do not have photocopiers (that outgas toxic VOCs), many homes should be concerned with radon emissions (a toxic "natural" gas emission from the Earth) from their basements. The modern home can be just as much a source of SBS symptoms as the modern office building, school, or hospital (see figure 10-2).

One of the ways the "genuine concern" of facility managers and the increasing research data on sick building syndrome is being translated into the domestic front is through a discipline called Bau-biologie. A German-based initiative, the term means the living or biological house. More specifically, Bau-biologie (pronounced BOW-bee-oh-low-gee) is "the study of the impact of the building environment upon the health of people and the application of this knowledge to the construction of healthy homes and work places." It is also the science of the "holistic interactions between life and the living environment," according to The Institute for Bau-biologie, the American branch of this innovative movement, based in Clearwater, Florida.

The Institute's prime purpose, it states, is to help people realize that health hazards may exist in their homes and work-places even though they may not be aware of them, and that not knowing about these hazards can be harmful to one's health, even to the larger outdoor environment. Based on research developed since the 1970s, the Institute has trained and certified over seventy "environmental inspectors"—architects, builders, electricians, medical practitioners, engineers, and others—who can evaluate indoor living spaces for the numerous health hazards identified by Bau-biologie.[21]

Other individuals and groups are taking up the European cue as well. John and Lynn Marie Bower formed the Healthy House Institute in 1992 in Bloomington, Indiana, to spread practical knowledge about how to build nontoxic homes and how to detoxify already built ones. Through their books, workshops, and website, they provide information to homeowners, designers, architects, and contractors "interested in making houses healthy places in which to live."

Building a nonpolluting natural house requires considerable research and planning and, until recently, most people tended to think the issue involved whether to live in a city or the country, in an apartment or an A-frame in the woods. But it's not so much the structure of the new house that matters, as what it's built with, says Bower. Almost everything, formerly taken for granted as "standard" building materials and furnishings, must be rethought.

Particle board and interior plywood walls, for example, can outgas formaldehyde from their glues; new synthetic carpets emit toxic fumes, can become havens for microorganisms, and generate synthetic dust in the indoor air; indoor paints, varnishes, and clear finishes can also release minute amounts of toxic fumes (VOCs). Tighter construction for increased energy efficiency (with less fresh air circulation) and the use of synthetic building materials (that outgas dozens of chemical pollutants or release particulates) both contribute to poor indoor air quality, which becomes a vehicle for distributing many other toxic elements in the indoor living space. Studies have shown that indoor air may contain concentrations of air pollutants 100 times higher than found in outside air. "Your house is where you spend the most time, so it is important to build it so that it won't contribute to your ill health," comments John Bower.

Consider the data on pesticide pollution inside the home, for example. According to a 1997 study conducted by the Special Education Department at the University of South Florida in Tampa, the majority of U.S. homes emit the pesticide chlordane into the living air space. How is this possible? For about thirty years, up until 1988 when it was banned, chlordane (a potent nerve toxin) was routinely used on building foundations to kill termites. Typically, 100-200 gallons of chlordane were applied underneath the home's concrete foundation. The pesticide may have been banned, but the regulation didn't ban the possibility of outgassing from the long-lived chemical residues.

Studies now show that chlordane vapor is leaking upwards (through foundation cracks or around pipes that enter the home) and contaminating the indoor air. Researchers report that seventy-five percent of U.S. homes built before 1988 routinely contain air levels of chlordane; one study showed that thirty-four percent of homes built before 1982 had air chlordane levels beyond the safety limit. The University of South Florida research team estimated that 100-185 million U.S. residents "are breathing questionable levels of chlordane in their homes daily," and that 10-20 million could be living in homes where the indoor air levels of chlordane are "exceeding" the recommended safe limits.[22]

What can chlordane do to you? It can have a negative impact on many parameters of mental function, as demonstrated in 1987 when 250 adults and children were exposed to a toxic dose of chlordane at an apartment complex. The building surfaces and grounds were sprayed with chlordane, and its fumes entered the apartments for years afterwards, outgassing from the wooden surfaces of the apartment complex. Seven years later, scientists at the University of Southern California School of Medicine at Los Angeles ran a battery of neurological tests on 216 of the former residents of this building to determine if they showed signs of neurotoxicity, which would indicate the pesticide was toxic to the nervous system. It was.

Simple reaction time for the chlordane-exposed residents was thirty-four percent slower; memory recall was twenty percent diminished; digit symbol attention was nineteen percent slower; balance dysfunction was sixteen percent increased; vocabulary use was twelve percent slower; mood state/tension was seventy percent elevated; mood state/depression was seventy-four percent increased; mood state/anger was sixty-nine percent more prevalent; vigor was twenty-seven percent reduced; fatigue was seventy-five percent elevated; and confusion increased by eleven percent. It wasn't just the brain that was affected. Other symptoms traced to chlordane toxicity included asthma, allergies, excess phlegm, chronic bronchitis, wheezing, shortness of breath, headaches, and indigestion.[23]

The same researchers analyzed nine patients in depth in an attempt to profile "chronic neurobehavioral impairment" due to chlordane exposure. They administered various tests to the nine people and found abnormal balance with eyes closed in seven, abnormal color discrimination in six, verbal recall problems in five, and various other perceptual disorders in four patients. "These observations suggest that chlordane causes protracted neurotoxicity," the scientists concluded.[24]

Chlordane is only one of many toxic chemicals that are potentially inside our living space polluting our indoor air. Even the way we clean our indoor living space may actually contribute to its toxicity, explains Lynn Marie Bower, author of a 700-page guide to nontoxic home cleaning, *Creating a Healthy Household*. "Many of the cleaners, polishes, and waxes you've been using could be making you and your family sick." Bower, who states she has been hypersensitive for twenty years, explains that children, the elderly, pregnant women, and those who are already sick, asthmatic, or allergic "are especially at risk."[25]

The Healthy Living Space Expert Interview: Michael Riversong, Design Ecologist and Environmental Assessor

As the years progress, healthy living space experts like the Browers are gaining more colleagues across the spectrum of disciplines and applications.

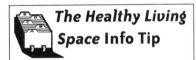

The Healthy Living Space Info Tip

For more information, including study materials, books, workshops, practitioner referrals, monitoring equipment, contact:
Bau-biologie USA,
1401A Cleveland Street,
P.O. Box 387,
Clearwater FL, 33755;
tel: 727-461-4371;
fax: 727-441-4373;
e-mail: baubiologie@earthlink.net;
website:
www.bau-biologieusa.com.
Also:
The Healthy House Institute,
430 N. Sewell Road,
Bloomington, IN 47408;
tel/fax: 812-332-5073;
e-mail:
healthy@bloomington.in.us;
website: www.hhinst.com.

One is Michael Riversong of Cheyenne, Wyoming, a multifaceted expert in creating healthy living spaces who calls his discipline Design Ecology.

Riversong combines the principles of Bau-biologie, feng shui (the ancient Chinese art of placement and energy relationships, discussed in chapter 11), and geobiology (the effect of Earth energies on humans, discussed in chapter 12). "Design Ecology is the process of addressing the effect of design on the physical, mental, and spiritual health of people," he comments in his book, *Design Ecology* (1996). His practice encompasses "the integration of music, environmental education, and advanced technology to create improvements in the living environment."

One of Riversong's specialties is an "environmental assessment," a thorough review of all aspects of a home or small business environment for the presence and influence of toxic elements, electromagnetic fields, radon, VOCs, and other toxins, followed by practical recommendations for eliminating these toxic factors. "I measure a lot of things with various instruments, all the while looking at the design of the place to see if there are communications being made by the design that are contrary to the goals of the people using the building."

For "communications" substitute the term "toxic factors" and you get an idea of what Riversong looks at when he's called in to evaluate an indoor living space. When Riversong refers to "various instruments," he is in part thinking of his handy threesome: a multifrequency gauss meter, a Geiger counter, and an electrostress meter. The gauss meter shows him the level of the magnetic fields present in an indoor environment, especially in the home's bedroom(s). Magnetic fields, says Riversong, can exert strong influences on humans, either healthy or toxic, depending on their type.

Relying on Swedish standards, Riversong says that magnetic fields higher than 2.5 milligauss (mG) are harmful to adults, and above 1.0 are "risky" for children. The combination of the human body's relatively high iron content, the possible iron content in the bed (metal spring mattress, metal bed frame), and an existing magnetic field can produce toxic effects in the bedroom. Let's say his gauss meter gives him a 4.0 milligauss reading in the bedroom. Sometimes the problem might be as simple as a miswired electrical junction box. One wire is misconnected, creating a "very heavy" electromagnetic field, Riversong notes. The remedy is simple: have an electrician fix the faulty wiring.

In other cases, an appliance, such as a television, can produce the problem. Say the head of the bed is up against a wall, on the other side of which sits the back of a television. The magnetic field emanated by that television goes through the wall and affects the sleeper in the bed. "The bed gets some electromagnetic interference from that television, especially as, even if the television is turned off, there is always current flowing through it." (For more on the subject of electropollution, see below.) "Home surveys should always start in the bedroom. This is vital because we depend on our nightly sleep for renewal of all biological systems," and disturbances in the electromagnetic fields can upset this crucial self-renewal mechanism of the body.

Riversong relies on another device for measuring electromagnetic disturbances—a surprisingly simple, low-cost approach developed by his mentor, the late Vince Wiberg, a healthy house wizard who practiced his trade for thirty years in Los Angeles. Get a cheap transistor A.M. radio and tune it to a high frequency range, such as 1500-1600, and in between stations, so you get only static. Walk around a building, or inside it, and listen to the sounds. "You can actually hear the electromagnetic disturbances," says Riversong. "You'll hear a buzzing type of sound, and different kinds of buzzes with different kinds of interference." This only works with an A.M. radio, he stresses.

Riversong emphasizes that the homeowner will get the best results by having an environmental assessment before the house is built. Then the various disciplines that comprise Design Ecology can have a *preventive* aspect—you can use health-promoting or at least nontoxic building materials to

Riversong takes the idea of preventive house design a step further and regularly consults with practitioners of alternative medicine. He encourages them to make it a standard procedure that an environmental assessment should be performed on the home of every new patient to see if whatever is bothering them has an environmental cause.

prevent illness in those who live within the indoor environment they create. "I encourage people to have me in on the planning stages of a remodeling job or new building construction, because if they do this, they will prevent so many problems later on." This is preventive medicine for a house; this is the way you produce a health house, says Riversong.

In fact, Riversong takes the idea of preventive house design a step further and regularly consults with practitioners of alternative medicine, such as naturopaths, acupuncturists, and chiropractors. He encourages them to make it a standard procedure that an environmental assessment should be performed on the home of every new patient to see if whatever is bothering them has an environmental cause. "The ideal scenario is to check the house to find out what's wrong with the patient."

Here are a few case studies from Riversong's practice that illustrate the point:

- The owner of a house with an attached office under construction was concerned with microwave contamination since his future home was near a large telephone and research installation. Riversong found a "microwave beam" in the owner's office (already completed); this beam was draining the man's energy and causing other health problems. Riversong had him redesign his office so that he was not sitting in the microwave beam, after which his health improved "and he found a whole new store of personal energy."

  When Riversong found another microwave beam going through what was to be the master bedroom, he was able to counteract this by installing microwave-blocking film on the bedroom windows. "A follow-up measurement after completion of the house showed microwave levels in the bedroom were very low, but right outside the window, levels were extremely high due to bouncing of the waves off the covering." The health of the occupants has been excellent since they moved in, says Riversong.

- Children who lived in a beach house were constantly coming down with colds and coughs. Riversong took a scraping of material from the bedroom carpet and examined it under the microscope. He found numerous insect parts, mostly from ultratiny creatures too small to be seen without a microscope. He recommended a thorough housecleaning (especially of the carpets, which harbor the numerous small insects found at the seashore) and a new air filtration system for the bedroom. The children's health began to improve after these changes were made.

- Residents of a home in Montana reported constant fatigue. Riversong notes that large parts of this state are underlain by high underground water tables, sometimes dangerously close to the surface. In this case, water regularly seeped into his clients' basement. Riversong, calling on his knowledge of dowsing and geobiology (see chapter 12 for details on these subjects), installed a length of thick copper wire in the ground near the house; this neutralized the energy-draining effect of the standing water. "The experiment worked, and they reported an immediate surge of personal energy."

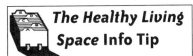

The Healthy Living Space Info Tip

For information about environmental assessments, music, books, devices, and other services, contact: Michael Riversong, P.O. Box 2775, Cheyenne, WY 82003; tel: 307-635-0900 or 303-829-0774; e-mail: MRiversong@earthlink.net; website: www.designecology.com.

HEALTHY LIVING SPACE DETOXIFIER #46
Get the Electropollution Out of Your Home

One of the pervasive features of modern technological society is the presence of electrical, magnetic, and electromagnetic fields[26] produced by human-made instruments and devices. While these fields are natural in the sense that all of nature, including the human body, runs on or emits differing energy fields of these types, they can be harmful to our health when they are too strong, when there are too many, or when we live too close to them.

The negative health influence of these invisible fields is now referred to variously as electropollution, electrosmog, EMF stress, or electrical hypersensitivity, and it's one of the prime contributing factors in SBS-type symptoms. Electrical hypersensitivity (or its variant, electrical sensitivity) is used to indicate a form of environmental illness, "specifically a chronic illness triggered by exposure to electromagnetic fields," according to Lucinda Grant, author of *The Electrical Sensitivity Handbook*.[27]

Grant says that being electrically sensitive means an illness you already have gets worse when you are near electrical

---

Figure 10-3. Typical Field Strengths for Common Appliances and Household Devices[28]

- Research has shown that the average refrigerator, measured at 10.5 feet away, has an EMF of 2.6 mG (milligauss); the worst designed model (tested in this particular study) had a field that measured 15.7 mG. "Healthy"—that is, well-designed and insulated—refrigerators typically emit a low intensity field of 0.1 mG, which is certainly a strength most people can handle.

- The average electric range at 10.5 feet has a field strength of 9 mG.

- The average fluorescent light fixture comes in at 5.9 mG.

- A typical nonelectronic analog clock is 0.8 mG.

- Televisions measure 7 mG.

- A typical microwave's EMF comes in at 36.9 mG.

- An electric radiant heating system, either ceiling or floor-mounted, emits a field strength of 26.6 mG at 10.5 feet.

- The average room in an American home has a background EMF of about 0.5 mG, although the typical kitchen has 0.7 mG. Distance from an EMF has a great deal to do with its biological effect, and the dependable thing about EMFs is that their effect drops off dramatically as you move only a short distance away from it. Consider the following examples:[29]

- Electric stove: at six inches, the EMF is 100 mG, at one foot it's 9 mG, and at three feet, <1 mG.

- Clothes dryer: 4.8-110 mG at four inches; 1.5-29 mG at one foot; 0.1-1 mG at three feet.

- Clothes washer: 2.3-3 mG at four inches; 0.8-3.0 mG at one foot; 0.2-0.48 mG at three feet.

- Electric can opener: 1300-4000 mG at four inches; 31-280 mG at one foot; 0.5-7.0 mG at three feet.

- Television: 4.8-100 mG at four inches; 0.4-20 mG at one foot; <0.1-0.11 mG at three feet.

- Fluorescent fixture: 40-123 mG at four inches; 2-32 mG at one foot; <0.1-2.8 mG at three feet.

- Portable heater: 11-280 mG at four inches; 1.5-40 mG at one foot; 0.1-2.5 mG at three feet.

- Hair dryer: 3-1400 mG at four inches; <0.1-70 mG at one foot; <0.1-2.8 mG at three feet.

appliances, power lines, or other significant sources of EMFs. Or you may experience symptoms *only* when in the presence of EMFs. The electrically sensitive (ES) person reacts sooner and more strongly to otherwise "normal" EMF fields that do not produce negative reactions in other people. ES people experience a "spreading" effect with sensitivity, in that their vulnerability to weaker, shorter EMF inputs increases and they get the reactive symptoms faster.

Typical ES symptoms include headache, nausea, fatigue, dizziness, tingling or prickling sensation on the skin, burning skin or eyes, memory loss, concentration difficulties, muscle or joint pain, fluctuations in heart rate, and sometimes paralysis, says Grant. "Electrical sensitivity has the great potential for being a missing link that uncovers explanations for many noticeable, recurring health problems people currently have no medical answers for and no long-term relief," comments Grant.

Sources of ES/EMF toxicity can include fields inside your house—generated by appliances, lighting, wiring, power panels, heating devices—or any electrical devices, or outside, such as the home's proximity to power lines.

A given home may have strong or weak EMFs depending on the situation. For example, if you use an electric hair dryer, you are generating a short-term EMF; it dissipates when the device is turned off. But your electric power panel emits a steady EMF regardless of which household appliance or other electrical device is operating (see figure 10-3).

Note that some household appliances, such as the electric can opener and hair dryer emit very high EMFs at close range. Unless one is already electrically hypersensitive, these short-term exposures to relatively high EMFs will not produce much harm to the body because the time of exposure is of such short duration: with a can opener; perhaps twenty seconds; a hair dryer, less than five minutes. But the clothes washer and dryer, television, and fluorescent fixtures can be more damaging depending on their location. If any of these items is situated on the other side of a bedroom wall (specifically, against the wall that abuts the head of the bed), or in the case of the fluorescent lights, directly over the bed, then their effect can be cumulative, even though their actual EMF strength is not as strong as the can opener. These are often called electromagnetic hot spots.

The constancy of human exposure is what produces the damage. What kind of damage? While this is a subject still under intense discussion and research, evidence is mounting suggesting causal links between EMF exposure and immune dysfunction, depression, childhood leukemia, central nervous system cancer, melanoma, and breast cancer.

For example, researchers at Pacific Northwest Laboratory in Richland, Washington, concluded that exposure to extremely low-frequency electric or magnetic fields (generated by typical 60-Hertz alternating electrical current found in U.S. households) can contribute to the onset of depression and depression-related suicide. They postulated that these fields disrupt the body's normal day/night rhythm (the circadian cycle) and the chemicals responsible for maintaining it, such as the neurotransmitter serotonin and the hormone melatonin. They further postulated that these low-frequency fields accomplished the disruption by negatively affecting the brain's pineal gland, which regulates the circadian rhythm and its chemicals.[30]

Other research since the mid-1980s has further substantiated the various negative health impacts of prolonged exposure to EMFs of varying strengths or duration. Documented effects include: alteration of brain waves from cell phone signals; increases in leukemia rates in adults and children; interference with hormone and intercell communication activity; a slowing of visual reaction time; impaired nervous system activity; changes in the brain's hippocampus; alterations in immune system function; significant reduction in REM sleep; decline in insulin levels; undesirable changes in the blood-brain barrier; changes in cell cycles and proliferation; decrease in appetite and ability to sleep; and tumor formation.

WaveGuide, a public interest website that summarized medical data on EMFs from dozens of studies, noted that these studies "indicate biological effects at exposure levels *far below* what would be explained by 'thermal effects' and well within the range people are commonly exposed to every day." Most of the exposures studied, commented WaveGuide, "lie *far below* the current advisory exposure standards in the United States."[31]

How does an EMF disturb human health? It may be harmful to human health in much the same way that free radicals[32] upset physiology, suggests Michael Riversong. Electropollution consists of a high level of positive ions in an environment, and positive ions, despite their confusing name, are bad for your health. Riversong suggests thinking of positive ions and free radicals as essentially identical, certainly in regard their biological effects.

A free radical, he explains, is "simply a piece of a molecule that is missing electrons, so it wants to 'eat' any electrons in the vicinity, and it will take them from living cells." A positive ion is also "hungry" for more ions, and it will take them from negative ions (the healthy, uplifting ones), which are "free" or in excess as electrons. Both positive ions and free radicals have been documented to contribute to the formation of numerous illnesses and bodily dysfunctions.

"Positive ions in a house result from many things. Any formaldehyde in the air, for example, is a bit of a free radical. This is one of the reasons it is harmful; it outgasses from wood products as a type of positive ion. Another source of positive ions in the house is plain old dust and grit because in many cases it has degraded to the point where it has positive ions on its molecules. And when your house is sealed in, as many modern houses are, you get positive ions from the lack of fresh air circulation. People (and pets) take in all the electrons they can inside a house, so that few are left in the air. What is left are insect parts, dust, and chemicals." Riversong explains that houses situated near busy roads are subject to indoor air pollution from the nitrous oxides from automobile exhaust. These, too, he says, are "essentially positive ions and will 'eat' electrons."

Here are some real-life case studies that show the effects of chronic EMF (and thus heightened positive ion) exposure. The first is provided by Veronica Strong, a British health-care practitioner and director of Dowsing for Health in the Vale of Evesham, England.[33] Strong consulted with a woman in her late forties who spent eighteen hours a day in bed, incapacitated. She had suffered from chronic fatigue for three years; she was unable to walk more than fifty yards without feeling exhausted; and she was getting worse every week. Strong determined that the woman's main problem was unrelieved electromagnetic stress. There was a television in her bedroom; its cable ran in the wall alongside her bed, and a TV booster was connected to it. Once these three factors were corrected and relocated, the woman started to recover rapidly, such that within only three weeks, she was able to go on long walks, and now puts in a twelve-hour workday.

Michael Riversong relates a case involving the staff of a small newspaper office. Several staff members had intermittent health problems. They would have mysterious pains that came and went and followed no pattern; the doctors attending these people were unable to make a diagnosis. The newspaper editor said he didn't like being in his office, and was concerned about the high turnover rate in his business. Previous employees and editors had resigned for health problems, and one had died. Riversong measured high magnetic field levels of 10 mG at the editor's desk. Remember, the Swedish standard for "acceptable" EMF exposure is only 2.5 mG, so this was four times the safe level.

The probable reason for the high EMFs, Riversong found out, was that the newspaper office was next door to an appliance store; the EMFs from TVs and refrigerators on display (and thus always on) came through the wall. The editor relocated his office and tried to work as much in other locations as possible.

In a second case, Riversong consulted with a woman who had severe headaches when she came home from college. A gauss mater reading of the woman's bedroom showed normal EMFs except at the head of her bed where it registered between 5-11 mG. The baffling thing was that there was nothing in her room to account for the high EMF, but when Riversong examined the room immediately on the other side of the wall, he found an old motorized clock on a shelf directly in line with the woman's headboard. The remedy was simple: Riversong moved the clock and the woman's headaches stopped.

"Sometimes simply moving appliances will take care of problems. We're lucky when we can get off that easily," comments Riversong. In other situations, you may need to turn off electrical power at night, or have an electrician install a special relay so that you can turn off the power by a bedside remote switch. "Many people have experienced sudden, dramatic improvements in health when taking control of their electrical environment in this way."

Here are some practical, fairly low-cost devices a householder can employ to minimize or neutralize electromagnetic field exposure. This is not meant to be a definitive list (nor an endorsement of any products), but merely a quick look at some available options.

Measure Your EMF Exposure

The more you know about your indoor electromagnetic environment the better informed you are for making a smart choice about a neutralization technique. There are a number of handheld consumer-oriented EMF-measuring devices (in a price range of about $19 to $140) called gauss meters that can be used to get EMF readings in various rooms of your home.

E.L.F.-Zone Gauss Meter: This unit has a minimum sensitivity of 0.25 mG, but reads EMFs from 20-20,000 Hz. Its three lights (red, yellow, green) are calibrated to come on when danger, caution, and safe thresholds, respectively, are reached in an environment.

Dr. Gauss: Called "The EMF Detective," this battery-powered device can measure magnetic field radiation from power lines, computers, and kitchen appliances, and other hidden sources of EMF radiation. Its measurement range works on two scales, from 0-1 mG and 0-10 mG.

Trifield Meter: This unit can measure magnetic and electric fields, EMF, and radio/microwave pollution across an "extremely wide frequency response," according to the manufacturer. Specifically, its magnetic readings range from 0.2 mG to 3.0 mG and 1 mG to 100 mg; electric from 1 kV/m-100 kV/m; and RF/microwave from 0.01 mVV/cm^2 to 1.0 mVV/cm^2.

Minimize or Neutralize Your Indoor EMF Exposure

Once you have identified the EMF "hot spots" in your home, you can take steps to reduce or eliminate their injurious effects on your health, using a variety of devices.

Magnetic Shielding Foil ("MuMetal"): This is an alloy of eighty percent nickel and fifteen percent iron (plus copper, molybdenum or chromium) used for years in industrial applications to shield delicate electronic components from EMFs. For consumer-household use, the material (in fifteen-inch-wide sheets) can be trimmed (in length) to fit the required size and form a magnetic barrier against emitters such as cell phones, microwave ovens, doorbell transformers, computer terminals, and buried wiring. According to the manufacturer, one thickness of the material (0.004 inches) draped over the offending object can shield its EMF emissions by seventy-five percent. Essentially, the MuMetal attracts and holds the magnetic field within its own molecular structure, preventing it from passing any further.

Mag-Stop Plates: These are thick magnetic alloy plates (made of MuMetal; twenty-four by thirty inches, weighing six pounds) used to shield EMF emissions from electric circuit boxes, side-by-side computer terminals (such as in an office), appliances on the other side of bedroom walls, or "any situation where you need a flat shielding material on a wall, floor, or ceiling."

Total Shield: This unit is designed to neutralize EMFs by producing a 7.83 Hz field capable of blanketing a 20,000 square foot area, according to its manufacturer. The 7.83 Hz field is considered beneficial because it is the Schumann Resonance, the "pulse rate" of the planet itself. By "blanketing" an indoor area with this frequency, the device is believed to overcome the negative effects of EMFs present.

Shield Your Body from EMF Exposure

It is now possible to enjoy EMF shielding in your personal body and auric space by portable devices, so that as you move around in your home, into different rooms, each with their own EMF problems, you are still protected.

QLink: One of the more popular of personal EMF shielding devices is called the QLink, a pendant made by Clarus Products, a company founded in 1992 and specializing in subtle energy devices based on a principle they call "Sympathetic Resonance Technology." According to Clarus, the QLink works like a tuning fork or permanent resonator, and can "mimic the harmonic energy range of a person who is balanced, in a state of well-being, and 'in the zone.'" Clarus further explains that the QLink requires no battery, but instead is powered by the wearer's own electromagnetic and other bioenergies when it is worn.

Wearing the pendant (made from lightweight, biocompatible acrylic) enables the wearer's energy systems to readjust to this example of physiological and energetic balance, and to "relax into" it. Its protective field is placed at about eighteen inches around the body. Clarus reports that user benefits include increased mental focus and concentration, heightened stamina and energy during the day, greater emotional balance, reduced emotional reactivity, less jet lag, and less of a "fried" feeling after extended computer use. According to Clarus, one-third of users who report noticeable benefits say they observe these positive changes within a week of using the QLink; the rest say it takes a month or so to register significant benefits.

Clarus also provides the same protective technology in a ClearWave digital clock, which shields EMFs for up to thirty feet in all directions (or 113,000 cubic feet), including up and down; other models of the ClearWave shield EMFs up to forty and fifty feet in all directions. Clarus' Portable Ally is a battery-driven tabletop device (4 by 2 by 0.75 inches high) that provides EMF shielding for up to 40 feet.

How Flower Essences Can Reduce Your EMF Stress

The next time overhead fluorescent lights irritate you, try taking a flower remedy to calm yourself. Research has documented that taking two flower essence formulas can reduce your system's reaction to the intense environmental stimulation produced by fluorescent lights and their accompanying electromagnetic fields. California researcher Jeffrey R. Cram, Ph.D., studied the benefits of using Yarrow Special Formula and Five-Flower Formula, two brand-name mixtures of different flower essences to reduce systemic EMF stress. A flower essence is a highly dilute infusion of flower blossoms taken as liquid drops, and available at most natural foods stores.

Dr. Cram monitored the brain waves and their changes in twenty-four subjects who took one or the other remedy in response to fluorescent light exposure. "The two flower essences were found to reduce physiological activation and stress on the human organism," concluded Dr. Cram. He theorized that these flower essences were able to "strengthen emotional equilibrium and equanimity in the face of stresses and environmental impacts, thus reducing the typical 'fight or flight' stress response." In other words, the flower essence formulas were able to address the person's physiological and emotional reaction to the stress of the electromagnetic fields of the lights.[34]

HEALTHY LIVING SPACE DETOXIFIER #47
Benefits of Nontoxic Carpets—Don't Let Your Carpets Kill You Softly

One common assumption is that if you keep an old carpet clean with regular vacuuming and occasional shampooing, you have eliminated the potential health hazards that rugs and carpets may bear. Another common assumption holds that a new carpet is the height of purity and cleanliness and surely a guarantee against the presence of germs and other possibly harmful residents of old carpets.

Neither assumption is correct. Let's start with the truth about new carpets. The alarming fact is that the newer the carpet the more toxic it might be. New carpets, because they are treated with a great number of chemicals and preservatives, can actually outgas toxic fumes and not only slowly but consistently pollute the indoor air quality of a house, but also generate allergies or seriously irritate those already overburdened with allergens. It's a distressing thought: here you are comfortably sitting in your apartment living room, enjoying the brand new plush rug underfoot, and now you learn this same rug might be continuously releasing into your indoor air molecules containing substances that might eventually make you sick.

Of the modern machine-made carpets made from synthetic fibers, ninety percent of these are tufted, with the tufts held in place by a latex substance. Further, the yarn fibers of such carpets tend to be treated to prevent stains and wear. The carpet's backing material often includes a vinyl coating or a layer of foam-cushioning made from a synthetic material. All of these materials are potential allergens and potentially toxic when outgassed into a room. More specifically, synthetic carpets may contain pesticides (antimicrobial substances), neurotoxic solvents (such as toluene and xylene), and benzene, a carcinogen.

Carpet toxicity is an increasingly serious problem, due to the high degree of carpeted interiors in the United States. In

1993, for example, it was estimated that seventy percent of the floors in the United States had a carpet, that 1.5 billion square yards of carpeting had been purchased in that one year (equivalent to 5.5 square yards per American), and that from 1960 to 1993, carpet purchases had grown by 654% in the United States.[35] So if carpets are a source of indoor toxic emission, a great number of households are potentially at risk, and the greater the amount of indoor carpeting in a home, the greater the chance that indoor air quality is polluted in every room.

New carpets, because they are treated with a great number of chemicals and preservatives, can actually outgas toxic fumes and not only slowly but consistently pollute the indoor air quality of a house, but also generate allergies or seriously irritate those already overburdened with allergens.

According to John Bower of the Healthy House Institute, in 1988 the United States Environmental Protection Agency had to remove 27,000 yards of new carpeting from EPA offices after they found that dozens of their employees (about ten percent in all) had become sick from being in contact with the new carpets.[36] EPA research revealed that a carpet substance called 4-phenylcyclohexene (found in the latex backing, abbreviated as 4-PC) was the main toxic substance sickening their employees. The chemical that gives carpets the "new carpet" smell, 4-PC has been found in concentrations of 20 ppb in new carpets, although the levels decline to 1-2 ppb by about two months after installation. This toxic substance has been linked to numerous respiratory and mucous membrane problems and allergic reactions, as well as nausea, fatigue, and memory loss.[37]

At least the EPA figured out it was their new carpets that were sickening their employees, and in fact this led to considerable scientific investigation of carpet toxicity. Unfortunately, in far too many cases, office managers and householders fail to make the connection and remain highly allergic, if not chronically sick or seriously incapacitated, from unsuspected toxic carpet gas emissions.

In 1995, Rosalind Anderson, Ph.D., a researcher at Anderson Laboratories in Dedham, Massachusetts, reported on her analysis of gas emissions (outgassing) from over 300 different carpet samples obtained from commercial outlets, carpet mills, or patients' homes. None of the carpet samples were older than 40 years and most had been in use from one week to twelve years. Dr. Anderson performed 500 different laboratory tests to measure the effect of carpet outgassing on laboratory mice.

Her results showed that the gas emissions from carpets decreased the breathing rate of mice immediately on contact, from a normal rate of 280 breaths/minute to 235/minute, after only 8 minutes of exposure. When Dr. Anderson removed the mice from contact with the gas emissions, their respiration quickly normalized. On further inspection of the mice, Dr. Anderson discovered that one or more exposures to the outgassing produced distress symptoms in the mice, including swelling of the face, bleeding beneath the skin surface, altered posture, balance problems, hyperactivity, tremors, convulsions, limb paralysis, and, in some cases, death.

Dr. Anderson next studied 125 carpet samples for neurotoxicity, that is, negative effects on the activity of nerve and brain cells. She found that ninety percent of these samples produced at least one toxic effect and that sixty percent produced three or more "severe neurotoxic effects" in at least twenty-five percent of the mice. In other words, nearly all of the carpet samples were able to sicken one-quarter of the mice population in the study.

Why are new carpets often killer carpets? Because over 200 different chemicals are now found in the typical modern carpet, and many of these chemicals are toxic to humans (and mice), capable of producing "diverse toxic effects," says Dr. Anderson, such as flu-like symptoms, muscle pain, fatigue, headaches (lasting for months after the initial exposure), memory loss, and concentration difficulties, among others.[38]

Even before Dr. Anderson's published research in 1995, evidence had been coming out, in part from her, linking carpet outgassing with illness. In 1991, the New York State attorney general released a consumer alert advising people who smoked, had allergies, or suffered from respiratory disorders that they would be "more prone to experiencing symptoms when exposed to new carpeting." The alert stated that the carpet chemicals were a serious risk for children and the fetuses of pregnant women. Notable symptoms produced by toxic emissions included flu-like feelings, rashes, asthma, respiratory conditions that worsen, and multiple chemical sensitivities.[39] The consumer alert was prompted by the fact that the United States Consumer Product Safety Commission had by 1991 received some 500 consumer complaints about suspected carpet toxicity. Individuals had reported a variety of symptoms, such as chills, fever, burning eyes, nausea, dizziness, vision problems, memory deficits, cough, numbness, depression, nervousness, concentration problems, and others.

Consumer advocate and health educator Debra Lynn Dadd relates a remarkable case study showing the health-damaging effects of new carpets on householders. A man installed seventy-nine yards of new synthetic carpeting in his home-based business and noticed that on the first day, not only was the indoor space filled with a pungent odor from the carpeting, but dozens of spiders had become immobilized on its surface. Formerly, they had been observed to crawl freely through the house. A few months later, the man and his family became sick, reporting headaches, nausea, concentration difficulties, unusual thirst, and mucous membrane burning, including of the eyes.

Soon the symptoms worsened, to include depression, skin rashes, and insomnia. The carpets were removed, but even after almost a year away from them, the family remained hypersensitive to many substances. A laboratory analysis of the carpet showed that it was outgassing at least six toxic substances including formaldehyde, and that another thirty-five toxic substances had been used in the carpet's manufacture.[40]

Of considerable toxicity are styrene (a carcinogen) and 4-PC, found in the styrene butadiene latex backing used on about ninety-five percent of carpets (applied in liquid form at the carpet mill). An estimated two-thirds of the 2.7 billion pounds of carpet yarns sold in the United States as of the mid-1990s were nylon, while only 0.5% were wool. The glue that holds the synthetic carpet fibers together contains 4-PC, the toxic substance discussed earlier.

Researchers writing in the British scientific journal *Nature* recently reported yet another toxic factor in modern rugs. Carpets can trap benzene from car exhaust and outgas this into the home's indoor air. Carpets (as well as wood and linoleum) are absorbent and can trap airborne benzene, a documented carcinogen, and eventually release it into the air.[41]

But it's not only new rugs that can trap airborne particles; in fact, old carpets can be troublesome as well. The carpet acts as a kind of floor-based air filter, collecting everything that's in the air, including, for example, hydrocarbons from car exhaust in the street or pesticides from a yard, tracked in by feet onto the rug. Airborne chemical compounds from sources other than carpets (such as paint fumes if a room is repainted while the rug is uncovered) can end up trapped inside the carpets to be released into the air later. Carpets also house dust mites (which leave highly allergenic excrement) and mold and mildew, allergens that can breed in damp carpets.

There is an additional problem with carpets and house dust. Dust and tracked-in soil accumulate in the carpets, then get released into the indoor air when people walk on them. Researchers examined the house dust collected from homes in North Carolina and found traces of fourteen pesticides and ten polycyclic aromatic hydrocarbons. They further discovered that the smaller the particle of house dust, the greater the concentrations of any of these twenty-four indoor air pollutants.[42]

Apparently it is possible to quietly sicken under the influence of toxic carpets without manifesting any overt symptoms for a long time, observes Cindy Duehring, research director for Environmental Access Research Network in Minot, North Dakota. "Lack of acute reactions to toxic carpeting are common, but the chemicals may be causing serious damage nonetheless," Duehring comments. "The lack of acute adverse reactions (e.g., headaches, breathing difficulties, seizures, etc.) does not mean that the chemicals coming off of the toxic carpet are not causing slow, silent damage." Duehring argues that carpeting can "make a person much more susceptible to getting a chronic illness in the future" and that sustained exposure to unhealthy carpets sets you up for future problems "by dosing yourself with dangerous chemicals on a regular basis with carpeting."[43]

As mentioned already, the main problem with synthetic carpets is their outgassing of toxic substances known as a group by the term volatile organic compounds, or VOCs. Technically, this group includes hundreds of organic compounds present in the Earth's atmosphere (containing hydrogen, carbon, and other elements); these compounds evaporate easily, hence the designation volatile. Outgassing refers to when VOCs evaporate or release gases from the substrate in which they are present (such as in the latex finish of carpet backings). Natural sources of VOCs include fossil fuel deposits, oil sands, volcanoes, trees, even bacteria. Human-made VOCs tend to be toxic, or more toxic than naturally emitted ones, and derive from motor vehicles, solvent use, industrial processes, and gasoline evaporation.

More specifically, toxic VOCs are found in—or outgassed from—carpets, photocopier machines, paints, solvents, varnishes, adhesives and glues, spray shoe polish, water repellents, dry-cleaning fluids and chemicals, underarm deodorants, and many others. Here are but a few examples of VOCs found in common household products: tetrachloroethylene (dry-cleaned clothes); chloroform (chlorinated water); benzene (tobacco smoke); formaldehyde (fabrics, pressed wood products, building insulation, even cosmetics); styrene (carpets, plastics); and para-dichlorobenzene (moth balls and deodorizers).

Given the nature of modern, tightly sealed homes and the lack of proper ventilation, it is not uncommon for a typical indoor air to contain VOC levels 100 to 1,000 times higher than outside air pollution levels. Put differently, the EPA reported that the average American home was likely to have VOC levels two to five times higher than outside, regardless of whether the homes were situated in a rural area or in cities. It is a shocking thought that the air outside the home may be less polluted than indoors.[44] Further, in 1989, based on a study of indoor air quality in ten newly constructed public access buildings, the EPA reported that over 900 VOCs were identified in the ambient indoor air.

As discussed previously, one of the new, serious, and medically vexing conditions to emerge as a result of prolonged exposure and allergic reaction to VOCs is multiple chemical sensitivity syndrome (MCS). This condition has multiple symptoms, affects multiple body organs and senses, and has multiple causes, thereby making it impossible for conventional medicine to diagnose according to its standard single-causative agent approach.[45]

Typically, MCS produces many symptoms involving the neurological, immune, respiratory, skin, gastrointestinal, and/or musculoskeletal systems. Medical studies show that about sixty-six percent of people suffering from chronic fatigue and fibromyalgia (chronic muscle pain)[46] also have MCS. Studies report that typical symptoms include all of the ones reported above (in connection with carpets) as well as sleeping and breathing difficulties, memory loss, mood swings, mental confusion, sneezing, itching, drowsiness, wheezing, runny or stuffy nose, muscle and joint pain, vaginal burning, frequent urination, constipation or diarrhea, joint and limb swelling, migraines, stomach pain, impaired balance, and increased sensitivity to odors, loud noises, bright lights, touch, extremes of heat and cold, and EMFs.

Usually, a person sustains an initial acute or chronic toxic exposure, which shocks the system and overloads the central nervous system and liver, then the initial sensitivity broadens or spreads to include reactivity to many more substances commonly found in the modern Western environment. It does not have to be a high dose once the system is overburdened with toxicity. Once the triggering sensitivity happens, low exposures to common chemicals can generate major allergic reactions, usually out of proportion to the dose of the exposure. Eventually, you become allergic (chemically sensitive) to seemingly everything chemical. Perhaps this is why some medical authorities think MCS would be better labeled Toxicant-Induced Loss of Tolerance to indicate a toxic exposure that leads to the loss of tolerance to widely encountered chemicals to which you would not expect a reaction.[47]

According to William J. Rea, M.D., director of the Environmental Health Center in Dallas, Texas, and for many years an expert in this field, chemical sensitivity is "an adverse reaction to ambient doses of toxic chemicals in our air, food, and water at levels which are generally accepted as subtoxic."[48] Another study (with mice) concluded: "A detailed chemical and microbial evaluation of the carpets and carpet emissions showed volatile organic compounds, pesticide residues, and microbiological flora, but at insufficient quantities to result in acute toxicity."[49]

Unfortunately, what is nontoxic and tolerable, or of "insufficient quantity" to one individual, can be quite toxic, sufficient, and intolerable to another. The trouble here is you can't know until your system has already reacted; another problem is that toxicity is cumulative and may take a long time to produce "acute" effects; a third problem is that not every individual corresponds to whatever norm for toxicity toleration is used in scientific studies from which safety standards are determined.

In fact, yet another study confirmed this effect. Scientists at the Centers for Disease Control and Prevention in Atlanta, Georgia, measured VOCs in human blood, noting that they are found in the general population at the high parts-per-trillion range, "but some people with much higher levels have apparently been exposed to VOC sources away from the workplace." Of especial significance here was the CDC's observation that while "most of the internal dose of these compounds is quickly eliminated [once they're in the blood], there is a fraction that is only slowly removed, and these compounds may bioaccumulate."[50]

The MCS-afflicted person becomes in effect allergic and potentially reactive to almost anything synthetic. In fact, the growing body of statistics on MCS is sobering: 17% to 34% of Americans report symptoms of chemical sensitivity.

The MCS-afflicted person becomes in effect allergic and potentially reactive to almost anything synthetic. In fact, the growing body of statistics on MCS is sobering: 17% to 34% of Americans report symptoms of chemical sensitivity; 6.3% of Californians have been given an MCS diagnosis; up to 80% of these also have chronic fatigue syndrome, 55% to 65% have fibromyalgia, and 50% have traditional allergies.[51]

In fact, there is such a degree of symptom overlap among MCS, chronic fatigue, environmental illness, fibromyalgia, and acute allergic reactivity that one wonders if there are real distinguishing differences between these conditions or if they are simply a variation on the same theme of sustained chronic toxicity. A study of 100 new MCS cases showed that 88% also had the symptoms of chronic fatigue syndrome, 49% had fibromyalgia symptoms, and 47% had all three. "These extensive overlaps highlight the need to screen patients for all three disorders whenever anyone is suspected," concluded Albert Donnay, executive director of MCS Referral & Resources in Baltimore, Maryland.[52]

Whatever the outcome of this question of overlapping disorders, the fact remains that, for the householder, uncorrected long-term exposure to toxic factors in the indoor living space can lead to any of these conditions in the extra-sensitive person or in one whose system is overburdened with toxicity from other sources. In fact, if you find yourself suffering from several of these conditions, it is worth considering that your house may be making you sick, that some element in your indoor living space is toxic.

One way to determine this possibility on a physiological basis is to have one of the many biochemical tests for toxicity detailed in chapter 3. Then if you test positive for toxic contaminants in your system, it is prudent to consider a comprehensive physiological detoxification program (see chapters 4-8) to flush the poisons out of your body and to help your liver regain its natural ability to detoxify your body. In the meantime, here are some practical steps to reduce your exposure to potentially toxic carpets.

Test Your Carpet for Toxicity

If you suspect your carpets are making you sick, you can have a professional toxicology laboratory test a sample to confirm or refute your suspicions. The same laboratory that produced the startling research by Rosalind Anderson in 1995 now offers product emissions testing of a range of items including carpets, mattresses, diapers, wallpaper, paint, adhesives, mothballs, insulation, air fresheners, perfumes, boots, even telephones.

A client sent in her telephone because she believed somehow it was making her sick. She was right: Anderson Laboratories found a cotton pad saturated with pesticide inside the mouth piece. The lab also reported that a survey of the first one hundred families who sent them carpets for emissions testing all had new symptoms arise after installing the carpets and these symptoms were consistent with those associated with sick building syndrome and multiple chemical sensitivity.[53] Laboratory analyses of product emissions range from $750 to $3500 depending on the extensiveness of the data requested.

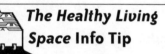

The Healthy Living Space Info Tip

For information about product emissions testing, contact:
Anderson Laboratories,
P.O. Box 323,
773 West Hartford Main Street,
West Hartford, VT 05084;
tel: 802-295-7344;
fax: 802-295-7648;
website:
www.andersonlaboratories.com.

For Nature's Carpet:
Colin Campbell & Sons Ltd.,
1428 West 7th Avenue,
Vancouver, BC, V6H 1C1, Canada,
tel: 800-667-5001 or 604-734-2758;
fax: 604-734-1512;
website: www.colcam.com.

For Hendricksen Natürlich, contact:
Natural Home,
P.O. Box 1677,
Sebastopol, CA 95473;
tel: 707-824-0914;
fax: 800-329-9398;
e-mail: nathome@monitor.net;
website:
www.naturalhomeproducts.com.

Do a "Bake-Out" on New Carpeting

If you are unable to remove new carpeting or must move into a new, renovated, or refurnished house or apartment with unremovable new carpets, one option is to do a carpet "bake-out." If the carpets have not yet been installed, ask the carpet provider to air the carpets in a well-ventilated area for seventy-two hours before bringing them to your home. Once the carpets are installed, stay away from your home for a few days. Before you leave, open all the windows, run the ventilation system (such as exhaust fans) at full capacity, and set the indoor heat at 100°F (38°C). The idea is to set the heat and ventilation systems to run at much higher than normal levels—overheating and overventilating. Let them run at that level for about forty-eight hours.

The theory behind the home bake-out is a bit like the self-cleaning oven: heat the house up and force the VOCs out of the carpets and, through the open windows, out of the house. It is believed that the high temperature forces the VOCs to be released quickly, compared to normal or ambient indoor conditions under which the VOCs are released more slowly and over a longer period, even up to years. Some studies have shown that a bake-out can reduce VOC emissions by sixty-five percent. However, other experts suggest that the bake-out may not have an effect on certain compounds such as formaldehyde, 4-PC, and BHT, which do not decay rapidly.[54]

After the bake-out, use a balanced mechanical home ventilation system, such as a heat recovery ventilator, that will continuously exhaust the indoor air (containing VOCs from all sources, including carpets) and replace it with fresh outside air. The recommended replacement rate of indoor with outdoor air is that thirty-three percent of the home's air should be exchanged every hour. This approach will reduce your exposure to airborne VOCs.[55] However, healthy building house expert John Bower comments: "Bake-outs aren't effective with long-term outgassing sources such as particle board and medium-density fiberboard."[56]

Do a Nontoxic Carpet Cleaning

A thorough cleaning of your carpets can reduce the likelihood of their contaminating your indoor space. Obviously a rigorous vacuuming is in order, followed by a hot water extraction and/or steam shampooing. Annie Berthold-Bond, an expert in environmentally safe options and author of *Better Basics for the Home*, recommends renting a steam-cleaning water-extraction machine and using your own nontoxic detergents for cleaning your carpets.

Almost always, commercial carpet cleaners will use detergents that have some amount of toxic substances such as perfumes, additives, or antimicrobial pesticides. As a nontoxic alternative, Berthold-Bond suggests mixing one-fourth cup of perfume-free, all-purpose liquid detergent (she advises using a product called Infinity Heavenly Horsetail, available at natural foods stores) with about four gallons of water. She also uses antifungal essential oils in the rinse water, notably tea tree oil (a natural essential oil known in aromatherapy as a powerful disinfectant; available at most natural foods outlets). Tea tree oil can also be applied as an antifungal carpet spray (not to be rinsed off) in a ratio of two teaspoons to two cups of water.[57]

Try Woven Wool Carpets

If your budget allows it, you might consider replacing your synthetic, allergenic carpets with a natural fiber alternative, such as woven wool carpets. Although woven wool carpets may still contain yarn that has been treated with pesticide mothproofing, it is possible that even if you react adversely to synthetic carpets you may be able to tolerate these. In addition, woven wool carpets use a great deal less latex than conventional synthetic latex-backed carpets; woven wool carpets also tend to have fewer outgassing VOCs than the average synthetic carpet with a glued backing.

A number of companies now offer natural woven wool carpets for the environmentally sensitive. One such firm is Colin Campbell & Sons of Vancouver, British Columbia, which has made their MCS-friendly "Nature's Carpet" since 1992. The company reports that their "clean scoured wool" is "totally biodegradable" and hasn't been subject to harsh chemicals during the mothballing stage of regular wool products; they apply a nontoxic latex made from a natural rubber base to the undersides of the carpets; no chemical dyes are used to color the yarns; and the dual backing of the carpet is made from natural jute (a hemp product).

"The complete absence of chemicals, at every stage of the carpet's manufacture and composition, means there is no toxic outgassing," explains Colin Campbell & Sons. An independent laboratory testing of Nature's Carpet in 1996 (by Anderson Laboratories) confirmed the company's claims. It found no evidence of sensory irritation or pulmonary iritation produced by a sample of the company's 100% wool carpet.

Another highly regarded source of natural carpets is Hendricksen Natürlich of Sebastopol, California. Since 1989, this company has been providing environmentally friendly carpets made from natural wool fibers. The carpets are free of formaldehyde, stain-repellents, flame retardants, and synthetic blends, and contain minimal outgassing glues.

Wool has many merits for the allergic, notes the company, for after all, it is the original that synthetics strive to copy. "Wool releases soil more easily than any other fiber, has the greatest resilience, absorbs noise and noxious gases from the air, and resists burns." In the warm months, it acts as a natural air conditioner by absorbing and releasing humidity and by definition is produced without hazardous chemicals, states Hendricksen Natürlich. According to a list they publish, obtained from a carpet manufacturer, at least forty-two potentially toxic chemicals are "commonly" used in carpet manufacture.

The Trouble with Indoor Air— Worse Pollution Indoors than Out

Ever since the outbreak of Legionnaire's disease in Philadelphia in 1976, attention has increasingly focused on the relationship between indoor air quality and human health. In that initially baffling outbreak in Philadelphia, a microbial contaminant was distributed throughout a hotel's interior by way of the ventilation system, sickening many of those guests who breathed the air. It's an extreme example that illustrates the need for fresh, pure, constantly ventilated indoor air, and the consequences of not having it.

As we discovered above, if you live in an apartment or a tightly sealed new home and have new or even recently installed wall-to-wall carpets, potentially you are breathing air contaminated with numerous VOCs outgassed from the carpets. However, carpets are not the only source of airborne pollutants found in the typical modern home, although they are certainly a vivid example of how the mechanism of indoor air pollution works. Unfortunately, there are a great number of things in the modern home that can poison you.

Indoor air quality can also be negatively affected by other factors including combustion gases, carbon monoxide, VOCs from other sources, formaldehyde, radon, biological contaminants, dust mite fragments and feces, molds, pollen, minerals and metals (notably asbestos, found in building materials; and lead, found in some paints, dinnerware, food cans, furniture, toys, dust, and soil), cleaning products made from synthetic chemicals, synthetic fibers and fabrics, household furnishings, pesticides, and tobacco smoke, among others.

For example, combustion gases (invisible gases left over from burning substances) can come from gas and oil furnaces, gas dryers, water heaters (gas or oil), and boilers (gas or oil). Carbon monoxide (formed as a result of the incomplete burning of carbon), can be released inside a home from fireplaces (wood, natural gas), stoves (coal or wood-burning), heaters (natural gas, propane, or oil), and hot water tanks. Radon, a radioactive gas from inside the Earth, can enter a home through cracks in the foundation and through well water.

Formaldehyde can outgas from urea-formaldehyde foam insulation, glues used in manufactured pressed-wood products (particleboard, plywood, fiberboard), clear finishes, resin treatments on fabrics, durable press drapes, environmental tobacco smoke, paint preservatives, veneered kitchen cabinets, and wet fingernail hardeners and polishes, among others. Symptoms of formaldehyde toxicity include watery eyes, a burning sensation in the eyes and throat, nausea, breathing difficulties, chest tightness, skin rashes, allergic reactions, and, for the extra-sensitive, asthma attacks; it is also regarded as a carcinogen.

A recent study of formaldehyde emissions from fifty-five domestic consumer and construction products measured over a twenty-four-hour period showed that among the high emitters are polyurethane floor finishings, wet fingernail hardeners and polishes, permanent press shirts and draperies, and pre-pasted wallpaper. They found that when wet, the polyurethane can emit one thousand times more formaldehyde than bare particleboard, usually considered a high emitter.[58]

Typically, formaldehyde is present in both indoor and outdoor air at an assumed "safe" level of less than 0.03 ppm, but it becomes problematic for humans when it reaches airborne levels greater than 0.1 ppm. The less circulation of indoor air there is, and the less an infusion of fresh outside air, the greater the chance that formaldehyde levels will build to toxic concentrations. Further, formaldehyde levels rise when the rooms are humid and hot, and drop when they are cool and dry, arguing for the desirability of indoor dehumidification.

For some people, a tiny amount of formaldehyde may be way too much. According to the EPA, ten percent of all individuals are hypersensitive to formaldehyde, reacting allergically at much lower concentrations than are generally considered safe. Hypersensitives can react severely to formaldehyde at a 0.1 ppm even though the "permissible" work place level established by OSHA (Occupational Safety and Hazard Administration) is much higher, at 0.75 ppm.

The above are only the most well-known offenders on the list of possible indoor pollutants. In fact, one researcher has tabulated seventy-nine different organic chemical compounds likely to be found in a typical indoor environment (home or office). You're likely to encounter these in: refrigerants, linoleum floor covering, epoxy paint, gypsum board, polyurethane wood finish, moth crystals/deodorizers, floor wax, cement flagstone, wallpaper, and plastics, among many other sources.[59] VOCs in indoor air can number from 20 to several hundred—1,000 different VOCs have been detected in indoor air altogether, drawn from many samples—and their concentrations inside tend to be larger than you would find outdoors, sometimes 100 times higher.[60]

Volatile organic compounds (VOCs) in indoor air can number from 20 to several hundred—1,000 different VOCs have been detected in indoor air altogether, drawn from many samples—and their concentrations inside tend to be larger than you would find outdoors, sometimes 100 times higher.

As mentioned earlier, studies have shown that indoor air can often be more polluted than outside air, containing a higher percentage of a variety of airborne contaminants. Using air conditioning rather than natural ventilation (open windows, fans) can make the situation worse, contributing to the onset of numerous sick building syndrome symptoms. Here's a look at some of the scientific findings on indoor air quality (IAQ) and illness:

- Researchers in France found exposure to air conditioning in offices (versus natural ventilation) was associated with an increased rate of SBS symptoms and sickness absence.[61]

- A study involving 2,761 office workers from five different buildings showed that SBS symptoms decreased by forty percent to fifty percent after the workers were relocated to a single new building with superior indoor ventilation. Their old building had relied on mechanical ventilation, air conditioning, humidification, and had sealed windows. Among the symptoms that improved with better indoor air quality were skin and eye irritations, respiratory problems, nose and throat irritations, fatigue, and headache. Even better, sixty percent of the workers who were originally symptomatic were free of all symptoms once they were in the new, properly ventilated building.[62]

- Taiwanese researchers looked at indoor air quality and respiratory illness symptoms in 264 nursing workers at 28 day-care centers and found a strong connection between dampness (indoor humidity) and SBS symptoms. The dampness concentrated airborne fungi and molds (notably *Aspergillus* strains), and those centers that had no air conditioning or air cleaning systems had higher concentrations.[63]

- Among 1,144 office workers, those working under ventilation conditions involving mechanical heating and ventilating, air conditioning, or fan coil units had a higher risk of experiencing SBS symptoms than those people working under conditions of natural ventilation. Symptoms included throat irritation, nasal discharges, blocked nose on awakening, migraines, and coughing.[64]

- German researchers studied the role of airborne dust and SBS symptoms in a group of 133 office workers who had complained of symptoms after sound-absorbing mineral fiber boards were installed as suspended ceilings in their work spaces. More than half the 133 employees (79 in all) had complained of itching, eye irritation (burning, reddening), and upper respiratory tract irritations, and 50% of the employees had consulted a doctor for treatment of their symptoms. It turned out the fiber content in the office air was quite high, sufficient for the researchers to link it with the health complaints.[65]

- Another Taiwanese study showed that inside building dampness is directly correlated with eye irritations, coughs, lethargy, and fatigue, based on a study of 1,237 workers in 19 air-conditioned offices. Reports of eye irritation were higher when stuffy odor or mold was present, still higher when both were present, higher still with the presence of water damage in the building, and the highest when all "dampness exposure" factors were present.[66]

- According to research at Texas Tech University Health Sciences Center in Lubbock, Texas, buildings with IAQ complaints often have high airborne concentrations of *Penicillium* strains (representing 89% to 100% of the total fungi), while buildings with a low incidence of IAQ problems have an indoor air "fungal ecology" (the overall balance of biological contaminants) similar to what's found outdoors. Fungal populations may vary outdoors, but the indoor fungal populations "tend to remain unchanged," researchers concluded.[67]

- An earlier study by the same group looked at forty-eight schools in which there had been concerns about indoor air quality and SBS symptoms. While five families of fungi (including *Penicillium*) comprise about ninety-five percent of the typical outdoor air, in twenty schools *Penicillium* was the dominant organism found in the indoor air and at rates higher than found outdoors. In eleven schools, significant amounts of *Stachybotrys atra* were isolated in the classrooms (under wet carpets, wet walls, behind vinyl wall coverings), leading researchers to conclude that SBS symptoms were associated with the presence of these two fungi.[68]

• On the positive side, researchers at McGill University in Montreal, Quebec, found that when office workers had a new ventilation system that allowed them to individually adjust the ventilation at their worksite, their productivity rose by eleven percent and SBS symptoms declined when measured sixteen months later. In other words, bad indoor air quality leads to lost productivity and illness, while proper indoor ventilation can lead to enhanced productivity and better health.[69]

As the research cited above suggests, molds and fungi are a big problem in the indoor environment. Experts are paying more attention to household fungi and toxigenic molds as possible main contributing factors in sick building syndrome and its many allergy-like symptoms. One fungus that is now particularly under study is called *Stachybotrys chartarum*, a toxic fungus that can cause health problems in humans and animals. For example, *S. chartarum* can produce skin rashes, nervous system complaints, nausea, vomiting, diarrhea, gallbladder-like colic pain, nosebleeds, and numerous respiratory problems typical of mild to strong allergic reaction.

How does it get into the house? It enters the indoor living space when the house has sustained water damage from broken pipes, flooding, roof leaks, sewage backups, or excessive condensation. These are ideal growth conditions for the fungus, which is present in soil, dust, dirt, the paper covering of sheetrock, wallpaper, ceiling tiles, various paper goods, natural fiber carpets, insulation material, wet cellulose products, and other organic debris. The fungus can grow in the damp conditions yet not be noticed by occupants; when observed, it is black, shiny if wet and powdery if dry.

Among the mostly commonly occurring microbes that can infest homes, offices, and schools are *Cladosporium*, *Alternaria*, *Fusarium*, *Penicillium* (4 species typically encountered), and *Aspergillus* (fifteen different species commonly encountered in homes). Often you can smell their presence before you actually spot them, in the form of a foul, musty odor when you enter the room. According to researchers at Georgia Tech's Indoor Environmental Research Program, in many respects the air pollution from molds and fungi is not much different than that generated by hazardous chemicals.

"Many of the volatile compounds produced by the cultured fungi are identical to those originating from solvent-based building materials and cleaning supplies."

In fact, the volatile organic compounds from molds and fungi can include hexane, methylene chloride, benzene, and acetone, thereby adding "heavily" to a building's existent level of toxic VOCs. In one case, the researchers found high levels of hexane in the indoor air but could not find an actual emitting source until they factored in the possibility of the ambient hexane levels being the result of microbiological contamination.[70]

One of the most likely places to find any of seventeen fungi growing indoors is in some part of the home's HVAC system (heating, ventilation, air conditioning). For example, *Acremonium spp.* grows in humidifier water and HVAC fiberglass insulation; *Alternaria spp.* in cooling systems, refrigerator coils, and on dust in ductwork; *Aspergillus spp.* in an evaporative air cooler, HVAC fiberglass insulation, cooling systems, coils, fans, filters, and dust in ductwork; *Fusarium spp.* in humidifier water; *Penicillium spp.* in air conditioners, HVAC ducts, filters, fans, and humidifier water. The same is true of at least eight harmful bacteria that grow indoors: *Micropolyspora faeni* flourishes in the humidifier; *Pseudomonas aeruginosa* in the evaporative air cooler, humidifier, and indoor dust; and *Thermoactinomycetes vulgaris* in air conditioners and humidifier water.[71]

HEALTHY LIVING SPACE DETOXIFIER #48
Filter Your Home's Indoor Air
to Remove Toxins and Allergens

The scientific reports give a vivid and sometimes chilling picture of the degree to which elements of our indoor living space can make us sick when we live in a home or work in an office that lacks good air circulation. Not necessarily every home or interior work or living space is toxic, or toxic to the degree that it guarantees some degree of illness. On the other hand, most of the VOCs are invisible, and many are odorless, so how can you tell if you're living under their baleful influence? One way is home testing.

Be a Professional House Doctor

A company in Iowa is now providing a set of seven inexpensive do-it-yourself Healthy Home Test Kits by which you can monitor indoor levels of molds and bacteria, lead, carbon monoxide, radon, asbestos, and formaldehyde. The kits range in price from about four dollars to forty dollars. No special knowledge of laboratory procedures or instrumentation is required to get reliable results, the company (Professional House Doctors, Inc., or PHD) explains.

For example, to test the levels of molds and bacteria, you expose a culture plate to the indoor air for fifteen minutes, store it in a dark place for seventy-two hours, then compare the results (that is, what has grown in the plate) against a chart to find out what contaminants you have. For formaldehyde, you expose the monitor to your indoor air for eight hours, then send it to the PHD laboratory for evaluation. For lead, you dip the lead test dauber in water and rub it on the item in question; if the item or dauber turns pink, the item contains lead. The carbon monoxide test is even easier: when the "CO Alert Badge" changes from tan to gray/black, it means you have too much carbon monoxide in your indoor air; the badge returns to its normal color when exposed to fresh air.

Monitors specifically for formaldehyde are available for home and office use as originally developed by Air Quality Research, an organization founded in 1982 at the School of Public Health at the University of California at Berkeley. One unit (PF-1) determines indoor levels of formaldehyde in work and home spaces; the second unit (PF-20) is a clip-on device to measure individual exposure levels for people in a work space.

The Healthy Living Space Info Tip

For information about Healthy Home Test Kits, contact: Professional House Doctors, Inc., 1406 E. 14th Street, Des Moines, IA 50316, e-mail: info@prohousedr.com; website: www.prohousedr.com.

For formaldehyde monitors, contact: Air Quality Research, 100 E. Main Street, Suite C, Carrborro, NC 27510; tel: 800-818-5894; e-mail: ppecevich@mindspring.com; website: www.airqualityresearch.com.

Decrease Your Mold Exposure

If you suspect mold in your indoor living space, a key preventive step to take is keep the indoor humidity level below forty percent and ventilate (with exhaust fans) all showers and cooking areas. Use a humidifier or air conditioner during the humid months; add mold inhibitors to indoor paints before applying to the walls if you are repainting; scour the bathrooms with mold-killing products (nontoxic, nonallergenic: see below); refrain from carpeting basement and bathroom floors; remove any carpets and upholstery that have sustained water damage.[72]

If your home has walls or floors that have sustained water damage, disinfect the surface with a chlorine solution of one cup of laundry bleach per gallon of water (provided you're not allergic to chlorine). It is prudent to do this with adequate ventilation, wearing goggles and rubber gloves.[73]

It is essential to regularly clean the water reservoir in humidifiers because they can act like "little mold factories . . . pools of standing stagnant water" that during a season can allow mold to grow, infiltrate the ducts, and get blown through the house.[74]

The most effective step to take to purify your indoor air of VOCs is air filtration, and here you have several choices. These include mechanical filtration by way of HEPA (high efficiency particulate air) filters, either whole house or individual room systems; electrostatic filtration, by electronically charged plastic panel filters inserted into a home's central heating system; ultraviolet radiation; and negative ion generators.

Before we review the different technological options for air filtering, let's get a sense for how fine the filtration mesh must be, which is to say, how small the toxic airborne particles are. The key measurement in this domain is the micron, which is equal to 1/25,000 of an inch. The HEPA systems are so called because they can deal with particles as small as 0.1-0.3 microns in diameter, but is that fine enough? Yes, for most microorganisms.

Among the airborne viruses, adenovirus (associated with the common cold) is 0.08 microns in width; rhinovirus (also with colds) 0.023; influenza (flu) is 0.1; respiratory syncytial virus (pneumonia) is 0.22; paramyxovirus (mumps) is 0.23; varicella-zoster (chickenpox) is 0.16; and mycobacterium tuberculosis (TB) is 0.86. Now for bacteria: *Acinetobacter* (opportunistic infections) is 1.3; *Corynebacterium diphtheriae* (diphtheria) is 1.0; *Klebsiella pneumoniae* (opportunistic infections) is 0.4; *Staphylococcus aureus* (opportunistic infections) is 1.0; and *Streptococcus pneumoniae* (pneumonia, otitis media [ear infection]) is 0.9. Among the fungi, *Cryptococcus neoformans* (cryptococcosis) is 5.5 microns wide, considerably larger than the viruses and bacteria.[75]

HEPA Mechanical Filtration

This approach is generally rated as capable of removing 99.99% of airborne particulates, such as dust, pollen, plant and mold spores, asbestos dust, animal hair, and tobacco smoke particles, if they are no smaller than 0.1 microns in diameter. There are *many* HEPA filters available, so the ones mentioned here are presented only to give the reader an idea of how a HEPA unit works and where to start looking for a suitable model.

The Safe Zone 2500 (weight: fifteen pounds) can handle a medium-sized room of about 300-650 square feet and uses both a carbon-activated and a HEPA filter. The activated carbon canister (weight: 8 pounds) is especially good at removing indoor odors, such as in a kitchen. One user stated that the unit "cut the dust buildup on our furnishings by probably 70%." The Safe Zone 3000 (weight: 22 pounds) air-cleans a 400-850 square foot room; one user employed it to ventilate her home nail salon business.

The Safe Zone 4000 is a whole-house, three-stage filtration unit that works with a home's HVAC system (heating, ventilation, and air conditioning) to clean and circulate indoor air. In addition to the HEPA and charcoal filters, the unit's third filter is a VOC cartridge capable of removing dangerous chemical gases outgassed from household products and fixtures. At 56 pounds, it is not as readily portable as the other Safe Zones, but is rated to air-filter 560-1100 square feet.

Activated Charcoal Air Filtration

In some instances, the hypersensitive person might require a non-HEPA indoor air filtering system. Chemical fumes and pollutants can contaminate the HEPA filter such that it begins to smell of them—a perfume, a new wall paint, or whatever chemical particulate it has absorbed. The Aireox Activated Carbon Air Purifier is recommended when a person could become allergic (chemically reactive) to the substances collected in the HEPA filter or when the primary offending substance is chemical fumes.

The carbon filter—the unit can be set unobtrusively on a desktop—can remove 99.95% of dust, pollen, and particulates to 0.5 microns, as well as most indoor fumes and odors. According to the manufacturer, "if your work place is loaded with VOCs, consider the activated carbon purifiers as the safest air purification."

Electrostatic Air Filters

The concept here is to remove particles from airstreams having large steady flow rates, such as you have with indoor heating or air conditioning. Air filters are placed within a home's central heating and/or air conditioning system to catch tiny airborne allergenic particles before (or as) they are blown through the ducts. In a sense, the furnace or air handling system becomes a whole-house air-cleaning device. The device is inserted in the place normally occupied by the filter in the existing furnace or air conditioner; the normal filter is usually fiberglass and removes only five percent to ten percent of particles.

The ElectroStatic Air Filter removes 99.97% of indoor air allergens of 1.3 microns in size and larger. Its surface has been treated with an antimicrobial substance to deactivate bacteria, molds, fungi, and other microbiological contaminants as they pass through it. The company also makes an OxyClean Air Filter, which they claim can remove foul odors and harmful gases present in indoor air. The filter can be used with activated charcoal pads to remove odors and gases.

According to the manufacturer, the filters use the magnetic effect of static electricity and special filtering media to attract and trap airborne particulates; in other words, the static electricity on the fibers of the filter attract the contaminants and, as the air blows across these electrically charged fibers, the static charge actually increases. The filter does not require replacement, but maintenance every thirty to sixty days (washing it out with a garden hose) is recommended.

Another brand called Dust Fighter 95 uses five layers of filtration media to trap about ninety-five percent of particulates passing through it. According to Dust Free, the manufacturer, numerous clients with allergy problems have reported improvement after using the air filters. A nurse (with allergies) who works with allergy patients found the filters "made a noticeable difference" in the amount of dusting she had to do in her home. A child with post-nasal

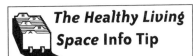

The Healthy Living Space Info Tip

For information about ElectroStatic Air Filter and OxyClean Air Filter, contact:

Crystal Enterprises,
770 Big Tree Dr., Building 114,
Longwood, FL 32750;
tel: 800-724-2220;
fax: 407-260-9690;
e-mail: webmaster@oxyfilters.com;
website: www.oxyfilters.com.

For Safe Zones 2500, 3500, and 4000:
AirFilters.net,
11905 NW 35th Street,
Coral Springs, FL 33065;
tel: 800-757-1836 or 954-752-1836;
fax: 954-752-0113;
e-mail: info@airfilters.net;
website: www.airfilters.net.

For Dust Fighter 95 and Bio-Fighter Anti-Microbial UV Light System (Nomad, Nomad 2, Triad):
Dust Free,
P.O. Box 519,
1112 Industrial,
Royse City, TX 75189;
tel: 800-441-1107;
fax: 800-929-9712;
website: www.dustfree.com.

drip and leg pain every morning found that these symptoms abated over the course of a few months once the unit was installed in his room.

An asthmatic child who started coughing the minute the home's central air conditioning blew dust through her room, had considerable reduction in her asthma attacks once a filter was in place. A woman said she no longer woke every morning with a sinus headache and dry sinuses; another user said the unit made it "so much easier to breathe" in her home; and still another said the filters reduced "moderately severe" allergies to house dust and animal fur.

Ultraviolet Light Air Purification

The idea behind this approach is to kill airborne pathogens with ultraviolet (UV) radiation, a naturally occurring frequency of light that has proven antimicrobial capabilities, especially against molds, bacteria, yeasts, and viruses. The Bio-Fighter Anti-Microbial UV Light System, for example, kills harmful microbes in the ductwork and air space of the home's HVAC system; it comes in four sizes, according to the size of the indoor environment needing purification. The device, which is installed in the ductwork or on either side of an A-coil, is meant to work alongside a dust filter or electrostatic air filter system already in place in a home. The UV light radiates a surface to prevent microbes from growing there, and it disinfects the airstream as it passes through the HVAC system. The "kill rate" for microbials passing through the UV light is fifteen percent to twenty percent with one UV lamp per single pass, according to the manufacturer, which adds that one lamp is normally enough to control microbial growth on the coils and drain pan of the HVAC system. Because indoor air is constantly recirculated, the kill rate is cumulative, and soon almost all the airborne pathogens are destroyed. UV light is basically safe for humans provided you do not look directly at the emitting source for more than five seconds; doing so can damage the eyes.

The Care 2000 Air Purifier is a device that combines HEPA air filtration and UV cleansing. It is billed as capable of removing mold, dander, odors, chemicals, dust mites, and virus and bacteria particulates with a system that changes the air six times an hour in a 1500-square-foot room. The UV features, says the manufacturer, make the unit especially advantageous for "vulnerable, immune-compromised, newborn, chronically ill, emphysemic, or bronchitic people."

The unit has five different filters, including a 10-micron particulate prefilter (to capture the big stuff, such as dust, pollen, dander, and mold particles); a fifteen-pound activated carbon filter (to absorb odors, gases, fumes, and VOCs); a 0.3-micron primary microfiltration 99.97% HEPA filter; a germicidal dual ultraviolet light, which constantly bathes the HEPA media, the other filters, and the air passing through them, killing any trapped microbes; and a carbon-impregnated post-filter, which reinforces the air cleansing performed by the first four filters.

HEALTHY LIVING SPACE DETOXIFIER #49
Install an "Indoor Waterfall" to
Add Negative Ions to Your Air

One of the popular ways of improving indoor air quality is through a negative ion generator, or what colloquially is referred to as an "indoor waterfall." Diffusing indoor ambient air with negative ions produces a refreshing, reinvigorating effect on the room's occupants similar to the excellent results you get from sitting before a plunging waterfall or breaking waves at the beach. Your body and its energy field are refreshed and healthfully stimulated with negative ions.

The term "negative ions" of course is confusing, for why is something with a positive value labelled negative? To answer that, we have to first understand what an ion is: a charged particle in the air produced when something forceful acts on a molecule (it could be carbon dioxide, nitrogen, water, or oxygen) such that it releases an electron. The molecule is now a positive ion, meaning, it's short an electron.

This now displaced electron attaches itself to the nearest available molecule, which becomes a negative ion—paradoxically now more than complete with the extra ion attached and thus capable of imparting a health benefit. It is the negative ions that exert the revitalizing effect, leading one commentator to dub them "vitamins of the air."

A negative ion generator takes advantage of this natural activity by emitting negative ions of oxygen, which once in the air collide with particulate matter (typically positive ions, such as dust, pollen, mold spores, bacteria, chemicals). The negative ions surrender their extra ions to the positively charged particles or positive ions (which, technically are deficient in ions, having lost some). Other positively charged particles start to surround this newly negatively charged particle, building up around it like a snowball. These react with dust and pollutants to form larger particles. Eventually, the "snowballs" of positive ions get too heavy to stay up in the air and fall to the floor where they can be vacuumed up.

The modern city and the tightly sealed office or apartment building act as "ion prisons," concentrating unhealthy levels of positive ions. Consider these sources of air pollution: car exhaust, factory fumes, dust, tobacco smoke, fumes from cooking and heating. All of these grab negative ions and either neutralize or convert them to positive ions.

The modern city and the tightly sealed office or apartment building act as "ion prisons," concentrating unhealthy levels of positive ions. Consider these sources of air pollution: car exhaust, factory fumes, dust, tobacco smoke, fumes from cooking and heating. All of these grab negative ions and either neutralize or convert them to positive ions. For example, the typical ion count of fresh country air is 2,000-5,000 negative ions per cubic centimeter (ccm); the negative ion count at big waterfalls, such as Yosemite Falls, is estimated to be 100,000 ccm. In contrast, indoor environments can have negative ion counts as low as 100 ccm.

Inside the buildings, the steel and concrete building materials also absorb all the negative ions, as do synthetic building materials, furniture coverings, clothing, metal ducts covering the ventilation outlets, and plastics (which emit a positive static charge). Air conditioned buildings and homes (as well as trains and planes) become laden with positive ions because the air conditioning system's metal blowers, filters, and ducts strip negative ions from the air before it is vented into the rooms.

You end up with an intensely positive-ion-dominated internal environment whose negative ion level may be below 100 ccm.

The minimum level considered supportive for top human functioning is about ten times that, or 1,000 ccm.

Positive ions exert numerous ill health effects. In a sense, they are the delivery system of the sick building syndrome and its effects. Research shows, for example, that they can alter the functioning of the human nervous system; induce a higher secretion of serotonin (the brain chemical associated with sleep, mood, nerve impulses); and slow down by thirty-three percent the sweeping action of tiny throat hairs and cut mucous flow, thereby lowering our resistance to airborne allergens.

Positive ions have been shown to raise blood pressure; decrease blood albumin; generate various allergy symptoms (dryness, burning, and itching of the nose, dry and scratchy throat, dizziness, breathing problems, eye irritations); decrease alertness; and increase depression, tension, irritability, and insomnia. Generally, the principal ill effects of positive ions are to produce tension and irritation, exhaustion, and an overstimulation of the thyroid gland (in the throat). The Santa Ana winds (the dry desert or sea winds, known by many different names worldwide) concentrate positive to negative ions at the rate of 33:1, producing numerous symptoms of physical and mental discomfort in people subjected to them.

Negative ions, in contrast, produce a great number of health benefits, according to more than 700 scientific papers. As early as 1932, researchers discovered that workers became ebullient when situated next to an electrostatic generator when it generated negative ions, but morose when it emanated positive ions. Subsequent research has shown that negative ions can reduce anxiety and neurosis, increase appetite and thirst, even stimulate sexual activity; they can sharpen reaction time, voluntary movement dexterity, and mental performance while reducing error rates.

Hyperactive children get calmer, students concentrate better, and teachers feel less fatigued when under the influence of negative ions. People report relief from allergies, migraines, and postoperative pains; infections and burns heal faster—apparently negative ions kill infection-propagating germs. Negative ions may also accelerate the blood's delivery of oxygen to the body's cells and enhance our ability to absorb and use oxygen.[76]

Other benefits of negative ions include reducing the severity of depression, counteracting the effects of tobacco smoke on mucous membranes, increasing work capacity, relieving allergy symptoms (such as sneezing, watery eyes, itchy nose, exhaustion from insomnia), providing an emotional lift, reducing germ counts (in one study, by fifty percent within six hours, by seventy percent in twenty-four hours), and disinfecting indoor air. Even better, houseplants growing under the influence of negative ions showed a marked increase in size and growth rate.[77]

There are numerous inexpensive portable or desktop-size negative ion generators now available on the consumer market. How do they work? Essentially, an extremely low current at a high voltage is applied to a group of sharp points known as the ion emitter within the device; electrons build up on these sharp points, then are ejected into the air and attach themselves to oxygen atoms. The electrons ejected have a negative charge, which means the oxygen molecules they attach to become negative ions. Here are some details on merely a few of the units available.

The Healthy Living Space Info Tip

For information about Electrocorp Zestron Ionair Ionizers, contact: Electrocorp, 595 Portal Street, Cotati, CA 94931; tel: 800-525-0711 or 707-665-9616, ext. 201; fax: 707-665-9620, ext. 201; e-mail: electrocor@aol.com; website: www.electrocorp.nu.

For IonAir Wein VI-2000 High Density Negative Ion Generator: The IonAir Company, Dept. Purify Online, 2574 North University Drive, Suite 201, Fort Lauderdale, FL 33322; tel: 800-478-7324; fax: 954-742-7882; website: www.purifyonline.com.

For Comtech Research units: Comtech Research, 4360 Walls Ford Road, Mansfield, MO 65704; tel: 417-741-6934; fax: 417-741-6056; e-mail: info@comtech-pcs.com; website: www.comtech-pcs.com/ions.

Electrocorp Zestron Ionair Ionizers

Various Electrocorp units may be used on a tabletop, in an automobile, greenhouse, laundry room, RV, truck, boat, or hotel room. The IG700 is a tabletop ionizer, but it can also be hung from a ceiling (IG1000). The IG200 works in a car and can be plugged into the cigarette lighter outlet. The IG300 and IG350 are fan-driven and work in a car or room. The IG900 is a desk model for use in an office or reception area. In terms of ion density emitted, the IG700, IG1000, and IG900 emit 4.5 million negative ions per ccm/second, measurable about three feet from the unit, while the IG300 and IG350 produce 500,000, and the IG200 produces 100,000. The units weigh between one and two pounds and can be purchased for around $150 each or less.

IonAir Wein VI-2000 High Density Negative Ion Generator

This unit is especially recommended (by its manufacturer) for relief of positive ion overload and radiation from working with computers and video displays. It is now scientifically recognized that long-term exposure to computer radiation and positive ion emission produces numerous symptoms, dubbed Video Operator Distress Syndrome. The symptoms include increased fatigue, eyestrain, blurred vision, rashes, headaches, back pain, irritability, depression, anxiety, and apathy. This unit covers a 400-square-foot area, plugs into any wall outlet, and can operate noiselessly on a desk next to the computer, emitting an estimated ion output of 70 trillion ions/second and an ion density of 1.6 trillion ions/cc at 2.5 cm from the device. The unit sells for about $110.

Comtech Research IG-033A

This unit, measuring 5 by 5 inches, can cover 400 square feet, or a room twenty feet by twenty feet, emitting an ion output estimated at 93 trillion ions/second and an ion density of 1.2 trillion ions/cc, and only 0.04 ppm of ozone close to the emitter. Comtech notes that it is safe to place the ionizer about four feet from your computer, safe in that it will not damage the computer yet still fill the air around it with negative ions.

HEALTHY LIVING SPACE DETOXIFIER #50
Use Houseplants to Filter Out Toxins from Your Indoor Air

One of the effective ways to improve indoor air quality may be something you already have in place in your home: houseplants. Joint research by the National Aeronautics and Space Administration (NASA) and the Associated Landscape Contractors of America beginning in the 1970s showed that common houseplants are capable of ridding indoor air of a variety of contaminants and VOCs. Somehow the plants are able to absorb the airborne toxins without ill effects to themselves and either deposit them in their leaves and roots, or in some cases, biodegrade the molecules into food.

In the NASA study, spider plants were placed in a closed chamber twelve cubic feet in size, the air of which contained either carbon monoxide at a concentration of 120 ppm or nitrogen oxide at a concentration of 50 ppm. NASA scientists observed that after twenty-four hours, the spider plants had removed ninety-six percent of the carbon monoxide and ninety-nine percent of the nitrogen oxide. They also found that the plant golden pothos was able to remove seventy-five percent of the carbon monoxide in the same time period.

Among the plants best suited for removing formaldehyde are aloe vera (ninety percent), elephant ear philodendron (eighty-six percent), and ficus (weeping fig, forty-seven percent). For removing benzene, there is English ivy (ninety percent), peace lily (eighty percent), Janet Craig (corn plant, seventy-nine percent), and golden pothos (sixty-seven percent). Also rated well for benzene removal are gerbera daisy and chrysanthemums. The peace lily can also remove fifty percent of the trichloroethylene from an indoor space in twenty-four hours, the study found.[78]

General Air Filtration

In terms of overall effectiveness in detoxifying indoor air, NASA ranks the houseplants in this order: heart leaf philodendron, elephant ear philodendron, green spider plant, lacy tree philodendron, aloe vera, golden pothos, Chinese evergreen, mini-schefflera, peperomia, and peace lily.

Formaldehyde

Plants with a large leaf surface area perform best in removing formaldehyde, the scientists found, and these include heart-leaf philodendron, elephant ear philodendron, green spider plant, lacy tree philodendron, golden pothos, Chinese evergreen, mini-schefflera, peperomia, peace lily, corn plant, snake plant, bromeliad, aloe vera, bamboo palm, pot mum, orchid, dumbcane, warneckii, Madagascar dragon tree, mass cane, poinsettia, weeping fig, variegated lily-turf, banana, azalea, Mother-in-Law's tongue, miniature umbrella plant, arrowhead plant, and oyster plant.

Small azalea plants can remove formaldehyde from a sealed chamber at the rate of about 1 ppm per hour, which is equivalent to 264 ug of formaldehyde. This means one azalea plant can remove 6,336 ug of formaldehyde per day from an office or home. To put this in perspective, the typical indoor air concentration of formaldehyde is about 5,436 ug, based on a contamination level of 0.2 ppm per 1,200 foot area.[79]

Toluene

Useful in removing this toxic chemical are Chinese evergreen and miniature umbrella plant.

Trichloroethylene

This toxic substance comes from dry cleaning, inks, paints, varnishes, lacquers, and adhesives, and can be effectively removed from indoor air by Gerbera daisy, chrysanthemum, peace lily, Warneckei, and marginata.

Benzene

This substance derives chiefly from tobacco smoke, gasoline fumes, synthetic fibers, plastics, inks, oils, and detergents. The following plants can help filter it out of your indoor air: English ivy, marginata, Janet Craig, chrysanthemum, Gerbera daisy, Warneckei, and peace lily.[80]

Carbon Monoxide

Spider plant and golden pothos can remove this toxic substance from indoor air.[81]

Orchids

The Dendrobium orchid can remove airborne pollutants such as acetone, methyl alcohol, and ethyl acetate as exhaled by humans. They can also remove xylene and carbon dioxide from indoor air and seem to be more effective at doing this when it is dark; they not only remove the toxins, but they also release oxygen. Used in conjunction with plants that filter air better during daylight hours (such as *Dracaena marginata*), the result is a stabilized day and night balance of carbon dioxide and oxygen in tightly sealed indoor environments.[82]

Hydroponically Grown Plants

As a variation on this approach, research developed at the University of Koln in Germany reports that plants grown by hydroculture (also called hydroponics, that is, in water, without any soil) are also effective in removing airborne toxins, notably formaldehyde, benzene, phenol, and nicotine.

Apparently, the plants are able to transform up to ninety percent of these pollutants into sugars, new plant material, and oxygen, rather than merely storing them in their own plant matter. Especially competent when used hydroponically are *Ficus benjamina* and golden pothos. Ficus and golden pothos together are effective against airborne nicotine, because the former removes nicotine and breaks it down (biodegrades it), while the latter stores nicotine in its growing leaves.

The German researchers said that you can "substantially" improve the plants' air-cleaning abilities by installing a special ventilator in their pots. This device acts as an air filter and draws indoor air over the roots for enhanced removal of toxins. The researchers further reported that one to two hydroponic plants can cleanse a room with an air space of 100 square feet. An additional advantage to using hydroponic plants used as air filters is that because they lack soil, they do not add fungus spores to the indoor air; this is a desirable factor for people with allergies. The plants also humidify the air, reducing the buildup of static electricity (or positive ions).[83]

Not everyone thinks plants are good toxic air filters. As a qualifying note, research since the NASA studies in the mid-1980s has challenged their findings, downgrading the ability of houseplants to filter out airborne toxins. Researchers at Ball State University in Muncie, Indiana, put plants in a sealed chamber and subjected the air to a continuously outgassing source of formaldehyde (particleboard). At the end of the trial, the ambient levels of formaldehyde were slightly lower, but nothing on the scale of the original NASA findings.

"The ability of over forty interior plants to remove various indoor air polluting chemicals from sealed chambers has been extensively tested and documented over the past ten years," declared B.C. Wolverton, Ph.D. in a 1992 report.

According to Lynn Marie Bower in *The Healthy Household*, if you have a great number of houseplants in a room or throughout your home, it raises the living space's relative humidity (from the regular watering), and insofar as formaldehyde outgasses faster in damp, high-humidity conditions, it may create suitable conditions for higher airborne concentrations of formaldehyde rather than lower. Further, it will probably take a lot of plants to duplicate NASA's botanical air filtering effect. In *Home Safe Home,* author Debra Lynn Dadd estimates that to get the same results that NASA reported you would need seventy-two plants for a nine-by-twelve-foot room.

Continuing research by B.C. Wolverton, Ph.D., director of Wolverton Environmental Services in Picayune, Mississippi, one of the NASA's principal researchers on this topic, tends to support the ability of plants to filter indoor air. He is the author of thirty-eight technical reports published by NASA and *How to Grow Fresh Air—50 Houseplants that Purify Your Home or Office*.

"The ability of over forty interior plants to remove various indoor air polluting chemicals from sealed chambers has been extensively tested and documented over the past ten years," he declared in a 1992 report. In 1993, Dr. Wolverton concluded that a low-light-requiring interior plant can remove "significant quantities" of formaldehyde, xylene, and ammonia from a sealed room. In 1996, one of his research colleagues reported that the accumulation of particulate matter (tiny particles of various chemicals) on horizontal surfaces inside a living space can be reduced by up to twenty percent by foliage plants.[84]

Even if the true air-filtering ability of plants is less than the NASA research indicates, your indoor air quality is bound to benefit considerably by having a fair amount of plant life around; the oxygen-releasing activity of houseplants in itself improves ambient air quality.

Clean Air Plant System

Here is a practical way to take advantage of the research linking indoor plants with air filtration. Sunshine Tropical Foliage in Homestead, Florida, has developed a combination houseplant, carbon charcoal filter, and small fan. The system uses one of five houseplants: White Bird of Paradise, Dracaena Marginata, Philodendron Xanadu, Spathiphyllum Supreme, or Golden Pothos Totem.

A small fan is placed inside a pot containing one of the plants. The filtration system draws room air down through the soil in the pot where the plant's roots trap the dust and particulate pollutants and, with help from the microorganisms in the soil, break them down into harmless substances. The air then passes through the charcoal filter and is exhausted back into the room as clean air.

According to Sunshine Tropical Foliage, if you run the unit twenty-four hours a day, it will change the indoor air in a typical 100-square-foot room about ten times. "That is more than adequate to give you good indoor air quality." The company claims the charcoal filter never needs to be replaced because the microorganisms around the plant's roots are "constantly eating the pollutants."

The Breathing Wall

This is a more ambitious, wall-sized solution to the problem of indoor air pollution and sick building syndrome, developed by Canadian scientist Wolfgang Amelung, director of Genetron Systems, Inc., of Downsview, Ontario. The Breathing Wall is an "indoor ecosystem" in the form of a sheet of moss and fern-covered lava rock, five feet high by fifteen feet long. It's kept constantly wet and is supported by an aquarium filled with fish and aquatic plants.

According to Genetron, there are fans behind the structure that draw the room's air across the plants and water, and through the "breathing wall," thereby absorbing the airborne pollutants. "Air passing nearby the continuously flowing water is filtered to remove water soluble pollutants and improve its overall quality," states Genetron. The Breathing Wall can be connected to a ventilation or air conditioning unit to distribute this plant-purified air throughout an entire building or home. The Breathing Wall is able to prevent unpleasant smells, allergens, and other contaminants (fumes, dust, fibers) from being released into a room's air.

As a filtration system, it "inhales sick air and exhales clean air." The Wall, says Dr. Amelung, is "a self-contained ecosystem in an enclosed space . . . like putting life on a planet that doesn't have life." The planet in this case is the sealed indoor living or work space.

The Breathing Wall was originally devised as a pilot project for a large Toronto-based insurance company's building. Called the Canada Life Environmental Room, it was an 1,100-square-foot meeting room featuring a Breathing Wall containing 8,000 different

---

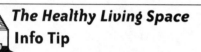

The Healthy Living Space Info Tip

For information about the Clean Air Plant System, contact:
Sunshine Tropical Foliage,
13805 SW 248 Street,
Homestead, FL;
tel: 305-251-6966;
fax: 305-257-1421;
e-mail: stf@netrus.net;
website:
www.zone10.com/tech/cleanair/cleanair.htm.

For information about the Breathing Wall, contact:
Genetron Systems, Inc.,
4801 Keele Street, Unit 34,
Downsview, Ontario M3J 3A4,
Canada;
tel: 416-665-8155;
fax: 416-665-8779;
website: www.flux.com/Genetron.

---

life forms, including mosses, ferns, orchids, and bulrushes, as well as frogs, insects, mollusks, salamanders, and fish. The wall was prepunctured with thousands of little holes through which ambient air could be drawn and filtered by the living organisms. The biological air cleaning system was later installed in other commercial settings and was studied by NASA for use in their proposed space station. Genetron reports that "the environmental quality in this partially sealed room is equal to that achieved by the most modern engineered system of air turnover."[85]

HEALTHY LIVING SPACE DETOXIFIER #51
Get the Radon Out of Your Basement

Not to be overlooked in our review of toxic elements in the home is radon, a gas derived from uranium and radium. Radon is a carcinogen linked with lung cancer, and it can enter a home through the basement or building foundation. Uranium, although it is found almost everywhere on the planet, is a radioactive element; it goes through a series of changes, changing into as many as a dozen other unstable elements until it settles into a stable form of lead. Radium is one of the in-between changes uranium makes, and radium, found in soil, emits a gas known as radon. While radon itself is a short-lived naturally occurring gas, sometimes existing for only a few days, it decays into various even more short-lived elements (or decay products) called radon progeny or "radon daughters," such as polonium, lead, and bismuth. You don't want these in your basement, and you definitely don't want to inhale them.

Radon is present in the outdoor atmosphere in highly dilute concentrations, so breathing it there causes no harm; but inside a building, its levels can concentrate to a toxic degree. Radon can be found in soil, rock under the home, well water, building materials, and loose underground pipe fittings; from any of these sources, it can enter the breathable air inside a living space. It seems that pressure differences between a home's interior (the inside of a tightly sealed construction) and the outside draws the radon gas into the home through existing cracks in the foundation. Then lack of adequate ventilation and fresh air circulation prevents the radon from getting diluted in the indoor air, and allows it to concentrate. Radon levels are usually higher below the ground than above.

It is helpful to think of radon exposure as somewhat akin to X-ray exposure. When the dangers of radon first came to national attention in the 1980s, it was through the unfortunate experience of a worker at a Pennsylvania nuclear plant who was triggering radiation alarms. What was puzzling was that his radiation exposure was not from the nuclear plant; rather, it came from a geologic formation called the Reading Prong, which had far higher than average radium concentrations, and the man's home sat over this radium factory. It turned out he and his wife were getting radon exposure at the equivalent of 455,000 chest X-rays per year—just by living in their home and breathing the radon-enriched indoor air.[86]

The cancer risk of radon exposure is well established. In fact, radon is now regarded as the second leading cause of lung cancer, the first being tobacco smoke. The National Cancer Institute (NCI) estimates that at least 15,000 people die of lung cancer due to residential radon each year. The NCI studied the morbidity data on 68,000 miners who were exposed to different levels of radon in their work and found they were dying of lung cancer at five times the expected rate for the general population. A 1998 mortality estimate by the National Academy of Sciences placed radon-caused cancer deaths at between 15,400 and 21,800 per year.[87]

According to a 1991 national residential radon survey conducted by the EPA, the average indoor radon level is 1.3 picocuries/liter (pCi/L) compared to 0.4 picocuries/liter outdoors. "Millions of homes and buildings contain high levels of radon gas," said the EPA in a 1996 fact sheet. How high is dangerous? The EPA says very high radon levels start at 10 pCi/L, and reports it has tested some homes at 30 pCi/L; levels between 2-10 pCi/L are "probably somewhat dangerous"; while "typical" indoor levels are 0.5-2 pCi/L, which might constitute a slightly increased risk. How dangerous is 4 pCi/L? If you're exposed to this level of radon, it's about thirty-five times as much radiation as the Nuclear Regulatory Commission would permit as a "safe" level if you stood at the fence of a radioactive waste site.

EPA advises that all homeowners should check their homes for radon, and homes in radon-intense regions of the country (with concentrations over 4 pCi/L) should not only test, but also take measures to correct the problem.

Regional Radon Reports

Want to find out if you're living in radon country? The Columbia University Department of Statistics and Lawrence Berkeley National Laboratory have prepared a highly detailed U.S. map of radon exposure levels, available on the following website: www.stat.columbia.edu/radon. Click on the part of the map corresponding to where you live, and the full-color map shows you the radon concentration in that area.

Another radon information database is offered by Air Check, Inc., which provides data per state, including the number of radon tests performed, average results, and a concentration report based on county. (See this website: www.radon.com/radon/radon_map.html; e-mail: info@radon.com) In Virginia, for example, 113,856 tests have been performed, with an average statewide radon level of 4.2 pCi/L, or "probably somewhat dangerous," according to EPA; 74.6% of the tests showed radon at less than 4.0 pCi/L and 19.5% of the results were 4.0-9.9 pCi/L. However, 73 tests (0.1% of total tests) showed radon levels above 100 pCi/L, indicating the state has some toxic radon neighborhoods.

Home Radon Testing

There are numerous local or regional radon testing services available for home radon monitoring, and simple home radon testing kits are available at hardware stores. Businesses that offer professional building inspections also may do radon tests. The tests may be based on short-term (a few days) or long-term (measured over many weeks) samples.

For an initial, short-term evaluation of your home's possible radon levels, AirChek offers a mail-in charcoal packet radon test, which they report has been used to determine radon levels in more than two million homes and 250,000 schoolrooms. The basic test takes ninety-six hours, but the company also has a long-term radon test kit (ninety days to one year). If your radon levels come in at the risk level, you might wish to proceed to a longer-term monitoring, or even to what is called a continuously operating radon gas monitor that provides you with "radon alerts" when ambient levels get too high.

If your radon level tests out above the EPA safety level, then you will need to engage professional radon

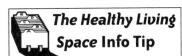

The Healthy Living Space Info Tip

For information about AirChek Radon Test kits, contact:
AirChek,
570 Butler Bridge Road,
Fletcher, NC 28732;
tel: 800-AIR-CHEK or
828-684-0893;
fax: 828-684-8498;
website: www.radon.com.

"mitigation" experts to develop a plan to rid your home of this gas; it may involve structural changes and/or the installation of specialized equipment. For example, you might need to install a radon ventilation system (to ventilate crawl spaces or the soil under the building's foundations) or to seal any foundation cracks that permit radon to enter the home's interior.

HEALTHY LIVING SPACE DETOXIFIER #52
Take the SADness Out of Your Indoor
Space with Full Spectrum Lighting

In thinking about the nontoxic, natural home and how to detoxify it, many people tend to overlook their lights. Light is a nutrient, and its absence can affect your health. The wrong kind of light can act as a toxin. Working indoors under standard fluorescent lights deprives you of the full spectrum light you need; living in an apartment in a big city also cuts down your exposure to natural sunlight. You get sunlight deprived as a result. You may know it as the winter blues, a season-long slump, a draining away of energy, vitality, and enthusiasm, and a corresponding desire for a quick—perhaps permanent—trip to the tropics.

The "winter blues" is now recognized as a legitimate medical condition known as seasonal affective disorder, or SAD for short (see figure 10-4). SAD refers to the measurable negative effect that a lack of natural sunlight has on the body and mind of the person deprived. Put simply, SAD is a light-mediated depression. The National Institute of Mental Health estimates that perhaps 10 million Americans suffer from SAD every year, while another 25 million are affected by a milder form of this dysfunction, which chiefly manifests as a seasonal depression and fatigue.

For example, an estimated one percent of people living in Florida experience SAD while ten percent of those living in Alaska have the problem. Other estimates place the incidence of SAD at ten percent of the general population of Northern New England, five percent of those living in the Baltimore-Washington, D.C., area and less than two percent of those living in Southern California.

Other symptoms of SAD include a desire for extra sleep accompanied by a failure to feel more rested from the expenditure under the covers; increased appetite and irresistible food

---

Figure 10-4. Typical Symptoms of SAD—Seasonal Affective Disorder

Depression	Memory loss
Increased appetite	Concentration problems
Need for extra sleep	Indecisiveness
Inability to feel rested	Low self-esteem
Irresistible food cravings	Thoughts of suicide
Weight gain	Anxiety
Menstrual discomfort	Irritability or violent outbursts
Social withdrawal tendencies	Sluggishness, tendency to being sedentary
Sadness to the point of grief	Feeling of hibernation
Diminished sexual drive	Season-long dose of jet-lag
Body aches and pains	

---

cravings, especially for carbohydrates (sugars, starches, alcohol), which lead to undesired, unneeded weight gain; diminished sex drive; body aches or pains; memory loss; concentration problems; indecisiveness; low self-esteem; suicidal thoughts; anxiety; and irritability, even to the extent of violent outbursts. Physical activity decreases, and one feels sluggish and sedentary. In women—seventy-five percent of SAD sufferers are female—SAD can produce a worsening of menstrual discomfort; in both men and women, it can create a desire to withdraw from the world and to avoid social contacts. SAD sufferers feel sad, sometimes to the point of grief.

You almost feel as if you have entered a period of winter hibernation—or would like to. Most people feel a diluted form of some of the SAD symptoms as a natural response to winter, but people with SAD are hypersensitive to these changes and suffer the physiological impact of reduced sunlight in a more intense form.

Another way to look at SAD is that it is a season-long dose of jet lag. Your body's internal clock gets thrown off by the steadily diminishing amount of daily sunlight (the shorter days of winter) and gets disoriented. Another way to put it is that the decreasing length of the "photoperiod," that part of the twenty-four-hour cycle in which natural sunlight is available, generates the symptoms of SAD.

SAD appears to deliver its negative effects through the hormonal system, specifically melatonin, a key player in the body's biological clock. People with SAD are said to have a disturbance in their biological clock; it runs slow—or too slow—in the winter. A sunlight deficiency leads to a reduction in the secretion of melatonin by the brain's pineal gland; melatonin is crucial to the body's sleep/wake cycle.[88]

The chief recommended therapy for SAD is called bright light therapy, which means being exposed to full spectrum bright lights from one-half hour to three hours daily during the winter months. The light is conveyed by way of full spectrum fluorescent bulbs or special light boxes. The concept behind light therapy is that the bright light helps to reset the biological clock and thereby restore normal physiological (and pineal gland-melatonin) function. For those with mild SAD symptoms, a device called a dawn/dusk simulator can be effective; this device gradually raises the light of a lamp over a preset time period, imitating the arrival of morning light.

It's important to realize that light is a nutrient, like food, air, and water, and that full spectrum light is the best photo-nutrient. "Our eyes are not only organs of sight, but they are also photo receptors for the brain glands," comments Nicholas Harmon, the president of Verilux, a company based in Stamford, Connecticut, that makes various full spectrum lighting devices (see below). "These glands produce hormones which affect our mood, health, and sense of well-being."[89]

Light Boxes

Typically, the therapeutic light exposure is at 2,500 lux (a technical measure of brightness), which is five times brighter than the average "well lit" office and twenty-five times brighter than the average living room, which can be as low as 100 lux (although normal indoor light is stated to be about 300-500 lux). Light boxes that emit 10,000 lux produce resolution of SAD symptoms even faster. To put this all in context, bright summer sunlight emits 100,000 lux.

The user sits or stands about two feet from the box; or you can place the light box in any part of the house where you are likely to perch for a time while awake, such as a home office, library, den, kitchen. "The light box provides a measured amount of balanced spectrum light equivalent to standing outdoors on a clear spring day."[90] The light enters the body through the eyes, which transmit the photonutrients to the brain where they help reset the body's internal clock. A typical self-treatment is thirty minutes at 10,000 lux or one hour at 5,000 lux once a day.[91] Generally, a SAD person begins to notice a response—many describe it as "energizing"—within two to four days of beginning light therapy, and the "cure" is often complete within two weeks.[92]

The North Star 10,000 Bright Light Box provides 10,000 lux at 26 inches, requiring the user to sit in front of it (the box measures 13" high by 24" long by 4" deep) for about thirty minutes daily to get the optimal benefit. The Ott-Lite, developed by pioneering "photobiologist" John Nash Ott, Ph.D., is a full spectrum device in the form of a desktop lamp, a clamp-on portable light, or a light box of 2,500 or 10,000 lux strengths.

Amjo Sunrise II and III are light boxes that have an adjustable lux strength; you can have 10,000 lux at 12 inches, 18 inches, or 24 inches, depending on how many bulbs are turned on inside the box. Amjo notes that they wrap a special tape around the base of the tubes to reduce or eliminate electrical, RF, or UV radiation from the cathode tubes, and that the tubes are hum and flicker-free. The Brite Lite IV from Apollo Light Systems provides 10,000 lux at 26 inches and has an electronic ballast on the tubes that eliminates the flicker and magnetic emissions typical of conventional tubes.

Full-Spectrum Fluorescent Tubes

If your home (or office) has conventional strip fluorescent lights, you might want to consider replacing them with full-spectrum lights. This way you eliminate a potentially toxic factor from your living space and introduce a health-promoting one at the same time.

Dr. Ott's early research on the relationship between light and human health revealed that standard partial-spectrum fluorescent lights were actually detrimental to health. He found that he

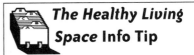

The Healthy Living Space Info Tip

For information about North Star 10,000 Bright Light box, contact: Alaska Northern Lights, P.O. Box 1801, Homer, AL 99603; tel: 907-235-6953 or 800-880-6953; fax: 907-235-7665; e-mail: nlights@xyz.net; website: www.alaskanorthernlights.com.

For Brite Lite IV: Apollo Light Systems, 352 West 1060 South, Orem, UT 84058; tel: 800-545-9667 or 801-226-2370; e-mail: info@apollolight.com; website: www.apollolight.com.

For Sunrise II, III, and Dawn Simulators: Amjo Corp., P.O. Box 8304, West Chester, OH 45069; tel: 513-942-2770 or 877-289-2656; fax: 513-942-2771; e-mail: support@sadlight.com; website: www.sadlight.com.

For Vita-Lite: Natural Lighting.com, 1939 Richvale, Houston, TX 77062; tel: 281-486-9583 or 888-900-6830; fax: 281-486-0352; e-mail: larry@naturallighting.com; website: www.naturallighting.com.

For Ott-Lites: Environmental Lighting Concepts, Inc., 3923 Coconut Palm Drive, #101, Tampa, FL 33619; tel: 800-842-8848 or 813-621-0058; fax: 813-626-8790; website: www.ott-lite.com.

The Healthy Living Space Info Tip

For Natural Spectrum light bulbs:
Verilux, 9 Viaduct Road,
Stamford, CT 06907;
tel: 203-921-2430 or 800-786-6850;
fax: 203-921-2427;
e-mail: verilux@ergolight.com;
website: www.ergolight.com.

could not successfully grow plants indoors under artificial lights and that the cathode radiation emitted by common fluorescent tubes made his plants mutate and form unnaturally.

Dr. Ott further discovered that artificial partial-spectrum light is another form of potentially dangerous indoor pollution. It illuminates more intensely on the yellow part of the color spectrum and can cause eyestrain and eye fatigue. Further, said Dr. Ott, light from fluorescent tubes (as well as from televisions and computer monitors) can cause red blood cells to clump together after a long-term exposure. The clumping then contributes to reduced mental alertness and a sense of chronic tiredness.

Natural sunlight, or full-spectrum lighting, in contrast, stimulates the red blood cells to unclump and does not strain or fatigue the eyes. Research suggests that full-spectrum lighting can improve your mood. When he installed radiation-shielded, full-spectrum lights in schools, Dr. Ott observed a significant reduction in behavioral problems and learning disabilities and an improvement in academic performance. Other research has supported Dr. Ott's findings. Canadian psychologist Warren E. Hathaway, Ph.D., studied 327 school children in five different elementary schools and found that under full-spectrum lighting they had fewer dental cavities, better attendance, higher rates of academic achievement, and greater physical development than students in classrooms with standard fluorescent tube lighting.[93]

"Full spectrum lighting, containing all wavelengths, sparks the delicate impulses which regulate brain and autonomic functions of the body, regulating these functions and maintaining health," comments John Downing, O.D., Ph.D., director of the Light Therapy Department at the Preventive Medical Center of Marin in Santa Rosa, California. "In order to maintain health, it is important to be exposed to light containing the full wavelength spectrum found in natural sunlight."[94]

Replacing conventional fluorescent tubes with full-spectrum, radiation-shielded ones can make simulated light a nutrient for your system. Vita-Lite, for example, "simulates the full color and ultraviolet spectrum of sunlight," according to the manufacturer who reports that these lights have been used in thousands of schools, medical care facilities, factories, banks, dental offices, retail establishments, grocery stores, and florist shops.

Healthy Light Bulbs

Verilux has developed Natural Spectrum light bulbs that they describe as "the closest replication of natural sunlight available." According to Verilux, their bulbs show the colors of the spectrum accurately in accordance with natural light, increase the contrast between black and white, and thereby reduce eye strain, glare, and ocular fatigue.

Dawn Simulators

These are programmable units (set to a specified wake-up time by the user) that can emit up to 400 watts of incandescent light. The Pi-Square SunUp and SunRizr by Amjo are examples of this approach, and are recommended for waking up refreshed on dark winter mornings.

The idea is to simulate the dawning and duration of natural sunlight so that your bedroom gradually brightens in the morning (presumably in the deep of SAD-flavored winter). The dawn-simulated light can either be directed at the user's pillow or indirectly elsewhere in the room; an ideal situation, says Amjo, is track lighting with three to eight 50-watt bulbs directly over, but about three to four feet above, the sleeper's head. The dawn simulator activates the lights according to its timer schedule, and you can set this timer so that the light reaches its full intensity in anywhere between one minute to three hours.

According to Sheri Lundstrom, founder of Light Therapy Products of Plymouth, Minnesota, and an admitted SAD sufferer, the dawn simulator prompts the brain's pineal gland to start stimulating the feel-good hormone, serotonin. Light is crucial in the production of serotonin, and serotonin is essential to the body because it influences numerous aspects of our physiology, such as pain,

Dr. Ott's research on the relationship between light and human health revealed that standard partial-spectrum fluorescent lights were actually detrimental to health. He further discovered that artificial partial-spectrum light is another form of potentially dangerous indoor pollution and can cause eyestrain and eye fatigue.

digestion, body temperature, blood pressure and clotting, immunity, sleep, and daily body rhythms.

But the shorter days of northern latitude winters, buildings with no outside windows, frequent cloudy skies, or not spending much time outside in the winter leads to a serotonin depletion and its host of symptoms. This is why Lundstrom characterizes light therapy as a "natural Prozac" for winter depression. She comments: "Research subjects have shown marked improvement in energy, mood, social interest, productivity, quality of sleep, and quality of awakening with dawn simulation."[95]

HEALTHY LIVING SPACE DETOXIFIER #53
Go Green with Your Household Products

From a certain perspective, it seems that most commercial products that are supposed to make our lives run smoother, more efficiently, and with more ease end up being potentially toxic for us. This is especially so if you are already allergic or chemically reactive to many of the fixtures of modern life, and it is acutely so if you have symptoms of sick building syndrome or multiple chemical sensitivities.

Many of the items we take for granted actually contain allergenic or toxic elements. These items household products (air fresheners, cleaners, bleaches, dishwashing detergents, floor wax, drain cleaners, carpet shampoos, laundry fabric softeners, oven cleaners, toilet bowl cleansers), paints, stains, thinners, home and garden pesticides, pet supplies (flea collars, cat litter, flea and tick products), auto products, art and craft supplies, cosmetics and personal care products, perfumes and colognes, hair conditioners and shampoos, dental and oral hygiene products, feminine hygiene products, nail polish, and skin products (deodorants, shaving creams).

The simple, possibly shocking, fact is that most of these products contain known toxins—some are poisons on purpose, such as disinfectants and pesticides—and when you use them you are exposing yourself to a poison, either through skin contact or by breathing in the product's vapors. Your exposure may be minimal and not necessarily produce an immediate or noticeable reaction, but you need to think in terms of long-range effects. Toxic exposure is often cumulative; the toxins remain in your system, and your liver is unable to remove them. Eventually your body is overloaded by a number of toxins, and you get sick. Perhaps you get an allergy first, then a gastrointestinal problem, then a hormonal imbalance, and eventually worse, more debilitating and chronic conditions emerge.

The matter of toxicity in common household and personal products is relative to the individual. Various governmental authorities, such as the EPA, have standards for "safe" levels of presumed or proven toxic elements in commercial products, but these standards are based on averages, norms for human biochemical tolerance. Your tolerance may fall above or well below these averages.

If you are healthy, detoxified, and fortified with nutrients, there is a strong chance your system can tolerate more exposure to toxins than the average. But if you are already allergic, and your immune system and liver are stressed by chronic exposure to toxic substances, one more toxin—from something as seemingly innocuous as your automatic dishwasher detergent—could send you down into a new level of dysfunction and ill health. You tolerated the first six toxic exposures, but the seventh made you sick. Your body's total toxic burden was exceeded.

Unfortunately, once you are chemically reactive or chronically allergic to human-made substances, it starts to extend to other items you wouldn't think could be harmful, yet, for you, they are. You need to concern yourself with furniture, upholstery, curtains, vacuum cleaners, bedding, clothes, even, in extreme cases, the ink used in books and magazines.

Given these physiological facts, it is prudent to carefully consider the products with which you customarily surround yourself in your home. Are they full of toxic chemicals? Do they contain known or suspected carcinogens? Is there evidence that they can produce allergies or symptoms that fall under the various medical categories of chronic fatigue, fibromyalgia, environmental illness, sick building syndrome, and multiple chemical sensitivity? If so, it's time to start thinking green—that is, thinking in terms of environmentally friendly products. But remember, there are two environments here: the outside world, which includes your home, and your body, which is your inner environment. An environmentally friendly, green product does not pollute either; many conventional household and personal products do.

The problem is the synthetic organic chemicals they contain. Today, an estimated 75,000 chemicals are in use in commercial products. Of these, only 1.5% to 3.0% (or 1,200 to 1,500) have been tested for carcinogenicity, that is, to see if they can cause cancer. So far, about 200 have been identified as carcinogens. But in 1995, the National Toxicology Program stated that somewhere between 5% and 10% of the existing industrially used chemicals could be carcinogenic, based on the 1.5-3.0% of chemicals they had tested. In other words, 3,750 to 7,500 chemicals found in products we might encounter or use could be carcinogenic.[96]

Since nobody knows yet which of the remaining 75,000 chemicals are carcinogenic, how will you know if you're using one? Worrying about cancer isn't even the chief concern here. The minute a chemical produces an allergic reaction, such as a sneeze, a rash, a gastrointestinal upset, your body is telling you—your liver actually—that it doesn't like this substance and considers it inappropriate for further contact. Either it doesn't want to or can't detoxify the substance and throws out an allergic reaction as notification of the fact. Allergies are the first act in a health tragedy that can lead to dozens of different dysfunctional conditions, including but not limited to cancer.

How can a chemical that's labeled "organic" be harmful to my health? It all comes down to petroleum, which, technically, is a natural, organic product, being derived ultimately from plant substances. Many of the toxic products contain petroleum as a base, employing its hydrocarbon composition (combinations of hydrogen and carbon atoms); hence the terms petrochemical and organic chemical. Yet these organic chemicals are synthesized, invented, as it were; hence the term synthetic.

In nature, for each compound there is an enzyme that can break it down and neutralize it, but in the case of synthetic organic chemicals, no balancing natural enzymes exist to break them down because the chemicals themselves have been added to nature, not derived from it. This means petrochemicals persist in the environment for a long time; it also means they can persist in the human body, producing illness.

"Organic chemicals are some of the most hazardous substances ever made," states a fact sheet published by Seventh Generation, a supplier of green products based in Burlington, Vermont. "The average household contains 63 different organic chemical products for a total of approximately ten gallons of hazardous petrochemicals . . . [and] most of them are found in an unlikely place—common household cleaners."

Here are a few examples of how common household products can be toxic. Window cleaners contain diethylene glycol, which depresses the nervous system. Toilet bowl cleaners contain chlorinated phenols, which are known to be toxic to the circulatory and respiratory systems. The phenols often found in disinfectants are harmful to these two systems as well. Laundry detergents and all-purpose cleaners often contain a chemical called nonyl-phenol-ethoxylate, which biodegrades slowly and into even more toxic compounds than itself.

You will find formaldehyde in some spray and wick deodorants; this chemical (discussed earlier) is a suspected carcinogen and a known irritant of the respiratory system. The petroleum solvents found in floor cleaners can damage mucous membranes. A substance commonly found in stain removers, called perchloroethylene, has been proven to cause damage to the kidneys and liver. Butyl cellosolve, a synthetic chemical you'll find in various cleaners, damages bone marrow, the kidneys, liver, and nervous system.[97] This is just the beginning of a long list of offenders.

Let's consider fabric softeners in detail. Thanks to EPA research collated by Julia Kendall (a multiple chemical sensitivity sufferer), former co-chair of Citizens for a Toxic-Free Marin (California), we know that at least nine toxic chemicals are found in many brands of this product.

A typical fabric softener can contain alpha-terpineol (causes central nervous system [CNS] disorders, irritates mucous membranes, can cause edema, loss of muscular coordination, headache); benzyl acetate (a pancreatic carcinogen that irritates eyes and breathing passages); benzyl alcohol (causes headache, vomiting, nausea, dizziness, blood pressure drops); camphor (causes CNS disorders, dizziness, confusion, nausea, twitching, convulsions); chloroform (a neurotoxin and carcinogen, vapors can cause headache, nausea, vomiting, drowsiness, kidney/liver damage); ethyl acetate (causes headache, stupor, anemia, liver/kidney damage); limonen (a carcinogen); linalool (a narcotic, causes CNS disorders, affects muscle and heart activity); and pentane (depresses the CNS, causes headache, nausea, vomiting, dizziness, eye irritation, skin rash). Incidentally, this is only a partial listing of the symptoms each of these nine substances can cause.[98]

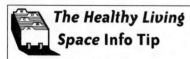

The Healthy Living Space Info Tip

For more information about and sources of environmentally-friendly, non-toxic, green household products: Seventh Generation, One Mill Street, Box A-26, Burlington, VT 05401; tel: 802-658-3773; fax: 802-658-1771; e-mail: recycle@seventhgen.com; website: www.seventhgen.com.

See also:
Real Goods, 200 Clara Street, Ukiah, CA 95482; tel: 800-762-7325, 800-994-4243, or 707-468-9292; fax: 800-508-2342; website: www.realgoods.com.

For information about and sources of products for environmentally safe and low-toxic building and interiors: Shelter Ecology, 43 Pine Ridge Road, Asheville, NC 28804; tel & fax: 828-251-5888; e-mail: sheltereco@aol.com; website: www.ioa.com/~shelterecology.

For information about household products from an advocacy organization: Environmental Health Network, P.O. Box 1155, Larkspur, CA 94977; tel: 415-541-5075; e-mail: wilworks@lanminds.com; website: www.users.lmi.net/wilworks.

Next consider the relationship between toxicity and the ingredients in various common fragrance-based (scented) household products. Examples of these are perfume, soap, shaving cream, deodorant, air freshener, hairspray, hand lotion, Vaseline lotion, after-shave, and many more similar products.

Acetone, found in cologne, dishwashing liquid, and nail polish remover, is a CNS depressant and can cause dryness of the mouth and throat, dizziness, nausea, slurred speech, even coma in severe cases. Benzaldehyde, found in perfume, cologne, hairspray, laundry bleach, deodorants, shaving cream, shampoo, and dishwasher detergent, is a CNS depressant, is irritating to all mucous membranes and the gastrointestinal tract, and can damage the kidneys. Even though FDA banned the use of methylene chloride in 1988, it can still show up in products because the chemical fragrance industry is protected by ingredient secrecy laws. Methylene chloride is a carcinogen, producing carbon monoxide in the body and reducing the blood's ability to transport oxygen. Again, this is just a brief review of the long list of toxic household products.[99]

Care for perfume? Perhaps you won't after reviewing some of the toxic constituents that may be found in various perfumes and fragrances. In general, perfumes may contain upwards of 5,000 natural or synthetic sources of sweet smells, of which, as of 1991, 84% have not been tested for toxicity to humans, or tested only minimally. Scents, incidentally, show up not just in perfume, but cosmetic and hygienic products, drugs, detergents, cleaning products, plastics, industrial greases, oils, solvents, and even foods. The National Academy of Sciences, back in 1986, targeted fragrances as one of six categories of chemicals requiring testing for neurotoxicity, that is, for their capacity to damage the nervous system. The other five groups included food additives, heavy metals, air pollutants, insecticides, and solvents.

Some of the chemicals found in fragrances have been identified as neurotoxic, carcinogenic, or capable of producing birth defects, while a few have even been designated "hazardous waste disposal chemicals," according to EPA standards. Of a list of 2,983 chemicals (a partial list) used by the fragrance industry, 884 of them were identified as toxic substances. Toluene, a chemical we first encountered earlier in this chapter in toxic carpets, is a big player in the fragrance industry, found in every fragrance sample in a 1991 EPA study, as well as in auto parts stores and in the fragrance sections of department stores. Toluene, among other things, is linked with asthma attacks, and it can trigger asthma episodes even in people who never previously had respiratory symptoms. Insofar as a 1986 study showed that seventy-two percent of asthma patients have adverse reactions to perfume, one reasonably wonders if the seeming ubiquity of toluene is a major factor in new cases of asthma.[100]

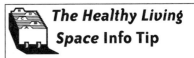

The Healthy Living Space Info Tip

For more on how-to recommendations for "less toxic living," see: www.betterbasics.com, edited by Annie Berthold-Bond.

In fact, the statistics on perfume and human health are very surprising, even the basis of advocacy movements to ban fragrances in public places. The American Lung Association states that 14.6 million Americans every year sustain a dangerous and/or painful reaction to fragrance chemicals in the form of an asthma attack; 5,000 of these people die from the effects of the asthma attack. Louisiana state medical officials reported that twenty percent of asthmatics in their state undergo an asthma attack as a result of exposure to perfumes or fragrances.

Rosalind Anderson, research director of Anderson Laboratories (visited above under toxic carpets) reports that laboratory mice experienced neurotoxic effects, pulmonary irritation, and airflow limitation as a direct response to being exposed to fragrances. In her view, this evidence was sufficient to advise humans to stop using fragrances, suggesting that sensitivity may be cumulative; you may not be chemically reactive today, but keep using the various scented household products for five or ten years (or months), and you may be.[101]

Don't stop your review of household toxins with the perfumes and scented products. There may be problems with your bedding. If your mattress is made of polyurethane foam plastic—your innerspring mattress can also be wrapped in this substance—this has most likely been sprayed with chemical fire retardants and has a covering of polyester plastic fabric. Exposure to polyurethane foam outgassing has been linked with bronchitis, skin and eye irritations, and coughing. This is probably due in large part to the fact that it outgasses toluene diisocyanate, a toxin known to produce respiratory problems. In effect, every time you lie down on your bed and, by your body weight, apply pressure on the mattress, you may be forcing the outgassing of this and other toxic chemicals into the bedroom's indoor air.

Further, if you have a polyester mattress pad, polyester pillow, polyester comforter, and if you use polyester sheets, you are exposing yourself to additional toxins. That's because the sheets may be treated with a permanent press finish based on formaldehyde. "Amid this cloud of plastic vapors, is it any wonder that millions of Americans take drugs to get to sleep at night?" comments nontoxic solutions expert Debra Lynn Dadd.[102] She might as well have added: Is it any wonder an estimated fifteen percent of Americans are hypersensitive to common household products?

The key principle with respect to toxic household products is simple and twofold: avoid and substitute. Don't use ones that contain synthetic chemicals (or at least reduce your use of them and thus your exposure to their contents) and find nontoxic green substitutes, of which there are many. When you have a choice between natural and nontoxic versus conventional and toxic, be prudent and go green. In many cases, you don't need to have a commercially prepared green substitute to go green; there are many homemade nontoxic solutions to standard household cleaning and personal care concerns.

This is by now a well-researched subject and a handful of excellent books detail your options. You might consider these as starters: *Home Safe Home*, by Debra Lynn Dadd (1997); *Better Basics for the Home*, by Annie Berthold-Bond, (1999), and *Clean House, Clean Planet*, by Karen Logan (1997).

CHAPTER 11

The Feng Shui of a Healthy Home:

Detoxifying the Energy Aspects of Your Living Space

As I write this, spring is imminent, and with it, the need to thoroughly air out my two-story home. As the weather warms up and the heater gets turned off for the season, all the doors and windows can be opened wide to encourage fresh spring air to rush through the interior space and blow out all the stagnant furnace-heated indoor air. My house has many windows, and they are situated in such a way that air can blow straight through the house, from the back porch to front garden. There are no troubling curves or strange corners or dead-end corridors where the air can get either trapped or slowed down. With all this fresh air cleansing my interior space, I am bound to feel invigorated every time I am inside now, and I will have more of a *feeling* for the outside while I'm indoors—I won't feel so shut in against the cold.

Airing one's house in the springtime of course is not a new idea, but it is a useful image to get across an idea central to the practical guidelines in this chapter: the role—and *circulation*—of energy in an indoor space. By energy, I don't mean gas, oil, electricity, or any other physically tangible form of energy; rather, I mean something more subtle, yet still one that can be sensed and adjusted.

In China, it's called *qi* (pronounced *chee*; also spelled ch'i), and in traditional Chinese medicine (and its vast philosophical foundations) it has a pivotal role as the prime agent of healing and health. In terms of a healthy living space, the circulation of *qi* in environments, both indoors and outdoors, is regulated by a practical discipline gaining increasing popularity and application in North America and known as feng shui (pronounced *fung schway*). This chapter will explore some of the many ways this vital energy can be used both to detoxify your indoor living space and to make it one that imparts health.

Charting the Movement of Life Force Energy

Before going any further, let's be sure we have a sense of the meaning of the two concepts of *qi* and feng shui.

The broadest observation we can make here is that both come out of a profound cosmological model put forth by classical China. This model encompassed heaven and earth, energy and matter, thoughts and emotions, health and illness, and had many practical applications including music, landscape utilization and architecture (feng shui), medicine (acupuncture), diet, herbology, physiology, meditation and "internal alchemy" (Taoism), philosophy (*I-Ching*, or the *Book of Changes*), and energy management on all levels. At the heart of all these applications is energy, or *qi*.

Qi is a Chinese word variously translated to mean "vital energy," "essence of life," and "living force." (In other cultures, it is known variously as *prana*, *dynamis*, od, orgone, and other names.) Generally, it's easiest to think of it as essential life force energy and to appreciate that it has a role in our body (managed through acupuncture) as well as our house and its surroundings (managed through feng shui).

In Chinese medicine, the proper (balanced) flow of *qi* along energy channels (meridians) within the body is crucial to a person's health and vitality. There are many types of *qi*, classified according to source, location, and function (such as activation, warming, defense, transformation, and containment). Within the body, *qi* and blood are closely linked, because each is considered to flow through the body along with the other. *Qi* may be stagnant (non-moving), deficient (partially absent), or excessive (inappropriately abundant) in a given organ system. *Qi* has two essential qualities: *yang* (active, fiery, moving, bright, energizing) and *yin* (passive, watery, stationary, dark, calming). The manipulation and readjustment of *qi* to treat disease and ensure maximum health benefit is the basic principle of acupuncture, although other remedies and therapies can be used to influence *qi*.

In a simplistic sense, feng shui is a form of acupuncture applied to environments, both interior and exterior. Feng shui means "wind" (*feng*) and "water" (*shui*), and evokes a sense of the constant movement and interplay of these two elements in a natural environment. In practical terms today, people tend to take the term to mean "the art of placement," in reference to designing interior spaces to maximize the health benefits. According to scholars, the term "feng shui" has been used only for the last one hundred years, and this complex science of energy and landscape was earlier known as *Kan Yu*, which means time theory (*kan*) and geographical theory (*yu*), and addresses the flow and change of *qi* through a landscape over time. *Qi* is a living, dynamic energy, constantly moving and changing.

Kan Yu, according to one expert, is about the study of the environment, both inside and out, both natural and constructed. The term evokes this state of mind: "Raise the head and observe the sky above. Lower the head and observe the environment around us."[1]

Kan Yu properly concerns itself with the location and orientation of a site, whether it is a room, home, garden, pagoda, city, or grave. The proper place for a site is dependent on "a complex interaction of location and direction of topographical and artificial features" as charted over time, explains another expert, Thomas Lee, a chartered land and hydrographical surveyor based in Hong Kong. "The technique of *Kan Yu* is mainly concentrated on the observation of surrounding features and understanding the flow of '*Qi*' in terms of time. Energy is therefore believed to flow periodically, cycling hourly, monthly, or annually, etc., under a rigid mathematical formula that has been applied for over thousands of years," explains Lee.[2]

The purpose of this energy flow is to balance and harmonize environments. "The degree of harmony in an individual place is solely dependent on the balance of Yin and Yang (Ch'i) in the theory," says Lee. Even though *qi* is invisible and hard to detect by conventional means, he adds, "it is an energy which brings good influence to the living organisms within its influence."[3]

The idea here is that *qi* not only flows through an environment (a landscape or a home), but it *changes*, with the seasons, the planetary influences, with the use given to that environment (e.g., a polluted landscape, a cluttered house or a clean, well-ordered one). The practical goal is to be aware of these flow changes and to utilize them for the health and well-being of those living in them. In the Chinese model, the benefits of maximizing the flow of *qi* include not only health, but prosperity, longevity, family and community cohesiveness, even political stability. "Utilizing these principles, people are creating comfortable, safe, and re-energizing environments for themselves and the people who visit their buildings or dwellings." When feng shui principles are applied, the results are "happier attitudes, more prosperity, more sense of harmony and balance, an improvement in health and well-being."[4]

Although this chapter focuses only on the movement of *qi* through a living space, it is instructive to appreciate the *wide* scope of Chinese thinking on energy flow, one that takes in the entire world, from bedroom to planet. Regarding the living space, feng shui looks at numerous factors, including the site; the orientation of the house (or apartment); the layout of the rooms; the qualities of light, air, and heat circulation; the placement of the furniture; the layout of individual rooms; and architectural shapes and angles within the house.

All of these factors, and many more not cited here, have marked health effects on the people living under their influence. These effects can be toxic or health enhancing. Recall, if you will, my opening example of airing the house in springtime. It is not only air that I invite to flow through

Regarding the living space, feng shui looks at numerous factors, including the site; the orientation of the house (or apartment); the layout of the rooms; the qualities of light, air, and heat circulation; the placement of the furniture; the layout of individual rooms; and architectural shapes and angles within the house. All of these factors have marked health effects on the people living under their influence.

my house when I fling open the windows and doors; *qi* will flow into the house with the air. If my house is laid out properly, the *qi* will reach every corner, flow through every room, and invigorate every aspect of my living space; but if my house is laid out poorly (as are many, if not most, modern North American homes), the *qi* flow will be blocked, compromised, curtailed, or rendered stagnant, and my living space will become a health-deteriorating one.

Bear in mind, because this is only an image to get an idea across, *qi* flows, or is blocked from flowing, in a house regardless of whether the windows and doors are open; everything in your house and the house itself either helps or hinders its flow on a moment-to-moment basis, and as the *qi* flows, so goes your health.

HEALTHY LIVING SPACE DETOXIFIER #54
Evaluate the Energy Flow in
Your Home with the Ba-Gua

How is one to know if one's house or apartment has good or bad feng shui, has *qi* flowing or stagnating? Increasingly, North Americans are seeking the advice of qualified feng shui advisors to evaluate their living spaces to answer this precise question.

One of the evaluation tools commonly used by feng shui practitioners is a standardized energy template or blueprint called the *Ba-Gua* (also spelled *Pa-Kua*). It is a kind of generic map of the ideal flow of *qi* through an interior environment, dividing this space into eight sections. Fortunately, you don't have to be a feng shui expert to compare the layout of your living space with the ideal *qi* template of the *Ba-Gua*.

The *Ba-Gua* is a complex symbol, based on complex ideas. In a simplistic sense, suitable for our purposes of home detoxification, it's useful to know that at its core is the yin/yang symbol, representing the basic twofold polarized nature of energy as active and passive, hot and cold, dry and wet.[5] The eight figures consisting of solid (yang) and broken (yin) thick lines are called trigrams; these are taken from the classic Chinese book of divination and philosophy, the *I-Ching* (which contains sixty-four trigrams) and represent different combinations of the five elements and the outcome of those combinations (see figure 11-1).

The five elements are in dynamic relationship with one another, subject to cycles of influence and passivity (see figure

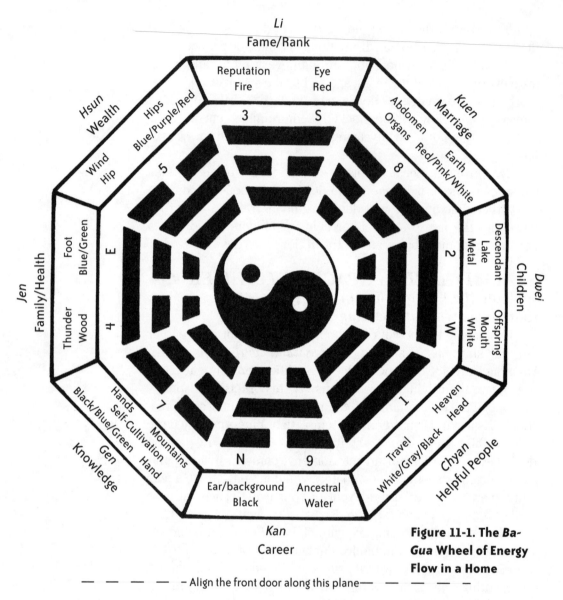

Figure 11-1. The *Ba-Gua* Wheel of Energy Flow in a Home

Reprinted with permission from Stanley Bartlett

11-2). The feng shui expert uses the five elements to restore energetic balance to a place.[6] As feng shui experts Sophia Tang Shaul and Chris Shaul, operators of the website *168 Feng Shui Advisors* and a feng shui consultancy in Burbank, California, note: "Used incorrectly, the elements can cause harm to relationships, health, or money prosperity. When used correctly, they can strengthen relationships, health, and money."[7]

According to the theory of feng shui, the way the elements are arranged (the variations on the trigrams) can be *predictive* of life situations, including health, prosperity, and longevity in a living space. You might think of the *Ba-Gua* template as a geometrical model of energy relationships with practical applications for how your house is laid out and how you are likely to fare living within this layout.

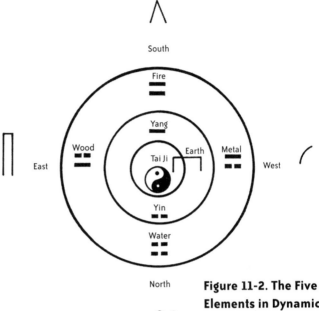

Figure 11-2. The Five Elements in Dynamic Relationship

Directions: Draw a floor plan of your house or apartment, showing all the different rooms and their compass orientation, windows, doors, and the placement of furniture. If your home has more than one story, make a separate diagram for each floor.

Mark the center point in your house diagram by drawing an "X" from opposite corners. If your house or apartment is not square, rectangular, or symmetrical, square it off on the diagram, then draw the two diagonal lines from the opposing corners to find the midpoint.

Next, align the *Ba-Gua* with your floor plan. Set the center of the *Ba-Gua* diagram on top of the midpoint on your floor plan, so that your front door corresponds to the bottom trigram of the *Ba-Gua*, marked "Career/Kan." This is called the "mouth of *qi*," and marks where the vital life energy enters the house, like a guest, and how it is "greeted" by the home's interior layout. It does not have to be the front door; if the main traffic pattern in your home is through a side or back door, then, functionally, this is the mouth of *qi* in your living space.

Now that you have matched the two diagrams, label your home floor plan with the terminology from the *Ba-Gua*. See where your bedroom, kitchen, living room, and other functional rooms show up in the ideal template. But first a quick word of clarification on the terms and concepts of this ideal template, starting with the mouth of *qi* then moving around the *Ba-Gua* clockwise.

- Career: Think of this first section as your financial livelihood and career path, your spiritual path, and generally the way you approach life.

- Knowledge: Matters of contemplation, introspection, meditation, study, and seeking guidance from within occur here.

- Family/Health: This area pertains to relationships with parents, authority figures, one's ancestors, and influences from the past.

- Wealth: Here we observe the flow of abundance and prosperity, but the blessings can take any form—money, materials, good will, good fortune.

- Fame/Rank: Your individuality and uniqueness of personal expression are grounded here.

- Marriage: This section of the house focuses on your primary relationships, such as with a partner, yourself, your friends, and colleagues.

- Children: Not only literally about children, this energy field deals with creativity, to anything that you can birth out of yourself.

- Helpful People: This points to the constellation of allies and supporters in your life, even helpful situations, such as finding answers from books; this section of the house connotes your relationship to philanthropy and generosity, and can be well used as an altar room.

- *Tai Ji:* The *Ba-Gua*'s central space is about health and vitality at the center of our living space.

This preliminary assessment of the layout of your living space contrasted with the ideal energy blueprint will give you ideas and insights as to how your house works, the degree to which it is in accord with the natural flow of energy, and the places where a feng shui adjustment would be advisable. Doing a *Ba-Gua* analysis of your domestic living space is analogous to doing a biochemical assay of your blood and your body's nutrition, as we explored in chapter 3. Both approaches give you a base line from which to evaluate your physiological and domestic status against a presumed ideal template, and to see to what degree your condition deviates from the optimal. As this chapter proceeds, the health significance of the deviation between your house and the *Ba-Gua* will become clear.

According to feng shui, a misalignment, such as having the bedroom in the career space, or the bathroom in the marriage space can be unfortunate; in fact, it can disturb or imbalance your life and possibly make you sick. In other words, it can be a toxic influence. Obviously, you cannot tear the house apart if the rooms are wrongly allocated, and in many cases this is not necessary, as feng shui offers many practical ways to alleviate the harmful influence of misaligned rooms. Nor is the *Ba-Gua* meant as an ultimate architectural authority; some feng shui experts see it as an interpretive overlay, while others see is as a tool for calculating the attributes of a building.

According to feng shui practitioner Terah Kathryn Collins, you can apply the *Ba-Gua* to individual rooms, taking the principal doorway into the room as the orienting "mouth of qi." While the *Ba-Gua* alignment of the entire house is of greater importance and holds more "structural qi" than that of individual rooms, it is still useful to chart the layout of individual rooms against the template. Once the evaluation and the practical feng shui adjustments are made, says Collins, "a positive change occurs that directly relates to the person's desires and goals in less than thirty days."[8]

The Healthy Living Space Expert Interview: Stanley Aaga Bartlett, Feng Shui Master

The *Ba-Gua* represents "an example of a perfect, balanced piece of the whole, a core template for understanding the flow of energy through a living space," observes Stanley Aaga Bartlett, a feng shui practitioner based in East Burke, Vermont. After twenty years in the real estate business, Bartlett shifted his professional interests to the use of feng shui for improving residential and commercial properties, and now consults nationally as a feng shui expert. "The *Ba-Gua* is a playful tool of discernment, a tool to better understand the clues as to what your environment is telling you about your life and a tool with which to change your reality. You can even carry the *Ba-Gua* configuration around with you and check out various environments, looking for clues as to what is going on." The *Ba-Gua's* eight sides correspond to the various central aspects of our lives, and when each of the eight sides of the *Ba-Gua* is in balance, then the whole is in balance, and our living space can fully support our well-being, Bartlett explains.

Foremost in Bartlett's approach to living space is the following principle gleaned over his years of feng shui practice: *As our environment goes, so go we.* In other words, our living space can either support our health and psychological well-being, or hinder them, Bartlett explains. "There is a direct relationship between what happens in our environment and what happens in our lives, and the reverse, too. So if there is some imbalance in our living environment, whether it is physical or nonphysical, it affects our health, our mental and emotional attitudes."

To truly achieve domestic balance, you must deal with both the obvious and the subtle, with the "practical/tangible issues and the transcendental/intangible aspects," Bartlett says. "On the physical level, you have the obvious issues such as color, lighting, floor plans, electrical pollution, air quality, the placement of objects, furniture, and doorways. On the non-physical side, you have electromagnetic influence, Earth energy imbalance, predecessor and lingering energies from previous occupants of the space."

It is crucial to use a feng shui approach that integrates both aspects, Bartlett says. "Considering only the practical aspects of feng shui might be 40% effective in creating harmonious space, but when the practical is combined with the transcendental, then it may have a 140% effectiveness. Knowledge of these transcendental aspects allows a feng shui practitioner to see through our environment what we are unable to see in our selves."[9]

Everything in our living space has an effect on us in some way, even the angles of the furniture, the geometric shapes that surround us. Further, how our living space is situated with respect to its environment also has a pronounced effect on our well-being, says Bartlett. In other words, how our house or apartment building sits on the landscape, the direction it faces, the houses or other buildings that face it, even the angles of those neighboring houses and which part of our home they face—all these factors and more come into play when a feng shui expert looks at a living space with a view to making health-supporting adjustments.

Heightened sensitivity certainly comes in handy in this kind of work. "When I walk into an environment, I see a panoramic view, a holographic pattern, if you will, of what is happening in that environment," Bartlett says. Somehow, his "internal computer gathers vast information" about the conditions of the immediate environment. Bartlett senses the subconscious of the living space, the influences that, perhaps not consciously known to the space's inhabitants, nonetheless are subtly shaping their lives, thoughts, feelings, and health.

He might hear an almost inaudible sound from an electrical transformer or power line nearby that is out of balance and creating a "gnawing, annoying, or irritating vibration" that affects the occupants of the house, even though they are not consciously aware of the origin of the toxic energy. "Perhaps the environment is telling me that the front door entrance is constricted and dark, the colors inside are dark and not very balanced and the wall is too close to the entrance as I walk in and it is compressing my energy field. You might also notice that the Earth energies are depleting your *qi* on one side of a room, but on the other side of the room you sense that the Earth energies are much more supportive." Bartlett says he often gets distracted by "another irritant" when he realizes the energy of the space suggests there must have been an argument in that room recently.

"I see the history of what has happened in a space. There are energies that linger—they're called *ling* energies in Chinese thinking, and mean the energies of the preceding occupants. For example, if there was an argument in this space yesterday or even a traumatic event one hundred years ago in this house, the energy *patterns* of that experience will sometimes remain, or linger, in that environment.

"Our environments have an energy consciousness to them, and there is a lot we can do to create a different reality in our lives and in our environment by using the tools of feng shui wisely," Bartlett says. "The goal of feng shui is to help us use this information to arrange our reality in more harmonious ways. Many wonderful stories exist of how people have used these teachings to bring health, prosperity, and good fortune to their lives."[10] Even though feng shui often deals with the highly subtle energy influences in our environment, it is also deeply practical, never overlooking the obvious, such as the effect of chronic clutter in a living space.

HEALTHY LIVING SPACE DETOXIFIER #55
Tidy Up All the Cluttered Areas in Your Home

Unattended clutter has repercussions in our life. "I look for clues in the environment on a physical level to see what is going on in one's life and what one is (sometimes unconsciously) creating," says Bartlett. A cluttered living space is often at the root of many dysfunctional aspects of a person's life, and clearing out clutter can be "one of the most powerful, yet unglamorous solutions to feng shui issues. When you are feeling stuck in life, start getting rid of clutter and watch how quickly new possibilities surface."

A dense, cluttered environment most definitely affects us. Not only do cluttered areas attract dust, but they become sites of stagnant qi, places around and through which invigorating qi cannot flow. Areas of stagnant qi then attract other energies, thoughts, objects that are in agreement with that level of stasis and stagnation.

Directions: Examine your living space with a neutral, detached, objective eye. Is it cluttered? Are there piles of old stuff, debris, unused possessions, clothes, books, postcards that only gather dust, closets bursting with forgotten objects, stacks of old magazines, crates of glass bottles, or too much furniture in too small a space? Probably few people can truthfully say there are no clutter zones in their homes. So start throwing stuff out, winnowing out what you do not need any more, and recycling, giving away, or selling the rest. Keep only those things "you truly love and need in your environment."

A dense, cluttered environment most definitely affects us, says Bartlett. "We say in feng shui, less is more, get rid of the old to make room for the new, and cluttered closets are like cluttered minds." Not only do cluttered areas attract dust, but they become sites of stagnant qi, places around and through which invigorating qi cannot flow. Areas of stagnant qi then attract other energies, thoughts, objects that are in agreement with that level of stasis and stagnation and these merely strengthen this stagnant quality, heightening the attraction for what Bartlett calls the "transcendental/intangible aspects" of a living space, in this case, negative, toxic aspects (discussed below).

Bartlett offers a vivid case study from his practice that illustrates the life-hindering effect of unattended clutter. Bartlett consulted with a woman named Joan who was having health, relationship, and career problems. "She was experiencing health issues, relationship deprivation, a lack of money, and an inability to achieve success in her career as an actress and theater director. She was stuck in survival and forced to accept menial jobs and was even experiencing difficulty securing regular menial work."

Her house was full of too many beautiful antiques, books, baskets, and other objects such that the overall visual impact was one of intense clutter. "Joan thought she was simply going to have a feng shui expert come in and help her arrange all her things, move her furniture into the correct feng shui positions, and that this would resolve all her problems," says Bartlett. But that would have been fruitless unless she made a substantial reduction in her clutter. Bartlett agreed to return for more consultation after she had cleaned up some of the clutter. "Joan began to understand that on some level she was surrounding herself with things out of a deep fear of lack. Somehow it felt safer if she kept lots of things around her. It also became clear to her that there were emotions hidden behind all these things that she had not been willing to look at for a long time."

A short while later, Joan called him up, saying she had thrown out, sold, or given away a fair amount of her stuff. She said: "I don't know what's going on but ever since you were here and I started clearing the clutter, I've been getting a lot of job offers."

Bartlett visited Joan again, and suggested another round of clearing, this time focusing on dense, old energies lingering in the house and how those energies were associated with Joan herself. "We did a healing of her environment to fill her home with loving light."

Bartlett left Joan a second time to complete the deeper housecleaning. This time, she threw out more stuff, cleaned the windows and walls, dusted everything, gave the place a proper scrubbing. Joan called back again. "I told you I hadn't been in a relationship for 19 years [since the death of her husband] and that I had some health issues. But all of a sudden, I'm getting inquiries from men." A few weeks later, Joan called Bartlett again. "This is really the ultimate," she told him. "I just had a call from a woman I knew well years ago; she had a very successful theater company. She made it big then lost everything, but now she's getting ready to make it big again and invited me to be her assistant director. So I'm selling my house and moving to the city." Joan's life continued to improve. "Romance is in, career is great, and the body is much healthier," comments Bartlett.

In a sense, the ultimate (and a little amusing) result of Joan's rigorous clutter-removing work was to get rid of her house. This of course is not always required. The essential point in this case study is that Joan had a high level of clutter and thus stagnant energy in three areas of her living space: Career ("mouth of qi"), Marriage, and Family/Health. As a result, her career was stalled, she had no love relationships, and her health was deteriorating.

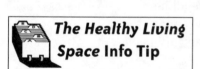

The Healthy Living Space Info Tip

Stanley Aaga Bartlett can be contacted at
Bartlett Designs,
P.O. Box 119,
East Burke, VT 05832-0119;
tel & fax: 802-626-9492;
e-mail: stanlu@aol.com;
website: www.bartlettdesigns.com.

When the clutter was removed and the stagnant energy exorcised from these domestic spaces, these three factors in her life reconfigured because she had reenergized their correlates in her living environment. "For Joan, by clearing her attachments to physical things and clearing out her clutter, it allowed new possibilities to enter her life. This is such a powerful thing to do for one's health and well-being because when one is stuck emotionally, energetically, one tends to be stuck in one's environment, and that's when things do not happen very well in our lives."

HEALTHY LIVING SPACE DETOXIFIER #56
Repaint All the Interior Walls with Your Color of Happiness

Before addressing any of the specifics of individual room layouts and alignments, there is a simple but powerful way to impart fresh qi to every inch of your living space. This is especially advised if you are moving into a new home or apartment because this detoxifying step is one you can—and should—do immediately upon taking possession of the place, even before you bring in your belongings.

Essentially you want to expunge the physical residues of all previous occupants *and* impart the unique stamp of your own energy and well-being. There are three interlinked cleaning tasks you can perform in your new space: repainting the walls, cleaning the carpets, and washing all the windows. While these are obvious hygienic, house-warming measures, they can become powerful feng shui tools by adding a special element: your *intention*.

I will illustrate this point with an example from my own experience. My wife and I once rented a fairly new home for a year. The owner gave us a reduction in the first month's rent in exchange for our repainting the interior. This suited us fine, not only for the cost savings, but because we could impart our own energy to the walls that would surround us for the next twelve months.

With every slap and swish of the brush, we imparted a sense of peace, stillness, and spiritual presence to the fresh white paint, gradually filling our interior environment with a new vibration—ours. We happened to be in pretty good spirits at the time—dare I say happy?—so this emotional quality flavored our intentions and whatever other qualities we sought to impart to the paint. Sometimes we played music to accompany the brush strokes, such as a Mozart sonata or vocal music of a gentle lilting quality, knowing that whatever vibrations we surrounded ourselves with during the "thoughtful" painting, along with the quality of our own internal state, the fresh paint (the "inner skin" of our living space) would "remember" and reflect back to us. We had a wonderful year within those newly painted walls.

Directions: "Embrace your environment as if it were a part of you, which it is," says Bartlett. He suggests that even before starting your thoughtful painting that you hold "the image of the perfect environment in your mind." This image, Bartlett explains, "might elicit a feeling of love, protection, and perfect harmony from all around you." It should be so strong that "when you near the entrance to your driveway, you begin to get this feeling that it is really good to be coming home." Then when you open the front door, "your heart opens wide with this overwhelming feeling of love and harmony."

The remarkable property of energy is that once you have formed this intention, once you have evoked this sense of heart-opened harmony and balance, you can impart it to your living space, through the paint, the substance with which you wash the windows, and the substances you use to clean your carpets. As long as you hold this feeling quality of the image, you can imbue everything around you with it—putting a little white magic spell on your walls, so to speak.

Bartlett recommends lightly sanding all the wall surfaces and cleaning them with soap and water before painting. This is another level to clearing out the old, dense energies of the space and bringing the environment up to a level of purity and neutrality upon which you can now impart your own intention and vibration. If your floors are carpeted, Bartlett advises vacuuming then cleaning them thoroughly with a nontoxic carpet-cleaning solution. You may need to use Clorox bleach to remove the residual mildew in and underneath the carpets. (Be careful, though: you don't want to bleach the color out of your rugs.) Similarly, scrub and sanitize all windows, both inside and outside, removing all traces of dirt and residue. "Windows are the eyes of the *qi* (life force energy) and affect one's clarity, so replace any broken panes and clean all the windows."

"Do this with clear intention, that you are clearing out older, denser energies, and filling your home with loving light," says Bartlett. "Intention is very important. Your thought-energy is crucial in creating a new reality for you." Once you have evoked a sense of your ideal living environment and the feeling-quality associated with it, try to stay in this meditative space throughout your housecleaning work. The positive, life-affirming vibrations you impart to your walls, paint, windows, and floorings, will return to nourish and support you throughout your stay in that home.

HEALTHY LIVING SPACE DETOXIFIER #57
Clear Your Space of All Predecessor Energy

Thoughtful painting and imparting the color of happiness to your interior walls is the outer, physical aspect of clearing out old, dense energies of former occupants of your living space, says Bartlett. But you also need to address the subtler aspects of having had former residents in your living room and bedrooms. The central idea here is that the older, denser energies of former residents will interrupt or contribute to the stagnation of *qi* in your house, unless you take steps to remove them.

"If you were to examine these dense, old, stuck energies with Kirlian photography, using a camera that takes pictures of energies in color, you would see these as a kind of clouded, murky fog," says Bartlett. "On the other hand, a light-filled energy would be very clear and crystalline-like. That's what we want to create in our environment because the denser energies tend to keep us stuck."

Let's ground this observation with some examples. Eira Hellberg, a Swedish collector of occult lore, remarked some years ago that often when examining an apartment with the intent to rent, she might discern "something unpleasant in the walls . . . an atmosphere that exhales something distinctly human." Even though the physical details of the room—wallpaper, carpets, furniture, the colors and layout—seem congenial and hygienic, there is still something off, exuding "an uncomfortable sense of oppression." The person showing the apartment may be friendly, but your feeling of unease does not go away.

Hellberg comments: "If our amiable hosts in their comfortable room cannot overcome our uneasiness, the reason is that the room and the objects in it are *saturated* with the mental activity of the occupants, their will- and thought-waves, which are beamed back on any receptive individual who comes within range of them."[11]

In other cases, intense feelings, such as of despair or violence, can remain in a room or "in" the former occupant's furniture (in the case of a furnished rented room) and exert a harmful, if unsuspected, influence on the new tenants of the living space. For example, French occult scholar Paul Sedir noted in 1923 that "human beings exercise a real influence on the objects in their environment. A chair that has been flung across the room in a rage stores anger inside it; the things used by a niggardly housewife make subsequent owners stingy."[12]

A feng shui expert echoes this observation: "If the last tenants' marriage ended in divorce, or someone was very sick, patterns of this energy stay with the house until it is cleared." Similarly, if a particular room had formerly been given over to young children with the intent of their having great fun in it, "lingering childish energy might impede your plans for a tranquil retreat."[13]

Stuck energy and "psychic debris" can accumulate in all rooms in a home, but especially in corners, nooks, and crannies, comments another expert. Many people, unknowingly, live in the "psychic equivalent of a garbage dump." Everything that happens in a room is recorded in all of its structures; "repetitive patterns get deeply imprinted, as do moods and atmospheres." Further, it is conceivable that if previous persons living in a house, or room, had health problems and were, for example, overweight, or had eating disorders, the energy supporting this, or associated with its expression, is still present in the house and may influence a new generation of weight disorders.[14]

Stuck energy and "psychic debris" can accumulate in all rooms in a home, but especially in corners, nooks, and crannies, comments another expert. Many people, unknowingly, live in the "psychic equivalent of a garbage dump." Everything that happens in a room is recorded in all of its structures.

German occult researcher Willy Schrödter relates how a Viennese family "suffered inexplicable health" for two years. It turns out an oil painting that hung in their living room was, according to a clairvoyant who discerned this, "a hate radiator." Once the painting was removed and *burned*, all occupants of that household regained their health. In other words, the painting radiated energy that acted as an unrelieved toxin to all those in its sphere. Schrödter cites the examples of others for whom hygiene encompassed the realm of subtle influences. One man surrounded himself only with new furniture and objects, so as "not to have any old thoughts or feelings hanging about him."

The reality of "mental atmospheres" and their effects on consciousness must be accepted, Schrödter and many other esotericists state, thereby confirming what feng shui has always said about *ling* energies, or predecessor energies. Schrödter comments that according to the Tibetans, "the Earth's atmosphere is injured by unkind thoughts" and that when people send out bad thoughts, they collect in a manner similar to water vapor condensing into rain, and fall down on people in the form of diseases.[15] This phenomenon of "raining toxicity" can happen at any level of residence—country, city, community, neighborhood, single house, or single room.

Directions: There are many practical steps for clearing an interior space of lingering predecessor energies, according to feng shui.

Remove Old Energies with an Energy Blanket

This is a practical step advised by Carol Bridges, an instructor at the Nine Harmonies School of Feng Shui in Nashville, Indiana. Bridges suggests visualizing that you wear "energy gloves," and that if you stretch your arms before you, you can send "strands of light" across your property (including your home or apartment). Imagine that a "team of spirit energies" (or helpful forces) are cooperating with you in this space-clearing work (that is, cleaning the subtle "airs" around you), and that they occupy the basic compass directions.

Next, visualize that you and the helpers hold an "energy blanket" underneath the entire property, so that it is twelve feet underground. Asking that the blanket collect all foreign, inimical, and predecessor energies from this site, raise the blanket up through the house until you and the helpers are holding it twelve feet above the top of the room, house, or apartment building, says Bridges. Coming up through the house, the blanket would have collected all these energies, which may or may not present themselves to you in a variety of displeasing forms. Bundle up and tie the blanket and ask the spirit team to take it away.[16]

Use Incense, Candles, and Expelling Mudras

One way to remove older, denser energies is to burn a strong-smelling incense such as frankincense, sage, or other pungent incense while walking through each room and allowing the smoke to infiltrate the air and furnishings, recommends Bartlett. As you fill each room with the aromatic fumes, visualize the older, denser energies clearing out and "loving light" filling the room throughout. You can also burn candles in each room to "burn off the old and symbolically fill your home with loving light," Bartlett adds.

Among the "transcendental cures" Bartlett uses in his feng shui practice is the expelling mudra. This is a special hand gesture meant to change the energy field in a room. Curl the middle and ring finger of each hand toward your palm while keeping the index and pinky fingers pointing straight out. Hold the backs (nails) of the middle fingers with the ball of your thumb. Flick the two middle fingers upward "expelling all older, denser energies." According to Bartlett, this mudra can be used to clear the aura, the land, an automobile, an airplane, and any room, including a motel room or a doctor's office, among many other venues.

Other simple but effective ways to change the energy of your interior space include singing, dancing, chiming bells, drumming, ringing gongs, striking cymbals, toning (emitting tones or other nonverbal sounds), or playing music in each room, says Bartlett. According to Celtic folklore, one of the principal reasons church bells were tolled frequently in villages, especially on Sundays, was to drive away all the lingering spirits, both good and bad. The spirits could not abide the sound of the bells and considered it "poison."

While performing these space-clearing exercises, it is important, says Bartlett, to visualize your living space "filled with loving light and that only those energies that are harmonious to your being are present."

Keep the Lights On

Most people think it is energy-efficient to keep only the minimum of lights on in a house in the evening. However, from a feng shui viewpoint, this is not advised. It is better for the circulation of qi through an interior environment if a light is left on in each room, preferably twenty-four hours a day, says Bartlett. "During the evening hours or on cloudy days, leave a light on for twenty-four hours in the basement to keep the qi active.

"It is not advisable to keep all the lights turned off, other than the one area you are currently in, as this can cause the energy in the rest of the house to become tired. This is especially important in the winter, as it helps to avoid winter blues and depression. A small light left on twenty-four hours a day in the basement will also help keep the foundation of your home activated." If the qi is moving and the foundation "activated," there is no room for energy stagnation, which is a reservoir for predecessor energy. "Carefully positioned lighting can cause stuck energy areas to flow. When we keep the qi flowing, that tends to be an environment where lingering energies choose not to hang out."[17]

On a practical level, Bartlett recommends conserving electricity (since he's advising to keep all the lights on) by using energy-efficient, full-spectrum fluorescent bulbs in each area of the house and by designating these as the lights that are kept on in the evenings. You can use 12-volt halogen track lighting in the kitchen instead of fluorescents, if desired, Bartlett adds.

Clapping in Every Room

According to "space-clearing" expert Karen Kingston, you can disperse static energy in a room by clapping your hands loudly in every corner, crevice, and closet in that room. After clapping, be sure to wash your hands under running water to clear away "any bits of psychic debris that may have clung to you" while clapping.[18]

Purify Secondhand Furnishings

Despite the fantastic bargain you may have achieved on that antique coffee table or Spanish clothes dresser or sofa-bed, it is quite likely that these furnishings bear energy residues of their former owners and users and that these residues, if not expunged, will visit your energy field and produce discomfort. Let's reprise a technique introduced in chapter 9 as Healthy Living Space Detoxifier #40, Scrub Your Aura Clean with a Golden Sponge.

First, apply this golden energy sponge to the furnishing in question, mentally swabbing all its surfaces and interior, visualizing that this golden energy field is absorbing the toxic residues. Then imagine that there is a drain under the table, dresser, or sofa-bed, and that this drain goes all the way to the center of the Earth. Instruct the drain to draw to it all the negative, foreign, toxic, predecessor energy presently within the object. You may get a visual impression of sludge or mucus flowing slowly out of the furniture and down the drain. Continue with this draining until no further exudate is visible, or for at least five minutes if you don't have any visuals on the proceedings. Then visualize a bright golden Sun over the furniture and slowly bring it into the object so that sunlight permeates every molecule of its structure. These steps should make the table, dresser, or sofa-bed fit for your aura.

HEALTHY LIVING SPACE DETOXIFIER #58
The Health Benefits of Ghost-Busting

Predecessor energies may involve more than the residual thought patterns and energy waves of previous occupants of your living space. They may involve the purely "transcendental" aspects of energy imprints, a term Bartlett uses to refer to "the realm beyond our current intellectual understanding." But what we cannot understand with our minds, our bodies and auras can nevertheless register, even if it is possible ghosts in the house.

According to the classical description of *ling* energies from the feng shui canon, the life force energy, or *qi*, of a deceased person may return to their familiar earthbound haunts, such as a former living space and inadvertently (or sometimes purposefully) annoy, irritate, or deeply trouble the current living occupants, says Bartlett.

He was recently asked by some householders to remove the influence of a former occupant who had died twelve years earlier and whose lingering presence was producing "weird ghostlike events" and other negative energies for the new owners. To some, the return of a deceased former resident—perhaps he is a relative or parent—can be perceived as a pleasant event, but for others it can be quite disruptive. In either case, it can be confusing and intrusive to one's own *qi* to be visited by the *ling* energy of a deceased being.

In ghost-busting cases such as these, Bartlett relies on his various space-clearing techniques, as described above. In some instances, occupants with no previous training or experience in metaphysical matters may be able to expel the foreign energies, or they may have to engage a consultant, says Bartlett. If you possess any physical objects belonging to the former and now deceased occupants, it is helpful to purify these of all energy residues of the previous owners, using the techniques described above in "Purify Secondhand Furnishings." Otherwise, these residues act as magnets or homing signals, enabling the deceased to find a familiar landmark in an otherwise troubling (because no longer "physical" the way it used to be) environment.

If it is the case of a lingering ghost, in most cases, the intelligence inhabiting the ghostly form does not know it is dead and no longer lawfully associated with the physical plane. Or if they know they're dead, sometimes they don't know what to do next, or feel a strong gravitational pull towards both their former domicile and the Earth plane in general, almost out of habit.

"It is appropriate to lovingly invite these *ling* particles [or spirits of the deceased] to return to the light for completion of their soul's journey," comments Bartlett. It may sound ridiculously simple, but often telling them these facts is sufficient to move them on their way. The hard part may be *believing* that the ghosts are really there in your house and are capable of exerting toxic effects on you.

Here are two examples from my experience as a house-holder that help to illustrate this possibly challenging, unsettling observation.

Once I stayed at a small ranch in New Mexico and found I couldn't sleep in the appointed guest room. I tossed and turned, and strange thoughts ran through my mind. I perspired, fretted, worried, got irritated, and got up. I usually fall asleep within five minutes of my head reaching the pillow, and if I don't, I figure it's because I went to bed too early. But this was different. My wife was unable to sleep, either. The next morning we learned from the owner that generally nobody was able to sleep well in the room.

Between the three of us, we mustered enough psychic power to investigate the problem. The impression we gathered was that underneath the room in question was a casket contain-ing the remains of a teenage Native American girl who had been buried there some two hundred years earlier. She had lived in the space where the ranch house now stood and had died young and under considerable trauma, due to a severe sudden illness. Our impression was that "she" didn't approve of where she was buried and was still traumatized by the events, which to us were several centuries ago, but to her, were the eternal present, hav-ing happened only "minutes" ago.

As we were not about to excavate the ground under the room, not to mention tear up the floor to get to it, we called on higher authorities for help. To the extent we were capable, we counseled the girl and advised her to move on, and let the spiri-tual helpers do the rest. That night we slept wonderfully in the room, as if it had never been the site of insomnia for many.

In this example, had someone taken over this room as a bed-room and not been aware of the possibility of *ling* energies, quite likely, physical, emotional, and mental symptoms would have developed in accordance with the "fault lines" of that person's con-stitution. The toxic emanations of the restless dead girl could have produced irritation, chronic sleeplessness or broken sleep, night-mares, foreign dreams, paranoia, despair, fear, panic, headaches, elevated blood pressure—any of a long list of possible symptoms.

In the second example, I once rented a home in coastal California. There was a two-car garage, which I appropriated as my office and filled with bookshelves and a large worktable. However, I soon noticed that every time I spent more than ten minutes in the garage, I became irritated, even angry. Even though that is my "fault line" psychologically, I have learned to use it as a dowsing rod to detect foreign, inimical energies. Feeling irritation is one way I receive information from my aura that there is an energy imbalance in my immediate environment; of course other times it's just because I didn't get my way.

My wife and I isolated the toxic energy influence to an area of about three feet square in the central part of the garage. It looked like a vertical column of energy, like a smoky quartz crystal column—nothing I'd want to have on my coffee table to be sure. Using a pendulum, we could chart where the field started and stopped; even so, being within ten to fifteen feet of it was enough to irritate me and drive me from the garage. We placed a very large clear quartz crystal on the edge of this toxic field to deflect the energy somewhat, but I still felt it anywhere I stood in the garage. Soon I stopped working in the garage and even avoided going into it unless I had to.

The day before we moved out of the house—we lived there only one year and did not like it at all—we discovered what the problem was in the garage. We saw two men lying on the garage floor, dead of knife wounds; police cars were parked in the driveway. The events took place approximately in the mid-1950s, which meant their toxic influence had lingered in the garage for more than forty years. Again, we asked for "backup" from the spiritual world, and watched as "they" escorted the lingering souls of the slain men off into the light. As soon as they were gone, the vertical column shattered into a thousand pieces and the vile energy spot was purified. The garage was now fit for human occupation, although I suspect the next residents used it for their car.

The lesson in this garage haunting is the same as with the dead girl under the floorboards. The toxic emanations were capable of producing no end of unfortunate effects on those within their field of influence. In matters like these, unless you can discern what is self and not-self as far as thoughts and inclinations go, you are likely, regrettably, to act out as your own, to some degree, the baleful influences your aura is registering. Sufficient immersion in that angry, literally murderous energy field in the garage could have provoked somebody to a significant outburst of rage, or worse. This is the kind of *ling* you don't want lingering under any circumstances.

Even *ling* energies of a more benign nature are not to be encouraged. "These energies disturb your *qi*, producing interference with your energy, so that things get too crowded energetically," explains Bartlett. "Unless these spirits are personal spirit guides, they are best not kept around your living space for long periods of time because then it becomes a case of too much interruption, too much interference." They become an additional toxic element in your living space, and can distract you from your focus on positive activities and your own creativity, says Bartlett. "In my experience, when your environment is free and clear of entities and ghosts, then you are allowed to co-create in more ease-filled and perfect ways."

Ghost-busting of course is not something everyone will feel comfortable undertaking, nor is it particularly advisable to try to remove restless spirits if you are just beginning to acknowledge subtle energies. Often in such cases, it is prudent to engage the services of a qualified feng shui practitioner, a dowser, or a psychic trained in this particular type of space clearing. It is not unusual for a well-seasoned dowser to be skilled in all three of these practices.

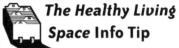

The Healthy Living Space Info Tip

For information about dowsing, including books, practitioner referrals, educational conferences, and publications, contact:
The American Society of Dowsers,
P.O. Box 24,
Danville, VT 05828;
tel: 800-711-9530 or 802-684-3417;
e-mail: ASD@Dowsers.org;
website: www.dowsers.org.

HEALTHY LIVING SPACE DETOXIFIER #59
Eliminate Poison Arrows and Cutting Qi

It sounds strange at first hearing, but according to feng shui practitioners, the quality of your life within your house can be affected, for better or worse, by the way other houses face yours. Obviously noisy neighbors can be irritating even when you are indoors, but this is different.

The way other houses *face* your house can be an energy toxic element. Face means the orientation of the other houses, their geometry with respect to yours, the angles and corners and how they're situated in relation to your house and particular sections (as defined by the *Ba-Gua*) of your house. When these geometric features of neighboring houses are injurious, they fall into the category feng shui terms "poison arrows" and "cutting *qi*," and this becomes something you need to address for your long-term well-being in your home.

Qi flows best and is most supportive of health when it can always move in gentle, meandering curves, but not in straight lines, and it should always be able to keep moving. When it enters a house, *qi* must be able to depart from a different door; it can't flow backwards. But you don't want the *qi* rushing into your house like an assault team, which can be the energy effect of an unchecked poison arrow.

A poison arrow (also called a "secret arrow") is any straight line or sharp angle that heads directly for you, like an energy arrow shot from the bow of an opposing architectural structure. Here's how feng shui practitioner Angel Thompson explains it: "When it is forced into straight lines or sharp angles, instead of gently falling and rising like the tummy of a sleeping baby, *chi* compresses into a barb, like an arrow, as sharp as the tip of a knife. . . ." She adds that no matter where you live, "there are many secret arrows around you."[19]

Here is a way to gain a visceral sense of the problem of poison or secret arrows. Sit before the corner of a rectangular table so that your eyes are about six inches from and level with the right angle. Observe how this makes you feel. It is very likely that within a matter of minutes, or less, your eyes will feel uncomfortable, as if assaulted, or even penetrated; you may feel that spears are piercing your eyes and you want to pull your face away from the line of vision. But what has happened? The table hasn't attacked you—or has it? In terms of feng shui, it has: it has thrown poison arrows at you by virtue of its geometrical relationship to you. On an energy level, the two lines that form the right angle continue through space, beyond the confines of the physical table, and pass through whatever is before it, in this case, your eyes.

You can expand the example to the sphere of an entire house. Say a neighboring house is situated at right angles to your front door, so that when you stand at your open door, you are confronted by the right-angle corner of that house. It doesn't matter if it's fifty or 100 feet away; you'll still get the poison arrow effect, just as you did when sitting before the table. Your energy field will register it as a hostile, even aggressive energy focus.

Other examples of poison arrows can include T-intersections on roads, driveways, sidewalks, rooflines, corners, streetlights, walls, signs, porches, pillars, clock towers, statues, any very large imposing object, the sharp edge of any nearby building, sharply defined hills and landscape contours—essentially any straight line, extended from an architectural or landscape feature, that comes right at you or at your front door. Other toxic situations include having your house at the center of a fork in two roads, at the outside of a bend in the road, or in the center of a circular traffic pattern, such as a rotary or roundabout. Remember, in and of themselves, each of these features is not necessarily harmful, but when placed in the wrong geometrical relationship to your house, they become toxic.

Poison arrows are harmful for your health because they embody "cutting qi," which is also known as noxious qi, "the cutting breath." They interrupt, distort, divert, or pollute the natural, health-promoting flow of basic life force energy through an environment, in this case, your home through its front door, the "mouth of qi." "All these structures give out an energy that is too strong and will overwhelm your home, often with sad or tragic consequences," explains Lillian Too, a well-known feng shui expert and author. Poison arrows can block the good, healthy qi from flowing into your home, leading to energy stagnation. Poison arrows generate *shar qi*, says Too, "the killing breath," capable of producing every type of misfortune and ill luck, especially disease and fatal illness.[20]

Some feng shui experts say the reason poison arrows are harmful is that they project "high-velocity qi," basic energy that's moving too fast (because it's moving in a straight line) to be health promoting. Qi is supposed to flow in curves, but when it is forced to move in a straight line, it gathers in power and acts like a speeding projectile or flying arrow. Others note that one main reason they're called "secret" arrows is that most people are not immediately aware of their effects, which build over time, from minor irritations to major disturbances. But meanwhile your energy field, or aura, feels as if it is facing directly into a sharpened knife point, or as if it is the stationary target receiving arrows in its body from an expert bowman.

Poison arrows are harmful for your health because they embody "cutting qi," which is also known as noxious qi, "the cutting breath." They interrupt, distort, divert, or pollute the natural, health-promoting flow of basic life force energy through an environment, in this case, your home through its front door, the "mouth of qi."

"A secret arrow is like having a stick stuck in your side: not only can it be annoying, but eventually it can also cause harm," notes Nancilee Wydra, founder of the Pyramid School of Feng Shui in Vero Beach, Florida. She adds that even a person with a normally positive, uplifted temperament can gradually be worn down by this "insidious or subtle pressure."[21] Secret arrows can distort your own *qi* field, and make you feel unsettled, confused, disoriented, and as if you have lost your grounding and sense of life direction.

Here's a practical way to visualize the probable effect of poison arrows. Imagine you stand within a large inflated balloon that extends perhaps three or four feet away from your physical body in all directions. Next, imagine all the poison arrows you documented on your list (see below) come at this balloon from the outside and cause indentations, punctures, and disfigurations. Now imagine that this balloon around you can transmit its energy to your physical body, and you are *feeling* the effects of these dents, holes, and distortions in your physical organism.

This "imagination" is actually not too far off the mark from what actually happens. The balloon corresponds to your aura, or energy field, which surrounds you and transmits energies to your physical body. Sooner or later, depending on your inherent vitality, your body will register the effects of these distortions in its energy envelope and will manifest this registration in the form of symptoms and, if unchecked, eventual health problems. Just to be precise, even though your aura can sustain punctures and holes, it does not "deflate," although its local integrity collapses inward to an extent at the site of the injury.

The feng shui answer to poison arrows is deflection. In nearly all cases, you won't be able to move the offending object or source of poison arrows, but you can effectively block their energy effects.

Directions: There are many ways to deflect or calm the incoming toxic *qi*, according to long-established principles of feng shui.

• Before we get into the practical steps, here is a preliminary exercise. Open your front door, stand in the doorway, and survey your environment. Look for poison arrows. Examine the buildings nearby: do they have sharp angles projected at your front door?

Repeat this exercise by standing before every window in your house, looking out at your neighbors from inside. Make a list of all possible secret and poison arrows, no matter how slight or inconsequential they may seem. Contemplate for a moment the combined effect of these poison arrows on your energy field, using the simple example of the effect of a table's corner on your eyes to get a visceral sense of the assault on your aura.

• Plant bushy trees, shrubs, or a dense hedge to block off the poison arrow. This is like placing a shield between yourself, your front door, or window, and the source of the poison arrows. The natural foliage will absorb the toxic energy stream of the poison arrow, so that it does not reach your house.

• Employ mirrors, shiny reflective surfaces, or plaques, even polished brass doorknobs, orienting these towards the source of the poison arrows. If a poison arrow from an abutting house is focused through a window, hang a reflecting mirror inside your window but facing outwards towards the arrow. (For more on mirrors, see Healthy Living Space Detoxifier #60, below.)

• Calm the incoming qi according to Five Element theory. This approach is typical of feng shui's marvelous sense of using restored balance as a way of eliminating problems. Simon Brown, a design engineer and feng shui consultant, explains that insofar as the *Ba-Gua* gives the orientation for the five elements (according to Chinese philosophy), you can use the interrelationships of these elements to deflect poison arrows and "calm" or "drain" their effect. For example, earth drains fire, metal drains earth, water drains metal.

Say you have an incoming poison arrow from the southwest, which is the orientation for earth, which is "drained" by metal, explains Brown. To calm or drain the cutting qi from the southwest, place an object associated with metal qi, such as a gold or silver disc in the southwest corner of your house. "Alternatively, place a large statue made of cast-iron, bronze or other metal, which includes circular shapes, in the garden between your house and the corner."[22] The same applications can easily be worked out with the other elements and compass directions, according to the *Ba-Gua*.

- If your home is disturbed by traffic patterns or is at the end of a T-intersection or other toxic traffic arrangement, hanging wind chimes in your hall, just outside the front door, or in your backyard can help cleanse and purify the *qi* around your house so that it no longer transmits disturbed energy patterns into your living space.

- If you have a tree, post, or pole directly facing your front door, the ideal solution is to remove the tree, because it blocks the flow of *qi* into your living space. If you can't remove the *qi*, Angel Thompson recommends placing a small mirror in the middle of the tree (or post or pole) so that it faces your front door. This mirror acts as a "symbolic hole," says Thompson, and absorbs the noxious *qi*.[23]

- If your walkway leads directly in a straight line from the road or driveway to your front door (thereby generating a poison arrow), arrange bricks, stones, or potted plants on the edge of the path along its course to deflect and soften the *qi* flow and to break up its straightness.

HEALTHY LIVING SPACE DETOXIFIER #60
Pacify Your Neighborhood with Feng Shui Mirrors

Probably most people have experienced obnoxious, noisy, or irritating neighbors whose lifestyle activities we wish we could curtail or eliminate. Or maybe our neighbors don't like us, or don't like anybody, and transmit a steady field of ill will and negativity in our direction. Or their back porch faces our back porch and they are too close for comfort. Or your house abuts a funeral parlor or cemetery.

There are many scenarios, both mild and serious, in which the presence of neighboring houses (and their occupants) sometimes exceeds our ability to cope. Short of moving away to live somewhere else, there are some palliative steps you can take using feng shui principles.

Directions: One of the simplest of these methods is the mirror, which some practitioners refer to as "the aspirin of feng shui." Specifically helpful here is the *Ba-Gua* mirror, an octagonal piece of reflecting mirror set inside an octagonal frame with some of the traditional *Ba-Gua* signs and traditional colors of red, green, and gold. If you have troubling neighbors, place a series of these mirrors (they're about four inches in diameter) around the outside of your house and facing the direction of the irritation.

Use the *Ba-Gua* mirror to redirect intrusive energies such as from an intrusive neighbor, says Stanley Bartlett. "Simply point the mirror with loving intention towards the intrusive energy and it will lovingly redirect it back to the source of the intrusion. That will redirect the intrusive energies as if to say 'return to sender.'" Using mirrors to deflect threatening *qi* achieves two purposes at once, according to Sarah Rossbach, author of *Interior Design with Feng Shui*. "The mirror both offensively reflects back malignant ch'i and defensively provides protection. Any size will do."

Using mirrored glass walls (such as you see on many urban skyscrapers) is also effective if you care to spend the money to refit your windows or redo one side of your house. Further, Rossbach suggests, as a way of removing "the overbearing forces altogether," a convex mirror that reflects the images upside down.[24] However, Bartlett cautions against over-using mirrors or using them randomly (especially inside the house), as "they are powerful remedies and can cause chaotic energies when misused."

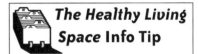

The Healthy Living Space Info Tip

For a source of practical feng shui devices, objects, mirrors, and other feng shui tools, as well as books and practitioner listings, contact:
Feng Shui Warehouse,
P.O. Box 6689,
San Diego, CA 92166;
tel: 800-399-1599 or 619-523-2158;
e-mail: fengshuiWH@aol.com;
website:
www.fengshuiwarehouse.com.

In terms of influencing your neighbors, there is more you can do than setting up effective defense perimeters against their noisy intrusions, explains Bartlett. You can send them nice vibrations. The simplest way to do that is by purifying your space; this change in the energy pattern of the neighborhood gets registered, at some level, by your neighbors. If they are sensitive, they may detect that somehow the change came from your house, and they may want to make changes themselves, says Bartlett.

"Because everything affects everything, if you focus on your environment, and make that as whole and healthy and clearly aligned as possible, then you immediately affect your neighbors," Bartlett says. "Inevitably, after doing a house clearing, sometime later—a week, a month or two—I'll get a call from somebody a street or two away in that same neighborhood asking me to do feng shui on their house. As I understand it, on some level, they *felt* the positive changes. They heard, felt, or sensed the energetic change in their neighborhood and it sparked them and woke them up, and now they want some of it, too. That's one way to affect your neighbors in a positive way."

HEALTHY LIVING SPACE DETOXIFIER #61
Optimizing the Mouth of Qi *at Your Front Door*

One of the most important elements of your living space to check and correct is your front door, or whichever entrance you use most frequently. This is your point of transition from outer to inner world, from the external environment into your private domestic space. The threshold into your home, and to a lesser extent, the threshold into any room in the house, is where the life force energy enters like an exhaled breath. Feng shui calls it "the mouth of *qi*," and if your home's "mouth" is unclean or obstructed, your health will suffer.

"The way *qi* flows throughout the house is important," explains Bartlett, and the front door can be the key to a healthy flow. Your home's mouth of *qi* represents your relationship with the outer world, both natural and social: energy, money, opportunities, good health, well-being, friends, and good fortune flow in through the front door, but if the flow of this energy (and its numerous expressions) is blocked, the *qi* cannot get to your marriage corner, or prosperity section, or any of the other six *Ba-Gua* life divisions, and your life, correspondingly, will be negatively affected.

You need to think about the matter of *qi* flow in both a symbolic and practical sense, because both realms will help you detoxify your home using feng shui principles. How the *qi* flows, or doesn't, affects the parts of your life that correspond to the parts of your house where the *qi* is obstructed. The front door is like a *qi* valve, which can let in positive energy and block out negative energy. "Inhibited, obstructed, or confused flow of chi is probably the number one problem to solve with feng shui," comments Angel Thompson. There are numerous ways in which the *qi* flow can be blocked, compromised, or diverted, and any of these arrangements can "frustrate, anger, even enrage the chi," with the result that the occupants feel the same way. "Tension, poor health, and bad luck await those who occupy the space."[25]

"What you see first upon entering a house is important, as this creates your first subconscious experience of its atmosphere," observes Bartlett, and this is especially true of your own living space. Preferable is a view of a foyer or vestibule or living room with its evocation of rest, leisure, and quiet entertainment; not preferable, for example, is a view of a bathroom or kitchen, says Bartlett. Particularly undesirable in a two-story home is a direct alignment of second-floor toilet, staircase, and front door; in the symbolic energy calculus of feng shui, your wealth (an expression of qi) flows right out the front door and/or down the toilet.

A first view of a kitchen is undesirable, says Bartlett, because the first thought you get upon entering your home is food. The result may be eating or bingeing tendencies, which lead to weight problems. Feng shui consultant Terah Kathryn Collins relates a case study of a woman who was unable to overcome her bulimia. Collins, upon visiting the woman's house, found that her front door opened directly into the kitchen. The solution was to transform the kitchen (at least what could be seen from the home's threshold) into an atrium, with palms, bromeliads, and a flowing water and rock feature. The kitchen functions were moved down to one end of the room and redesigned as a kitchen nook. The woman thereafter found it much easier to correct her unbalanced eating habits since her home (and its mouth of qi) was not constantly stimulating her to overeat.[26]

You can get a sense of the flow of energy through your home's mouth of qi by standing at the threshold of your home, facing in. Imagine a gently forceful breeze flowing into your house through this open front door; it is a breeze that brings all good things, invigorates everything it contacts, clears out stagnation, and brings well-being—*provided* its flow is unobstructed. Follow this flow of energy through your house: what path does it take? What gets in its way? Where does it get stuck? Is there an exit point, a back door, out of which it can flow when it's finished inside your home?

The information you gather from this simple exercise can be the basis for applying feng shui "remedies" to improve the qi flow in your living space. The key point to remember is this: obstructed qi flow produces energy stagnation, and this negatively affects the health of the home's occupants.

- Keep hallways and access areas free of clutter and unnecessary objects, says Bartlett. If possible, avoid zigzagging flows (such as multiple L-layouts in hallways and attached rooms) from one section of the house to another. These "twist up your energy field, causing confusion and an uncentered feeling, which can be quite exhausting." Further, it makes it hard for the qi to flow smoothly, or at all, through the house, says Bartlett.[27]

- Make sure your front door opens fully and is not obstructed by anything behind it. The hindrance in opening fully obstructs the qi flow and it can chronically provoke a reaction of annoyance and irritation by those who open the door, expecting it to yield fully. "When doors are allowed to open fully, the people walking through them can open fully to promising opportunities, resources, and circumstances in their lives."[28]

- Another typical and undesirable feature at the entrance is constriction, such as if there is a wall close to the entrance on the inside. "If upon entering you come to a wall close to the entrance, then this would be said to limit your opportunities in life," says Bartlett. It inhibits qi and, according to traditional feng shui thinking, it guarantees you a life of struggle, if not failure within three years.

  If this is the case in your home, place a mirror (not a feng shui mirror but a conventional larger reflecting mirror) on the wall to face the door, "thereby expanding the reflected image so that the wall feels more expansive." Alternatively, you can hang a picture or photograph of an outdoor scene, "featuring a stream flowing down through a valley, thereby allowing your sensitivities to go beyond the wall in front of you," says Bartlett.

- If you live near a place of excellent qi, such as by the ocean, a park, a river, lake, mountain view, or other natural setting of high quality qi, there is a simple way to invite this qi to flow into your home. Place a feng shui mirror outside your front door (or the door or window facing the auspicious scene) in such a way that it reflects the scenic environment into your house. You should be able to see the scene reflected in the outside mirror as you stand at your front door (or window).[29]

• If the immediate space inside your front door is dark or constrained, this oppresses the mouth of qi and "chokes" the occupants' good luck. Or if the entrance is a narrow hallway, this can generate health problems such as respiratory problems and difficult births; further, the psychological impact of such a darkened entryway is depressing and can lead to melancholy moods. The feng shui "cure" is to install a very bright ceiling light (at least 100 watts) and a mirror on the opposite wall; both will invigorate the qi and create a sense of depth.[30]

• Feng shui offers other practical low-cost devices either to ward off harmful qi or to maximize inflowing positive qi. Wind chimes, hung under eaves, can temper and redirect malignant energy or summon positive qi into a living space. Rounded prisms or small-faceted crystal balls can convert overly strong qi and disperse it throughout an interior space.

HEALTHY LIVING SPACE DETOXIFIER #62
Setting Up a Feng Shui-Friendly Bedroom

Possibly of equal importance to your home's mouth of qi is the disposition of your bedroom, where you spend up to one-third of your life. There are many key factors to consider in applying feng shui to your bedroom, including the following recommendations about bed placement:

•Do not situate your bed such that your feet, as you lie in bed, face the bedroom door. In classical Chinese thinking, this is the "death position." In old China, corpses were laid out with their feet pointing towards the door to facilitate their passage into the next world. *Do* situate your bed so that the bed faces the door but displaced to the side. In other words, your feet face the same wall that contains the door, yet none of the bed directly faces the door opening. Remember, that on a smaller scale, the door into your bedroom is the mouth of qi for that room and its function, so the same principles apply here as they do for your home's main front door.

• Put the bed against a solid wall if possible, but not a window because your qi can escape through the window while you sleep, leaving you depleted in the morning.

- Regarding bed placement, the important principle is to have the correct relationship with your bedroom's mouth of *qi*, explains Bartlett. Ideally, you want to be in a "commanding position," he says, so that "when you're lying in bed on your back, you can clearly see the doorway to the bedroom. This gives you a feeling of being in control, of having power over your environment." If anything enters the bedroom, you will see it as it enters and not be taken by surprise by its unannounced entry. "On a subconscious level, if you are not able to see the bedroom's doorway at night when you sleep, this might create a feeling of uncertainty and insecurity."

One long-term consequence of having your bed positioned wrongly with respect to the bedroom's mouth of *qi* is that "your opportunities in life might be limited," says Bartlett. "You might find that you're not easily manifesting and creating things that you want and need." Bartlett cites an example from his case records.

One long-term consequence of having your bed positioned wrongly with respect to the bedroom's mouth of qi is that "your opportunities in life might be limited," says Bartlett. "You might find that you're not easily manifesting and creating things that you want and need."

He consulted with a woman who lived in an apartment; she told Bartlett she felt stifled in her career and wanted to establish a relationship with someone. "Her bed was placed in such a way that it was not in the commanding position, yet when I explained this to her, she was resistant to changing it." She told Bartlett she felt comfortable being "tucked away" into the room's corner; he countered by suggesting that it was perhaps "part of her subconscious need to protect herself." He encouraged her to try moving the bed as an experiment, to see how she felt under the new conditions. "She did this, then all those difficult aspects immediately changed in her life."

- Do not place your bed under an exposed beam or low slanted ceiling. "These angular protrusions are carriers of sha [negative *qi*] and can cause headaches, confused thinking, and even financial and career problems." An exposed beam that runs the length of the room, bisecting the bed from above, can provoke marital discord, literally by placing an energy barrier between the partners. Beams that cross the bed horizontally can generate aches, pains, even diseases in the body regions under the crossing influence, such as a beam across the abdomen leading to digestive disorders.[31]

• Do not place mirrors facing the bed. If you wake in the middle of the night and see your reflection, it can be very unsettling, even shocking.

• Generally, it is not advisable to place electronic equipment in the bedroom, such as computers, televisions, fax machines, or radios. These generate a constant electromagnetic field, which can negatively affect you while sleeping, and they can confuse the function of the bedroom (rest and regeneration) with profession and career (such as using the computer for writing, bookkeeping, or Internet research). They serve as continual reminders of work obligations, and this is contrary to the state of mind that induces relaxation and rest.

• There are two ways to minimize or eliminate the effect of electromagnetic fields upon you as you sleep at night, says Bartlett. First, if your head is near an electrical outlet (not desirable but often unavoidable), you can install a switch in the circuit box that shuts off all electrical power to the bedroom at night. Second, you can place a flat spiral dielectric resonator under your bed. "This device balances the energetic field under a bed and will neutralize most noxious zones. Aside from improved sleep, many people report they suddenly feel more comfortable."[32]

• Don't use the bedroom as a storage facility. Piles of materials, such as books, clothes, boxes, or other objects in corners of the room or under the bed lead to areas of stagnant, nonflowing qi, and these conditions will eventually have a negative impact on the health of the room's occupants. These piles can also produce jumpiness and disturb one's sleep.

• Don't situate the head of your bed against a wall that abuts the bathroom. Feng shui consultant Angel Thompson relates a case in which a woman consulted her for relationship help, reporting that her affairs were constantly falling apart and "going down the toilet." Thompson found that the head of the woman's bed was against the same wall that abutted the toilet. So symbolically and energetically, her relationship/marriage section of the *Ba-Gua* was in the toilet space, which flushed away all the marriage *qi* generated or cultivated in the bedroom.

Thompson recommended moving the bed to another wall; this apparently worked as, soon after, the woman got married. If you can't move your bed, place a mirror in the bathroom on the wall opposite the toilet to deflect the toilet energy from entering the bedroom, Thompson suggests. Alternatively, place a mirror on the bedroom wall opposite the bed "to symbolically move the bed to the opposite side of the room" and away from the toilet wall.[33]

- There are several ill-advised locations within the house for a bedroom, according to feng shui practitioners: under a toilet, a washing machine, or stove (on the next floor up); over a garage; at the end of a long corridor. The flow of *qi* down a long corridor is too fast and strong and can attract health problems over time; it's even more harmful if your bed faces the door that opens into the corridor. The situation of a bed over a garage leads to an inability to develop foundations in your life, to the sense of rootlessness and a transitory residence in the home.

HEALTHY LIVING SPACE DETOXIFIER #63
Setting Up a Feng Shui-Friendly Bathroom

Feng shui experts agree that a key principle with bathrooms is that the *qi* must be able to flow in and out of this room without any obstruction or any place in which it can get stuck and produce stagnation. They also agree that feng shui imbalances in this section of the house can produce health problems, as this case study from the practice files of Terah Kathryn Collins vividly shows.

Collins was called in to consult with a woman who had moved into a new house only nine months previously. During that short stay, she had sustained an inexplicable sudden bout of clumsiness and three falling injuries. She had tripped or fallen as many times in nine months as she had in her entire life of forty-five years, so she suspected something in her environment might be stimulating this. Collins determined that while most of the woman's house was in good feng shui balance, there was a significant problem with the bathroom. For one thing, it was in the wrong place—that is, the home's sole toilet was situated between two bedrooms, both of which opened into it with their doors in direct opposition to each other.

This configuration speeded up the flow of qi as it passed through the bathroom and into the bedrooms, especially as their doors were usually left open, says Collins. "Living with the rushing Ch'i can cause you to move too quickly," she told the homeowner, who admitted that in the three falling incidents, in which she was injured, she was "rushing to do something." In other words, her own actions were influenced by the imbalanced flow of qi: it rushed through, and so did she, except she got off balance each time and fell.

Once Collins had identified the source of the problem, she was able to apply effective feng shui solutions. Keep the bathroom doors closed whenever possible; keep the bathroom drains closed and the toilet lid down; hang two round faceted crystals in the bathroom, one by the window (to draw the qi into the bathroom from outside), the other in the middle of the bathroom (to balance the flow from the two bedrooms when both doors were open).

Collins further recommended that the woman hang in the bathroom a piece of art that to her symbolized good health, and also hang a large wardrobe mirror on the outside of the bathroom door leading into the bedroom currently being used as an office to increase productivity in that room. A few months after the changes were completed, the woman reported that ever since the changes, she had been healthy, calmer, and had not fallen or tripped.[34]

As mentioned above, qi needs to move easily and briskly in and out of the bathroom, but water is another element of crucial importance to this room. Sink, toilet, shower stall, bathtub—from out of the bottom of each flows water. Feng shui experts counsel that it is vital to observe the energy symbolism here so that water does not get equated with money, and as your bathroom goes, so goes your prosperity. It is a truism—yet true nonetheless—that if your toilet faces your mouth of *qi* (your home's main entrance), you run the real risk of having your good fortune (incoming *qi*) flushing down the toilet every day. Here are some additional tips for the feng shui-friendly bathroom:

- A potted plant can encourage *qi* to flow into the bathroom, and blue is an excellent color for the walls or fittings because this color relates to the water element, advises feng shui advisor Richard Webster.

- However, he counsels if your bathroom is located in the middle of your home, in the good luck area (the center of the *Ba-Gua* octagon), this is most unfortunate because "it will send negative ch'i throughout the house" and your good luck down the toilet. Obviously it is not practical to rip out the toilet and move it, so Webster suggests placing *Ba-Gua* mirrors on all four walls of the bathroom to produce the effect of making the room symbolically disappear. In a sense, its otherwise negative energy gets trapped and neutralized in an infinite hall of mirrors, and becomes incapable of escaping this energy matrix to exert an influence on the rest of your home.

- Webster also says it is unfortunate if your bathroom is located at the end of a long corridor, because this sends a *shar* (poison arrow) heading directly into it, and beneficial *qi* entering your house through its mouth of *qi* goes down the toilet and is lost to the home's occupants. The solution is to keep the toilet lid down when not in use, to keep the bathroom door closed, and to place a mirror on the outside of the bathroom door— again to make the room "symbolically" disappear and at least to disarm the poison arrow flying down the corridor.[35]

- Another problem with the bathroom is if it is located in the wealth section of the *Ba-Gua*, as this is likely to produce financial or abundance problems. Again, the issue is one of flushing your wealth down the toilet. If your toilet is located in this section, Australian architect, engineer, and feng shui consultant George Birdsall advises placing a crystal in the bathroom window to attract incoming *qi* from outside, keeping the toilet lid down and the bathroom door closed, and placing a feng shui (*Ba-Gua*) mirror on the outside of the bathroom door to "seal off this room's energy from the rest of the home or business."[36]

The Health Costs of Having an Energy-Imbalanced Home

At first glance, many of the feng shui observations and recommendations cited here and throughout the burgeoning literature of the ancient art of placement seem odd, perhaps ridiculous, and surely impossible according to our general sense of the way the world works. How can a toilet flush affect our well-being? But feng shui describes the world and its workings at a subtler level of operation than we are accustomed to credit it as having; it works in a sphere of influence about which we are normally oblivious. Feng shui deals with causes, and we are usually aware only of the effects, in the form of dysfunction, ill health, or misfortune.

Even though it seems hard to grant that your prosperity can be symbolically flushed down the toilet if your bathroom is situated in the wrong part of your house, this eventuality has been demonstrated empirically in hundreds of documented case studies reported by feng shui practitioners. The *Ba-Gua* is not an arbitrary or fancifully contrived scheme; it is, according to feng shui, a true-to-life model of energy relationships at any level of reality—a hologram of the cosmos, if you will—and especially at the level of a residence. Functions within each of its eight sections are influenced, if not directed, by that section's symbolic role within the overall energy configuration and the dynamic interplay of the five elements during the course of the year.[37]

Perhaps the best way to demonstrate this point is to relate the following remarkable case study of the terrible effect of bad feng shui arrangements in a home upon its occupants, as explained by Jenny Liu, an environmental designer and feng shui professional. Liu relates the extreme toxic effects a house had on its teenage resident and how she corrected the bad feng shui.[38]

A woman called Liu and said her teenage son was rebellious, having "mental problems," and generally driving her crazy. Visiting the woman's house, Liu immediately saw that the orientation of the house itself was highly unfavorable. It was a "backwards-sitting house," which means a hill rises in front of the house, and behind the home, the ground slopes downward. For well-being, the arrangement should be the opposite, Liu says. The hill before the house blocks the inflow of good energy into the house, while the incline out back allows energy to drain away from the house.

There were other more arcane aspects to the home's orientation—its orientation and energy style were contrary to that of its occupants—that ensured that the home itself would produce internal trouble for its occupants, especially any males living within it. It would weaken their health (producing head colds and respiratory problems) and generate unstable relationships. Inspecting the interior of the home, Liu found that a fireplace directly faced the main entrance (mouth of *qi*). "Having a major circulation path where people are constantly coming into conflict with fire energies is a potential cause of family arguments," Liu told the woman, who confirmed that her family members had many disagreements.

Further, a stove and an exposed overhead beam were located in the center or "heart" of the home. This spelled further trouble, because the stove produced temper, while the exposed beam "suppresses heart energies that can cause family members to feel congested and stifled." Both features were triggers for constant quarrels among family members. The son's bedroom door was directly in line with that of his parent's master bedroom, a configuration that set the stage for conflicts between the occupants of both rooms. Further, the two bedrooms were separated by a bathroom, which faced the *Ba-Gua* direction associated with the liver and eldest son, in classical Chinese thinking. Functionally, this meant that the bathroom's inherently "degrading energies" would conflict with the son's liver energies, and make him moody and easily tired, and hinder his body's ability to detoxify itself.

Liu found the bedrooms to be dark, poorly ventilated, and intensely cluttered, and the teenage son's room had numerous wall posters depicting violent images. Just to complicate matters further, the home's previous owner had died in the house and the present owner's teenage son had tried to commit suicide three times already. Liu's overall assessment was that this house was a "container of *sha qi*," or harmful, negative, health-dampening energies. Anyone living in such a house, she added, "is bound to get very sick, have abnormal behavior, mental problems, and suffer a great deal of trouble and money loss."

Astonishingly, the woman's family had endured this "sick house" for ten years, although she had tried on occasions to move; failing this, she admitted her family was "slowly falling apart."

Liu's main recommendation was to move out of the home immediately. It was too full of negative, stagnant energies for her family to cope any longer; already the males had succumbed to its bad influence. Liu noted that the woman's husband's aura was extremely dark and that his face showed signs of kidney exhaustion; even so, he was unaware that the house was having a bad influence on him, and he denied that there were any problems afoot inside his home at all, so he refused to move.

Liu set out to purify the *sha qi*, or negative energies. She advised the family to clean up the clutter and get rid of everything they didn't need; to cover the fireplace with a screen to hide it; to hang crystal balls and place living green plants on either side of it to neutralize the fire energy; to place a mirror behind the stove to reflect negative energies away from the home's center; and to hang a wind chime between the son's room and that of his parent's to disperse some of the conflicted energy between them. Liu further instructed the son to take down all the violent posters and put in their place images of nature and uplifting themes related to his personal goals.

"These are temporary means of ameliorating some of the negative energies, so that they may live a bit more comfortably while they search for a new home," observes Liu, noting that the father finally consented to move. These measures would not, she added, change the bad effects of the land and home's structural configuration, but they would help the family enhance their own positive energies so as to resist the debilitating effect of their home. These measures would help them "break the cycle of having the house's energies constantly degenerating their well-being." While the combined toxic elements of this *sha qi* house did not entirely produce all the ill-health and poor results in this family, they *amplified* the residents' latent vulnerabilities, tendencies, and unresolved conflicts to the extent that they became almost unbearable and lethal.

With the exception of the issue of the home's orientation, most of the health-destroying toxic elements in this "sick house" existed inside the house. In the next chapter, we take a look outside the house to see what effect subtle exterior environmental influences and toxic agents can exert on our health.

CHAPTER 12

Cleansing the Home's Exterior Environment:

Neutralizing the Effects of Geopathic Stress

It comes as an alarming discovery to many to learn that after having removed all the toxic elements in the home to make it a bau-biologie-friendly residence, as discussed in chapter 10, and having arranged the home according to feng shui principles to make it a *qi*-friendly living space, as in chapter 11, there may still be another underlying toxic element, one of equal if not greater potency to produce ill health. This one literally *under-lies* the home.

The influence is called geopathic stress, or geopathogenic stress, and refers to the ability of the Earth to produce illness or pathology. It isn't that the planet itself is inherently toxic, but that in certain places, the combination of natural and/or human-made elements can produce toxic effects. If your home is situated over such a confluence of potentially toxic energies, you may develop any of a wide range of illnesses and physical dysfunctions, including chronic fatigue syndrome, cancer, and multiple sclerosis. It gets worse if your bedroom, or merely your bed, sits over such an underground field of noxious influence, principally because most people spend one-third of their lives here.

Typically, the term geopathic stress encompasses the health-altering effects of underground water streams (50-450 feet below the surface and 10-20 inches wide, although they can be any width), mineral and ore deposits and concentrations, caves, geological faults, underground cavities, or specially "disturbed" places within various energy "grids" purported to exist on or below the Earth's surface. It can also include human-made features such as mining installations, foundations for tall buildings, underground transport systems such as subways, sewers and drains, and public utility installations.

These various geobiological influences, according to the researchers, emit what have variously been described as "noxious fields," "earthrays," "Earth radiations," and "black streams" that penetrate everything above them, destabilize the electromagnetic fields of living organisms, compromise immune function, and produce illness. The key is that various factors can distort the Earth's natural, and usually beneficial electromagnetic field (EMF); in fact, the planet's EMF is subject to natural gradients, of variations of stronger or weaker strengths. As one expert puts it, "Geopathic stress occurs when the Earth's magnetic field is disturbed, either naturally or artificially, and the background field we normally experience is changed."[1]

Once the natural radiation is disturbed, it can become harmful to biological life, including ours as humans, if we spend a lot of time over it. If you spend enough time over a geopathic stress zone (and the amount of time can vary dramatically from hours to years), some form of illness or dysfunction is likely to develop, according to the Dulwich Health clinic in London, one of England's premier geopathic stress (GS) and treatment facilities. "By diagnosing well over 40,000 people, we have found GS in people with most types of serious and long-term illnesses."

The effect is especially enhanced if we sleep over it, because while relaxed, the body is more susceptible to the harmful influences, and the brain and nervous system must spend some of their energy dealing with the noxious influence instead of resting. Normally during sleep the brain accomplishes the body's "housekeeping," creating some eighty percent of required new cells and directing the body to absorb nutrients and adjust its hormone levels. "GS will interfere with this process and leave your immune system weak. Geopathic stress does not cause any illness, but lowers your immune system and your ability to fight off viruses and bacteria." Dulwich Health emphasizes that usually all these body functions return to normal once GS is removed from the environment and its effects cleansed from the body.[2]

Put more technically, advocates of the discipline of geopathic stress explain that harmful Earth energies, in the form of ionizing and nonionizing electromagnetic radiation that emanates[3] naturally from the planet's "geophysiology," rise upwards to the surface of the planet and can negatively affect all life living over and in its influence. Fortunately, geopathic stress, once detected, can be minimized, reversed, or eliminated according to a variety of simple but effective techniques.

Disease Can Be a Problem of Location

Knowledge of geopathic stress emerged in Germany in the early days of the twentieth century when a researcher named Baron Gustav Freiherr von Pohl discovered a link between cancer clusters and the patients' homes. In 1929, working in Vilsbiburg, Germany, a village of 3,300 people and 565 houses, von Pohl correlated the addresses and sleeping locations of 54 people who had died of cancer with the existence of noxious underground water streams that passed beneath the homes or bedrooms of the cancer victims.

Von Pohl was acting on a hunch inspired by the earlier Winzer-Melzer survey of Stuttgart in the 1920s, which had determined that major geological faults in that city traversed the districts that had the highest cancer mortality rates. The tentative conclusion was that an unknown but noxious radiation emanating from the earth faults might be an important and overlooked contributory cause of the cancers.

Through dowsing, von Pohl located all the major subterranean water veins (lying at a depth of forty-four to fifty meters with a width of three to four meters) under Vilsbiburg, then mapped their courses on the city street plan. Next he crosschecked this with the residences of the fifty-four recent cancer fatalities and arrived at a startling conclusion. "The completed check of my map confirmed all the beds of the 54 cancer deaths were where I had drawn the radiation currents," von Pohl wrote in 1932 in his now classic *Earth Currents: Causative Factor of Cancer and Other Diseases*.

Von Pohl concluded that those who died from cancer had "slept in a strongly ray-infected place" at the time of their diagnosis. In fact, he declared: "All diseases of human beings, animals, trees and plants are actually caused by earth currents; the currents weaken the organism and make it more vulnerable to disease." Von Pohl was confident about his discoveries but tended to take a conservative stance regarding developing a hypothetical model. "My observations set down in this book about negative electrical earth currents are in the main virgin territory for medical science. We not only hope but expect that more doctors will research and advance this new knowledge for the benefit of mankind."

Eighteen months later, von Pohl returned to Vilsbiburg and found that the beds of another ten cancer mortalities were situated directly over the intersection of underground streams. Following von Pohl's indications, another researcher named Dr. Hager investigated the residences of 5,348 people who had died of cancer over a 21-year span in the town of Stettin; he found that in all cases "strong earth rays" and a subterranean water vein had intersected underneath their homes. "Medical science has now a preventative measure which did not exist previously," noted von Pohl. "If one makes sure one's bed does not stand above a strong underground current and one tries not to work above these underground currents, one should not get cancer."[4]

There are very few people whose constitution is robust enough to permit sleeping "in a bed full of radiation" without some form of adverse health effect, von Pohl added. In fact, von Pohl documented the direct relationship between sleeping in a bed situated over Earth currents and numerous health complaints: nervous itching, insomnia, abdominal pains, asthma, shivers, headaches, migraine, gallbladder dysfunction, rheumatism, heart spasms, tuberculosis, heavy menstruation, thrombosis, mental illness, and epilepsy, among others. Not only did von Pohl describe the correlations between bed location and noxious underground emissions, he demonstrated the curative benefit of simply moving the bed to avoid the geopathogenic zones. He thereby produced remarkable reversals in numerous immedicable health conditions.

Von Pohl had determined the existence of the underground streams using the services of professional dowsers, which to most scientists was not a "legitimate" methodology. In 1960, another German researcher named Jacob Stangle replicated von Pohl's research using sophisticated geomagnetometers and confirmed von Pohl's 1929 findings. Since von Pohl's day, a host of researchers from Germany and other countries have confirmed and considerably extended his model of "cancer houses" and "cancer beds."

For example, in the 1930s, Swiss researcher Dr. S. Jenny studied the effects of geobiological faults and subterranean water streams on the health of laboratory mice. He documented these geopathic effects on 25,000 mice over a period of twelve years of study. Dr. Jenny found that when the cage of the mice was placed over a disturbance in the geomagnetic field, the mice grew agitated, gnawed their own tails, and sometimes ate their offspring; they also often developed cancer. When they were moved to a neutral zone, free of geopathic stress, the mice settled down. Given the choice, the mice chose to stay over the neutral (healthy) zone rather than over the geopathically stressed one. Not long after, Professor K.E. Lotz of the School of Architecture of Biberach, Germany, analyzed 400 cancer deaths and found that 383 were related to beds situated over geological faults, underground water veins, or disturbances in the natural geomagnetic field.[5]

Austrian researchers found that when a person was exposed to the noxious energy emissions of the Earth there were measurable changes in a majority of the twenty-three biochemical factors considered, such as the blood values of serotonin and melatonin as well as levels of important minerals such as zinc and calcium.

In 1989, Austrian researchers finished a twenty-four-month study on the short-term effects of geopathogenic sites on human health. Researchers led by Otto Bergsmann, M.D., a specialist in internal medicine at the University of Vienna in Austria, tested 985 sites with 462,421 different measurements included within 6,943 individual tests. They found that when a person was exposed to the noxious energy emissions of the Earth there were measurable changes in a majority of the twenty-three biochemical factors considered, such as the blood values of serotonin[6] (an important brain chemical, or neurotransmitter) and melatonin[7] (the sleep-regulating hormone) as well as levels of important minerals such as zinc and calcium. "There were many other altered states to biological functions noted as a result of short-term exposure to these forces."[8]

Hans Nieper, M.D., another noted German researcher and former director of the Paracelsus Silbersee Hospital in Hannover, Germany, concluded on the basis of his clinical obser- vations that seventy-five percent of his multiple sclerosis patients spent too much time over a geopathogenic zone. He found similar correlations for cancer, reporting that ninety-three percent of people with malignancies acquired them as a result of residing over "a crossing in a geopathogenic zone."

Dr. Nieper explained that the geopathogenic zone did not necessary produce the cancer all by itself, but the incidence of cancer cases is certainly higher in correlation with such zones than otherwise, and the effect of living or sleeping over these noxious zones "increases the risk of gene lability," which becomes a biochemical foundation for the emergence of cancer. Dr. Nieper characterized the "geopathically stressed zone" as "the ultimate push button" that makes the cancer happen.[9] Like von Pohl, Dr. Nieper strongly advised those suffering from the ill effects of geopathically stressed areas to remove themselves from the site of geopathogenic exposure.

HEALTHY LIVING SPACE DETOXIFIER #64
When Nothing Else Heals, Try Moving Your Bed

Despite the complexity of the geopathic stress theory and its dismaying illumination of another toxic environmental energy, often the solution is radically simple. Move your bed, even a few feet, and you may get well. While the subject of geo- pathic stress and geopathogenic zones is still practically an unknown medical category in North America, in Europe, espe- cially Germany and England, it has been recognized to a far greater extent by physicians as a factor in illness and its rever- sal. In fact, some physicians now state that as a rule of thumb if a patient fails to respond to the indicated therapies (either con- ventional or alternative), it is possible that a geopathogenic influence exists in their living space.

In an influential article in the British *Journal of Alternative and Complementary Medicine*, physician Anthony Scott- Morley of the Institute of Bioenergetic Medicine looked at how geopathic stress might block natural therapeutics. He proposed that habitual exposure to "geopathic disturbance" produced by "localized variations in the geomagnetic flux of the earth" might be a basic reason why natural therapies like acupuncture and homeopathy fail to provide a definitive cure in some patients. He reasoned there must be other mitigating factors that compromised what was otherwise "excellent and appropriate therapy."

Scott-Morley reported that according to "experienced practitioners who are aware of these stresses," thirty percent to fifty percent of chronically sick patients exhibit some degree of geopathic stress. "A geopathic stress may be defined," wrote Scott-Morley, "as a geomagnetic disturbance which is geographically localized and which disrupts the homeostatic mechanisms of the sensitive patient. It does seem that geopathic stresses energetically weaken the body so that the patient may be more prone to disease-forming processes."[10] A more recent study concluded that geopathic stress can undermine "both the body's subtle energy system (the etheric body, chakras, and meridians), and the body's electrical system (brain, heart, and muscles), thus delaying healing and recovery."[11]

Von Pohl produced stunning turnabouts in clinical conditions merely by moving the patient's bed out of a dowsed geopathogenic zone in the bedroom. Since his time, other practitioners have applied his insight and helped many suffering individuals reverse their otherwise intractable health conditions. Notable among these practitioners has been Kathe Bachler, an Austrian dowser who investigated over 3,000 homes and 12,000 cases of geopathic stress among individuals in fifteen countries. Bachler concluded that toxic underground energy emissions— she called them "noxious Earth energies"—represent a major contributing factor in the emergence of many health problems.

"*All* serious illnesses I have found up to now occur above interference crossings: twitching, tinnitus, facial paralysis, angina, asthma, heart attacks, strokes, inflammation of the kidneys, cancer (in more than 700 cases without exception). Doctors say that our immune system is weakened by constant radiation so that, depending on one's constitution and the prevalent influences, different diseases can develop."[12] Bachler specialized in correlating poor school performance in children and children's health problems with geopathogenic zones or what she refers to as "interference zones." Below is a sampling of her empirical field results.

- A young mother had two boys with serious behavior problems. Every night, one of the boys, depending on which bed he was sleeping in, would toss and turn, and throw his arms about as if he were having a fit. Bachler found he was sleeping over an interference zone that got activated every night when the boiler on the other side of the bedroom wall was turned on. She moved both beds and the children slept soundly thereafter.

- A boy was a chronic bed-wetter and, after seven years, no physician could provide an answer to the embarrassing problem. Undersized for his age, nervous, and irritable in the morning, he was sleeping on a crossing of two interference zones. "With other bed-wetters—all of whom lie on interference zones—a cure can often be immediate and often achieved simply by moving the bed at random," says Bachler.

- Poor school performance is often linked with "geobiological influences." Bachler found that students who were always tired, were the slowest in doing school work, had the greatest difficulty in concentrating, were the most forgetful or the worst behaved, or were frequently ill "were all victims of interference zone crossings."

- A twelve-year-old girl developed a severe backache during a gym class, and the pain did not go away afterwards. She was confined to her bed for eight weeks with cramp-like pain, but no physical cause could be identified for her discomfort. Bachler found she was sleeping over an interference zone. The girl's bed was moved immediately and in a few weeks the mother reported her daughter's back problem had healed.

In the cases above, and in the thousands of others treated by Bachler, moving the bed of the one who was ill reversed the health problem, usually in a dramatically brief period. In every house, even in every room in a house, "there are also good places where we all have the chance of becoming healthier in body, mind, and spirit," she concluded.[13]

During the last three decades of the twentieth century, as the concept of geopathic stress gained currency in the progressive flanks of American research and alternative medicine, dowsers independently verified and extended the original findings. For example, Vermont dowser Herbert Douglas stated that based on ten years of research and investigation of sixty cases of arthritis, twenty of cancer, and nine of cataracts, in every case, intersecting lines of energy passed under the bedroom in direct relation to the affected part of the body.

In almost all the cancer cases, Douglas found "a network of water veins creating anywhere from thirty to fifty crossings." In some cases, clefts or breaks in a subterranean rocky ledge underneath the ground (but directly underneath the bed) created the harmful energy emissions, he said. Douglas said the easiest way to visualize this hidden but measurable effect was to lay a series of wooden laths across the patient's bed, to correspond with the dowsed underground energy lines. With actual clients, Douglas laid the laths on the bed, according to his dowsing indications, then had the patient assume their customary sleeping position on top of them. "Repeatedly, the crossing of the laths indicates precisely where the person is afflicted," states Douglas.[14]

French research in the 1940s demonstrated the connection between subterranean energy emissions (ionizing radiation) and the incidence of cancer. Pierre Cody made a seven-year study in the French city of Le Havre using an electrometer to measure air ion concentrations at various locations in the cellars underlying 7,000 "cancer beds" in the homes of people who had died of cancer. Cody discovered that the air ion concentrations were ten times higher when measured on the spot in the cellar directly under the bed than at spots even a few feet away; he further found that the typical width of the band of toxic radiation was about four and one-half feet. His study also showed that the radiation was capable of rising vertically, up from within the ground and through the patient's bed, without spreading out horizontally.[15]

British dowser and geopathic stress investigator Alf Riggs also built an impressive empirical base for his conclusions about geopathogenic zones. He studied the energy emissions in 14,000 homes in fifteen countries for correlations between noxious underground radiation and illness. Among the health problems, he studied 2,200 cases of chronic fatigue syndrome (myalgic encephalomyelitis, as the British call it) and found that one of the two major causes of chronic fatigue is exposure to specific types of Earth radiation, the other being energy depletion due to viruses.

"As a result of these observations, I contend that chronic fatigue syndrome is initially a bioelectric problem," says Riggs. This illness often results "from an imbalance in the value of bioelectric fields at cell level caused by the invasion of specific electromagnetic fields" from the outside edges of the underground water stream. Riggs further concludes that disease is, in fair measure, "a problem of location, with the fields generated from Earth and manmade sources having the ability to invade the cell, altering the values of the bioelectric systems within."[16]

As a subterranean water stream flows under a house (or simply under the Earth's surface), it interacts with the geological strata present and creates a positive electrical field, more specifically, a direct-current-generated magnetic field, Riggs explains. Small bands of energy appear on both outside edges of the flowing water and radiate upwards. According to Riggs, most of the biological damage caused by geopathogenic zones produced by underground water is due to these two outside bands. Riggs estimates it is the chief factor in seventy-two percent of cases.

He reports that after moving a patient's bed into a neutral zone in the bedroom, "away from the harmful Earth rays and manmade radiation," chronic fatigue patients "often enjoy a measurable improvement," although they do not always have a full recovery from this intervention alone. Usually what completes the recovery is some form of energy therapy or "bioelectric treatment" by a skilled practitioner. This combination of approaches has resulted in significant improvement in over eighty percent of the cases Riggs has overseen, including many long-term cases involving severe disabilities.

Riggs further explains that these frequencies have deleterious effects on women by interfering with their estrogen cycle. Riggs investigated 1,600 cases of energy depletion, and found that young girls can sleep in beds positioned over the outside edge lines of underground streams for years without being noticeably affected until they reach puberty, when without exception they develop chronic fatigue. Boys may sleep on such noxious lines without ill effect, but adolescent girls always suffer far worse because of the negative interaction between the emitted electromagnetic fields and estrogen, says Riggs.

Not only can the position of the bed be a negative health factor when it sits over a geopathogenic zone, but sometimes the composition of the bed itself can relay the noxious energies to the sleeper, says Riggs. In one case, he found that the geomagnetic field under and around a single bed was within normal range (that is, the bed lay over a zone, but the zone exerted only a minor influence), but the mattress springs and the metal in the headboard increased the field by ninety percent, rendering it toxic to the person in the bed.

This person had been ill for six years with a variety of problems including chronic fatigue, depression, mental confusion, and candidiasis (systemic yeast infection). The occupant's health problems had begun right after she had bought the bed six years before. Riggs recommended getting rid of this bed, and using instead one made entirely of wood with a nonspring mattress; the bed was also moved elsewhere in the bedroom to a neutral zone. Once she made these changes, the woman's health started to return, even though she had received no therapeutic benefit from years of consulting a list of qualified health practitioners.

HEALTHY LIVING SPACE DETOXIFIER #65
Scan Your Home and Environment for Signs of Geopathic Stress

The evidence continues to mount linking bed location and noxious underground emissions with health problems. But how can you tell if your bedroom, or the location of your bed, is making you sick because it sits over a geopathogenic zone? British natural health practitioner and geopathic stress educator Jane Thurnell-Read offers the following "do-it-yourself" indicators:

- Look for places of persistent dampness in your house. Even though physical factors such as poor ventilation may seem to be the cause, the reason the damp flourishes may be due to an unsuspected geopathic zone.

- Often your pulse rate (measured at the wrist) rises significantly when you spend time in the influence of a geopathic zone.

- Bees, ants, and cats flourish over geopathic energy zones that are harmful to humans. If you have these animals in your environment, study their behavior; wherever they congregate, you should not. Thurnell-Read notes a curious correspondence between high levels of geopathic stress and homes that have cats that were once strays. She adds that in many cases the homeowners had discouraged the strays from staying, but they had remained nonetheless, probably because of a preference for the noxious (to humans) geopathic zones. Further, look for where your cat sleeps; some cats often choose drafty, unpleasant (to humans) areas, preferences that might indicate the presence of harmful Earth energies.

- Most trees will tend to lean away from negative Earth energies, with the exception of oaks, ash, willows, elder, and elm, which like geopathogenic zones. If you can discern this botanical behavior on your property, see if the tree leaning fits a generic pattern of distortion and if this pattern can be traceable or definable to a particular area of ground, such as the ground under which a water vein might pass. Also look for cancerous-like growths on apple trees, abnormal sap increase in cherry trees, and plum and pear trees that rot or wither. These phenomena indicate geopathic stress, says Thurnell-Read.[17]

- Other techniques may be used, but they require a little advanced training or, in some cases, a little enhanced sensitivity. You can dowse your environment, using rods or a pendulum, asking the device to indicate a "yes" or "no" answer to designate the presence or absence of geopathic stress. You can use muscle testing or kinesiology to measure your body's response (or that of someone else) to different energies and locations in your environment; here, typically, a muscle goes weak when the body is in contact with something unbeneficial to it.

Another way to determine if your house sits over a geopathogenic zone is to fill out the following questionnaire (see figure 12-1), developed by professional dowsers and geopathic stress educators Tom Passey and Robert D. Egby.[18] These are some indicators of probable geopathogenic zones in your bedroom.

If you answer yes to at least one third of these, it is worth considering calling in an expert to investigate your house for possible geopathogenic zones. It certainly can't hurt things to move your bed provisionally to a different spot in your bedroom and observe the results in your health and well-being over the next two weeks.

Figure 12-1. 13 Telltale Signs that You're Probably Living in a Geopathic Zone

If you experience at least one third of these symptoms, it's quite likely you are exposed to a geopathic zone in your home:

- strong resistance to going to bed
- insomnia and it takes hours to fall asleep
- nightmares, and/or feeling a "presence" in your bed
- an aversion to lying in certain spots in your bed
- the feeling of falling out of your bed, even though you don't
- sleepwalking
- sweating while sleeping
- feeling cold or shivering while sleeping
- waking up tired, unrested, and apathetic most mornings
- waking up feeling nauseous or actually vomiting
- a feeling of despondency, stress, or depression
- often crying when you wake in the morning
- rapid heart beat or cramps while lying motionless in bed

Another approach is to get a geopathic survey performed on your house. One organization that provides this service is the Geo Group, based in Medina, Washington. "A geopathic (*geo*-Earth, *pathic*-disease) survey determines if there are Earth energies . . . under a home or office and if they are neutral or negative (polluted or potentially harmful)," the organization explains. All the Geo Group requires from a homeowner in order to prepare a geopathic survey is a map of the home, its interior layout and how it sits on its property; the location and types of furniture in each room; a listing of known problems or unusual conditions; and the names of the people living in the home.

Based on twenty years experience, the Geo Group's founder Chuck Pettis recommends a geopathic survey if someone in your family is hyperactive, cranky, or moody for no discernible reason; a place in your home doesn't feel right, or feels scary or evil; you feel energy is being drained from you or pulled out of you; you feel someone or something is watching you; you feel unproductive; there is someone in the house with a history of illness or a disease that doesn't improve; there is a feeling of unease; strange things happen in your home.

The Geo Group notes that while geopathogenic zones can produce these effects, the effects can be exacerbated or complemented by the presence of "human entities (ghosts) and non-human entities (invisible malevolent beings)."[19] (See chapter 9.)

Pettis, an expert in creating "sacred space," comments: "Entities tend to take up residence around water lines or springs. They seem to be attracted to the field that the moving water gives off." Although he does not mention this, it is logical to presume that if you have, without knowing it, unwholesome energies or beings in your aura, by a kind of negative resonance this in itself can attract you to live in an environment that has corresponding geopathogenic energies.

That there is a kind of feedback loop or field of resonant attraction between your energy field, entities, and sites of geopathic stress is confirmed by Australian psychic practitioner, Samuel Sagan, M.D., whose views on auric pollution we visited in chapter 9. Living in a house full of noxious lines, also called earth ray lines or black streams, "often leads to catching multiple perverse energies and, possibly, entities," he says. (Perverse energies are not entities as such, but discordant nonsentient energy fields.) Dr. Sagan notes that if you meditate for long periods over noxious lines you may "catch" an entity; similarly, sleeping or meditating above a sewage pipe, a tank of stagnant water, or an underground creek can lead to entity attachment. Any mass of stagnant water, including a water bed, "can attract several 'unattached' entities."

Further, it is prudent to be aware, to whatever degree possible, of the potential presence of "spirits of the place" or nature spirits at your living location, advises Dr. Sagan. He notes that the Australian city of Sydney has many sacred sites with heightened "land energies." Some of these sites are uplifting and beneficial to humans, but others are not, and are "completely incompatible" with healthy human life. Some buildings have been unadvisedly constructed at such heightened land energy sites, Dr. Sagan comments. He says "unadvisedly" because they are sites where no human dwelling should ever be situated. Such places "will attract fragments [perverse energies] like sticky paper attracting flies." Architects usually design homes on paper only and are "completely insensitive" to land energies; if they unknowingly pick the wrong place, it is a losing proposition. Remove one entity, and ten more will come back within the week, says Dr. Sagan.

He has witnessed homes where the residents and their animal pets were constantly attacked by entities and perverse energies, and where the "spirits of the place were constantly waging war on them." The residents became depressed, mentally disturbed, even severely ill as a result. In such cases, it is better to move than to try to combat or remove the spirits of the land.[20] Lest this seem too fantastic a scenario, one needs only remember the plot line of Steven Spielberg's film *Poltergeist* (1982), in which the troubled spirits of Native Americans made the life of a California family unbearable because their home, while being constructed, had disturbed an ancient burial ground. Of course, nobody removed the spirits; rather they removed the house by imploding it.

This is why Dr. Sagan, like other experts in geopathology, recommends that before moving into a house, you have the house and its surrounding land dowsed for negative energies. If there are traces of previous residents or lingering "ghosts" in the land, in many cases these can be removed, if done expertly. In ancient Indian culture, for example, recognition of this was commonplace. When a person moved into a new dwelling, the local priests would perform a *yajna*, or fire ceremony, including a *bhuta-shuddhi*, or entity-clearing and purification ritual, to cleanse the energy field of the home and its surroundings, making it fit for human habitation.[21] Something in the spirit of this approach is still recommended today by geopathic practitioners.

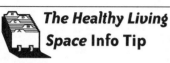

The Healthy Living Space Info Tip

For information about a geopathic survey of your home, contact:
The Geo Group,
P.O. Box 602,
Medina, WA 98039;
website: www.geo.org/dowse1.htm;
e-mail: chuckp@geo.org.

Also:
For information about dowsing, including books, practitioner referrals, educational conferences and publications, contact:
The American Society of Dowsers,
P.O. Box 24,
Danville, VT 05828;
tel: 800-711-9530 or 802-684-3417;
e-mail: ASD@Dowsers.org;
website: www.dowsers.org.

The Healthy Living Space Expert Interview:
Patrick MacManaway, M.D., Ch.B., Geomancer

Scottish-born physician Patrick MacManaway has made a career out of treating sick homes, a discipline he dubs "whole Earth geomancy." With offices both in Shelburne, Vermont, and Strathmiglo, Scotland, Dr. MacManaway operates on the principle that ill effects in a building's residents may be (and often are) traceable to harmful energies emanating from the ground over which they live or work.

Dr. MacManaway goes to homes and figures out the sources of geopathic stress that hinder the residents' health. He does this through a process he calls "therapeutic dowsing," which is dowsing with a medical focus; once he has identified the problem—geopathic zone, underground water, radioactive fields, disturbed energy flows, "lines of various Earth grids or traumatized psychic energies"—he uses a variety of techniques to neutralize the ill effects.

For him, geopathic stress denotes a place where the energy relationship between people and environment has become toxic. "Often there is a great deal of associated emotional trauma and dissonance held in the energy field, with or without the presence of disturbed and disoriented spirits. Geopathic stress may be first experienced as a disturbed, heavy, cold or unfriendly atmosphere in a place, and it progressively gives rise to emotional fatigue and a sense of being overwhelmed, difficulty in human communication and relationship, and it leads to depleted physical health. This energetic soup of trauma and dissonance can be very disturbing to attune to, and I typically know how bad the problems are by how tightly I feel myself contract and tighten as I arrive on the site. The tension that develops in my body, most noticeable in and around my gut and abdomen, gives me a feel for how the people resident in that building feel most of the time."

He defines whole Earth geomancy as "a holistic environmental health service that is committed to teaching and providing healthy solutions for homes, work environments, and landscapes." But what is geomancy? It is a science barely known in North America, but one that is widely employed by practitioners in the British Isles and Northern Europe. "Geomancy," says Dr. MacManaway, "is the study of the dynamic and interwoven relationship between human consciousness and its subtle energetic matrix with the consciousness and subtle energetic matrix of the Earth." Both humans and planet, Dr. MacManaway explains, exist in a perpetual "dynamic interdependent relationship," and geomancy is the discipline that both explains and rebalances this relationship.[22]

One's ties, both emotional and energetic, to one's house are often more profound than people think, says Dr. MacManaway. "The human relationship with a place is the primary relationship a human being has. Stress questionnaires have shown that the most stressful thing you can do to yourself is to move; this is an even stronger influence than changing your job, which is second, and getting married, which is third. I think this speaks to the primacy of the relationship between a person and place. Almost in the same way as coming into mood with a piece of music played in the background, humans tend to be primarily reactive to the subtle energetic environment they find themselves in."

The trouble is that our system may be "reactive" to an environment, but we are not necessarily aware of it. Most of the time the effect is "off our radar screens," says Dr. MacManaway. The body recognizes the influence—geopathic stress—but the mind doesn't know how to interpret it, so in a sense, it minimizes or even ignores it. "How rare this is, and how little we notice—so much of our time we are in landscapes of place and of people that are woven with pain and fear, anxiety and hurt. We may notice the initial contraction, but once pulled in to ourselves, we no longer notice how small we have become. We have simply adapted to our environment, and in our adaptation, defined limits to our energetic and emotional availability. We've been taught to disbelieve our imagination, so the place from which we get this level of geomantic information is locked away for many people."

"Geopathic stress may be first experienced as a disturbed, heavy, cold or unfriendly atmosphere in a place, and it progressively gives rise to emotional fatigue and a sense of being overwhelmed, difficulty in human communication and relationship, and it leads to depleted physical health," says Patrick MacManaway, M.D.

Locked for many, but fortunately not for Dr. MacManaway. In his process of therapeutic dowsing, he scans a residence or its surroundings for evidence of geopathic stress. "The first layer I scan for is the basic nature and health of the Earth's energies themselves, including water veins and any other detectable lines or pockets of energies. The next layer I look for is the accumulated psychoemotional residue that 'floats' in that first energy layer." This residue can include what feng shui characterizes as *ling* or "predecessor energy" (discussed in chapter 11), the presence of discarnate spirits, the residues of human trauma, or imbalances in the subtle energies of nature, what mystics and clairvoyants call the "elemental and devic kingdoms"— nature spirits to the rest of us. All of these factors can have a bearing on human health, and when they are disturbed, the effect can be harmful.

The most direct physiological effects come from prolonged human exposure to underground water streams or veins, says Dr. MacManaway, to which he attributes eighty percent of geopathic stress. "Underground water is a passive receptive energy form; it absorbs energy into itself. It will drain psychic and emotional energy out of a living space so that a room above it may feel cold or appear darker than it actually is, measured objectively." It has a kind of vampiric effect, producing a sensation not unlike having a hole in your energy field, he explains.

"People residing over such a water stream will tend to get very sleepy and lethargic." And if it drains energy, the immune system is likely to suffer, he adds, and when that happens, any of a long list of possible health problems may develop and persist until the Earth energy cause is resolved. The data from the Bergsmann study, cited earlier in the chapter, testifies to this observation. "That study showed shifts in plasma immunoglobulins, changes in the EKG, EEG, and quite a variety of both blood-based and electrophysiological measurements, and both specific and nonspecific measurements of immune function."

The biggest shift noted was in serotonin, which affects mood and the biological measuring of time (as discussed previously). "That's one of the key factors that one sees with geopathic stress—a disorientation in time sense. A body will tend to sleep heavily, sleep long, but wake unrefreshed. Many times you find gynecological dysfunction, problems with the menstrual cycle and with conception, both in animals and humans. One of my observations from working with geopathic stress is that it is quite frequent in women of menstruating age who are exposed to underground water to have menstrual irregularities for a month or so *after* I've rectified the geopathic stress. There seems to be a resetting of the pineal measurement of time when the geopathic imbalance is resolved."

Of special interest here, says Dr. MacManaway, is the fact that all of the physiological parameters studied by Dr. Bergsmann in relation to geopathic stress would also shift under direct electromagnetic field exposure. But this fact does not take us away from geopathogenic zones at all, because, as Dr. MacManaway explains, "geopathic stress is related to geomagnetic anomaly (disturbances or imbalances) and to the physiological pathway for naturally occurring electromagnetic disturbance, which affects the energy of geopathic stress. EMF problems of human-made origin go through the *same* physiological pathway."

Not only do they share the same pathways, but they interact; further, geopathic zones with their associated EMFs also interact with atmospheric phenomena. "Lightning tends to strike where underground water veins cross under the Earth, particularly where you have a deeper, faster flowing vein that is crossed at a shallower level by a weaker one. All of atmospheric radiation and pollution grounds itself in a more intensely focused way over underground water veins. So if there are local EMF sources and you're on a water vein, then you are probably getting a double dose of geopathic stress."

Let's see how these models of geomancy, therapeutic dowsing, and neutralization of geopathic stress play out in actual case histories drawn from Dr. MacManaway's files. "The most florid and exciting stories are those involving psychic disturbance. Psychic disturbance is very depleting of the energy field and leaves people drained, lethargic, irritable, and, if sensitive, psychically manipulated and physically quite unwell. Some degree of psychic involvement is classic in chronic conditions such as chronic fatigue, although whether the energy depletion or psychic attachment comes first can be hard to sort out."

A woman named Patty contacted Dr. MacManaway after thirteen years of "one disaster after another," as she told him. She lived in a 400-year-old house on the border of Wales and England. The house sat in the "Y" of a lane that came down from a church at the base of a hill, which meant it was "almost certainly" situated on what British dowsers call a "ley line."[23] Dr. MacManaway found that behind the church and up on the hill was a big boulder—a "glacial erratic"—which marked the border between Wales and England. "It was known locally as a magic stone, and if you went around it three times and made a wish, your wish would come true. It had also been the site of incredible atrocities." In the old days, anyone found on the wrong side of the border was subject to having his hands chopped off at this stone, says Dr. MacManaway.

Factoring the influence of the stone and its conduit, the ley line, Dr. MacManaway concluded that "there was significant psychic and emotional trauma here as well as a very strong energy in the house." Patty did not have any physical health issues, "but her whole life was miserable." Lots of bad things had happened in it—the list of phenomena is startling:

Three businesses that Patty opened in the house failed; she was a painter, yet shortly after moving into the house, her creative energy dried up and she wasn't able to sell any of her work either. Her neighbors treated her with hostility; several parts of the house felt cold, appeared dark, and felt fearful to her. There were certain rooms she would not enter at night. The plumbing in one of the bathrooms was always breaking down. Patty said she was aware of ghosts in the house; friends and family who visited the house hated it, and all had terrible nightmares when they slept over. Her mother came to visit, got ill, and eventually died in the house; two infants almost died while staying there. Patty's neighbors redug a drain and caused very expensive flooding and water damage in her house, such that she had to wage a six-year legal battle with them for reparations.

Even though she had a large garden with fruit trees, in the thirteen years she lived there, no birds ever visited the property. Dr. MacManaway found this fact alone highly suggestive of major geopathic stress, as birds do not like geopathic zones. When Patty would try to sell the property, major problems would erupt and require up to two years to set right before the house was marketable again. In fact, nobody ever made a bid on the house.

In desperation, Patty went to the magic stone, circumambulated it three times, and fervently wished to be rid of her house. Three nights later, reality obliged and her house almost burned down, generating thousands of dollars of repairs and many months' delay before the house could go back on the real estate market. All told, there were two floods and two fires.

The "magic stone" seemed to be the focal point for the disturbances at Patty's house, Dr. MacManaway concluded. "It was the focal point for a lot of the psychic trauma this house contained." Dr. MacManaway performed what he calls "Earth acupuncture" around the house (described in more detail

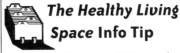

The Healthy Living Space Info Tip

Patrick MacManaway, M.D., may be contacted at:
Westbank Natural Health Centre, Strathmiglo, Fife, KY14 7QP, Scotland, UK;
tel. & fax: 01337-868-945.

Also at: Whole Earth Geomancy, 4076 Shelburne Road, Suite 6, Shelburne, VT 05482;
tel. & fax: 802-985-2266;
e-mail: PatchMac@aol.com;
website:
www.geomancy.org/patrick/patrserv.html.

below). He burned the aromatic herb sage in the house, and daubed the interior of the home with water from a holy spring. He assembled seven other people and together they did a "collective blessing" on the house, ringing bells, lighting candles, offering prayers, and focusing love and attention on the situation. Basically, he was attempting to detoxify the geopathogenic zone and neutralize its harmful effect on Patty's life and fortunes.

Just as a structured physical detoxification program produces a healing crisis for the body and a temporary worsening of symptoms, eventually yielding to greatly improved health and well-being, so too does a geomantic housecleaning. Patty went through a few weeks of "very intense and unpleasant withdrawal experiences, gastric upset, heavy flu-like symptoms and emotions that were all over the place," says Dr. MacManaway. Why did Patty get the brunt of the geopathic detoxification?

For years, her physiology and energy body had been living within the disturbed matrix of the geopathogenic zone and its harmful radiations. "There is a constant interchange between us and our environment with every breath, every heartbeat—it's a two-way flow of energy. So whatever dissonance is present in our environment, depending on how strong a personality and constitution we have, we will react to its influence like a thermometer reacting to heat." In a sense, Patty's body had grown accustomed to this toxic energy milieu and to an extent reset itself to the imbalanced biological parameters. But once the geobiological parameters were corrected and restored to normal (or at least their effects were neutralized), Patty's system was allowed to go back to normal; getting there was what caused all the detoxification reaction she experienced.

Does everyone who wants a detoxified home have to go through what Patty did? Not necessarily. "Not everybody is equally sensitive and not everybody has been chronically exposed," says Dr. MacManaway. "In extreme cases, I observe in clients two or three nights of very vivid dreaming and restless and disturbed sleep, followed by seven to ten days of detoxification symptoms typical of withdrawal from the harmful energies." These can include flu-like symptoms, gastrointestinal upset, excess mucus and phlegm, and "a fragile emotional state."

Often Dr. MacManaway uses his body's own reaction to the change in environment to give him reliable feedback that the geomantic work has been successful. "As my work proceeds on site and the healing process goes along—Earth acupuncture easing qi flow and restoring vitality, psychic intervention allowing the release and easing of long-stored hurts—the pain, dissonance, and trauma are gently brought to a harmony of peace and balance. A state of grace often descends upon the place. The way I generally notice that my work is taking effect is that my body starts to relax and my mood to lighten. This is for me a most interesting phenomenon, and one that is so repeatable that it has become predictable. I never know which stage in the process of healing is going to bring the energy field into peace and balance, but I know that creeping feeling of ease that accompanies it, almost like the relaxing warmth of easing into a hot bath."

Once her body had detoxified and adjusted to the new energy parameters of the geobiologically balanced house, things started to clear and get better for Patty. About four weeks after the geomantic work, her neighbors started treating her more cordially; she resumed painting; she sold some paintings; she received a statement of interest in the house. "The house felt lighter and brighter," says Dr. MacManaway. "Since your visit, the birds are everywhere in the front garden and back. The house is now peaceful and no longer has an icy feel to it," Patty told Dr. MacManaway. The flocks of finches and a fair number of robins visiting Patty's property perhaps made it a little easier to sell, which she did a few months later.

Dr. MacManaway relates another case in which geopathic stress produced constant migraine headaches in a resident. The client had noticed that along with the onset of his migraines, a number of newly planted shrubs and trees on his property were not thriving, and some had died. Dr. MacManaway found that "harmful Earth rays" crossed the client's bed. As a remedy, he placed copper rods in the ground around the house to neutralize the rays. As the client testified afterwards, "He told me I might have some withdrawal symptoms that first night in the form of a headache, which I did, but soon I was waking up with no more migraine headaches and with much more energy."

Another case shows how both humans and plants can be affected by geopathogenic zones. Dr. MacManaway was called in to consult with a woman who had been diagnosed with Hodgkin's disease, a form of cancer. He found a harmful ray at chest level going across the woman's bed. She remarked that her husband suffered a chest disease. His placement on the bed corresponded to where the harmful ray crossed the bed. In the couple's garden, an apple tree that was falling over and had to be supported and two azaleas that hadn't bloomed in seven years were both situated over a harmful energy line. "The results of Dr. MacManaway's work is the azaleas look healthier and one has flowered," the woman commented. "The apple tree is firmer in the ground. My husband's health is much better and his sleep is less restless. I, too, am feeling much healthier."

Very often fruit trees affected by geopathic stress "pick up tremendously and put out much greater blossom and fruit after the Earth energies are 'sweetened' for them," says Dr. MacManaway. "I 'rescued' one plum tree which had never had any fruit on it and heard that next season it had a bumper crop of plums." He also rescued a warren of commercially grown rabbits, as his next case highlights.

Dr. MacManaway was called in to help a rabbit breeder whose Angora rabbits were not doing well. For months, all of the rabbits born in one hutch at the end of the barn (out of seven hutches) died soon after birth. "Three post-mortems had been performed by the veterinarian who was unable to explain the deaths. I found a toxic line running under the hutch and balanced it with simple Earth acupuncture techniques." The litter of rabbits being carried by the doe in that hutch at the time of Dr. MacManaway's visit died shortly after birth, but subsequently there were no further problems or unexplained mortalities.

"Interestingly for me, this would suggest that the problems had been intra-uterine, affecting the mother rather than primarily affecting the baby rabbits. Pineal function is greatly responsible for governing the fertility and childbearing cycle, and, as discussed by Dr. Bergsmann, it can be disordered by exposure to geopathic stress."

HEALTHY LIVING SPACE DETOXIFIER #66
Take Your Energy Body Out
of the Curry-Hartmann Grid

The majority of research in the field of geopathic stress for the past one hundred years has come out of Germany. An additional element was added to the theoretical model of geopathogenic zones by the complementary work of two German researchers, Ernest Hartmann, M.D.,[24] and Manfred Curry, M.D.[25]

In the late 1940s, Dr. Hartmann described a tightly woven checkerboard energy grid comprised of naturally occurring charged and magnetically oriented lines running North-South and East-West across the entire surface of the planet. According to Dr. Hartmann, alternate lines are positively or negatively charged, and where N-S and E-W lines meet, there can be double positive charges, double negative charges, or a mix of both charges. It is the intersections that are problematic and that figure into the expanded model of geopathic stress. "At the more powerful crossing points of this system, there is a fifty percent increase of radioactivity," and the grid of Hartmann lines are distorted during earthquakes and take thirty minutes to return to normal.[26]

According to one commentator, the Hartmann network "appears as a structure of radiations rising vertically from the ground like invisible, radioactive walls" nine inches wide. The lines are spaced about six feet, six inches (north to south) by eight feet, two inches (east to west). A crossing of the rays in this "terrestrial grille" is called a Hartmann knot, and here "there is very frequently found a geopathogenic point having great importance for the health of a human being, even to the point of chronic illness."

Remaining for any length of time over a Hartmann knot, either in a bed or at a desk, is considered unhealthy. The new discipline of "geocancerology" has demonstrated that when a bed is situated over a Hartmann knot and a subterranean water vein, the deleterious effect is amplified. "Cells located on a geopathogenic point become tired or, contrarily, defend themselves by multiplying."

Remaining for any length of time over a Hartmann knot, either in a bed or at a desk, is considered unhealthy. The new discipline of "geocancerology" has demonstrated that when a bed is situated over a Hartmann knot and a subterranean water vein, the deleterious effect is amplified. "Cells located on a geopathogenic point become tired or, contrarily, defend themselves by multiplying." The Hartmann grid "penetrates everywhere, whether over open ground or through dwellings."[27]

Dr. Manfred Curry, in turn, described a global gridwork of electrically charged lines, also naturally occurring, that run diagonally to the north and south poles—NE-SW and SE-NW. The lines are believed to be about nine feet (three meters) apart, although the width can vary; the medically significant "Curry crossings" occur as double lines about forty-seven yards apart. Again, the problematic area is where the lines crisscross.

Dr. Curry contended that positively charged spots on his "Curry Net" can cause cells to proliferate, and potentially lead to cancerous growths, while the negatively charged points at the intersections can produce inflammations. So confident was he of the etiological role of his gridwork, that Dr. Curry claimed he could forecast which part of a patient's body would be the most affected by knowing where the subterranean rays crossed the bed.

The geomancer who seeks to neutralize areas of geopathic stress at a residence must take into consideration the combined effects of these two energy grids, says Dr. MacManaway. Researchers in the field of geobiology generally contend that in some way the Curry-Hartmann grid (a meshwork of intersecting lines) represents an interface between incoming cosmic rays (whose existence is well-documented and confirmed by astronomers and astrophysicists) and the Earth's various layers and types of energy (see figure 12-2).

One theory is that the combined webwork is an "earthing grid for cosmic rays" subject to distortion by geological fault lines and underground mining. Another interpretation is that the Curry-Hartmann grid describes the planet's geomagnetic field with "its active and neutral zones, the active areas being lines 21 cm wide with the neutral zone lying between the lines."[28]

Whatever the Curry-Hartmann energy grid proves to be, for geomancer Dr. MacManaway it has a certain experiential validity. "Certainly a lot of dowsers, and I myself, find energy grids in the ground. My observation is that as far as geopathic stress goes, these grids tend more to be carriers of energy than causative problems. They are usually never problematical unless there is underground water present, too." It's like a fish net, and unless there is a fish in the net, the net itself is not a problem.

**Figure 12-2.
Pictures of Hartmann
Net and Curry Grid**

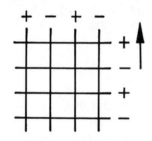

Hartmann Lines run 6'6" apart North-South,
and 8'2" apart East-West.

Curry Lines run 9' apart Northeast-Southwest,
and 8'2" apart Southeast-Northwest.

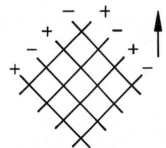

"These carrier grids definitely hold any psychoemotional residue of previous occupants of that space, so if there has been emotional trauma expressed in the landscape, it will get held in this grid which is analogous to the human nervous system." Dr. MacManaway notes that when there is unresolved trauma in the land, the grid lines will tend to compact and draw themselves close together, "almost like forming a scar in the lattice work where the land has been wounded." When the psychoemotional tension is released at a location, the lines tend to space themselves further apart again. He also says that when working with the grids, he often observes them clearing within twenty minutes, while energy residues in the home may take up to two weeks to fully be purged.

But how do human emotional residues get into this energy grid in the first place? Dr. MacManaway explains that there is a constant transfer of subtle information between the human energy body, or aura, and the equivalent energy "body" of the landscape. Human traumas might include domestic quarrels or violence, traffic accidents, sudden intense emotional experiences, former military battles, or forgotten burial grounds. "Patterns will tend to repeat themselves over and over again as people just express the energies that are there." Let's take a moment to amplify the idea of toxic residues of psychological and emotional trauma in the landscape. "The land has memory and therefore every act of violence is registered on Mother Earth," explains English spiritual teacher and dowser, Reshad Field in his book, *Here to Heal.*

He notes, for example, that when he goes to a place where strip mining has been done, he gets a tingling in his solar plexus and a desire to leave the place immediately. There is a place in the Scottish Highlands called Glencoe where a massacre once occurred; few people ever stop there, Field says, because "they can sense the smell of blood." Something nasty still remains from the terrible events that happened there many years ago.

Near Sedona, Arizona, Field was asked to consult on the possible reasons for the strange atmosphere around a creek that flowed through a canyon. For the most part the land held great charm, he noted, except for one area. There the temperature of the air was colder, people didn't talk to one another, and something was clearly amiss. Finally, Field identified the source of the disturbance. According to dowsing vocabulary, it was a negative energy spiral, which means, the energy was flowing in the wrong way. But the reason it did was that there was "the most terrible atmosphere of grief and violence present," as it were, trapped in the landscape. It was Field's impression that somebody had been either raped or murdered on this spot.

In a manner similar to acupuncture, the geomancer can "aid in bringing back harmony to the land by redeeming the long-lasting effects of man's mistakes," Field says. In this case, he inserted three rods into the ground to release the stuck, traumatized energy. People accompanying Field said they felt "a tremendous sense of relief," and Field noted that the air temperature rose an estimated ten degrees, leaving a warm, inviting warmth where there had been a chill.[29]

The Curry-Hartmann grid lines are like "capillaries in the Earth's subtle, energy body; they are its warp and woof," says Dr. MacManaway, as if the combined effect of the Curry-Hartmann grid lines were a globally encompassing energy carpet (see figure 12-3). Fortunately, any carpet can be cleaned. Here are two

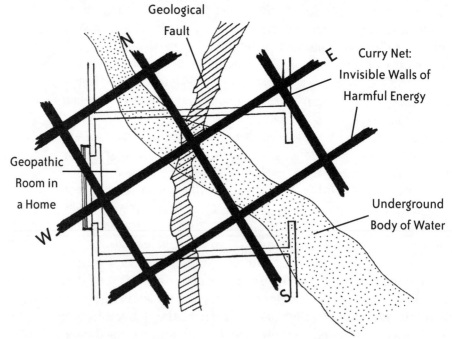

Figure 12-3. The Geopathic Room: Layers of Energy Disturbance

of the techniques Dr. MacManaway uses to neutralize geopathic stress and to remove psychoemotional residues from the Curry-Hartmann energy grid:

Eliminating Detrimental Energy from an Underground Stream

Dowsers commonly employ a rebar, which is a steel or iron reinforcing rod used with concrete pouring for house foundations. Once you, or a dowser, geomancer, or psychic has identified the location of an underground stream and found the place and angle at which it passes underneath your home, hammer the rebar (it should be several feet in length) into the ground over the water vein upstream, says Dr. MacManaway.

Typically, this will be ten to twenty feet away from the house, and depending on the size of the metal and the strength and volume of the water vein, "you can clear a 150-300 yard section of vein by doing this." He calls this "staking the heart of the vampire," referring to fact that the underground vein can literally suck energy out of people who live in a house situated over its "mouth." On certain kinds of water veins, it is better to situate the rebar over the edges of the current, while in other cases, it works better if you pin the center of the vein with the rebar.

More often than not, Dr. MacManaway locates the rebar upstream, sometimes at the edge of the property line, sometimes leaving a small part of the bar above the ground's surface. "I tend to sink most of mine under the surface although the occasional practitioner will leave part of the bar protruding. Doing this is like putting an antenna in the ground. You ground the atmospheric electromagnetic field and you allow an ion exchange from the Earth upward so that it is locally concentrated. That way you change the water vein's radiating effect, even though you are not actually moving its physical course." More traditionally, other dowsers tend to hammer the rebar all the way into the ground. In any event, be sure there are no electric cables, cable lines, sewer pipes, or other necessary human-placed pipes or conduits under the ground where you propose to place a rebar.[30]

Space-Clearing a Hartmann-Curry Knot

Here Dr. MacManaway uses what he calls "an Earth acupuncture technique." He finds a nodal point in the energy web then inserts long copper needles (fifteen inches long by one-half-inch wide) into the ground, leaving them in place for twenty to forty minutes. He inserts these either into the "knot" in the Hartmann or Curry grid, as close to it as he can get, or at the appropriate distance to be able to affect it. Somehow the copper "acupuncture" needles "release and disperse the energy held there."

HEALTHY LIVING SPACE DETOXIFIER #67
Five Simple Techniques for
Detoxifying a Room or Environment

Here are several simple, do-it-yourself techniques for cleansing an interior space or local outdoor environment, derived from the experiences of two seasoned geopathic stress experts:

Salt

Dr. MacManaway may also use table salt placed in an open dish for a few days in the room of the house where the problem is most acute. The salt absorbs the toxic energy during this time; in fact, it is well recognized as capable of absorbing heavy or depressed vibrations out of the atmosphere in a room. Leave the bowl of salt exposed in a targeted room; after a few days, dump the salt in a compost heap outside the house or dissolve it in water and sprinkle it around the edge of the property. Repeat as needed, or do this regularly if you desire. "Salt is a wonderful cleanser of atmospheric influences," he notes.

Burning Cauldron of Salt

As a variant, try burning salt. This is a technique borrowed from magical rituals, where the salt (Epsom salt, not sodium chloride) is used to purify the local atmosphere of inimical influences. Use a fireproof container, such as a metal cauldron, and fill it with two cups of Epsom salt. Just before lighting, coat it with one to two cups of ninety-nine percent alcohol (found at drugstores). Light with a long fireplace match. The fire should burn yellow and produce almost no smoke; be sure to keep the cauldron away from any flammable materials. The more alcohol you use, the longer the salt will burn. You can employ this technique when you have a particularly disturbed room or if you are planning on dedicating a room to a pursuit, such as art or meditation that requires a clean energy field.[31]

Sound

Dr. MacManaway also uses sound, delivered by a set of tuning forks, to help release trapped emotions from a knot in the energy grid of a property. Similarly, he might assemble a group of men and women and have them stand over the troubled area (or as close to it as they can get) and then have them "just express themselves with a tone or sound." People express grunts or tones, but it tends to be very dissonant and chaotic as they release the stored energy through themselves. But gradually the noise becomes more harmonious and congruent. Once the group is in harmony, then that is generally a sign that the space has been cleared." He adds that prayer and "focused loving attention to channel healing" to a site may be what does the real work.

Rock the Walls with Wagner

In chapter 9, British psychic protection expert William Bloom showed us how to use physical vibration, or shaking, to release stuck energy from our bodies. The same technique can be used to clear a room of baleful influences. Here vibration, from music or sound, dislodges the toxic traces from the room's atmosphere. "Vibration is naturally created by sweeping, mopping, beating, wiping, and vacuuming, all of which work directly into the fabric of the floors and walls," Bloom comments.

With regard to sound, Bloom advises filling a troubled room with loud music that has a strong bass vibration, such as Johannes Brahms or rock music. (My preference is some of the stirring, high-decibel moments in Richard Wagner's operas.) Also useful, if available, are Scottish bagpipes, drums, cymbals, bells, vibrant chanting, or even trumpets. The Tibetans traditionally used ten-foot long trumpets to cleanse the atmosphere; Christian churches have relied on full-strength organ bass notes and clanging bells to shake the toxic energies out of a space.

Bloom advises playing your music system full blast for five minutes every few weeks to vibrate your house as a kind of interior energy cleansing, an approach bound to please most teenagers and the recidivistic Woodstockers in many of us. While the music is vibrating the room, air all blankets and coverings, and thump, shake, and thwack—a tennis racket is helpful here— all chairs, sofas, mattresses, and cushions, says Bloom.[32]

Flower Essences

Often Dr. MacManaway pours drops of flower essences (in liquid form) in the ground at the site where he would place copper needles, in other words, at the troubled zone. Or he might dilute them in water and sprinkle the mixture around the site, much as one applies plant food in water; or he may put the essences in an aerosol mister and spray the area this way. There are some 1,600 commercially available flower essences, so Dr. MacManaway typically dowses for the appropriate ones, finding "they tend to be specific to the kind of trauma that occurred at the site." However, he finds that often he uses a preparation called Rescue Remedy or Five Flower Formula as a "safe first aid catch-all essence."[33]

Further, he often gives the same essences to the house's occupants, so they can make the same shift as their property and home. "This minimizes their withdrawal symptoms—that is, the transitory healing crisis—and it minimizes their likelihood of recreating the same problem just because they have become habituated to it, as this can sometimes happen. People can recreate the original trauma that you've cleared because it has become an established pattern of their own behavior."

HEALTHY LIVING SPACE DETOXIFIER #68
Put in an Energy Drainage Pipe from Your House to the Center of the Earth

Do you happen to remember the movie by Steven Spielberg called *Poltergeist*? A California family found their house had been built over native burial grounds and the spirits were intensely restless. In fact, they were so disturbed by the placement of the house (part of a hillside housing development) that after they had finished frightening and even abducting the occupants, they caused the house to implode and effectively cease to exist. It was their retribution for the obliviousness of the builders and residents and for the continuing desecration of their sanctified land that the presence of the house represented.

This is a dramatic and of course exaggerated scenario of what can happen when the house and its occupants are out of harmony with their immediate environment and when they are unaware of (initially) and ineffectual against (later) the existence of and incursion by nonphysical beings and energies into their domestic terrain. The energy field of the house or apartment is in many respects similar to that surrounding the human being. Foreign, inappropriate, and/or generally unhealthy or unwholesome energies may reside in it, or pass through, or squat uninvited in it for a time, contributing their influences and "flavors" to the overall energy mix of the home. In most cases, the presence of such beings or nonphysical energies is not beneficial to the residents in terms of physical and mental well-being.

In Healthy Living Space Detoxifier #43: Ground Yourself to the Center of the Earth (chapter 9), we reviewed the benefits of establishing a kind of master energy drainage pipe between your physical body and the center of the planet. The same can be done for a home. Why not let the planet itself absorb the negativity or toxic energy from a room or given locality?

It may seem counterintuitive, but energetically, the planet is well equipped to absorb negativity flushed down an energy drainage pipe; in many respects, it can handle it easier than physical toxicity. Even though it is toxic to the Earth when we dump physical chemicals and poisons into the landscape, it is different when we "drain" toxic energies into the Earth. It is capable of absorbing and transmuting much of our local accumulation, suggests William Bloom. We often forget "what a huge and magnificent creature of energy she is," he says, referring to the planet in its energy aspect.

Bloom recommends visualizing a "spinning plug-hole" directly under the toxic place in question, and seeing the vortex spin itself down to the center of the Earth, carrying the toxins with it like grey water down a sink drain. In a sense, you can "instruct" the "spinning plug-hole" to collect and remove the toxic energies you have identified or sensed in a room or local environment, seeing the drain as a kind of vertical vacuum cleaner. This technique is especially useful if you need to drain the energy out of a room in which a group has discharged "a load of emotion and pain," says Bloom.[34]

In terms of specific recommendations, the idea is to visualize the drainage pipe as being set under a specific room or, better, under the entire house. Imagine there is a drainage pipe with an open diameter as wide as you house. Set your house, room, or apartment on it, or set the pipe under it, and make sure the connection is secure. Make sure the pipe connects firmly to the center of the planet as well. You could visualize a name plate "down there" that says "my house" or "the house (or room, or apartment) of the so-and-so family."

Once you have the drainage pipe in place, you tell it to release and drain the toxicity from the room or house. You could visualize a lever at the top of the pipe marked "release"; set the lever on release. All this may seem a bit like magic, but because you're affecting energy with energy—the toxic residues in a space with a mentally energized construct—it works. The bad energies will drain out. It is advisable to renew this pipe every day. You can do this by refreshing the visualization: go through the steps again, making the image stronger and more vivid, and instruct it again to release toxic energies from the living space.

This drainage pipe will release a fair amount of unpleasant energy from your living space. It will work even better if you put into play many of the suggestions in chapter 9, even, ideally, having at least one psychic reading or energy clearing session with a qualified psychic practitioner. Remember, you and your living environment are in a perpetual feedback loop. Events and toxic exposures in one will affect the other.

If it is physically toxic, and you are trying to detoxify your body, the toxins in the home will come into you. If your home is detoxified, chemically and energetically, but you are not, the toxic energies in your own energy field or aura may contribute to a retoxification of your living space. As I have stressed throughout the book, it is essential to detoxify both aspects of your living space—body and home—at the same time to get the best results.

There is another benefit to putting in an energy drainage pipe for your living space. It grounds the living space. It gives the space an energy center, a calm, focused midpoint. When you are in this space, you will feel more grounded yourself. You will feel calmer, more centered, relaxed, less reactive, less emotionally volatile, and less mentally agitated. You are sitting in a living space that is grounded to the center of the planet. That has a wonderful psychic and psychological effect on everyone in that space. It also acts as a subtle protection device for your home, discouraging robbers or others that might be otherwise motivated to damage, vandalize, or rob the home. As an energy equation, groundedness equals strength, much like having a strong, vital immune system is the best protection against infectious disease.

Every time you are able to drain off residual toxic energy, you are helping the energy situation of the entire planet or what might be called the planet's "psychic ecology," Bloom suggests. A great deal of the planet's vibrational pollution comprises negative attitudes and stuck energy, he says. Energy is stuck in the body and the home—in both aspects of our living space. There is in fact a "huge amount of invisible psychic pollution floating around the whole planet," and it might be a major contributing factor, even a root cause, of the ubiquitous toxic pollution, creating the disturbed energy framework that makes it possible for toxic substances to accumulate.[35]

HEALTHY LIVING SPACE DETOXIFIER #69
How to Take the Stress Out of a Geopathic Zone

As the role of geopathic stress in human health becomes gradually accepted and more widely studied, low-cost neutralizing devices are now appearing on the market to enable individuals to clear suspected geopathic stress out of their homes. The following is a review of a few of the units available and some of the health claims put forward by their manufacturers or distributors.

RadiTech

This a device that comes in four sizes, according to the size of the geopathically stressed area. It plugs into a wall socket yet draws almost no current. Physically, the device is an unassuming thin white canister varying in height (according to the model) from about six inches to a little less than two feet tall. It operates on the principle of "stabilizing multiwave oscillators," by which it neutralizes the electromagnetic field (which causes the geopathic stress in the first place) of an entire building, apartment, house, hospital room, or office, and removes the effects of geopathic stress from the individuals within its radiating field. There is also a portable RadiTech unit that one can carry into an office, supermarket, or other environment for "moving" protection.

Further, the device apparently adjusts the balance between positive and negative ions in an environment, so that negative ions predominate, producing an effect similar to fresh mountain air, which is high in healthful negative ions. The manufacturer (Dulwich Health clinic of London) claims that the RadiTech works at maximum efficiency within a few moments of installation and that as the geopathic stress is cleared out of a person, one is likely to experience transitory withdrawal symptoms as the body releases toxins. These symptoms typically include brief headaches, irritability, flu-like feelings, upset stomach, and disturbed sleep.

The affidavits for the RadiTech are copious and impressive, illustrating its positive effects on numerous health conditions as well as further exemplifying the multiple ways in which geopathic stress can compromise your health, according to Dulwich Health. The following are examples of how RadiTech has helped relieve health problems:

- Prominent among the health conditions benefited has been chronic fatigue. A woman who suffered from "tremendous limitations in energy levels" and a "mystery paralysis" for thirty years found she could now clean her house again, go out shopping, and resume seeing clients. Another chronic fatigue sufferer—ill for six years and diagnosed with chronic fatigue for the previous two—was able to discontinue use of her wheelchair.

- A woman experienced her first pain-free menstruation in over a year.

- Old injuries tend to start to heal suddenly. A man's old leg sore started to heal within seven days. Another elderly man with long-term open leg sores found they started to heal and close up.

- A woman installed a RadiTech in her house after she tried to commit suicide. After six weeks with the unit, "she . . . [was] a changed person, optimistic, and making plans for her future." She went out dancing (before she never wanted to leave the house); she ate well for the first time in years; and she went off her tranquilizers and antidepressants.

- People with chronic migraines have benefited. One man who had endured migraines for twenty years found that they virtually ceased, with only one minor attack in five months. Another man who for twenty-seven years had food-allergy-related migraines found he could now eat all his formerly allergenic foods with no resulting migraine. A woman used to wake up at night with an "oppressive feeling and a splitting headache"; in fact, she had suffered from migraines since childhood and was unresponsive to conventional pain-killing drugs. After a few days with the unit in her bedroom, she felt much "brighter and ha[d] more energy . . . and no longer . . . [got] up five or six times a night."

- Other conditions that improved include asthma; eczema; hyperactivity; arthritis; neck, back, and leg pain; nervous stomach; neck gland swelling; and moodiness, among many others. Speaking of the device's effect on an entire home, one user commented: "It feels as if my house has been spring-cleaned."

Energeia

This device, which bills itself as a geopathic stress neutralizer and is plugged into a wall socket, can clear a home of distorted energies, raise the occupants' energy levels, put a "protective field" around them, and enhance one's sense of harmony and well-being, according to its British manufacturer, Geomack Products. The Energeia device comes in three sizes, one of which is portable. It weighs from between one and eight pounds (depending on the model), and can reduce the harmful electromagnetic field emitted from household appliances, computer equipment, or electric utility poles.

According to Geomack, "Harmful energy fields are emitted from the Earth, electrical products, and transmitters. Energeia works in conjunction with a property's electrical wiring system to convert detrimental distorted energy fields into well-balanced beneficial energies."

One application of the Energeia that has drawn positive response is its use in British natural health clinics.

- Dr. Laurent Bannock of the Nutrafit Clinic in Wimborne, Dorset, reported noticing a "distinctive difference in the 'feel'" of his building's atmosphere after installing two units. Various unexplained headaches and migraines that had bothered staff members disappeared, and when Dr. Bannock used a portable Energeia with his laptop computer, he found it "made a tremendous difference in my ability to concentrate at the screen for long periods of time, without feeling ill or suffering from a bad headache."

• Liz Morris of the Heavenly Bodies Therapy Clinic in South Wonston, Winchester, Hantshire, reported that prior to using the unit she had been unable to sleep well at night, and that for the previous thirty months, three to four hours a night was the best sleep she could expect. She also suffered from depression and was on antidepressants, but once she started taking these, she slept so well that she had trouble waking in the morning. She developed irritability, self-doubt, concentration problems, and lethargy, among many other symptoms. Three months after using the Energeia, Morris reported being "a different person"; her symptoms had abated and she was "back at the top of the hill instead of at the bottom."

The Healthy Living Space Info Tip

For information about RadiTech, contact:
Dulwich Health,
130 Gipsy Hill,
London SE19 1PL,
England;
tel: 0181-670-5883;
fax: 0181-766-6616;
website: www.dulwichhealth.uk.com.

For Energeia, contact:
Geomack Products,
P.O. Box 519,
Southampton SO16 7RW,
England;
tel: 23-8076-0100;
fax: 23-8076-0200;
e-mail: mail@geomack.com;
website: www.geomack.com.

For products available in the United States from:
The Healing Center,
1924 Juan Tabo NE, Suite E,
Albuquerque, NM 87112;
tel: 505-292-222, ext. 1;
fax: 505-821-2325;
e-mail: add1easy@aol.com.

• Mayne Sundewall-Hopkins, a therapist in Looe, Cornwall, with more than twenty years' practice, reported that ever since she moved into her house seven years ago, her health started to deteriorate. "Something didn't feel right, but I couldn't put my finger on what or why," she said. She had problems upon problems: aching muscles, digestive disturbances, allergies, joint stiffness, mood swings, concentration difficulties, constant flu/cold symptoms, fatigue, stress. "It was as though something like a leech was continually emptying me of energy," she said, adding that even regular acupuncture and other natural healing modalities failed to improve her condition. This, as we saw above, is a classic indicator of geopathic stress.

By good fortune, Sundewall-Hopkins came across the Energeia device and installed one in her home and realized she had identified the source of all her problems: geopathic stress. "The distorted energies in the house prevented me from getting well. My immune system suffered and thus everything gradually worsened," she explained. "With the unit in the house, I felt better within hours."[36]

HEALTHY LIVING SPACE DETOXIFIER #70
Selecting Energy Wells in a
Geography of Enlightenment

One of the most practical steps you can take, suggests Samuel Sagan, M.D., is to become sensitive to Earth and ambient energies in local environments, even in as small a space as a single room in a house. Many living spaces are crisscrossed with toxic energy lines and geopathogenic zones, as discussed above, yet they often present positive Earth energies, too. Dr. Sagan calls these positive, uplifting sources energy wells. Both rooms and landscapes have energy wells, and if you can identify them, they can help restore your health by reestablishing energetic balance, he says.

If you are gifted with clairvoyance, an energy well resembles "a little fountain of energy, a little 'geyser,' a column of light," says Dr. Sagan. Even if you cannot see one, you may be able to sense the presence of an energy well. You may find your thoughts uplifted, more positive, exalted, happy, or inspired, or you may experience some degree of healing of a discomfort as you reside, even for just a few moments, within an energy well. Dr. Sagan reports that typically an energy well is quite small, perhaps one or two feet in diameter.

How do you sense an energy well? Listen to the "belly signal," advises Dr. Sagan. The solar plexus, and especially navel area, has a keen ability to act as a dowsing rod for sensing ambient energies, he says. This is the energy basis of the folk wisdom about having a "gut feeling." Once you know what neutral feels like in your "gut" or solar plexus, you can sense energy changes in that region in response to sensing new environments. In fact, when sensing for energy lines, geopathic or otherwise, it is more helpful to think in terms of "walls" not "lines," Dr. Sagan comments. He makes the interesting observation that what you will feel is more like a "wall of vibration" or "a wall of etheric smoke" than a two-dimensional line.

Developing a sensitivity to energy wells within your home, property, or immediate landscape can have a definite practical value. It could lead you to completely reorganize how you use and allocate living space, suggests Dr. Sagan. "All this means that you have to reconsider your habits and to start using the space in harmony with the energy of the house." You may wish, to the degree it is possible, to redesign the interior of your home so that you sleep, meditate, eat, work, think on energy wells to get their maximum benefit for consciousness and the functions of your mind and body.

Doing this, suggests Dr. Sagan, provides "immense" benefits for your physical, mental, and spiritual health. "By systematically choosing spots of high-quality energy, we can influence our state of health and consciousness positively." Dr. Sagan notes that people often select an environment, even which chair to sit on in a room, based on resonant vibrations. There is a correspondence between one's energy quality and that of a room or environment, and thus we are drawn (or repelled) accordingly.

For example, in his experience, many people unconsciously select toxic spots in which to sit in a house, movie theater, or other enclosed space; this selection is energetically appropriate (but not therapeutic) because it reinforces, or is in resonance with, the quality of their own energy imbalances. Modifying the principle of homeopathy: like draws like.

But once you have detoxified a certain amount of your mental, emotional, psychic, and physiological toxins, you will start being in resonance with the health-affirming energy wells rather than the geopathic spots. You will start moving within what Dr. Sagan elegantly calls "a geography of enlightenment," selecting your every environment—the seat in a movie theater, the table in a restaurant, the plush chair in a living room—based on your sensing of energy qualities and high and low points in a given living space. You will avoid the toxic sites and gravitate toward the healthy ones. It is possible, Dr. Sagan assures us, to so fine-tune this sensing ability that standing in the doorway of a new interior living space, you can detect the toxic sites and the energy wells, and thereby avoid the first and move towards the second.[37]

Life in a Healthy Living Space

So what happens next? What is life like after detoxification? How can we use detoxification as a foundation for further exploration in our lives and the world?

In a sense, the experience of detoxification can be like a re-entry into the physical world, and even into our own bodies. This is especially so if we undertake our first detoxification intensive in our forties or fifties. Purging ourselves of half a lifetime of toxic accumulation can be acutely stimulating. It's as if we are free to think, feel, and sense anew, if for the first time. Our life works better in all its aspects.

Perhaps as a result of following the seventy detoxifying steps in *The Healthy Living Space* you are considering the matter of medicine and health care. The mental clarity produced by your detoxification gives you the "space" to consider some interesting questions. Perhaps alternative medicine and its non-toxic worldview is new to you; maybe you never critically examined the principles and practices of conventional medicine even though you have been a recipient of its "products" all your life.

Conversely, maybe you are an "old hand" at alternative medicine and in agreement with its principles. Either way, it is important to note that medicine is not neutral: it embodies a philosophy of matter, a way of looking at and understanding the physical world. It expresses an orientation toward the body and the environment. It invades and attacks; or it supports and nurtures. It has ramifications in the world, and affects our total environment. Your choice of medicine—essentially it comes down to conventional and alternative systems—affects how you relate to your body. It is quite likely that the detoxification experience has given you a new perspective on this.

You might ask yourself three questions: Does a given medical approach or an entire field contribute to or diminish my existing level of toxicity? Does it stimulate my waking up to my role and responsibility in the physical world, or does it keep me in the dark as a nonplayer? Does it make me more conscious or less? Many of these matters are discussed in my book *Physician: Medicine and the Unsuspected Battle for Human Freedom*.

After detoxifying ourselves, we have a new understanding of our relationship to the world, and our responsibility for that relationship. We as consumers participate in the pollution of the planet and the sickening of human bodies by all our choices in the marketplace. Now we have woken up to that responsibility and we are making new, more informed consumer choices. But there's more.

We have a new sense of how our physical well-being influences our psychological and emotional well-being, and vice versa. We no longer divide our life into categories, each separately treatable. Now we see they are interconnected. So, too, we see our home afresh. Our body and home form a living system, and this living system itself has a relationship to the larger environment.

It is quite likely that the detoxification experience has given you a new appreciation of how you relate to your living space, your home. You may see the need to adopt a new style of relationship consistent with the conclusions you reached about how you will treat your body from now on.

How we relate to either our body or our home represents a philosophy of matter, represents a definition we have formed of both. Are things living or inert? Is consciousness important? Does it have a role in the world? Do our decisions really affect the planet? The detoxification experience may open up some large questions for you and encourage you to consider big subjects that previously you had neglected or thought too remote from your interests. The matter of toxicity and detoxification is one way you can see your inter-relatedness with the entire planet and all of matter. It's a doorway, and once through it, you will have a vista of far more than free radicals, organochlorines, and the liver's two-phase detoxification pathway.

Perhaps some of the ideas in chapter 12 were provocative. The concept that subtle, technically "invisible" energies from the landscape can affect how we feel and how our bodies function is certainly a different perspective than that offered by conventional science and medicine. In this book, for the most part, we focused on those landscape energies that were harmful to health. But are there Earth energies that are good for us, that elevate consciousness and improve our health just by our being in proximity to them? Yes, there are.

Just as many traditional societies routinely practiced detoxification, they also knew about beneficial Earth energies and used them in their rituals, placement of holy buildings, and other aspects of their lives. Such places are known today variously as sacred sites, holy places, power points, vortexes, and pilgrimage destinations, among other names. Such places have a definite "energy" to them, but it is subtle.

Detoxification actually prepares you to be more sensitive and receptive to beneficial Earth energies in much the same way as ritual purification and detoxification were employed in traditional societies for the purposes of preparing people for spiritual experiences. Detoxification frees you up to consider the concept of Earth energies, and it fine-tunes your senses so you can make some discoveries on your own. This field is called geomancy, and many aspects of this subject are discussed in my forthcoming book, *The Galaxy on Earth: A Traveler's Guide to the Planet's Visionary Geography*.

Taking the large view, we can say that the planet itself is our total living space. Do we want it to be toxic or healthy? Detoxification of the planet truly starts at home with the choices we make. When we choose to detoxify, it has a global impact. One person detoxifying affects everything. It may seem like a minute influence, but big effects are compounded by many minute influences working together. The detoxification experience itself shows us convincingly that our seemingly inconspicuous efforts to purify ourselves of toxicity can change the world and help make it the healthy living space it was always meant to be.

Endnotes

Chapter 1

1. Theo Colborn, Dianne Dumanoski, and John Peterson Myers, *Our Stolen Future. Are We Threatening Our Fertility, Intelligence and Survival—A Scientific Detective Story* (New York: Dutton/Penguin Book, New York, 1996): 106.

2. For more information about POPs, see: www.stoppops.org. This is a politically active organization working to eliminate POPs in the world environment and food supply. See also: www.ewg.org (Environmental Working Group, 1718 Connecticut Avenue, N.W., Suite 600. Washington, D.C., 20009; e-mail: info@ewg.org).

3. Eric Dewailly et al., "Concentration of Organochlorines in Human Brain, Liver, and Adipose Tissue Autopsy Samples from Greenland," *Environmental Health Perspectives* 107:10 (October 1999): 823-828.

4. "Alpine Lake Traps 'Dirty Dozen' Poisons," Reuters Limited, 11 April 2000, EnviroLink News Service www.envirolink.org/environews.

5. Sandra Steingraber, *Living Downstream. An Ecologist Looks at Cancer and the Environment* (Reading, Mass.: Addison-Wesley Publishing Company, 1997): 177.

6. Some experts now use the term "toxics" to distinguish toxic substances from "toxins," which, technically, are poisons from plants and animals, and from "toxic substances," which tend to indicate only chemicals and not radiation. "Toxics" thereby refers to chemicals, nuclear radiation, and even electromagnetic fields and noise. See: John Harte et al., *Toxics A to Z. A Guide to Everyday Pollution Hazards* (Berkeley: University of California Press, 1991): xiv.

7. "Enjoy Vibrant Health in a Toxic World," Health Designs International (1997) www. healthdesigns.com.

8. Iris R. Bell, *Clinical Ecology: A New Medical Approach to Environmental Illness* (Bolinas, Calif.: Common Knowledge Press, 1982).

9. Sherry A. Rogers, *Tired or Toxic? A Blueprint for Health* (Syracuse: Prestige Publishing, 1990): 5,10,11.

10. This list of toxicity symptoms is adapted from several sources, including a detailed toxicity screening questionnaire published by Health Designs.com. To take the test and get numerical toxicity rankings of the results, see: www.healthdesigns.com/DetoxificationTest.html.

11. Catherine Hoffman, Dorothy Rice, Hai-Yen Sung, "Persons with Chronic Conditions," *The Journal of the American Medical Association* 276 (November 13, 1996): 1473-1479.

12. Peter Bennett, Stephen Barrie, and Sara Faye, *7-Day Detox Miracle: Restore Your Mind and Body's Natural Vitality with This Safe and Effective Life-Enhancing Program* (Rocklin, Calif.: Prima Health/Prima Publishing, 1999): 30-33.

13. W. John Diamon, W. Lee Cowden, with Burton Goldberg, *An Alternative Medicine Definitive Guide to Cancer* (Tiburon, Calif.: Future Medicine Publishing, 1997): 545.

14. The EHIS has been publishing its chemical profiles since 1978 by Congressional mandate. The full text of the *9th Report on Carcinogens, 2000*, is available at http://ntp-server.niehs.nih.gov/ NewHome Roc/9RocFacts/html. You can also contact them at: National Toxicology Program-RoC, MD EC-14, P.O. Box 12233, Research Triangle Park, NC 27709; tel: 919-541-4096; email: jameson@niehs.nih.gov.

15. Philip J. Landrigan, "Commentary: Environmental Disease—A Preventable Epidemic," *American Journal of Public Health*, 82 (July 1992): 941-943.

16. Philip J. Landrigan, *Environmental Neurotoxicology* (Washington, D.C.: National Academy Press, 1992): 2.

17. Robert W. Pinner et al., "Trends in Infectious Diseases Mortality in the United States," *Journal of the American Medical Association*, 275:3 (January 17, 1996): 189-193.

18. David W. Talmage et al., *Biologic Markers in Immunotoxicology* (Washington, D.C.: National Academy Press, 1992): 1.

19. Cynthia Wilson, "Chemical Sensitivities: A Global Problem," *Earth Island Journal,* Spring 1998 www.earthisland.org/ejournal/spring98.

20. Richard Leviton, "Environmental Illness—A Special Report," *Yoga Journal*, November/December 1990.

21. William J. Rea, "Chemical Hypersensitivity and the Allergic Response," *Ear, Nose, and Throat Journal* 67 (January 1988). William J. Rea and Monte J. Mitchell, "Chemical Sensitivity and the Environment," *Immunology & Allergy Practice* (September/October 1982). William J. Rea and Alfred R. Johnson, "20th Century Illness," *Total Health*, December 1986. Yaqin Pan, Alfred R. Johnson, and William J. Rea, "Alipathic Hydrocarbon Solvents in Chemically Sensitive Patients," *Clinical Ecology* V, no. 3 (1987).

22. John L. Laseter, Ildefonso R. DeLeon, William J. Rea, and Joel R. Butler,, "Chlorinated Hydrocarbon Pesticides in Environmentally Sensitive Patients," *Clinical Ecology* II, no. 1 (Fall 1983).

23. Janette D. Sherman, *Chemical Exposure and Disease. Diagnostic and Investigative Techniques* (Princeton: Princeton Scientific Publishing, 1994): 88, 91, 97,101-102, 118-119.

24. Agrow Reports, "World Non-Agricultural Pesticides Markets," March 2000; data summarized in "Non-Ag Pesticides Market Growing," September 12, 2000, by Pesticide Action Network North America (49 Powell Street, Suite 500, San Francisco, CA 94102; tel: 415-981-1771; fax: 415-981-1991; e-mail: panna@panna.org; website: www.panna.org). The organization offers a free weekly e-mail newsletter called PANUPS, available on their website.

25. Joel Grossman, "Dangers of Household Pesticides," *Environmental Health Perspectives* 103:6 (June 1995): 550-554.

26. The National Library of Medicine offers a searchable online database for toxic substances and their effects, including toxicology, lists of hazardous substances, and carcinogens. See http://toxnet.nlm.nih.gov.

27. Sherman, Chemical Exposure and Disease, 223, 230.

28. EPA, Office of Toxic Substances, "Broad Scan Analysis of the FY82 National Human Adipose Tissue Survey Specimens," EPA-560/5-86-035 (Washington, D.C.: 1986).

29. P.A. Stehr-Green, "Demographic and Seasonal Influences on Human Serum Pesticide Residue Levels," *Journal of Toxicology and Environmental Health* 27 (1989): 405-421.

30. F. Adeshina, E.L. Todd, "Organochlorine Compounds in Human Adipose Tissue from North Texas," *Journal of Toxicology and Environmental Health* 29 (1990): 147-156.

31. J.L. Jacobson et al., "Determinants of Polychlorinated Biphenyls (PCBs), Polybrominated Biphenyls (PBBs), and Dichlorodiphenyl Trichchloroethane (DDT) Levels in the Sera of Young Children," *American Journal of Public Health* 79 (1989): 1401-1404.

32. Walter J. Crinnion, "Environmental Medicine, Part 1: The Human Burden of Environmental Toxins and Their Common Health Effects," *Alternative Medicine Review* 5 (February 2000): 53-54.

33. Benjamin C. Blount, et al., "Levels of Seven Urinary Phthalate Metabolites in a Human Reference Population," *Environmental Health Perspectives*, 108 (October 2000): 979-982.

34. Kenneth Bock and Nellie Sabin, *The Road to Immunity. How to Survive and Thrive in a Toxic World* (New York: Pocket Books/Simon & Schuster, 1997): 81.

35. Al Meyerhoff, "We Must Get Rid of Pesticides in the Food Supply," *USA Today Magazine*, November 1993, 51-53.

36. Peter Montague, "Illegal Poisons in Our Food," *Rachel's Environment & Health Weekly* 9 May 1996, www. rachel.org.

37. J.E. Davies, "Changing Profile of Pesticide Poisonings," *New England Journal of Medicine* 316:13 (March 26, 1987): 807-808.

38. James Liebman et al., "Rising Toxic Tide: Pesticide Use in California, 1991-1995," 1997, Pesticide Action Network & Californians for Pesticide Reform, San Francisco, CA. For more information, see www.igc.org/cpr; see also www.panna.org. Both organizations, based in San Francisco, are coalitions of numerous citizens groups around the world working to oppose the misuse of pesticides and to promote sustainable, ecologically-based agriculture.

39. "EWG Air Monitoring Finds Toxic Pesticides Drifting from California Farm Fields," Environmental Working Group, Washington, D.C., 13 January 1999 www.ewg.org.

40. Robert Repetto et al., *Pesticides and the Immune System: The Public Health Risk* (Washington, D.C.: World Resources Institute, 1996): 3, 9-16, 18, 21, 56, 46-48.

41. "Technical Report," Beyond Pesticides/National Coalition Against the Misuse of Pesticides 15:7 (2000). 701 E. Street SE, Suite 200, Washington D.C., 20003; tel: 202-543-5450; fax: 202-543-4791; website: www.beyondpesticides.org. This organization is a good source of information about the hazards of pesticides and the means of taking advocacy action to limit their use.

42. Jacqueline D. Savitz et al., *Factory Farming: Toxic Waste and Fertilizer in Virginia*, 1990-1995, Environmental Working Group, Washington, D.C. (n.d.) www.ewg.org. EWG offers a free downloadable report on toxic wastes used in fertilizer for each of the fifty states.

43. John Cary Stewart, *Drinking Water Hazards: How to Know If There are Toxic Chemicals in Your Water and What to Do If There Are* (Hiram, Ore.: Envirographics, 1990): 158.

44. "Tap Water in Central Valley Tainted With Banned Pesticide," Environmental Working Group, Washington, D.C., 15 November 1999 www.ewg.org.

45. "Government Underestimates Infant Exposure to Toxic Weed Killer," Environmental Working Group, Washington, D.C., 28 July 1999 www.ewg.org.

46. Although arsenic is a naturally occurring element (the 20th most common in the Earth's crust), it can be toxic to humans. High-dose exposure to arsenic can produce gastrointestinal irritations, problems in swallowing, abnormally low blood pressure, excessive thirst, even convulsions and cardiovascular collapse in cases of acute exposure. Arsenic has also been linked to cancer and diabetes. In addition to ingesting it in water, people consume arsenic through fish and seafood.

47. MSNBC Staff and Wire Reports, "How Much Arsenic in Our Water?" MSNBC News/Environment, 25 February 2000 www.msnbc.com/news.

48. Butch Kinerney, "New Map Shows Arsenic in Nation's Ground Water," UniSci, Daily University Science News, 10 May 2000 www.unisci.com/stories.

49. Denise Riedel Lewis et al., "Drinking Water Arsenic in Utah: A Cohort Mortality Study," *Environmental Health Perspectives* 107 (May 1999): 359-365.

50. Päivi Kurttio et al., "Arsenic Concentrations in Well Water and Risk of Bladder and Kidney Cancer in Finland," *Environmental Health Perspectives* 107 (September 1999): 705-710.

51. "Update 1. U.S. Toxic Pollution 3 Times Worse Than Thought—EPA," Reuters Limited, 12 May 2000, EnviroLink News Service www.envirolink.org/environews.

52. Steingraber, *Living Downstream*, 197-202.

53. Hans-Rudolf Buser and Markus D. Muller, "Occurrence of the Pharmaceutical Drug Clofibric Acid and the Herbicide Mecoprop in Various Swiss Lakes and in the North Sea," *Environmental Science and Technology*, 32:1 (1998): 188-192. Janet Raloff, "Drugged Waters," *Science News*, 153:12 (March 21, 1998): 187-189. Peter Montague, "Drugs in the Water," *Rachel's Environment & Health Weekly*, September 3, 1998.

54. Christian G. Daughton and Thomas A. Ternes, "Pharmaceuticals and Personal Care Products in the Environment: Agents of Subtle Change?" *Environmental Health Perspectives* 107: supp. 6 (December 1999): 907-938. Also: Peter Montague, "Pay Dirt from the Human Genome," *Rachel's Environment & Health Weekly*, #702, 6 July 2000 www.rachel.org.

55. Other toxic substances are emitted from motor vehicles or formed as byproducts of incomplete combustion, contributing to air pollution. These substances include benzene, toluene, xylene, formaldehyde, acetaldehyde, and 1,3-butadiene. Some of these are known or suspected carcinogens.

56. W.S. Linn and H. Gong, Jr., "The 21st Century Environment and Air Quality Influences on Asthma," *Current Opinions in Pulmonary Medicine* 5 (January 1999): 21-26.

57. William S. Linn et al., "Air Pollution and Daily Hospital Admissions in Metropolitan Los Angeles," *Environmental Health Perspectives* 108 (May 2000): 427-434.

58. South Coast Air Quality Management District, "Smog and Health," July 1996 www.aqmd.gov. The South Coast AQMD is the smog control agency for Los Angeles and three neighboring counties.

59. S. Takafuji and T. Nakagawa, "Air Pollution and Allergy," *Journal of Investigative Allergology and Clinical Immunology* 10 (January-February 2000): 5-10.

60. G. D'Amato, "Outdoor Air Pollution in Urban Areas and Allergic Respiratory Diseases," *Monaldi Archives of Chest Diseases* 54:6 (December 1999): 470-474.

61. Rob McConnell et al., "Air Pollution and Bronchitic Symptoms in Southern California Children with Asthma," *Environmental Health Perspectives* 107 (September 1999): 757-760.

62. Joachim Heinrich et al., "Respiratory Diseases and Allergies in Two Polluted Areas in East Germany," *Environmental Health Perspectives* 107 (January 1999): 53-62.

63. Bart D. Ostro et al., "Air Pollution and Health Effects: A Study of Medical Visits Among Children in Santiago, Chile," *Environmental Health Perspectives* 107 (January 1999): 69-73.

64. South Coast Air Quality Management District, "Smog and Health" www.aqmd.gov.

65. Annette Peters et al., "Associations Between Mortality and Air Pollution in Central Europe," *Environmental Health Perspectives* 108 (April 2000): 283-287.

66. Joe Thornton, *Pandora's Poison: Chlorine, Health and a New Environmental Strategy* (Cambridge, Mass.: MIT Press, 2000).

67. Ibid., vii.

68. The production of chlorine gas is the "single root cause" for all the pollutants known as organochlorines, says Thornton. A powerful electric current is passed through a saltwater solution (sodium chloride plus water). This changes sodium chloride, entirely natural and a part of nature and our body, into chlorine gas, "a heavy, violently reactive, greenish gas." Most of the chlorine gas is then used as the "feedstock" or base material for making 11,000 organochlorines, also foreign to nature. The chlorine industry produces about 40 million tons of chlorine gas annually, most of which is used to make chlorinated organic chemicals.

69. Some organochlorines can persist a very long time in the atmosphere. The half-life of chloropentafluoroethane is 381 years; of dichlorotetrafluoroethane, 152 years; of dichlorodifluoromethane, 69; and of trichlorotrifluoroethane, 58. A half-life means how long it takes for a substance to degrade to 37% of its original concentration—in other words, for about two-thirds of it to degrade. The half-lives of 20 other organochlorines range from 0.4 years (chloroform) to 31 years (trichlorofluoormethane). The persistence of organochlorines in water involves unbelievable stretches of time. Scientists estimate that 1,2-dichloroethylene found in water will require 21 billion years to degrade; heaxachloroethane will take 1.8 billion years; perchloroethylene, 990 million years; 1,1-dichloroethylene, 120 million; and trichloroethylene, 1.3 million years. (Data from Thornton, *Pandora's Poison*, 27, 33.)

70. Ingrid Gerhard et al., "Chlorinated Hydrocarbons in Women with Repeated Miscarriages," *Environmental Health Perspectives* 106 (October 1998): 675-681.

71. A. Mayani et al., "Dioxin Concentrations in Women with Endometriosis," *Human Reproduction* 12 (1997): 373-375.

72. It is shocking to learn, as Thornton documents, that the global organochlorine problem and the entire chlorine industry were the

result of trying to find a use for a chemical byproduct. In the late 19th century, German chemists found a faster way to make alkali, needed for the manufacture of paper, soap, glass, textiles, and other products. They introduced an electrical current into brine and got alkali, hydrogen, and chlorine gas. The trouble was they got a lot of chlorine gas: to make one ton of alkali, nine-tenths of a ton of chlorine gas was generated. It was dangerous to store and impossible to get rid of, so new markets and applications had to be found for it. These included, during the 20th century, bleaching powder; chemical weapons and war gas; degreasing solvents; and PCBs, DDT and other pesticides.

73. Jay M. Gould, *The Enemy Within: The High Cost of Living Near Nuclear Reactors* (New York: Four Walls/Eight Windows, 1996): 15-56. See also Ralph Graeub, *The Petkau Effect. The Devastating Effect of Nuclear Radiation on Human Health and the Environment* (New York: Four Walls/Eight Windows, 1994).

74. Interference with the functioning of the thyroid gland is a serious matter. The thyroid gland, one of the body's seven endocrine glands, is located just below the larynx in the throat, with interconnecting lobes on either side of the trachea. The thyroid is the body's metabolic thermostat, controlling body temperature, energy use, and, in children, the body's growth rate. The thyroid controls the rate at which organs function and the speed with which the body uses food; it affects the operation of all body processes and organs. Of the hormones the thyroid synthesizes and releases, T3 (triiodothyronine) represents seven percent and T4 (thyroxine) accounts for almost ninety-three percent of the thyroid's hormones active in all of the body's processes; T4 is converted into T3 outside the thyroid gland. Iodine is essential to forming normal amounts of thyroxine. The secretion of both these hormones is regulated by the thyroid-stimulating hormone, or TSH, secreted by the pituitary gland in the brain. The thyroid also secretes calcitonin, a hormone required for calcium metabolism.

75. Jay M. Gould, "The Current Cancer Epidemic and the Baby Boom Generation," *Nuclink. The Journal of Current Radiation and Public Health and Issues* 17 February 1999 www.radiation.org.

76. Joseph J. Mangano, "Improvements in Local Infant Health After Nuclear Power Reactor Closing," *Environmental Epidemiology and Toxicology* 2:1 (March 2000): 32-36.

77. Jay M. Gould, "Why Cancer Rates in the Hamptons Are So High," *Nuclink. The Journal of Current Radiation and Public Health and Issues,* 14 September 1998 www.radiation.org.

78. Russell L. Blaylock, *Excitotoxins—The Taste That Kills* (Santa Fe, N. Mex.: Health Press, 1994).

79. For a comprehensive list and discussion of the toxicity of each food additive, see "Chemical Cuisine: CSPI's Guide to Food Additives," Center for Science in the Public Interest www.cspinet.org. Address: CSPI,

1875 Connecticut Avenue, NW, Suite 300, Washington, D.C. 20009; tel: 202-332-9110; fax: 202-265-4954; e-mail: cspi@cspinet.org. CSPI also publishes *Nutrition Action Healthletter*, a monthly nutrition newsletter.

80. Doctor's Guide to the Internet (Medical & Other News), "Food Additive Can Cause Severe Allergic Reactions," 5 November 1997 www.docguide.com.

81. Carol Simontacchi, *The Crazy Makers. How the Food Industry is Destroying Our Brains and Harming Our Children* (New York: Jeremy P. Tarcher/Putnam, Penguin Putnam, Inc., 2000): 35, 93.

82. Marc Kaufman, "Antibiotics in Animal Feed—A Growing Public Health Hazard, Worries Rise Over Effect of Antibiotics in Animal Feed," *The Washington Post*, March 17, 2000.

83. Kirk E. Smith et al., "Quinolone-Resistant *Campylobacter Jejuni* Infections in Minnesota," *New England Journal of Medicine*, 340:20 (May 20, 1999): 1525-1532.

84. M. Kathleen Glynn et al., "Emergence of Multidrug Resistance *Salmonella Enterica* Serotype Typhimurium DT104 Infections in the United States," *New England Journal of Medicine* 338:19 (May 7, 1998) 1333-1338. Also Denise Grady, "A Move to Limit Antibiotic Use in Animal Feed," *The New York Times*, March 8, 1999.

85. Food poisoning from bacterially-tainted food is a serious matter: about 76 million cases are reported annually in the United States, of which 5,000 result in fatalities.

86. Shannon Brownlee, "Agribusiness Threatens Public Health with Antibiotics in Animal Feed," *The Washington Post*, May 21, 2000.

87. Michelle Allsopp et al., "Recipe for Disaster. A Review of Persistent Organic Pollutants in Food," Greenpeace Research Laboratories, March 2000 www.greenpeace.org.

88. Environmental Working Group, "Moms . . . and POPs" www.ewg.org.

89. Allsopp et al., "Recipe for Disaster" www.greenpeace.org.

90. Environmental Working Group was founded in 1993 and is today, with its staff of eighteen researchers, a leading source of information for public interest groups campaigning to protect the environment. Its website (www.ewg.org) offers a searchable database on numerous environmental issues.

91. Environmental Working Group, "Moms . . . and POPs" www.ewg.org. EWG compiled this information based on the FDA "Total Diet Study, 1991-1997" and USDA "Continuing Survey of Food Intake by Individuals, 1994-1996."

92. EPA, "EPA's Agency-Wide Multimedia Persistent, Bioaccumulative, and Toxic Pollutants Initiative, 1999 Accomplishments Report," EPA 743-R-00-003, July 2000 www.epa.gov/pbt/accomp99.htm.

93. Joe Thornton proposes that it will take six human generations, or about 150 years, before all the PCBs and the other organochlorines

have been removed from human fat cells—even if no further organochlorines were introduced into the global environment starting today. In other words, we may be contaminated for centuries, he says. Thornton further suggests that our natural detoxification mechanisms may be ineffective against many organochlorines, although they are able to degrade some of them into more easily excreted chemical forms. (Thornton, *Pandora's Poison*, 43, 215).

Chapter 2

1. Peter Bennett, Stephen Barrie, and Sara Faye, *7-Day Detox Miracle: Restore Your Mind and Body's Natural Vitality with This Safe and Effective Life-Enhancing Program* (Rocklin, Calif.: Prima Health/Prima Publishing, 1999): 113-114.

2. Rudolph M. Ballentine, *Radical Healing. Integrating the World's Great Therapeutic Traditions to Create a New Transformative Medicine*, (New York: Three Rivers Press, 1999): 294-297.

3. Frank Edward Allen, "One Man's Suffering Spurs Doctors to Probe Pesticide-Drug Link," *The Wall Street Journal*, October 14, 1991.

4. Kenneth Bock, and Nellie Sabin, *The Road to Immunity: How to Survive and Thrive in a Toxic World* (New York: Pocket Books/Simon & Schuster, 1997): 34-36.

5. There are six types of free-oxygen radicals, including superoxide, hydroxy radical, lipid peroxy radical, singlet oxygen, hydrogen peroxide, and hypochlorous acid.

6. Stephen B. Edelson, "Free Radical Pathology: A Unified Cause of Chronic Illness," Environmental and Preventive Health Center of Atlanta, 1995 www.ephca.com.

7. Genox Corporation, Baltimore, Md., providers of Oxidative Stress Profile www.genox.com.

8. D. Harman, "Free Radicals in Aging," *Molecular Cell Biochemistry* 84:2 (December 1998): 155-61; "Aging: Phenomena and Theories," *Annals of the New York Academy of Sciences* 854 (November 20, 1998): 1-7; "Extending Functional Life Span," *Experimental Gerontology* 33:1-2 (January-March 1998): 95-112; "Free Radical Involvement in Aging: Pathophysiology and Therapeutic Implications," *Drugs Aging* 3 (January-February 1993): 60-80.

9. J.E. Gallagher et al., "Comparison of DNA Adduct Levels in Human Placenta from Polychlorinated Biphenyl Exposed Women and Smokers in which CYP 1A1 are Similarly Elevated," *Terato Carcino Mutagen* 14 (1994): 183-92.

10. Joseph Pizzorno, *Total Wellness. Improve Your Health by Understanding the Body's Healing Systems* (Rocklin, CA: Prima Publishing, 1996): 99.

11. Ibid., 101-102.

12. Toluene, a hydrocarbon distilled from crude oil, is a common additive in gasoline. It is vented into the air every time a car, truck, bus, or airplane is driven. A catalytic converter can remove about ninety-five percent of toluene from automobile exhaust. Toluene is also an additive in model glues, paints, inks, resins, and adhesives; and is found in dyes, detergents, linoleum, perfumes, lacquers, prescription drugs, and saccharin, among other products. You will also encounter toluene in tobacco smoke from cigarettes. For more information about toluene, and other toxic substances, see John Harte et al., *Toxics A to Z: A Guide to Everyday Pollution Hazards* (Berkeley: University of California Press, 1991).

13. Bennett, Barrie, and Faye, *7-Day Detox Miracle,* 99-101.

14. Since the Center was founded in 1974, more than 30,000 patients have passed through its bio-detoxification program or have received treatment for toxicity-related illness. "We analyze difficult cases from all angles using environmental, nutritional, allergy, medication, and surgical strategies tailored to the individual patient," states an information release by the Center. Reknowned for its carefully executed, chemically-reduced indoor environment for sensitive patients, the Center has also consulted on "less-toxic building technology" for 17,000 private and public buildings. Dr. Rea is the author of two books, the medical textbook *Chemical Sensitivity*, Vols. 1-5 (CRC Press-Lewis Publishers, 1992-1997), and coauthor of *Your Home, Your Health and Well-Being* (Ten Speed Press, 1988) as well as over 100 peer-reviewed medical articles.

15. W.J. Rea and G.H. Ross, "Food and Chemicals as Environmental Incitants," *Bol Asoc Med P R* 83 (July 1991): 310-315.

16. W.J. Rea et al., "Confirmation of Chemical Sensitivity by Means of Double-Blind Inhalant Challenge of Toxic Volatile Chemicals," *Bol Asoc Med P R* 83 (September 1991): 389-393.

17. Sherry A. Rogers, *The E.I. Syndrome: An Rx for Environmental Illness* (Syracuse: Prestige Publishing, 1986); *Tired or Toxic: A Blueprint for Health* (Syracuse: Prestige Publishing, 1990); *You Are What You Ate: An Rx for the Resistant Diseases of the 21st Century* (Syracuse: Prestige Publishing, 1988). Also Richard Leviton, "Environmental Health—Sherry Rogers, M.D.," *East West Journal,* July/August 1991.

18. Walter J. Crinnion, "Environmental Medicine, Part 1: The Human Burden of Environmental Toxins and Their Common Health Effects," *Alternative Medicine Review* 5:1 (February 2000): 52-63.

19. W. Crinnion, "Results of a Decade of Naturopathic Treatment for Environmental Illnesses: A Review of Clinical Records," *Journal of Naturopathic Medicine* 7:2 (1998): 21-27. See also W. Crinnion, "Chronic Fatigue Syndrome and Environmental Overload," (n.d.) www.naturopathic.org/Library/articles.lay/WC.CFS.html.

20. M.S. Wolff et al., "Blood Levels of Organochlorine Residues and Risk of Breast Cancer," *Journal of the National Cancer Institute* 85 (1993): 648-652.

21. J.R. Davis et al., "Family Pesticide Use and Childhood Brain Cancer," *Archives of Environmental Contamination and Toxicology* 24 (1993): 87-92.

22. Crinnion, "Environmental Medicine, Part 1" 57.

23. C.G. Ohlson and L. Hardell, "Testicular Cancer and Occupational Exposures with a Focus on Xenoestrogens in Polyvinyl Chloride Plastics," *Chemosphere* 40 (May-June 2000): 1277-82.

24. Ted Schettler et al., *In Harm's Way: Toxic Threats to Child Development* (Cambridge, Mass.: GBPSR, 2000): 1-8. This report is available in full online at www.igc.org/psr/ihw.htm. Or by mail: Greater Boston Physicians for Social Responsibility, 11 Garden Street, Cambridge, MA 02138; tel: 617-497-7440; fax: 617-876-4277; e-mail: psrmabo@igc.org.

25. Peter Montague, "Dumbing Down the Children-Part 1," *Rachel's Environment & Health Weekly*, #687, February 17, 2000 www.rachel.org.

26. Peter Montague, "Dumbing Down the Children-Part 3," *Rachel's Environment & Health Weekly*, #687, March 2, 2000.

27. Ibid.

28. Peter Montague, "Toxics and Violent Crime," *Rachel's Environment & Health Weekly*, #551, June 19, 1997.

29. Peter Montague, "Toxics Affect Behavior," *Rachel's Environment & Health Weekly*, #529, January 16, 1997. See also Herbert L. Needleman et al., "Bone Lead Levels and Delinquent Behavior," *Journal of the American Medical Association*, 275 (February 7, 1996): 363-369.

30. Roger D. Masters, "Environmental Pollution, Toxic Chemicals, Crime and Disease," at www.dartmouth.edu/~rmasters/research.html.

31. Crinnion, "Environmental Medicine, Part 1," 60.

32. The thyroid gland is located just below the larynx in the throat, and has interconnecting lobes on either side of the trachea, giving it the effect of a bowtie on the trachea. This gland is the body's metabolic thermostat, controlling body temperature, energy use, and, in children, the body's growth rate. The thyroid controls the rate at which organs function and the speed with which the body uses food; it affects the operation of all body processes and organs. Of the hormones the thyroid synthesizes and releases, T3 (triiodothyronine) represents seven percent and T4 (thyroxine) accounts for almost ninety-three percent of the thyroid's hormones active in all of the body's processes. The thyroid also secretes calcitonin, a hormone required for calcium metabolism and for satisfactory digestion. Conventional medicine tends to downplay, if not ignore, the importance of the thyroid in many health problems, and it tends to use inadequate laboratory tests to measure thyroid hormone levels, thereby giving, in many cases, a false picture of thyroid hormone status. The thyroid gland also is one of the first of

the endocrine glands to be damaged by exposure to nuclear radiation, indicating its sensitivity to environmental poisons.

33. M.H. Li and L. Hansen, "Enzyme Induction and Acute Endocrinic Effects in Prepubertal Feamel Rats Receiving Environmental PCB/PCDF, PCDD Mixtures," *Environmental Health Perspectives* 104 (1996): 712-722.

34. J.F. Leatherland, "Changes in Thyroid Hormone Economy Following Consumption of Environmentally Contaminated Great Lakes Fish," *Toxicology and Industrial Health* 14 (1998): 41-57.

35. Susan Porterfield, "Vulnerability of the Developing Brain to Thyroid Abnormalities: Environmental Insults to the Thyroid System," *Environmental Health Perspectives* 102:2 (1994): 125-130.

36. There are five main groups or categories of endocrine-disrupting chemicals: 1) phthalates (used as plasticizers; can imitate estradiol, a type of estrogen); 2) alkylphenols (used in industrial and domestic detergents); 3) bisphenol A (found in dental lacquers and used to coat the interior of metal food cans; estrogenic to breast cancer cells); 4) organochlorine pesticides (lindane, DDT, altrazine; may increase breast cancer risk; DDT can block the action of male hormones); 5) polychlorinated biphenyls (PCBs) and dioxins (dioxins are produced during incineration and industrial processes; PCBs were once used in electrical equipment, and still present in transformers and capacitors); and 6) others (the cosmetics preservative parabens; food antioxidant BHA; fungicide vinclozolin; and a group of natural plant compounds called phytoestrogens). From research provided by Dr. A. Michael Warhurst, "Introduction to Hormone Disrupting Chemicals," Friends of the Earth, London, England, 1998 www.website.lineone.net/~mwarhurst.

37. Dieldrin is an organochlorine insecticide, used extensively in agriculture since the 1940s. "It is one of the most persistent of all pesticides, remaining for years in soils, accumulating in the fatty tissues of living organisms, and consequently, concentrating in the food chain." Dieldrin is no longer used in the United States on food crops, yet dieldrin residues continue to be detected in foods, especially carrots, corn, cucumbers, and sweet potatoes. It is highly persistent in water, more so than other organochlorines, and enters the human body through the skin, eyes, lungs, and gastrointestinal tract. (Harte et al., *Toxics A to Z*, 207-208.)

38. A.P. Hoyer et al., "Organochlorine Compounds and Breast Cancer—Is There a Connection Between Environmental Pollution and Breast Cancer?" *Ugeskr Laeger* 162 (February 14, 2000): 922-926.

39. S.A. Ahmed et al., "Gender and Risk of Autoimmune Diseases: Possible Role of Estrogenic Compounds," *Environmental Health Perspectives* 107, supp. 5 (October 1999): 681-686.

40. N. Olea et al., "Inadvertent Exposure to Xenoestrogens in Children," *Toxicology and Industrial Health* 15 (January-March 1999): 151-158.

41. J.P. Sumpter, "Xenoendocrine Disrupters—Environmental Impacts," *Toxicology Letters*, 102-103 (December 28, 1998): 337-42.

42. Gina M. Solomon, "Endocrine Disruptors. What Should We Do Now?" Natural Resources Defense Council, 1997 www.nrdc.org.

43. Theo Colborn, Frederick S. vom Saal, and Ana M. Soto, "Developmental Effects of Endocrine-Disrupting Chemicals in Wildlife and Humans," *Environmental Health Perspectives* 101 (October 1993): 378-384.

44. OCCs are synthetic, organic, chlorinated chemicals—in other words, industrially produced chemicals (synthetic) based around carbon (organic), to which chlorine has been added (chlorinated). Examples of OCCs are chloroform, DDT and PCBs, certain pesticides, and dioxin. Normally carbon and chlorine are not found bound together into a molecule in nature, other than as a byproduct of volcanic eruptions and forest fires, and as a natural exudate of marine algae.

45. Peter Montague, "Dangers of Chemical Combinations," *Rachel's Environment & Health Weekly*, #498, June 13, 1996. See also Steven F. Arnold et al., "Synergistic Activation of Estrogen Receptor with Combinations of Environmental Chemicals," *Science* 272 (June 7, 1996): 1489-1492.

46. Montague, "Dangers of Chemical Combinations."

47. It is encouraging to note that in Massachusetts it is now a law that certain chemicals may not be used in schools and day-care centers, and any use of pesticides requires parental notification first. Although thirty other states have some form of chemical regulation, the Massachusetts law, passed in June 2000, is considered the most far-reaching. Other states, such as California, New York, and Wisconsin, are attempting to pass similar laws. For more information about pesticides and schools, contact: Beyond Pesticides/NCAMP (National Coalition Against the Misues of Pesticides), 701 E. Street SE, Suite 200, Washington, D.C., 20003; tel: 202-543-5450; fax: 202-543-4791; e-mail: info@beyondpesticides.org; website:www.beyondpesticides.org.

48. Kagan Owens and Jay Feldman, "The Schooling of State Pesticide Laws: Review of State Pesticide Laws Regarding Schools," *Pesticides and You* 18:3 (1998): 9-23. Published by Beyond Pesticides/NCAMP (National Coalition Against the Misues of Pesticides), 701 E. Street SE, Suite 200, Washington, D.C., 20003; tel: 202-543-5450; fax: 202-543-4791; e-mail: info@beyondpesticides.org; website: www.beyondpesticides.org.

49. World Resources Institute, "Threats from Environmental Estrogens," 1995 www.wri.org.

50. Theo Colborn, Dianne Dumanoski, and John Peterson Myers, *Our Stolen Future: Are We Threatening Our Fertility, Intelligence, and Survival?—A Scientific Detective Story* (New York: Dutton/Penguin Group, 1996): 187-209.

51. Clinical molecular medicine is so named, says Dr. Edelson, because it integrates environmental medicine, which assesses the effect of the environment on human illness, and applied immunology (how the immune system functions), toxicology (how toxins make us sick), and clinical nutritional biochemistry (the scientific way of using nutrients to improve health based on an understanding of cellular chemical processes that are not working optimally).

52. Stephen B. Edelson, "Requirements for Chemical Detoxification," 1998, The Edelson Center for Environmental and Preventive Medicine, 3833 Roswell Road, Suite 110, Atlanta, GA 30342; tel: 404-841-0088; fax: 404-841-64156; website: www.ephca.com; also: www.edelsoncenter.com.

53. Elson M. Haas, "Detoxification and the Detox Diet: An Important Healing Process," 1999 www.elsonhaas.com.

54. Elson M. Haas, M.D., "General Detoxification and Cleansing," (n.d.) HealthWorld Online www.healthy.net. See also *The Detox Diet: The How-to and When-to Guide for Cleansing the Body* (Berkeley, Calif.: Celestial Arts, 1996): 21-32. Elson Haas, M.D., may be contacted at Preventive Medical Center of Marin, Inc., 25 Mitchell Blvd., Suite 8, San Rafael, CA 94903; tel: 415-472-2343; fax: 415-472-7636; e-mail: lora_pmc2000@hotmail.com; website: www.elsonhaas.com.

55. Elson M. Haas, "Spring Cleansing," 2000 www.elsonhaas.com.

56. Strictly speaking, for some, especially Westerners raised on animal protein, soybeans are not easy to digest and can produce gastrointestinal discomfort. However, for the purposes of this example, the statements made about soybeans are accurate.

Chapter 3

1. Natural killer (NK) cells are central to the immune system's ability to withstand toxins and potential disease. They are a type of nonspecific, free-ranging immune cell produced in the bone marrow and matured in the thymus gland, located behind the sternum. NK cells can recognize and quickly destroy virus and cancer cells on first contact. "Armed" with an estimated 100 different biochemical poisons for killing foreign proteins, they can kill target cells without having encountered them previously. As with antibodies, their role is surveillance, to rid the body of aberrant or foreign cells before they can grow and produce cancer or infection.

2. Symptoms of mercury toxicity make a very long list: anorexia, depression, fatigue, insomnia, arthritis, multiple sclerosis, moodiness, irritability, memory loss, nausea, diarrhea, gum disease, swollen glands, headaches, and many more. Mercury toxicity has been shown to have a destructive effect on kidney function and to contribute to cardiovascular disease, neuropsychological dysfunction, reproductive disorders, and birth defects.

Mercury fillings, or amalgams, have been used in dentistry since the 1820s, but not until 1988 did the routine use of mercury raise serious enough questions for the Environmental Protection Agency (EPA) to declare scrap dental amalgam a hazardous waste. Even so, the majority of dentists routinely install mercury fillings in patients' mouths, despite the fact that it is a certified poison. Evidence now shows that mercury amalgams are the major source of mercury exposure for the general public—at rates six times higher than those found in fish and seafood. Studies by the World Health Organization show that eight amalgams in a single mouth can release 3-17 mcg of mercury per day. A Danish study of a random sample of 100 men and 100 women showed that increased blood mercury levels were related to the presence of more than four amalgam fillings in the teeth.

3. DMPS stands for 2,3-dimercaptopropane-1-sulfonate. It is a substance used by progressive physicians as an evaluation tool to measure suspected mercury levels in a patient. DMPS is the chelating (binding-up) agent of choice for the removal of elemental mercury from the human body. It can be given orally, intravenously, or intramuscularly, and is useful for people who have been exposed to mercury amalgam through their dental fillings, or for those who show evidence of or suspect heavy metal toxicity from other sources.

4. The pivotal concept in EDS is that an energetic event transfers its signal through an acupuncture meridian to the nervous system, with the end result being a cellular pathology, or some kind of organic disturbance. Essentially, a trained practitioner conducts an "interview" with the patient's organs and tissues, gathering information about the basic functional status of those systems and their energy pathways. Not only can EDS show the degree of stress affecting an organ, it is able to monitor the progress of therapy. EDS practitioners assert that this enables them to avoid the trial and error and general guesswork that often accompany difficult diagnoses.

As a form of computerized information gathering, EDS places a blunt, noninvasive electric probe at specific points on a person's hands, face, or feet, corresponding to acupuncture points at the beginning or end of energy meridians. The theory behind EDS is that very small electrical discharges from these points serve as information signals about the condition of the body's organs and systems, useful for the physician in evaluation and developing a treatment plan. EDS uses a scale of 0 to 100, with 45-55 being "normal" or "balanced." Readings above fifty-five are interpreted as indicating an inflammation of the organ associated with the meridian tested, while readings below forty-five to fifty suggest organ stagnation and degeneration.

5. Fats and oils are made of building blocks called fatty acids. A fatty acid is made of a chain of carbon atoms with hydrogen atoms attached, and an acid group of atoms at the end able to combine with

glycerol. When three fatty acids attach to one molecule of glycerol, this makes a simple fat called a triglyceride. The chain of carbon atoms can be short (two to six atoms), medium (eight to ten), or long (twelve to thirty). Butyric acid, found in milk fat, butter, and cream, is a short-chain fatty acid. A fatty acid that has its full quota of hydrogen atoms is a saturated fatty acid (animal fats and hardened fats, solid at room temperature); a fatty acid with less than its full allotment of hydrogen atoms is an unsaturated fatty acid (many plant and fish oils, liquid at room temperature). When a fatty acid lacks only two hydrogen atoms, it is a monounsaturated fatty acid (such as oleic acid); a fatty acid lacking four or more hydrogen atoms is a polyunsaturated fatty acid (linoleic acid). Unsaturated fats required in the diet are called essential fatty acids and include linoleic acid (an omega-6 oil), found in corn, beans, and some nuts and seeds; and alpha linolenic acid (an omega-3 oil), found in fish, flaxseed, and walnuts.

6. Dr. Robert C. Greenberg, "Biological Terrain," Biological Technologies International, 1998 www.bioterrain.com.

7. King James Medical Laboratory, Inc., "Frequently Asked Questions Regarding the Analysis of Metals in Hair Specimens," 1998 www.kingjamesomegatech-lab.com.

8. Affinity Labeling Technologies specifies five proteins found in gingival crevicular fluid, each indicating a different aspect of possible (or probable) dental infections under way. 1) Human alkaline phosphatase: Normally found inside the body's cells, when this protein is present in the gingival fluid, it indicates inflammation or tissue destruction at the sampling site. It will not be found around a healthy tooth; also, the higher the level of this protein, the greater the degree of periodontal disease. 2) Bacterial alkaline phosphatase: This protein is produced by various species of anaerobic (not requiring oxygen) bacteria in the mouth and associated with dental disease. This substance, used by bacteria for their own growth, is not found around healthy teeth; thus its presence indicates infection. 3) Human serum albumin: This protein normally appears only in the blood; when it is encountered in the mouth, it means the blood vessels in the mouth have become permeable, allowing this protein to "leak" out. Its presence usually indicates inflammation. 4) Bacterial proteases: These are enzymes that break down other proteins and are secreted by various bacteria found in the mouth. They are responsible for a fair amount of the connective tissue damage that happens with periodontal disease. 5) Human antibodies: The immune system releases specific immune cells (antibodies) in response to the presence of pathogenic microorganisms present in the mouth in the case of dental infection. See "GCF Components: Proteins Present in Gingival Crevicular Fluid (GCF) Samples (Not Added by ALT, Inc.) and the Possible Reason(s) for Their Presence," Affinity Labeling Technologies, 2000 www.altcorp.com.

9. The term intestinal dysbiosis refers to an imbalance of intestinal flora, or the total microbial population of the large and small intestines. Specifically, these flora are friendly, beneficial bacteria, such as *Lactobacillus acidophilus* and *Bifidobacterium bifidum*, and unfriendly bacteria such as *Escherichia coli* and *Clostridium perfringens*. In dysbiosis, the unfriendly bacteria predominate; they begin fermentation, producing toxic byproducts, such as ammonia, amines, nitrosamines, phenols, cresols, indole, and skatole, which interfere with the normal elimination cycle. Dysbiosis is considered a primary cause or major cofactor in the development of many health problems, such as acne, yeast overgrowth (by *Candida albicans*), chronic fatigue, depression, digestive disorders, bloating, food allergies, PMS, rheumatoid arthritis, and cancer.

10. Richard S. Lord, "Dysbiosis Metabolic Markers," MetaMetrix Clinical Laboratory, 2000 www.metametrix.com.

11. Gary Kaplan, "Chronic Pain, Fatigue, and Sinus Headaches," *Alternative Medicine Digest*, October/November 1997, 56-63.

12. James Braly, "Detecting Hidden Food Allergies," *Alternative Medicine Digest*, June/July 1998, 30-34.

13. Ibid.

14. Richard Leviton, "The Allergy-free Body," *Alternative Medicine Digest*, April 1995, 8-13.

Chapter 4

1. Peter Bennett, Stephen Barrie, and Sara Faye, *7-Day Detox Miracle: Restore Your Mind and Body's Natural Vitality with This Safe and Effective Life-Enhancing Program* (Rockland, Calif.: Prima Health/Prima Publishing, 1999): 164.

2. Ibid.

3. F. Batmanghelidj, *Your Body's Many Cries for Water*, Global Health Solutions, Inc., P.O. Box 3189, Falls Church, VA 22043; tel: 703-848-2333; fax: 703-848-2334; website: www.watercure.com.

4. Terry Grossman, *The Baby Boomers' Guide to Living Forever: An Introduction to Immortality Medicine* (Golden, Colo.: The Hubristic Press, 2000): 53.

5. You can be exposed to VOCs in your drinking water even if you rely on untreated (unchlorinated) well water. In 1999, the United States Geological Service (USGS) reported that about 42 million Americans were consuming water from an untreated groundwater aquifer containing at least one VOC. Out of 3,000 water sources tested, VOC levels in 6% of urban wells and in 1.5% of rural wells exceeded the established safety levels for VOCs, said USGS. In urban areas, about fifty percent of the wells had at least one VOC, and thirty percent had two or more, while in rural areas, fifteen percent of the wells had one VOC, and six percent had two or more. The four most commonly

detected VOCs in wells were chloroform, methyl-tert-butylether, tetra-chloroethene, and trichloroethene. See "About 42 Million Americans Drink Water Containing at Least One VOC," Earth Vision Reports, 12 October 1999 www.earthvision.net; this is a publication of Global Environment & Technology Foundation, at: www.getf.org

6. M. Thomason et al, "Study of Water Treatment Effects on Organic Volatiles in Drinking Water," *Journal of Chromatography* 158 (October 1, 1978): 437-47.

7. *Cryptosporidium parvum* is a parasite capable of causing human disease. It is generally not removed or deactivated when water is chlorinated. In 1993, 400,000 people in Milwaukee, Wisconsin, developed diarrhea (the disease is called cryptosporidiosis) after drinking municipal water contaminated with this microorganism, a single-celled protozoa. The parasite is transmitted through the stool of an infected person or animal. The presence of chlorine in water actually makes the parasite enter a self-protective cystic form, in which it surrounds itself with a hard impermeable shell, like an egg, which is chlorine resistant and very hard to destroy. Thus, chlorination supports the toxicity of *Cryptosporidium* in water. Chlorine is also ineffective against *Giardia lamblia*, another hard-shelled cyst that produces human illness.

8. G.A. Boorman, "Drinking Water Disinfection Byproducts: Review and Approach to Toxicity Evaluation," *Environmental Health Perspectives* 107, supp. 1 (February 1999): 207-17.

9. T.F. Lin and S.W. Hoang, "Inhalation Exposure to THMs from Drinking Water in South Taiwan," *Science of the Total Environment* 246 (January 31, 2000): 41-49.

10. Kirsten Waller et al., "Trihalomethanes in Drinking Water and Spontaneous Abortion," *Epidemiology* 9 (March 1998): 134-140. Shanna H. Swan et al., "A Prospective Study of Spontaneous Abortion in Relation to Amount and Source of Drinking Water Consumed in Early Pregnancy," *Epidemiology* 9 (March 1998): 126-133.

11. R.D. Morris et al., "Chlorination, Chlorination By-Products, and Cancer: A Meta-Analysis," *American Journal of Public Health* 82 (July 1992): 1347-1348.

12. M. Wrensch et al., "Spontaneous Abortions and Birth Defects Related to Tap and Bottled Water Use in San Jose, California, 1980-1985," *Epidemiology* 3 (March 1992): 98-103.

13. L. Fenster et al., "Tap or Bottled Water Consumption and Spontaneous Abortion in a Case-Control Study of Reporting Consistency," *Epidemiology* 3 (March 1992): 120-4.

14. M.D. Gallagher et al., "Exposure to Trihalomethanes and Adverse Pregnancy Outcomes," *Epidemiology* 9 (September 1998): 484-489.

15. L. Dodds et al., "Trihalomethanes in Public Water Supplies and Adverse Birth Outcomes," *Epidemiology* 10 (May 1999): 233-7.

16. Judith B. Klotz and Laurie A. Pyrch, "A Case Control Study of Neural Tube Defects and Drinking Water Contaminants," Agency for Toxic Substances and Disease Registry, Atlanta, Ga., January 1998.

17. Frank. L. Bove et al., "Public Drinking Water Contamination and Birth Outcomes," *American Journal of Epidemiology*, 141 (May 1, 1995: 850-862.

18. Andrew T.L. Chen et al., "Re: 'Public Drinking Water Contamination and Birth Outcomes,'" *American Journal of Epidemiology* 143 (June 1, 1996: 1179-1180.

19. P. Magnus et al., "Water Chlorination and Birth Defects," *Epidemiology* 10 (September 1999): 513-17.

20. P. D. Lilly et al., "Trihalomethane Comparative Toxicity: Acute Renal and Hepatic Toxicity of Chloroform and Bromodichloromethane Following Aqueous Gavage," *Fundamentals of Applied Toxicology* 40 (November 1997): 101-110.

21. Kenneth Cantor, "Bladder Cancer, Drinking Water Source, and Tap Water Consumption: A Case-Control Study," *Journal of the National Cancer Institute*, 79 (December 1987): 1269-1279. See also Peter Montague, "Chlorine Chemicals in Our Water Linked to Human Bladder Cancer," *Rachel's Environment & Health Weekly*, #84, July 4, 1988 www.rachel.org.

22. R.J. Bull et al., "Use of Biological Assay Systems to Assess the Relative Carcinogenic Hazards of Disinfection By-products," *Environmental Health Perspectives* 46 (December 1982): 215-27.

23. M.S. Kanarek and T.B. Young, "Drinking Water Treatment and Risk of Cancer Death in Wisconsin," *Environmental Health Perspectives* 46 (December 1982): 179-86.

24. J.K. Dunnick et al., "Bromodichloromethane, a Trihalaomethane that Produces Neoplasms in Rodents," *Cancer Research* 47 (October 1, 1987): 5189-93.

25. J.K. Dunnick and R.L. Melnick, "Assessment of the Carcinogenic Potential of Chlorinated Water: Experimental Studies of Chlorine, Chloramine, and Trihalomethanes," *Journal of the National Cancer Institute* 85 (May 19, 1993): 817-22.

26. R.D. Morris, "Drinking Water and Cancer," *Environmental Health Perspectives* 103, supp. 8 (November 1995): 225-31.

27. W.D. King and L.D. Marrett, "Case-Control Study of Bladder Cancer and Chlorination By-products in Treated Water (Ontario, Canada)," *Cancer Causes Control* 7 (November 1996): 596-604.

28. T.J. Doyle et al., "The Association of Drinking Water Source and Chlorination By-products with Cancer Incidence Among Postmenopausal Women in Iowa: A Prospective Cohort Study," *American Journal of Public Health* 87 (July 1997): 1168-76.

29. K.P. Cantor et al., "Drinking Water Source and Chlorination By-products. I. Risk of Bladder Cancer," *Epidemiology* 9 (January 1998): 21-28.

30. M.E. Hildesheim et al., "Drinking Water Source and Chlorination Byproducts. II. Risk of Colon and Rectal Cancers," *Epidemiology* 9 (January 1998): 29-35.

31. K.P. Cantor et al., "Drinking Water Source and Chlorination Byproducts in Iowa. III. Risk of Brain Cancer," *American Journal of Epidemiology* 150 (September 15, 1999): 552-60.

32. KDF uses high-purity copper-zinc granules to remove heavy metals, microorganisms, and chlorine from water. KDF has been demonstrated to remove ninety-nine percent of free chlorine from water, ninety-five percent of chlorine in municipal water, and ninety-eight percent of water-soluble, positively charged ions of lead, mercury, copper, nickel, chromium, mercury, and other dissolved metals. For more information, contact KDF Fluid Treatment, Inc., 1500 KDF Drive, Three Rivers, MI 49093; tel: 616-273-3300; fax: 616-273-4400; website: www.kdfft.com.

33. "News You Can Use: Everybody Out of the Pool," *Non-Toxic Times*, 1 (August 2000): 4-5, published by Seventh Generation, One Mill Street, Box A26, Burlington, VT 05401; tel: 802-658-3773; fax: 802-658-1771; e-mail: recycle@seventhgen.com; website: www.seventhgen.com. Seventh Generation is also an online source of "environmentally conscious products," including alternatives to chlorine-based products.

34. A.R. Hinman et al., "The U.S. Experience with Fluoridation," *Community Dental Health*, 13, supp. 2 (September 1996): 5-9.

35. Toxic waste remaining from the manufacture of phosphate fertilizer is the source of a large portion of the fluorides dumped in American water. The waste left over from making phosphate fertilizer contains about nineteen percent fluorine. Municipalities all over the United States purchase "fresh pollution concentrate" in the form of fluorosilicic acid from Florida companies. This acid is composed of tetrafluorosiliciate gas and other types of fluorine gases collected by pollution scrubbers in the manufacture of phosphate fertilizer. Fluorosilicic acid would otherwise be classified as a hazardous waste if governmental and industry "health" authorities hadn't set it up to be used to fluoridate public drinking water. Fluorosilicic acid contains at least two radionuclides (radiation products): polonium-210 and radon-222; both are decay products of uranium, which is found in phosphate rock used to make the fertilizer. When we talk about radionuclides, we're talking about carcinogens. See George C. Glasser, "Fluoride and the Phosphate Connection," *Earth Island Journal*, Summer 1998, 12.

36. Fluoride has always been the aluminum industry's "most devastating pollutant," and in 1938, when the aluminum industry had to step up production to meet wartime demands, it had to find new ways to deal with its toxic byproduct. Ironically, the industry sustained a number of damage suits claiming damage to human health from exposure

to fluoride wastes. Conveniently, the aluminum industry found a way to dump its toxic waste product into America's public drinking water in the 1940s under the guise of dental benefits, even though very little hard evidence had been generated to support the contention. See Joel Griffith, "Fluoride: Industry's Toxic Coup," *Earth Island Journal*, Spring 1998 www.earthisland.org.

37. Richard Leviton, "The Fluoride Lie—Santa Cruz Refuses to Comply with State Law," *Alternative Medicine*, August-September 1998, 105-109.

38. Gar Smith, "Why Fluoride Is an Environmental Issue," *Earth Island Journal*, Summer 2000 www.earthislandjournal.org.

39. L. Seppa et al., "Caries in the Primary Dentition, After Discontinuation of Water Fluoridation Among Children After Receiving Comprehensive Dental Care," *Community Dental and Oral Epidemiology* 28 (August 2000): 281-8.

40. B.A. Burt et al., "The Effects of a Break in Water Fluoridation on the Development of Dental Caries and Fluorosis," *Journal of Dental Research* 79 (February 2000): 761-9.

41. W. Kunzel and T. Fischer, "Caries Prevalence After Cessation of Water Fluoridation in La Salud, Cuba," *Caries Research* 34 (January-February 2000): 20-5.

42. J.J. Warren et al., "Fluorosis of the Primary Dentition: What Does It Mean for Permanent Teeth?" *Journal of the American Dental Association* 130 (July 1999): 922.

43. K.E. Heller et al., "Dental Caries and Dental Fluorosis at Varying Fluoride Concentrations," *Journal of Public Health Dentistry* 57 (Summer 1997): 136-43.

44. R.H. Selwitz et al., "Dental Caries and Dental Fluorosis Among Schoolchildren Who Were Lifelong Residents of Communities Having Either Low or Optimal Levels of Fluoride in Drinking Water," *Journal of Public Health Dentistry* 58 (Winter 1998): 28-35.

45. L. Morgan et al., "Investigation of the Possible Associations Between Fluorosis, Fluoride Exposure, and Childhood Behavior Problems," *Pediatric Dentistry* 20 (July-August 1998): 244-52.

46. D.G. Pendrys et al., "Risk Factors for Enamel Fluorosis in Optimally Fluoridated Children Born After the U.S. Manufacturers' Decision to Reduce the Fluoride Concentration of Infant Formulas," *American Journal of Epidemiology* 148 (November 15, 1998): 967-74.

47. A. Bardsen et al., "Dental Fluorosis Among Persons Exposed to High and Low-Fluoride Drinking Water in Western Norway," *Community Dental and Oral Epidemiology* 27 (August 1999): 259-67.

48. A.E. Villa et al., "Dental Fluorosis in Chilean Children: Evaluation of Rsik Factors," *Community Dental and Oral Epidemiology* 26 (October 1998): 310-15.

49. A. Bardsen and K. Bjorvatn, "Risk Periods in the Development of Dental Fluorosis," *Clinical Oral Investigations* 2 (December 1998): 155-60.

50. Morton Walker, "Fluoridation Brings Hazards to Human Health," *Townsend Letter for Doctors & Patients*, No. 202, May 2000, 30-36.

51. G.J. Judd, "Mass Fluoridation Causes Alarming Rise in Cancer Deaths," *Health Freedom News*, May 1995, 10.

52. E. Tohyama, "Relationship Between Fluoride Concentration in Drinking Water and Mortality Rate from Uterine Cancer in Okinawa Prefecture, Japan," *Journal of Epidemiology* 6 (December 1996): 184-91.

53. W. John Diamond, M.D., and W. Lee Cowden, M.D., with Burton Goldberg, *An Alternative Medicine Definitive Guide to Cancer* (Tiburon, Calif.: Future Medicine Publishing, 1997): 580-582.

54. Collation of published researched provided by Health and Longevity Resource Center, 1998 www.all-natural.com.

55. S. Hillier et al., "Fluoride in Drinking Water and Risk of Hip Fracture in the UK: A Case-Control Study," *Lancet* 355 (January 22, 2000): 265-9.

56. John R. Lee, "Fluoridation and Hip Fractures," *Earth Island Journal*, Summer 2000 www.earthisland,org.

57. M. Diesendorf et al., "New Evidence on Fluoridation," *Australian New Zealand Journal of Public Health* 21 (April 1997): 187-90.

58. J.K. Maurer et al., "Two-Year Carcinogenicity Study of Sodium Fluoride in Rats," *Journal of the National Cancer Institute* 82 (July 4, 1990): 1118-26.

59. Richard G. Foulkes, "The Fluoride Connection," *Townsend Letter for Doctors & Patients*, April 1998, 11.

60. Leviton, "The Fluoride Lie," 107.

61. Bob Woffinden, "A Clear and Present Danger," *Earth Island Journal*, Summer 2000 www.earthisland.org.

62. P.J. Mullenix et al., "Neurotoxicity of Sodium Fluoride in Rats," *Neurotoxicology and Teratology*, 17 (March-April 1995): 169-177.

63. Joel Griffith, "Fluoride: Industry's Toxic Coup," *Earth Island Journal*, Spring 1998 www.earthisland.org.

64. Gar Smith, "Why Fluoride Is an Environmental Issue," *Earth Island Journal*, Summer 2000 www.earthislandjournal.org.

65. Joseph Dispenza, *Live Better Longer: The Parcells Center Seven-Step Plan for Health and Longevity* (San Francisco: Harper San Francisco, 1997): 38-45.

66. Research summarized from C.H. Van Middelem, "Fate and Persistence of Pesticides," presented at Pesticides in the Environment, a 1965 symposium, reprinted at www.veggiewash.com.

67. For a good review of the subject and its ramifications, see Martin Teitel and Kimberley Wilson, *Genetically Engineered Food:*

Changing the Nature of Nature (Rochester, Vt.:Park Street Press, 1999). See also the author's website, the Council for Responsible Genetics: www.gene-watch.org.

68. Richard Leviton, "Bioengineered Foods—Putting Consumer Health and Safety Last," *Alternative Medicine*, November 1998, 104-110.

69. Ibid., 108.

70. Julie A. Nordlee et al., "Identification of a Brazil-nut Allergen in Transgenic Soybeans," *New England Journal of Medicine* 334 (March 14, 1996): 688-692.

71. "Frequently Asked Questions About Genetically Engineered Food," Summer 1999, The Council for Responsible Genetics, 5 Upland Road, Suite 3, Cambridge, MA 02140; tel: 617-868-0870; fax: 617-491-5344; website: crg@gene-watch.org.

72. Francesca Lyman, "'Transgenic' Pollution a New Concern," MSNBC News, 28 September 1999 www.msnbc.com.

73. Rich Charnes, "Genetically Altered Food: Myths and Realities," EarthSave, 2000 www.earthsave.org. Earth Save International, 1509 Seabright Avenue, Suite B1, Santa Cruz, CA 96062; tel: 831-423-0293 or 800-362-3648; fax: 831-423-1313.

74. Joe Cummins, "Gene Tinkering Blues: Allergy," *Gene Tinkering Blues*, February 1997 www.holisticmed.com/ge/allergy.html.

75. Marion Nestle, "Allergies to Transgenic Foods—Questions of Policy," *New England Journal of Medicine*, 334 (March 14, 1996): 726-728.

76. Ronnie Cummins, "Son of Frankenfoods: GE Trees, Fish, and Functional Foods," *BioDemocracy News* #28, July 2000 www.purefood.org.

77. "Summary of U.S. Consumer Polls on GE Foods," Center for Food Safety, 666 Pennsylvania Avenue, SE, Suite 302, Washington D.C., 20003; tel: 202-547-9359; fax: 202-547-9429; website: www.centerforfoodsafety.org.

78. Peter Montague, "Genetically Altering the World's Food," *Rachel's Environment & Health Weekly*, #639, February 25, 1999.

79. Richard Leviton, "The Tainted Milk Mustache—How Monsanto and the FDA Spoiled a Staple Food," *Alternative Medicine*, January 1999, 94-108.

80. Samuel S. Epstein, "Unlabeled Milk from Cows Treated with Biosynthetic Growth Hormones: A Case of Regulatory Abdication," *International Journal of Health Sciences* 26:1 (1996): 173-185.

81. Steve Emmott, "EU Scientific Committee Warns of Human Health & Cancer Hazards of Monsanto's Recombinant Bovine Growth Hormone (rGBH)," March 1999 www.purefood.org.

82. Susan E. Hankinson et al., "Circulating Concentrations of Insulin-like Growth Factor 1 and Risk of Breast Cancer," *The Lancet* 351 (May 9, 1998): 1393-1396.

83. June M. Chan et al., "Plasma Insulin-like Growth Factor 1 and Prostate Cancer Risk: A Prospective Study," *Science* 279 (January 23, 1998): 563-566.

84. "Summary of U.S. Consumer Polls on GE Foods," Center for Food Safety www.centerforfoodssafety.org.

85. For a complete list of labeling requirements and loopholes, see "Background and Status of Labeling of Irradiated Foods," BioDemocracy and Organic Consumers Association, 28 June 2000 www.purefood.org.

86. See John W. Gofman, "Preventing Breast Cancer: The Story of a Major, Proven, Preventable Cause of this Disease" (Committee for Nuclear Responsibility, San Francisco, Calif., 1996). "Radiation from Medical Procedures in the Pathogenesis of Cancer and Ischemic Heart Disease" (Committee for Nuclear Responsibility, San Francisco, Calif., 1999). "Radiation-Induced Cancer from Low-Dose Exposure" (Committee for Nuclear Responsibility, San Francisco, Calif., 1990).

87. Richard Leviton, "FDA's Mission Impossible—Selling the American Public the Food Irradiation Safety Con," *Alternative Medicine*, May 1998, 103-108.

88. Jeffrey Reinhardt, "Liver Cancer: Danger of Radiolytic Products in the Diet," BioDemocracy and Organic Consumers Association, 26 June 2000 www.purefood.org.

89. Wenonah Hauter, "Overview of Food Irradiation Reports," *Public Citizen*, 28 December 1999 www.citizen.org.

90. See Gary Gibbs, *The Food That Would Last Forever* (Garden City Park, N.Y.: Avery Publishing Group, 1993).

91. S.G. Srikantia, Professor of Food and Nutrition, University of Mysore, India, in testimony before U.S. Congressional hearings on Food Irradiation, June 19, 1987. Published at www.citizen.org.

92. "Memorandum, Irradiation and the New Proposed National Organic Program Area of Concern," Center for Food Safety, 5 April 2000 www.centerforfoodsafety.org.

93. "How It Hurts: Key Research on the Unwholesomeness of Irradiated Foods," Public Citizen, 2000, www.citizen.org.

94. Wenonah Hauter, "Food Irradiation: Do You Know Where Your Dinner Has Been?" Public Citizen, 1999 www.citizen.org.

95. Patricia Kane, "Lifting Depression with Nutrition," *Alternative Medicine Digest*, March 1998, 64-70.

96. A. Ascherio et al., "Trans-fatty Acids and Coronary Heart Disease," *New England Journal of Medicine* 340 (June 24, 1999): 1994-8.

97. Research compiled and summarized by Mary G. Enig at www.enig.com. Dr. Enig is a nutritionist, former faculty research associate with the Lipid Research Group at the University of Maryland, director of nutritional sciences at Enig Associates, Inc., and the author of two books on fats.

98. For more information, see: Mary G. Enig, *Trans-Fatty Acids in the Food Supply: A Comprehensive Report Covering 60 Years of Research*, 2d ed. (Bethesda, Md.: Bethesda Press, 1995): available from www.enig.com; e-mail: marye@enig.com. Also Mary G. Enig, *Know Your Fats: The Complete Primer for Understanding the Nutrition of Fats, Oils, and Cholesterol* (Bethesda, Md.: Bethesda Press, 2000): Bethesda Press, Suite 340, Meadows Park Building, 12501 Prosperity Drive, Silver Spring, MD 20904; tel: 301-680-8800; fax: 301-680-8100; website: www.bethesdapress.com.

99. Mary G. Enig, "Published Estimates of Trans-Fatty Acid Availability and Consumption in Various Countries," (n.d.) www.enig.com.

100. Bruce Fife, *The Detox Book. How to Detoxify Your Body to Improve Your Health, Stop Disease, and Reverse Aging* (Colorado Springs, Colo.: Health Wise, 1997): 99.

101. Elson M. Haas, *The Detox Diet. A How-To & When-To Guide for Cleansing the Body* (Berkeley, Calif.: Celestial Arts, 1996): 119.

102. Lewis Harrison, *30-Day Body Purification. How to Cleanse Your Inner Body & Experience the Joys of Toxin-Free Health* (Paramus, N.J.: Reward Books/Prentice Hall, 1995): 80-81, 83.

103. Jacquelin Krohn, M.D., Frances Taylor, and Jinger Prosser, *The Whole Way to Natural Detoxification. Clearing Your Body of Toxins* (Point Roberts, Wash.: Hartley & Marks, 1996): 132-33.

104. Fife, *The Detox Book*, 93.

105. John Updike, *Rabbit Redux* (New York: Alfred A. Knopf, 1971): 194.

106. Charles Tart, quoted by Ralph Losey in "The Problem of the Subtle Sybil Effect," www.sun-angel.com.

107. [Untitled, unsigned editorial], *Cogenesis Journal*, Eos Co-Creations, P.O. Box 483, Cave Creek, AZ 85327; tel: 602-502-0686; website: www.cogenesis.com.

108. Also known as bitter salts or heptahydrate, Epsom salt is a naturally occurring mineral called epsomite, with a high magnesium sulfate content. For commercial use, it is made through the action of sulphuric acid on magnesite (magnesium carbonate/oxide). During the bath, the high magnesium concentration in the salt enables water to be pulled out through the body's skin pores and, with it, toxins capable of excretion through the skin. It is not uncommon for the bath water to turn a light grey color after one has been soaking for twenty minutes or so; this is an indication that toxins have been excreted through the skin. Epsom salt is also an effective, safe, nontoxic laxative, taken as a drink, mixed with water, per instructions on the package. As a topical agent, Epsom salt is recommended for providing some relief from stiffness, soreness, joint tightness, arthritic pain, discomfort from tender

muscles, bruises, sprains, or strains, and to improve sleep and increase the body's energy levels through deep relaxation.

109. Valerie Ann Worwood, *The Fragrant Mind. Aromatherapy for Personality, Mind, Mood, and Emotion* (Novato, Calif.: New World Library, 1996): 131-132.

110. Ibid., 193-194.

111. Chrissie Wildwood, *The Encyclopedia of Aromatherapy* (Rochester, Vt.: Healing Arts Press, 1996): 83.

112. The approach was developed in 1954 by Dr. John C. Lilly, a pioneer in brain and behavioral research and later famous for his work with dolphins. Dr. Lilly experimented with the effects on the brain of restricting external sensory stimulation; he thought it would put the brain to sleep. Instead, it woke it up. Using himself as his first test subject, Dr. Lilly removed all visual, sound, tactile, and temperature stimuli, and found his brain operated independently of external sensory data, and functioned at an even higher level as a result. He found that the greatest benefit to floating in salt in a sensory deprivation chamber was the profound state of relaxation it induced. He stated that two hours in the flotation tank is equivalent to eight hours of restful sleep and that floating is an excellent way to destress after an overloaded work day.

113. The autonomic nervous system (ANS) can be likened to your body's automatic pilot. It keeps you alive through breathing, heart rate, and digestion, without your being aware of it or participating in its activities. The ANS has two divisions: the sympathetic nervous sysyem, which expends body energy; and the parasympathetic nervous system, which conserves body energy. The sympathetic nervous system is associated with arousal and stress; it prepares us physically when we perceive a threat or challenge by increasing our heart rate, blood pressure, and muscle tension. The parasympathetic nervous system slows heart rate and increases intestinal and most gland activity.

114. According to information provided by ThinkTank International Pte. Ltd. (Singapore) about the PathFinder floatation tank; website: www.thinktank.com.sg.

115. Thomas H. Fine and Roderick Borrie, "Flotation REST in Applied Psychophysiology" (paper presented at the Sixth International Conference on REST, San Francisco, Calif., April 17, 1997) International REST Investigators Society (IRIS) www.concentric.net/%7Etfine/flotrest.shtml.

116. According to information provided about Oasis Flotation Systems by Biofeedback Instrument Corporation, New York, N.Y.; website: www.biof.com/oasis.

117. According to information provided by Samadhi Tank Corporation, Nevada City, CA; website: www.samadhitank.com.

118. Comments by Steven Halpern drawn from "Push-Button Relaxation," 1997 www.stevenhalpern.com; from an interview by

Richard Leviton, 1992; and from Richard Leviton, "Healing Vibrations," *Yoga Journal*, January-February 1994.

Chapter 5

1. First developed by 19th-century European physicians, naturopathy is an umbrella term to describe the original basis of natural, holistic, and alternative medicine. A naturopath understands that Nature heals and that the body is inherently self-healing when given the appropriate support therapies, such as diet; herbs; nutritional supplementation; detoxification and internal cleansing regimens; exercise; heat and water therapy; massage; bodywork; counseling; and relaxation. Naturopathy emphasizes disease prevention and health promotion. It is currently licensed as a medical profession in at least eleven U.S. states, with the number of new states accepting naturopathy growing steadily. In a few states, naturopaths function as primary care physicians, and insurance companies cover their services. There are several accredited four-year naturopathic medical colleges now in operation.

2. These cruciferous vegetables all contain a nutritionally valuable component called glucosinolates. Studies have shown that these compounds can increase the body's detoxification activities and help protect against the effects of carcinogens. According to nutritionist Jeffrey Bland, Ph.D., the beneficial activity of cruciferous vegetables may be due not only to glucosinolates, "but to the synergistic interaction of many substances inherent in cruciferous vegetables." Dr. Bland further notes that it is important not to overcook this type of vegetable, because the heat destroys or denatures the enzymes, thereby diminishing their benefit. See Jeffrey S. Bland, *The 20-Day Rejuvenation Diet Program, With the Revolutionary Phytonutrient Diet* (New Canaan, Conn.: Keats Publishing, 1997): 65-66.

3. Bile is a thick, viscous, straw-colored fluid produced by the liver, from which it passes into the common bile duct and then into the small intestine as needed. Bile is also stored in the gallbladder and discharged as needed. It is typically produced at the rate of a pint to a quart per twenty-four hours, although during fasting, little bile is formed. Bile functions as a digestive juice and emulsifying agent, facilitating the digestion of oils and fats in the small intestine. Essentially, bile emulsifies the fats so that digestive enzymes from the pancreas can break them down. When consumed food (especially fats) reaches the first part of the small intestine (duodenum), it triggers the liver and gallbladder to release bile into the intestine. Bile also stimulates peristalsis, or the rhythmic contractions of the intestines that move fecal matter along to its final elimination. Normally bile is ejected from the liver or gallbladder storage only during small intestine digestion.

4. Laurel Vukovic, *14-Day Herbal Cleansing. A Step-by-Step Guide to All Natural Inner Cleansing Techniques for Increased Energy, Vitality and Beauty* (Paramus, N.J.: Prentice Hall, 1998), 73, 145-6.

5. Carolyn Reuben, *Cleansing the Body, Mind, and Spirit* (New York: Berkley Books, 1998): 178.

6. P.R. Bradley, ed., *British Herbal Compendium*, Vol. 1 (Bournemouth, Dorset, U.K.: British Herbal Medicine Association, 1992): 112-114. J. Yamahara et al., "Gastrointestinal Motility Enhancing Effect of Ginger and Its Active Constituents," *Chemical Pharmacology Bulletin* 38 (1990): 430-1.

7. Paul Pitchford, *Healing with Whole Foods. Oriental Traditions and Modern Nutrition* (Berkeley, Calif.: North Atlantic Books, 1993): 497.

8. Helene Silver. *Rejuvenate. A 21-Day Natural Detox Plan for Optimal Health* (Freedom, Calif.: The Crossing Press, 1998), 42.

9. Donald J. Brown, N.D., *Herbal Prescriptions for Better Health. Your Everyday Guide to Prevention, Treatment, and Care* (Rocklin, Calif.: Prima Publishing, 1996): 151-158.

10. Vukovic, *14-Day Herbal Cleansing*, 75.

11. Daniel B. Mowrey, *Herbal Tonic Therapies* (New Canaan, Conn.: Keats Publishing, 1993): 239-241.

12. Marie Nadine Antol, *Healing Teas. How to Prepare and Use Teas to Maximize Your Health* (Garden City Park, N.Y.: Avery Publishing Group, 1996): 122-123.

13. David Hoffmann, *The Holistic Herbal. A Herbal Celebrating the Wholeness of Life* (Shaftesbury, Dorset, U.K.:Element Books, 1988): 62.

14. Bennett, *7-Day Detox Miracle*, 187-88.

15. Ibid., 179-186.

16. Carol A. Newall, Linda A. Anderson, and J. David Phillipson, *Herbal Medicines. A Guide for Health-Care Professionals* (London: The Pharmaceutical Press, 1996): 60-61.

17. Michael Tierra, "How to Do a Liver Flush," 1999 www.planet herbs.com.

18. Silver. *Rejuvenate*, 51,49.

19. Christopher Hobbs, L.Ac., *Healing with Herbs & Foods* (Loveland, Colo.: Botanica Press/Interweave Press, 1994).

20. Serafino Corsello, M.D., "Reversing Lupus and Diabetes," *Alternative Medicine Digest*, February-March 1998, 44-53.

21. William Lee Cowden, M.D., "Health Hazard in Your Intestines," *Alternative Medicine Digest*, November 1996, 26-29.

22. W.C. Willett et al., "Relation of Meat, Fat, and Fiber Intake to the Risk of Colon Cancer in a Prospective Study Among Women," *New England Journal of Medicine* 323 (December 13, 1990): 1664-72.

23. B. Trock et al., "Dietary Fiber, Vegetables, and Colon Cancer: Critical Review and Meta-Analyses of the Epidemiologic Evidence," *Journal of the National Cancer Institute* 82 (April 1990): 650-61.

24. E. Benito et al., "A Population-Based Case-Control Study of Colorectal Cancer in Majorca," *International Journal of Cancer* 45 (January 15, 1990): 69-76.

25. C.F. Babbs, "Free Radicals and the Etiology of Colon Cancer," *Free Radical Biological Medicine* 8:2 (1990): 191-200.

26. "The Colon: Sewer or Cesspool?" Angel Healing Center, 1999 www.cyberport.net/angel.

27. Dr. Bernard Jensen, *Dr. Jensen's Guide to Better Bowel Care* (Garden City Park, N.Y.: Avery Publishing Group, 1999): 27, 37-38, 51-54.

28. "Medicinal Activated Charcoal Tablets and Biscuits," J.L. Bragg (Ipswich) Ltd., Suffolk, England www.users.globalnet.co.uk.

29. Robert C. Atkins, M.D., *Dr. Atkins' Vita-Nutrient Solution. Nature's Answer to Drugs* (New York: Simon & Schuster, 1998): 237-238.

30. Richard C. Kaufman, "The Universal Antidote and Detoxifier That Extends Life: Activated Charcoal," *Journal of the Megahealth Society*, July 1989 www.healingtools.tripod.com.

31. S.M. Lipson and G. Stotzky, "Specificity of Virus Adsorption to Clay Minerals," *Canadian Journal of Microbiology* 31 (January 1985): 50-53.

32. M.D. Sobsey and T. Cromeans, "Effects of Bentonite Clay Solids on Poliovirus Concentration from Water by Microporous Filter Methods," *Applied Environmental Microbiology* 49 (April 1985): 795-8.

33. V.M. Illrin et al., "A New Sorbent for Concentrating Viruses from an Aqueous Medium," *Lik Sprava*, May-June 1995, 5-6, 177-9.

34. W.A. Hartman and D.B. Martin, "Effect of Suspended Bentonite Clay on the Acute Toxicity of Glyphosate to Daphnia pulex and Lemna minor," *Bulletin of Environmental Contamination and Toxicology* 33 (September 1984): 355-361. And R.D. Fairshter and A.F. Wilson, "Paraquat Poisoning: Manifestations and Therapy," *The American Journal of Medicine* 59 (December 1975): 751-753. D. I. Blodgett, et al. "Adsorption of Aflatoxin with Feed-Approved Clays," Virginia Corn Board Project Progress Report (n.d.) www.yerbaprima.com/bentproc.htm.

35. J.M. Santurio et al., "Effect of Sodium Bentonite on the Performance and Blood Variables of Broiler Chickens Intoxicated with Aflatoxins," *British Poultry Science* 40 (March 1999): 115-9.

36. M.A. Abdel-Wahhab et al., "Effect of Aluminosilicates and Bentonite on Aflatoxin-Induced Developmental Toxicity in Rats," *Journal of Applied Toxicology* 19 (May-June 1999): 199-204.

37. T.C. Schell et al., "Effects of Feeding Aflatoxin-Contaminated Diets with and without Clay to Weanling and Growing Pigs on Performance, Liver Function, and Mineral Metabolism," *Journal of Animal Science* 71 (May 1993): 1209-18.

38. R.A. McKenzie, "Bentonite as Therapy for Lantana camara Poisoning of Cattle," *Australian Veterinary Journal* 68 (April 1991): 146-8.

39. Ran Knishinsky, *The Clay Cure* (Rochester, Vt.: Healing Arts Press, 1998). See also "Cleanse Yourself Internally with Liquid Clay—The Bentonite Cure," *Alternative Medicine* (December 1998-January 1999), 14-15.

40. "Chlorella Q & A" www.earthrise.com.

41. W. John Diamond, M.D., Lee W. Cowden, M.D., and Burton Goldberg, *An Alternative Medicine Definitive Guide to Cancer* (Tiburon, Calif.: Future Medicine Publishing, 1997): 809-811.

42. "Greater Health and Longevity: Chlorella, the Green Algae Superfood, May Be the Answer," *Alternative Medicine Digest* 12 (1996): 56.

43. Information provided by Taiwan Chlorella Manufacturing Co., Ltd., Taipei, Taiwan; website: www.taiwanchlorella.com.

44. Randal Merchant, M.D., "1999: Research Update," Health & Happiness Publishing, The Press Room, 2435 E. North St., #116, Greenville, SC 29615; tel: 800-694-2774; e-mail: info@health-books.com; website: www.health-books.com/PressRoom.

45. Randal Merchant et al., "Dietary *Chlorella Pyrenoidosa* for Patients with Malignant Glioma: Effects of Immuno-Competence, Quality of Life, and Survival," *Phytotherapy Research* 4:6 (1990): 220-231.

46. R.S. Pore, "Detoxification of Chlordecone Poisoned Rats with Chlorella and Chlorella Derived Sporopollenin," *Drug and Chemical Toxicology* 7:1 (1984): 57-71.

47. I. Hagino, "Effect of Chlorella on Fecal and Urinary Cadmium Excretion in 'Itai-Itai,'" *Japan Journal of Hygiene* 30:1 (1975): 77.

48. T. Nagano et al., "Absorption and Excretion of Cadmium by the Rat Administered Cadmium-Containing Chlorella," *Eisei Kagaku* 24:4 (1978): 7182-7186.

49. Randal Merchant et al., "Nutritional Supplementation with *Chlorella pyrenoidosa* for Patients with Fibromyalgia Syndrome: A Pilot Study," *Phytotherapy Research* 14 (May 2000): 167-73.

50. Merchant, "1999: Research Update."

51. Ayurveda is the traditional medicine of India, based on many centuries of empirical use. Its name means "end of the Vedas" (which were India's sacred scripts), implying that a holistic medicine may be founded on spiritual principles. Ayurveda describes three metabolic, constitutional, and body types (doshas) in association with the basic elements of Nature. These are vata (air and ether, rooted in intestines), pitta (fire and water/stomach), and kapha (water and earth/lungs). Ayurvedic physicians use these categories (which also have psychological aspects) as the basis for prescribing individualized formulas of herbs, diet, massage, breathing, meditation, exercise and yoga postures, and detoxification techniques.

52. Dr. Michael Tierra, L.Ac., O.M.D., "The Wonders of Triphala: Ayurvedic Formula for Internal Purification," Online Articles, 1996 www.planetherbs.com.

53. Rudolf M. Ballentine, M.D., *Radical Healing. Integrating the World's Great Therapeutic Traditions to Create a New Transformative Medicine* (New York: Three Rivers Press, 1999): 306.

54. Jacqueline Krohn, M.D., Frances Taylor, and Jinger Prosser, *The Whole Way to Natural Detoxification. Clearing Your Body of Toxins* (Point Roberts, Wash.: Hartley & Marks, 1996): 17.

55. L.J. Cheskin et al., "Mechanisms of Constipation in Older Persons and Effects of Fiber Compared with Placebo," *Journal of the American Geriatric Society* 43 (June 1995): 666-9.

56. J. Stevens et al., "Comparison of the Effects of Psyllium and Wheat Bran on Gastrointestinal Transit Time and Stool Characteristics," *Journal of the American Dietetics Association* 88 (March 1988): 323-6.

57. M. Tomas-Ridocci et al., "The Efficacy of Plantago ovata as a Regulator of Intestinal Transit. A Double-Blind Study Compared to Placebo," *Rev Esp Enferm Dig* 82 (July 1992): 17-22.

58. W. Ashraf et al., "Effects of Psyllium Therapy on Stool Characteristics, Colon Transit and Anorectal Function in Chronic Idiopathic Constipation," *Alimentary Pharmacological Therapy* 9: (December 1995): 639-47.

59. All cholesterol is not unhealthy; some is required for the body's metabolic and hormonal functions; but one form of cholesterol is believed to be injurious. To understand this, we need to discuss lipoproteins. These are found in two principal forms: low- and high-density. Low-density lipoproteins (LDLs), which are made from protein and fat molecules, circulate in the blood and act as the primary carriers of cholesterol to the cells of the body. An elevated level of LDL, often called "bad" cholesterol, contributes to atherosclerosis, a circulatory system disease that leads to a buildup of plaque deposits on the inner walls of the arteries. These plaque deposits can eventually cause heart attacks, stroke, and other illnesses. A diet high in saturated fats can increase levels of LDLs in the blood. In contrast, high-density lipoproteins (HDLs) contain a larger amount of protein and less fat than LDLs. HDLs readily absorb cholesterol and related compounds in the blood and transport them to the liver for elimination. A higher ratio of HDL to LDL cholesterol in the blood is associated with a reduced risk of cardiovascular disease.

60. J.W. Anderson et al., "Cholesterol-Lowering Effects of Psyllium-Enriched Cereal as an Adjunct to a Prudent Diet in the Treatment of Mild to Moderate Hypercholesterolemia." *American Journal of Clinical Nutrition* 56 (July 1992): 93-8.

61. W.L. Haskell et al., "Role of Water-Soluble Dietary Fiber in the Management of Elevated Plasma Cholesterol in Healthy Subjects," *American Journal of Cardiology* 70 (September 15, 1992): 840.

62. Technically, this physiological experience, or sensation, is called the Jarisch-Herxheimer reaction or effect, or sometimes "herx," for

short. It is named after the Austrian dermatologist, Jarisch Adolf Herxheimer, who identified it in 1895; the effect was confirmed by his brother, Karl Herxheimer, M.D., also a dermatologist but working in Germany. Originally it was used in reference to syphilis, but doctors found it accurately described the phenomena of other illnesses, such as tuberculosis, arthritis, and candidiasis (yeast infestation by *Candida albicans*). The term refers to a temporary increase of symptoms under the influence of treatment; in the case of syphilis, it referred to the temporary worsening or intensification of symptoms as a result of administering anti-syphilitic drugs, or antibiotics. In that case, the syphilis organisms were literally dying off at a rate faster than the body could clean up and remove their toxic debris. The term is now being used in the context of Lyme disease, caused by the spirochete *Borrelia burgdorferi*, related to *Treponema pallidum*, the organism responsible for syphilis. But it is also being used even more generally for comparable experiences during detoxification. Although the experience is unpleasant, it is a sure sign that the detoxification protocols are working. It demonstrates the ironic truth of the following statement: You wouldn't feel this miserable if you weren't actually getting better.

63. Thomas Fleming, ed., *PDR® for Herbal Medicines* (Montvale, N.J.: Medical Economics Company, 1998): 1090.

64. Mowrey, *Herbal Tonic Therapies*, 215-218.

65. Richard Anderson, N.D., N.M.D., "The Key to Excellent Health: Cleansing the Colon," *Alternative Medicine*, March 1999, 18-22. *Cleanse & Purify Thyself*, Book 1.5, Richard Anderson (publisher), 1998, 48-49, 66-67.

66. Anderson, "The Key to Excellent Health: Cleansing the Colon," 21-22.

67. Ann Louise Gittleman, *Guess What Came to Dinner: Parasites and Your Health* (Garden City Park, N.Y.: Avery Publishing Group, 1993): xiii.

68. An immunoglobulin is one of a class of five specially designed antibody proteins produced in the spleen, bone marrow, or lymph tissue and involved in the immune system's defense response to foreign substances. The main types of immunoglobulins, grouped according to their concentration in the blood, are: IgG (80%), IgA (10-15%), IgM (5-10%), IgD (less than 0.1%), and IgE (less than 0.01%). Technically, all antibodies are immunoglobulins.

69. Silena Heron, N.D., and Eric Yarnell, N.D., "Treating Parasitic Infections with Botanical Medicines," *Alternative & Complementary Therapies* 5 (August 1999): 214-224.

70. Leo Galland, M.D., "Persistent GI Upset a Signal of Hidden Giardiasis," *Cortlandt Forum* (1990):120-21.

71. Leo Galland, M.D., et al., "*Giardia lamblia* Infection as a Cause of Chronic Fatigue," *Journal of Nutritional Medicine* 1 (1990): 27-31.

72. "Results of Testing for Intestinal Parasites by State Diagnostic Laboratories," United States, 1987, *Morbidity and Mortality Weekly* 40 (SS-4) (1992): 25-30.

73. J. Lee, G.M. Park et al., "Intestinal Parasite Infections at an Institution for the Handicapped in Korea," *Korean Journal of Parasitology* 38 (September 2000): 179-81.

74. K.J. Lee, Y.K. Ahn, and T.S. Yong, "A Small-Scale Survey of Intestinal Parasite Infections Among Children and Adolescents in Legaspi City, the Philippines," *Korean Journal of Parasitology* 38 (September 2000): 183-5.

75. M. Youssef et al., "Bacterial, Viral, and Parasitic Enteric Pathogens Associated with Acute Diarrhea in Hospitalized Children from Northern Jordan," *FEMS Immunology and Medical Microbiology* 28 (July 2000): 257-63.

76. A.L. el Idrissi, M. Lyagoubi et al., "Prevalence of Intestinal Parasitic Disease in Three Provinces in Morocco," *Eastern Mediterranean Health Journal* 5 (January 1999): 86-102.

77. Joseph Pizzorno, N.D., *Total Wellness. Improve Your Health by Understanding the Body's Healing Systems* (Rocklin, Calif.: Prima Publishing, 1996): 215.

78. J. Flegr, P. Kodym, and V. Tolarova, "Correlation of Duration of Latent *Toxoplasma gondii* Infection with Personality Changes in Women," *Biological Psychology* 53 (May 2000): 57-68.

79. Pizzorno, *Total Wellness*, 79.

80. Michael Murray, N.D., and Joseph Pizzorno, N.D., *Encyclopedia of Natural Medicine*, rev. 2d ed. (Rocklin, Calif.: Prima Publishing, 1998): 436-437.

81. R. Sharma, C.K. Joshiu, and R.K. Goyal, "Berberine Tannate in Acute Diarrhea," *Indian Pediatrics* 7 (1970): 496-501.

82. V.P. Choudry, M. Sabir, and V.N. Bhide, "Berberine in Giardiasis," *Indian Pediatrics* 9 (1972): 143-6.

83. S.A. Kamat, "Clinical Trial with Berberine Hydrochloride for the Control of Diarrhea in Acute Gastroenteritis," *Journal of the Association of Physicians of India* 129 (1967): 525-9.

84. J. Lal, S. Chandra et al., "In Vitro Antihelmintic Action of Some Indigenous Medicinal Plants on *Ascardia galli* Worms," *Indian Journal of Physiological Pharmacology* 20 (April-June 1976): 64-68.

85. V. Munoz et al., "The Search for Natural Bioactive Compounds through a Multidisciplinary Approach in Bolivia. Part II. Antimalarial Activity of Some Plants Used by Mosetene Indians," *Journal of Ethnopharmacology* 69 (February 2000): 139-55.

86. A.D. Frame et al., "Plants from Puerto Rico with Anti-Mycobacterium Tuberculosis Properties," *Puerto Rican Health Science Journal* 17 (September 1998): 243-52.

87. A. Singh, S.P. Singh, and R. Bamezai, "Postnatal Efficacy of *Momordica charantia* Peel, Pulp, Seed, and Whole Fruit Extract in the Detoxification Pathway of Suckling Neonates and Lactating Mice," *Cancer Letters* 122 (January 9, 1998): 121-126.

88. P. Scartezzini and E. Speroni, "Review on Some Plants of Indian Traditional Medicine with Antioxidant Activity," *Journal of Ethnopharmacology* 71 (July 2000): 23-43.

89. O.V. Rybaltovskii, "On the Discovery of Cucurbitin—a Component of Pumpkin Seed with Antihelmintic Action," *Med Parazitol* (Mosk) 35 (July-August 1966): 487-8. R.J. Blagrove and G.G. Lilley, "Characterisation of Cucurbitin from Various Species of the Cucurbitaceae," *European Journal of Biochemistry* 103 (February 1980): 577-84.

90. S.J. Bhatia et al., "*Lactobacillus acidophilus* Inhibits Growth of *Campylobacter pylori* in Vitro," *Journal of Clinical Microbiology* 27 (October 1989): 2328-30.

91. M. Racccach, R. McGrath, and H. Daftarian, "Antibiosis of Some Lactic Acid Bacteria Including *Lactobacillus acidophilus* toward *Listeria monocytogenes*," *International Journal of Food Microbiology* 9 (August 1989): 25-32.

92. M.Y. Lin and F.J. Chang, "Antioxidative Effect of Intestinal *Bifidobacterium longum* ATCC 15708 and *Lactobacillus acidophilus* ATCC 4356," *Dig Dis Sci* 45 (August 2000): 1617-22.

93. O. Sreekumar and A. Hosono, "Immediate Effect of *Lactobacillus acidophilus* on the Intestinal Flora and Fecal Enzymes of Rats and the in Vitro Inhibition of *Escherichia coli* in Coculture," *Journal of Dairy Science* 83 (May 2000): 931-9.

94. N.M. de Roos and M.B. Katan, "Effects of Probiotic Bacteria on Diarrhea, Lipid Metabolism, and Carcinogenesis: A Review of Papers Published Between 1988 and 1998," *American Journal of Clinical Nutrition* 71 (February 2000): 405-11.

95. G.H. McInbtosh, P.J. Royle, and M.J. Playne, "A Probiotic Strain of *L. acidophilus* Reduces DMH-Induced Large Intestinal Tumors in Male Sprague-Dawley Rats," *Nutr Cancer* 35:2 (1999): 153-9.

96. L.I. Chernyshova, "Effects of Dysbacteriosis and Impairment of Immunity Formation in the Early Neonatal Period on Morbidity of Children During the 1st Year of Life and Ways of Its Reduction," *Pediatriia* 6 (1989): 24-29.

97. P.S. Moshchich, L.I. et al., "Prevention of Dysbactriosis in the Early Neonatal Period Using a Pure Culture of Acidophilic Bacteria," *Pediatriia* 3 (1989): 25-30.

98. H.S. Gill et al., "Enhancement of Natural and Acquired Immunity by *Lactobacillus rhamnosus* (HN001), *Lactobacillus acidophilus* (HN017), and *Bifidobacterium lactis* (HN019)," *British Journal of Nutrition* 83 (February 2000): 167-76.

99. Natasha Trenev, *Probiotics. Nature's Internal Healers* (Garden City Park, N.Y.: Avery Publishing Group, 1998): 74-75.

100. John Anderson, "*Acidophilus*—Why Your Intestines Need This Friendly Bacteria," *Alternative Medicine*, November 1998, 72-76.

101. Bennett, *7-Day Detox Miracle*, 192.

102. Diamond, *An Alternative Medicine Definitive Guide to Cancer*, 963-964.

103. T. May et al., "Effect of Fiber Source on Short-Chain Fatty Acid Production and on the Growth and Toxin Production by *Clostridium difficile*," *Scandinavian Journal of Gastroenterology* 29 (October 1994): 916-22.

104. R.K. Buddington et al., "Dietary Supplement of Neosugar Alters the Fecal Flora and Decreases Activities of Some Reductive Enzymes in Human Subjects," *American Journal of Clinical Nutrition* 63 (May 1996): 709-16.

105. Trenev, Probiotics. Nature's Internal Healers, 126-7.

Chapter 6

1. W. John Diamond, M.D., W. Lee Cowden, M.D., with Burton Goldberg, *An Alternative Medicine Definitive Guide to Cancer* (Tiburon, Calif.: Future Medicine Publishing, 1997): 968.

2. Morton Walker, D.P.M., "Jumping for Health," *Townsend Letter for Doctors* (July 1995): 42-48.

3. John Anderson, "Rebounders—Bounce Your Way to Better Health," *Alternative Medicine Digest* (October-November 1997): 42-46.

4. A. Bhattacharya et al., "Body Acceleration Distribution and 02 Uptake in Humans During Running and Jumping," *Journal of Applied Physiology* 49 (November 1980): 881-887.

5. Walker, "Jumping for Health," 42-48.

6. H. Erichsen and H. Bottcher, "Trampoline Therapy with Brain-Injured Children and Adolescents," *Rehabilitation* 15 (May 1976): 100-2.

7. J.K. Stanghelle et al., "Effect of Daily Short Bouts of Trampoline Exercise During Eight Weeks on the Pulmonary Function and the Maximal Oxygen Uptake of Children with Cystic Fibrosis," *International Journal of Sports Medicine* Supplement 1 (February 9, 1988): 32-36.

8. Helene Silver, *Rejuvenate. A 21-Day Natural Detox Plan for Optimal Health* (Freedom, Calif.: The Crossing Press, 1998): 128.

9. Farida Sharan, M.D., *Iridology. A Complete Guide to Diagnosing Through the Iris and to Related Forms of Treatment* (Wellingborough, U.K.: Thorsons Publishing Group, 1989): 141.

10. W. J. Evans, "Vitamin E, Vitamin C, and Exercise," *American Journal of Clinical Nutrition* 72 (supp.) (August 2000): 647S-52S.

11. D.A. Leaf et al., "The Exercise-Induced Oxidative Stress Paradox: The Effects of Physical Exercise Training," *American Journal of Medicine and Science* 317 (May 1999): 295-300.

12. M.C. Polidori et al., "Physical Activity and Oxidative Stress During Aging," *International Journal of Sports Medicine* 21 (April 2000): 154-7.

13. Bruce Fife, N.D., *The Detox Book. How to Detoxify Your Body to Improve Your Health, Stop Disease and Reverse Aging* (Colorado Springs, Colo.: HealthWise, 1997): 124.

14. Electrolytes are substances in the blood, tissue fluids, between the cells, or in the urine that conduct an electrical charge, either negative or positive. Specifically, potassium, magnesium, phosphate, sulfate, bicarbonate, sodium, chloride, and calcium are all electrolytes. These substances provide inorganic chemicals needed to run cellular reactions and to control mechanisms such as the conduction of electrochemical impulses to nerves and muscles. The body also requires adequate stores of electrolytes for crucial enzymatic reactions involved in metabolism.

15. Saunas come in two modalities: dry, radiant heat and wet heat, or steam. Most of the scientific studies of the benefits of sauna therapy or heat stress have been based on dry heat saunas. Similarly, most detoxification experts who discuss sauna therapy advise dry over wet heat. In a dry sauna, no moisture is introduced into the chamber, while in a wet sauna, moisture is introduced. A wet heat sauna is akin to the traditional Native American sweat lodge, where water is splashed on super-hot rocks inside a tightly sealed chamber to produce steam.

16. Blood pressure is the force of the blood against the walls of the arteries, veins, capillaries, and heart chambers as it is pumped through the body and as the heart beats. Two measurements are involved: systolic (the heart contracts and pumps blood) and diastolic (the heart rests and fills with blood). The ratio of systolic and diastolic equals blood pressure, as in an average or normative reading of 120/80.

17. J. Leppaluoto, M. Tuominen et al., "Some Cardiovascular and Metabolic Effects of Repeated Sauna Bathing," *Acta Phsyiologica Scandinavia* 128 (September 1986): 77-81.

18. K. Kauppinen, "Facts and Fables About Sauna," *Annals of the New York Academy of Science* 813 (March 15, 1997): 654-62.

19. A. Eisalo and O.J. Luurila, "The Finnish Sauna and Cardiovascular Diseases," *Annals of Clinical Research*, 20:4 (1988): 267-70.

20. T.A. Parpalei, L.G. Prokof'eva, and V.G. Obertas, "The Use of the Sauna for Disease Prevention in the Workers of Enterprises with Chemical and Physical Occupational Hazards," *Vrach Delo* 5 (May 1991): 93-95.

21. K.V. Sudakov, V.V. Sinitchkin, and A.A. Khasanov, "Systemic Responses in Man Exposed to Different Heating and Cooling

Treatments in a Sauna," *Pavlov Journal of Biological Science* 23 (July-September 1988): 89-94.

22. W. Dean, "Effect of Sweating [letter]," *Journal of the American Medical Association* 246 (August 7, 1981): 623.

23. "Have a Sauna At Home: Healing Benefits from a Plug-In Radiant Heat Sauna," *Alternative Medicine Digest* 17 (March 1997): 72-74.

24. Zane R. Gard, M.D., and Erma J. Brown, "Literature Review and Comparison Studies of Sauna/Hyperthermia in Detoxification," *Townsend Letter for Doctors and Patients* (August/September 1999): 76-86.

25. "Aromatherapy Spa—Detoxify, Relax Muscles, and Enhance Immunity," *Alternative Medicine Digest* 15 (November 1996): 57-58.

26. Laurel Vukovic, *14-Day Herbal Cleansing* (Paramus, N.J.: Prentice Hall, 1998): 209.

27. Joseph Dispenza, *Live Better Longer: The Parcells Center Seven-Step Plan for Health and Longevity* (San Francisco: Harper San Francisco, 1997): 31-34.

Chapter 7

1. Biological dentistry stresses the use of nontoxic restoration materials for dental work and focuses on the unrecognized impact that dental toxins and hidden dental infections can have on overall health. Typically, a biological dentist will emphasize the following: the safe removal of mercury amalgam; avoidance or removal of root canals; the investigation of possible jawbone infections (cavitations) as a "dental focus" or source of body-wide illness centered in the teeth; and the health-injuring role of misalignment of teeth and jaw structures.

2. Morton Walker, D.P.M., *Elements of Danger: Protect Yourself Against the Hazards of Modern Dentistry* (Charlottesville, Va.: Hampton Roads, 2000): 63-65.

3. Joachim Thomsen, D.D.S., "The Frequent Involvement of 'Vital' Teeth in Focal Disturbances," *American Journal of Acupuncture: Special EAV Issue* (1989): 94-99.

4. Richard Leviton, "Cancer, Miscarriage, and Your Teeth," *Alternative Medicine* (July 1998): 56-62.

5. Hal Huggins, D.D.S., M.S., "Dental Toxins. Your Teeth May Be Making You Sick," *Alternative Medicine* (May 1998): 48-54.

6. Burton Goldberg and the Editors of Alternative Medicine Digest, *Alternative Medicine Guide to Chronic Fatigue, Fibromyalgia, & Environmental Illness* (Tiburon, Calif.: Future Medicine Publishing, 1998): 191-192.

7. M.M. van Benschoten, "Acupoint Energetics of Mercury Toxicity and Amalgam Removal with Case Studies," *American Journal of Acupuncture* 22:3 (1994): 251-262.

8. Christopher Hussar, D.D.S., D.O., "No More Chronic Pain," *Alternative Medicine Digest* (November 1996): 30-34.

9. J.W. Osborne, "Dental Amalgam and Mercury Vapor Release," *Advanced Dental Research* 6 (September 1992): 135-8.

10. L.J. Hahn et al., "Dental 'Silver' Tooth Fillings: A Source of Mercury Exposure Revealed by Whole-Body Image Scan and Tissue Analysis," *FASEB Journal* 3 (1989): 2641-2646. Also Fritz Lorscheider et al., "Mercury Exposure from 'Silver' Tooth Fillings: Emerging Evidence Questions a Traditional Dental Paradigm," *FASEB Journal* 9 (1995): 504-508.

11. W. J. Crinnion, "Environmental Medicine, Part Three: Long Term Effects of Chronic Low-Dose Mercury Exposure," *Alternative Medicine Review* 5 (June 2000): 209-23.

12. J.W. Reinhardt, "Side-Effects: Mercury Contribution to Body Burden from Dental Amalgam," *Advanced Dental Research* 6 (September 1992): 110-113.

13. A. Jokstad, Y. Thomassen et al., "Dental Amalgam and Mercury," *Pharmacological Toxicity* 70 (April 1992): 308-13.

14. W. Melillo, "How Safe is Mercury in Dentistry?" *The Washington Post Weekly Journal of Medicine, Science, and Society*, September 1991, 4.

15. A. Lussi and V. Schoenberg, "The Mercury Release of Different Amalgams in Vitro," *Schweiz Monatsschr Zahnmed* 101:11 (1991): 1405-8.

16. H. Lichtenberg, "Mercury Vapor in the Oral Cavity in Relation to the Number of Amalgam Surfaces and the Classic Symptoms of Chronic Mercury Poisoning," *Journal of Orthomolecular Medicine* 11:2 Second Quarter (1996): 87-94.

17. Hal Huggins, D.D.S., M.S., and Thomas E. Levy, M.D., J.D., *Uninformed Consent. The Hidden Dangers in Dental Care* (Charlottesville, Va.: Hampton Roads, 1999): 170-171.

18. N. Galic et al., "Dental Amalgam Mercury Exposure in Rats," *Biometals* 12 (September 1999): 227-31.

19. E. Berdouses et al., "Mercury Release from Dental Amalgams: An *In Vitro* Study Under Controlled Chewing and Brushing in an Artificial Mouth," *Journal of Dental Research* 74 (May 1995): 1185-93.

20. Walker, Elements of Danger, 90.

21. For an excellent bibliography of published scientific articles documenting the effects of mercury, see "Our References" at www.iaomt.org.

22. R. L. Siblerud and E. Kienholz, "Evidence that Mercury from Silver Dental Fillings May be an Etiological Factor in Multiple Sclerosis," *Science of Total Environment* 142 (March 15, 1994): 191-205.

23. R.L. Siblerud, "A Comparison of Mental Health of Multiple Sclerosis Patients with Silver/Mercury Dental Fillings and Those with Fillings Removed," *Psychol Rep* 70 (June 1992): 1139-51.

24. S. Ziff, "Consolidated Symptom Analysis of 1,569 Patients," *Bio-Probe Newsletter* 9 (March 1993): 7-8.

25. Diana Echeverria et al., "Behavioral Effects of Low-Level Exposure to Elemental Hg Among Dentists," *Neurotoxicology and Teratology* 17 (March-April 1995): 161-168.

26. R.L. Siblerud, J. Motl, and E. Kienholz, "Psychometric Evidence that Mercury from Silver Fillings May be an Etiological Factor in Depression, Excessive Anger, and Anxiety," *Psychol Rep* 74 (February 1994): 67-80.

27. A. Kingman, T. Albertini, and L.J. Brown, "Mercury Concentrations in Urine and Whole Blood Associated with Amalgam Exposure in a U.S. Military Population," *Journal of Dental Research* 77 (March 1998): 461-71.

28. Walker, *Elements of Danger*, 138.

29. M.J. Vimy et al., "Maternal-Fetal Distribution of Mercury," G. Drasch, "Public Annoucement 25," *Bio-Probe Newsletter*, January 1994. M.J. Vimy and F.L. Lorscheider, "Intra-Oral Mercury Released from Dental Amalgams," *Journal of Dental Research* 64:8 (1985); 1069-71.

30. Huggins and Levy, *Uninformed Consent*, 172-175.

31. A.O. Summers et al., "Mercury Released from Dental 'Silver' Fillings Provoks an Increase in Mercury- and Antibiotic-resistant Bacteria in Oral and Intestinal Floras of Primates," *Antimicrobial Agents in Chemotherapy* 37 (April 1993): 825-34.

32. *Candida albicans* is a yeast-like fungus found widely in nature, in the soil, on vegetables and fruits, and in the human body. It is frequently present in small quantities in the intestines and in the vagina. Provided its population is small, *Candida* is generally not harmful to the human body. A *Candida* overgrowth, a condition called candidiasis, can become pathogenic and cause allergic reactions throughout the body. These reactions can lead to a wide range of symptoms, including depression, fatigue, weight gain, anxiety, rashes, headaches, and muscle cramping.

33. Richard Leviton, "Fibroids and Male Impotence," *Alternative Medicine Digest*, (August-September 1997): 46-53.

34. The peripheral nervous system (PNS) is a part of the central nervous system and consists of a network of about 93,000 miles of nerves and nerve channels inside the body. The PNS works with the five senses and motor branch of the body to translate sensory information from the outside world into appropriate muscle movements by the body.

35. L.J. Hahn et al., "Whole-Body Imaging of the Distribution of Mercury Released from Dental Fillings into Monkey Tissues," *FASEB Journal* 4 (1990): 3256-3260.

36. The sympathetic nervous system is involved with responding to stress or physical threats to the body. It prepares the body's systems by

increasing the heart rate, blood pressure, and muscle tension; it also controls the contraction and expansion of blood vessels; the activity of the connective tissue, a body-wide network; and the voltage (called membrane potential) that exists across the cell wall in every cell. So when a toxic substance starts affecting the sympathetic nervous system, it potentially affects every operation in the body.

37. Richard Leviton, "Migraines, Seizures, and Mercury Toxicity," *Alternative Medicine Digest* (January 1998): 60-66.

38. R.F. Kidd, "Results of Dental Amalgam Removal and Mercury Detoxification using DMPS and Neural Therapy," *Alternative Therapies* 6 (July 2000): 49-55.

39. Y. Omura et al., "Significant Mercury Deposits in Internal organs Following the Removal of Dental Amalgam," *Acupuncture Electrotherapy Research* 21 (April-June 1996): 133-60.

40. Y. Omura, S.L. Beckman, "Role of Mercury (Hg) in Resistant Infections and Effective Treatment of *Chlamydia trachomatis* and Herpes Family Viral Infections (and Potential Treatment for Cancer) by Removing Localized Hg Deposits with Chinese Parsley and Delivering Effective Antibiotics Using Various Drug Uptake Enhancement Methods," *Acupuncture Electrotherapy Research* 20 (August-December 1995): 195-229.

41. Maya Muir, "Current Controversies in the Diagnosis and Treatment of Heavy Metal Toxicity," *Alternative & Complementary Therapies* (June 1997), 170-178.

42. A.L. Miller, "Dimercaptosuccinic Acid (DMSA), a Non-Toxic, Water-Soluble Treatment for Heavy Metal Toxicity," *Alternative Medicine Review* 3 (June 1998): 199-207.

43. J. Forman, J. Moline, et al., "A Cluster of Pediatric Metallic Mercury Exposure Cases Treated with Meso-2,3-Dimercaptosuciccinic Acid (DMSA)," *Environmental Health Perspectives* 106 (June 2000): 575-77.

44. G. Englund Sandborgh et al., "DMSA Administration to Patients with Alleged Mercury Poisoning from Dental Amalgams: A Placebo-Controlled Study," *Journal of Dental Research* 73 (March 1994): 620-8.

45. P. Grandjean et al., "Placebo Response in Environmental Disease: Chelation Therapy of Patients with Symptoms Attributed to Amalgam Fillings," *Journal of Occupational Medicine* 39 (August 1997): 707-14.

46. H.V. Aposhian, "Mobilization of Mercury and Arsenic in Humans by Sodium 2,3-Dimercapto-1-Propane Sulfonate (DMPS)," *Environmental Health Perspectives* 106, supp. 4 (August 1998): 1017-25.

47. H.V. Aposhian et al., "Urinary Mercury after Administration of 2,3-Dimercaptopropane-1-Sulfonic Acid: Correlation with Dental Amalgam Score," *FASEB Journal* 6 (April 1992): 2472-6.

48. D. Gonzalez-Ramirez et al., "Sodium 2,3-Dimercaptopropane-1-Sulfonate Challenge Test for Mercury in Humans: II. Urinary Mercury, Porphyrins, and Neurobehavioral Changes of Dental Workers in Monterrey, Mexico," *Journal of Pharmacological Experimental Therapy* 272 (January 1995): 264-74.

49. R.K. Zalups, "Influence of 2,3-Dimercaptopropane-1-Sulfonate (DMPS) and Meso-2,3-Dimercaptosuccinic Acid (DMSA) on the Renal Disposition of Mercury in Normal and Uninephrectomized Rats Exposed to Inorganic Mercury," *Journal of Pharmacology and Experimental Therapies* 267 (November 1993): 791-800.

50. J. Nerudova et al., "Mobilization of Mercury by DMPS in Occupationally Exposed Workers and in Model Experiments on Rats: Evaluation of Body Burden," *International Journal of Occupational Medicine and Environmental Health*, 13:2 (2000): 131-46.

51. Hal Huggins, D.D.S., M.S., "Appointment Scheduling," Hugnet FAQs, 1997 www.hugnet.com.

52. Daniel F. Royal, D.O., "Health Hazard in Your Teeth," *Alternative Medicine Digest* (July 1996): 40-44.

53. Huggins and Levy, *Uninformed Consent*, 212.

54. Mark A. Breiner, D.D.S., *Whole-Body Dentistry. Discover the Missing Piece to Better Health* (Fairfield, Conn.: Quantum Health Press, LLC, 1999): 102-106.

55. Dr. Karen Evans and Dr. Stephen R. Evans, "Cavitations," 1999 by Affinity Labeling Technologies, Inc., 235 Bolivar Street, Lexington, KY 40508; tel: 606-388-9445; fax: 606-388-9645.

56. P. Schupbach, V. Osterwalder, and B. Guggenheim, "Human Root Caries: Microbiota of a Limited Number of Root Caries Lesions," *Caries Research* 30:1 (1996): 52-64.

57. K. Okuda, Y. Ebihara, "Relationships Between Chronic Oral Infectious Diseases and Systemic Diseases," *Bulletin of the Tokyo Dental College* 39 (August 1998): 165-74.

58. F.A. Scannapieco, "Position paper of the American Academy of Periodontology: Periodontal Disease as a Potential Risk Factor for Systemic Diseases," *Journal of Periodontology* 69 (July 1998): 841-50.

59. W.J. Loesche, "Association of the Oral Flora with Important Medical Diseases," *Current Opinions in Periodontology* 4 (1997): 21-8.

60. G.J. Debelian, I. Olsen, and L. Tronstad, "Systemic Diseases Caused by Oral Microorganisms," *Endodontics and Dental Traumatology* 10 (April 1994): 57-65.

61. V. Lucas and G.J. Roberts, "Odontogenic Bacteremia Following Tooth Cleaning Procedures in Children," *Pediatric-Dentistry* 22 (March-April 2000): 96-100.

62. R. Hayrinen-Immonen et al., "Oral Health of Patients Scheduled for Elective Abdominal Aortic Correction with Prosthesis," *European*

Journal of Vascular and Endovascular Surgery 19 (March 2000): 294-8.

63. I. Tar, K. Bagyi et al., "Screening of Patients Referred to Our Clinic for Odontogenic Focal Diseases," *Fogorv Sz* 92 (October 1999): 295-300.

64. X. Li, L. Tronstad and I. Olsen, "Brain Abscesses Caused by Oral Infection," *Endodontic Dental Traumatology* 15 (June 1999): 95-101.

65. B. Bertrand, P. Rombaux et al., "Sinusitis of Dental Origin," *Acta Otorhinolaryngol Belg* 51:4 (1997): 315-22.

66. Hubert N. Newman, "Focal Infection," *Journal of Dental Research* 75:12 (1996): 1912-1919.

67. J.H. Meurmann, "Dental Infections and General Health," *Quintessence International* 28 (December 1997): 807-11.

68. George E. Meinig, D.D.S., F.A.C.D., *Root Canal Cover-up* (Ojai, Calif.:, Bion Publishing, 1994): 7.

69. W.A. Price, "Dental Infections and Related Degenerative Diseases," *The Journal of the American Medical Association* 84 (January 24, 1925): 254-59.

70. Breiner, *Whole-Body Dentistry*, 99-100.

71. M. Georgopoulou, E. Kontakiotis, and M. Nakou, "In Vitro Evaluation of the Effectiveness of Calcium Hydroxide and Paramonochlorophenol on Anaerobic Bacteria from the Root Canal," *Endodontic Dental Traumatology* 9 (December 1993): 249-53.

72. N. Olea et al., "Estrogenicity of Resin-Based Composites and Sealants Used in Dentistry," *Environmental Health Perspectives* 104 (March 1996): 298-305.

73. H. Oysaed, I.E. Ruyter, T. J. and Sjovik Kleven, "Release of Formaldehyde from Dental Composites," *Journal of Dental Research* 67 (October 1988): 1289-94.

Chapter 8

1. Florinda Donner, *Being-in-Dreaming. An Initiation into the Sorceror's World* (San Francisco: Harper San Francisco, 1991): 126-127.

2. John Diamond, M.D., "Reversing Fibroids and Ovarian Cysts," *Alternative Medicine Digest* (January 1998): 98-102.

3. Norman Levin, M.D., "Rheumatoid Arthritis and Fibromyalgia," *Alternative Medicine Digest* (September 1997): 100-105.

4. Candace B. Pert, *Molecules of Emotion. Why You Feel the Way You Feel* (New York: Scribner, 1997): 187, 189, 192.

5. Joseph Riccioli, M.D., N.D., "Talking to Your Body," *Alternative Medicine* (March 1999): 72-80.

6. Christiane Northrup, M.D., *Women's Bodies, Women's Wisdom. Creating Physical and Emotional Health and Healing,* rev. ed. (New York: Bantam Books,1998): 19-21, 55-56.

7. Carolynn Myss, *Anatomy of the Spirit. The Seven Stages of Power and Healing* (New York: Harmony Books, 1996): 40.

8. W. John Diamond, M.D., and W. Lee Cowden, M.D., with Burton Goldberg, *An Alternative Medicine Definitive Guide to Cancer* (Tiburon, Calif.: Future Medicine Publishing, 1997): 616.

9. Dr. Arthur Janov, *Why You Get Sick and How You Get Well. The Healing Power of Feelings* (West Hollywood, Calif.: Dove Books, 1996) 5, 6, 8, 16, 141-143.

10. Others have followed suit to expand the original concept of flower essences. Today, an estimated 20 different brands of flower remedies, based on plants native to many landscapes, from Australia to India to Alaska, offer about 1,500 different blends for a diverse range of psychological conditions. Innovative remedies are now made from gems and crystals, certain types of sea creatures, even the essence of glaciers.

11. Patricia Kaminski and Richard Katz, *Flower Essence Repertory. A Comprehensive Guide to North American and English Flower Essences for Emotional and Spiritual Well-Being*, rev. ed.(Nevada City, Calif.: The Flower Essence Society, 1994): 26.

12. Patricia Kaminski, *Flowers That Heal. How to Use Flower Essences* (Dublin, Ireland: Newleaf/Gill & Macmillan, Inc., 1998): 27, 30, 104.

13. Kaminski and Katz, *Flower Essence Repertory*, 329.

Chapter 9

1. Willy Schrödter, quoting Henry Cornelius Agrippa, in *History of Energy Transference: Exploring the Foundations of Modern Healing* (York Beach, Maine: Samuel Weiser, 1999): 115.

2. Willy Schrödter, quoting Dr. Friedrich Markus Huebner, in *History of Energy Transference*, 116.

3. Willy Schrödter, quoting Hiro Hasegawa, in *History of Energy Transference*, 107.

4. Ruth Berger, *The Secret is in the Rainbow: Aura Interrelationships* (York Beach, Maine: Samuel Weiser, 1979): 47-57.

5. Walter J. Kilner, *The Human Aura* (Secaucus, N.J.: The Citadel Press, 1965): 160.

6. John C. Pierrakos, M.D. *Core Energetics. Developing the Capacity to Love and Heal* (Mendocino, Calif.: Life Rhythm, 1990): 73-74, 91.

7. Shafica Karagulla, M.D., and Dora van Gelder Kunz, *The Chakras and the Human Energy Fields* (Wheaton, Ill.: Quest Books, 1989): 207-208.

8. Shafica Karagulla, M.D., *Breakthrough to Creativity. Your Higher Sense Perception* (Santa Monica, Calif.: DeVorss & Company, 1967): 123-146.

9. Shakuntala Modi, M.D., *Remarkable Healings. A Psychiatrist Discovers Unsuspected Roots of Mental and Physical Illness* (Charlottesville, Va.: Hampton Roads, 1997): 295, 297, 334-336, 357-361.

10. Arthur Guirdham, *The Psyche in Medicine* (Jersey, U.K.: Neville Spearman, 1978): 44, 48, 73, 223.

11. Samuel Sagan, M.D., *Entity Possession. Freeing the Energy Body of Negative Influences* (Rochester, Vt.: Destiny Books, 1997).

12. William J. Baldwin, D.D.S., *Spirit Releasement Therapy. A Technique Manual*, 2d ed. (Terra Alta, W.Va.: Headline Books, 1992): 13, 15.

13. Modi, *Remarkable Healings*, 353.

14. Adapted from suggestions by Shakuntala Modi, *Remarkable Healings*, 290-291.

15. The Dead Sea in Israel is the world's lowest point, at 293 meters (approximately 900 feet) below sea level. It is considered a unique source of concentrated natural minerals and salts, which have been used over the centuries for cosmetic and therapeutic purposes.

16. Information provided by the manufacturer, Ashtar Natural Dead Sea Products; website: www.fjcc.com/amig/ashtar.

17. William Bloom, *Psychic Protection: Creating Positive Energies for People and Places* (London: Judy Piatkus Publishers, 1996): 70-72.

18. According to occult scholar Willy Schrödter, the nape of the neck, where the medulla oblongata passes through the occiput (at the base of the skull and the top of the neck), is important in occultism. It is a place of strong and easily detected psychic radiation, and is known by different names: *Uls* (ancient Egyptian magicians); *Lus* (Jewish Qabalists); "divine mouth" (Indian Kriya yoga); "and the exit-point of a hypothetical subtle meta-organism," says Schrödter. When you sense people behind you and it makes you uncomfortable, your psychic gate at the nape of the neck is registering an energy input from this other source. In Schrödter, *History of Energy Transference*, 31. Another writer, Peter Dawkins, calls this site the eighth or alta major or Pan chakra, and says it is associated with universal consciousness. "It acts as a control chakra and integrates the powers and qualities of all the other chakras. It is the primary gateway for divine inspiration . . . and is perhaps the most sensitive area of the whole body." In: Peter Dawkins, *Zoence—The Science of Life. Rediscovering the Sacred Spaces of Your Life* (York Beach, Maine: Samuel Weiser, 1998): 72.

19. Judy Hall, *The Art of Psychic Protection* (Forres, Scotland: Findhorn Press, 1996): 97-105.

20. Irene Dalichow and Mike Booth, *Aura-Soma. Healing Through Color, Plant, and Crystal Energy* (Carlsbad, Calif.:, Hay House, 1996): 23-24.

21. Heinrich Zimmer, *Philosophies of India*, ed. Joseph Campbell (Princeton: Princeton University Press/Bollingen Series XXVI, 1951): 231, 251.

22. Mona Rolfe, *The Sacred Vessel* (Sudbury, England: Neville Spearman Limited, 1978): 59-62.

Chapter 10

1. "Indoor Air Facts No. 4 (Revised): Sick Building Syndrome (SBS)," Office of Radiation and Indoor Air, Environmental Protection Agency, April 1991 www.epa.gov/iaq/pubs/sbs.html.

2. C.A. Redlich, J. Sparer, and M.R. Cullen, "Sick-Building Syndrome," *The Lancet* 349:9057 (1997): 1013-16.

3. Adrian Bejan, "A Cure for Sick Buildings," 1994 www.tc. cornell.edu/er/sci93/dis04sickb/dis04sickb.html.

4. J.E. Woods, G.M. Drewry and P.R. Morey, "Office Worker Perceptions of Indoor Air Quality Effects on Discomfort and Performance." In B. Seifert et al (eds): *Indoor Air '87. Proceedings of the 4th International Conference on Indoor Air Quality and Climate.* Berlin, Institute for Water, Soil and Air Hygiene, 1987.

5. "Bad Office Air, Not Bad Vibes, May Cause Many Symptoms of Sick Building Syndrome, a New Cornell Study Finds," Cornell University News, 24 Feb. 1998 www.news.cornell.edu/releases/Feb98/ sick.building.ssl.html.

6. O.A. Seppanen, W.J. Fisk, et. al., "Association of Ventilation Rates and CO_2 concentrations with Health and Other Responses in Commercial and Institutional Buildings," *Indoor Air* 9 (December 1999): 226-52.

7. Michael Hodgson, M.D., M.P.H., "The Medical Evaluation" and "The Sick Building Syndrome: Effects of the Indoor Environment on Health." Cited in *Occupational Medicine: State of the Art Reviews* 10 (January-March 1995): 167-194.

8. P. Skov, O. Valbjorn: Danish Indoor Climate Study Group. "The 'Sick' Building Syndrome in the Office Environment: The Danish Town Hall Study," *Environ Int* 13 (1987): 339-349.

9. S. Burge et al. "Sick Building Syndrome: A Study of 4373 Office Workers," *Annals of Occupational Hygiene* 31 (1987): 493-504.

10. P.O. Fanger, et al., "Air Pollution Sources in Offices and Assembly Halls, Quantified by the Olf Unit," *Energy Building*, 12 (1988):7-19.

11. P.L. Ooi, K.T. et al., "Epidemiology of Sick Building Syndrome and Its Associated Risk Factors in Singapore," *Occupational Environmental Medicine* 55 (March 1998): 188-193.

12. P.L. Ooi and K.T. Goh, "Sick Building Syndrome: An Emerging Stress-Related Disorder?" *International Journal of Epidemiology* 26 (December 1997): 1243-9.

13. L. Lundin, "Allergic and Non Allergic Students' Perceptions of the Same High School Environment," *Indoor Air* 9 (June 1999): 92-102.

14. E. Bjornsson et al., "Symptoms Associated to the Sick Building Syndrome in a General Population Sample: Associations with Atopy,

Bronchial Hyper-Responsiveness and Anxiety," *International Journal of Tubercular Lung Disease* 2 (December 1998): 1023-28.

15. R.A Phipps, W.E. Sisk, and G.L. Wall, "A Comparison of Two Studies Reporting the Prevalence of the Sick Building Syndrome in New Zealand and England," *New Zealand Medical Journal* 112 (June 25, 1999): 228-30.

16. Arnold Mann, "This Place Makes Me Sick. Modern, Airtight Offices are Causing More Cases of Sick-Building Syndrome, Just Ask Southwest Airlines." *Time,* December 21, 1998, 152-25.

17. M. Bullinger, M. Morfeld et al., "The Sick-Building Syndrome— Do Women Suffer More?" *Zentralbl Hyg Umweltmed* 202 (August 1999): 235-41.

18. Michael J. Hodgson, M.D., M.P.H., "Clinical Diagnosis and Management of Building-Related Illness and the Sick-Building Syndrome," *Occupational Medicine: State of the Art Reviews* 4 (October-December 1989): 602-603.

19. Burton Goldberg and the Editors of *Alternative Medicine Digest, Alternative Medicine Guide to Chronic Fatigue & Environmental Illness* (Tiburon, Calif.: Future Medicine Publishing, 1998): 251-255.

20. "Is Your Building Sick?" *TFM on-line, Today's Facility Manager* 18 July 1999 www.tfmgr.com.

21. An encouraging trend is found in the fact that the International Institute for Bau-biologie has established an affiliation with the University of Natural Medicine of Santa Fe, New Mexico. This will enable students of alternative medicine to include Bau-biological principles in their understanding of health and healing, and thus gain an additional therapeutic edge in treating clients. For more information, contact: The University of Natural Medicine, P.O. Box 4089, Santa Fe, NM 87502; e-mail:natmedu@aol.com; tel: 505-424-7800 or 800-893-3367; fax: 505-424-7878; website: www.unaturalmedicine.edu.

22. Richard W. Pressinger, M.Ed., "Environmental Causes of Learning Disabilities and Child Neurological Disorders," University of South Florida, 1997 www.chem-tox.com.

23. Kaye H. Kilburn,M.D., and John C. Thornton, "Protracted Neurotoxicity from Chlordane Sprayed to Kill Termites," *Environmental Health Perspectives* 103 (July-August 1995): 690-694.

24. K.H. Kilburn, "Chlordane as a Neurotoxin in Humans," *Southern Medical Journal* 90 (March 1997): 299-304.

25. Comments by John and Lynn Marie Brower derived from their website www.hhinst.com.

26. An electromagnetic field (EMF) is created by the interaction of an electric field (surrounding an electric charge) and a magnetic field (surrounding a source of magnetism), when an electric current passes

through a wire. Put slightly differently, an EMF is a biologically active but invisible energy field that accompanies electrical current flow. For ease of layperson understanding, you could think of an EMF as the energy aura emitted by the interaction of the electric and magnetic fields, and which surrounds the carrier of the electric current, such as a wire, appliance, electric panel, power line, etc. Electric fields are found around electric typewriters, lamps, digital clocks, heaters, and water pipes, among other objects.

27. Lucinda Grant, in *The Electrical Sensitivity Handbook*: *How Electromagnetic Fields Are Making People Sick*, Weldon Pub., 1995, reproduced in part at www.northlink.com/~lgrant/whatises.html. For further information (and a six-issue/year newsletter called *Electrical Sensitivity News*), contact: Electrical Sensitivity Network, P.O. Box 4146, Prescott, AZ 86302.

28. Lynn Marie Bower, quoting data provided by the Electric Power Research Institute study, in *The Healthy Household: A Complete Guide for Creating a Healthy Indoor Environment* (Bloomington: The Healthy House Institute, 1995): 383-384.

29. Ellen Sugarman, quoting J.R. Guager, "Household Appliance Magnetic Field Survey. IEEE Transactions on Power Apparatus and Systems," PA-104 (September 1985), in *Warning: The Electricity Around You May Be Hazardous to Your Health* (New York: Simon & Schuster, 1992) and reprinted at WaveGuide website www.wave-guide.org/exposure.html.

30. B.W. Wilson, "Chronic Exposure to ELF Fields May Induce Depression," *Bioelectromagnetics* 9:2 (1988): 195-205.

31. Data review provided by WaveGuide's "What Are the Studies Telling Us?" www.wave-guide.org/ccwti/studies.html.

32. A free radical is an unstable, toxic molecule of oxygen with an unpaired electron that steals an electron from another molecule and produces harmful effects. Free radicals are formed when molecules within cells react with oxygen (oxidize) as part of normal metabolic processes. Free radicals then begin to break down cells, especially the cell membranes, often in a matter of minutes to an hour. A single free radical can destroy a cell. Their work is enhanced if there are not enough free-radical quenching nutrients, such as vitamins C and E, in the cell. While free radicals are normal products of metabolism, uncontrolled free-radical production plays a major role in the development of degenerative disease, including cancer and heart disease. Free radicals harmfully alter important molecules, such as proteins, enzymes, fats, even DNA. Other sources of free radicals include pesticides, industrial pollutants, smoking, alcohol, viruses, most infections, allergies, stress, even certain foods, and excessive exercise.

33. Veronica Strong, "Biosensing to Counter Geopathic Stress," www.positivehealth.com/permit/Articles/Environment/strong33.html.

34. Jeffrey R. Cram, "Flower Essences Reduce Stress Reaction to Intense Environmental Stimulus," Flower Essence Society, 5 February 1999 www.flowersociety.org/DrZ.htm.

35. "Carpeting, Indoor Air Quality, and the Environment," *Environmental Building News* November/December 1994 www.environmentalbuilding.com/Archives/Features/Carpets/Carpets.html.

36. John Bower, "Healthy Construction Recommendations for Health People" (speech presented at the Energy Efficient Building Association Excellence in Housing Conference, Dallas, TX, February 1994) published at www.hhinst.com.

37. David Pearson, *The Natural House Catalog: Everything You Need to Create an Environmentally Friendly Home* (New York: Fireside/Simon & Schuster, 1996): 141.

38. Rosalind C. Anderson, "Toxic Emissions from Carpets," *Journal of Nutritional and Environmental Medicine*, 5:4 (1995): 375-386.

39. Robert Abrams, "Consumer Alert: Chemicals in New Carpets Pose Potential Health Hazard," April 1991, cited at www.holisticmed.com/carpet/tcl.txt.

40. Debra Lynn Dadd, *Home Safe Home: Protecting Yourself and Your Family from Everyday Toxics and Harmful Household Products* (New York: Jeremy P. Tarcher/Putnam, 1997): 316-319.

41. Merritt McKinney, "Home Carpets Catch & Hold Benzene from Car Exhaust," 9 March 2000 www.sightings.com.

42. Robert G. Lewis et al., "Distribution of Pesticides and Polycyclic Aromatic Hydrocarbons in House Dust as a Function of Particle Size," *Environmental Health Perspectives* 107 (September 1999): 721-726.

43. Cindy Duehring, "Carpet Concerns, Part Four: Physicians Speak Up as Medical Evidence Mounts," and "Toxic Carpeting: Important Points to Remember," Environmental Access Research Network, 1995 www.holisticmed.com/carpet/tc4.txt.

44. Maury M. Beecher, and Shirley Linde, *Healthy Homes in a Toxic World: Preventing, Identifying, and Eliminating Hidden Health Hazards in Your Home* (New York: John Wiley & Sons, 1992): 160-166.

45. For a comprehensive source of information about MCS and numerous sources of toxicity, as well as legal and political aspects, contact: Chemical Injury Information Network (CIIN), publishers of the monthly newsletter, *Our Toxic Times*. P.O. Box 301, White Sulphur Springs, MT 59645; tel: 406-547-2255; fax: 406-547-2455; website: ciin,org/newsletter.htm. CIIN was founded in 1990 as an advocacy organization run by chemically injured persons primarily for the benefit of other chemically injured individuals. It is considered a major clearinghouse for information on the adverse effects of chemical exposures.

46. Fibromyalgia is a multiple-symptom syndrome primarily involving widespread muscle pain (myalgia), which can be debilitating in its severity. The pain seems to be caused by the tightening and thickening

of the myofascia, the thin film or tissue that holds the muscle together. Typical tender sites include the neck, upper back, rib cage, hips, and knees. Other symptoms include general fatigue and stiffness, insomnia and sleeping disorders, anxiety, depression, mood swings, allergies, carpal tunnel syndrome, headaches, the sense of "hurting all over," tender skin, numbness, irritable bowel symptoms, dizziness, and exercise intolerance. Post-traumatic fibromyalgia is believed to develop after a fall, whiplash, or back strain, whereas primary fibromyalgia has an uncertain origin. The majority of fibromyalgia sufferers are women between the ages of thirty-four and fifty-six.

47. Peter Montague, "A New Mechanism of Disease," *Rachel's Environment & Health Weekly*, February 12, 1998.

48. William R. Rea, M.D. et al, "Considerations for the Diagnosis of Chemical Sensitivity," in D.W. Talmage et al.: *Biologic Markers in Immunotoxicology* (Washington, D.C.: National Academy Press, 1992): 169. See also Thomas Orne and Paul Benedetti, "Multiple Chemical Sensitivity," American Council on Science and Health. 1991 www.hcrc.org/contrib/acsh/booklets/mcsdoc.html.

49. J.S. Tepper, V.C. Moser et al., "Toxicological and Chemical Evaluation of Emissions from Carpet Samples," *American Industrial Hygiene Association Journal* 56 (February 1995): 158-70.

50. D.L. Ashley, M.A. Bonin et al., "Measurement of Volatile Organic Compounds in Human Blood," *Environmental Health Perspectives* 104, supp. 5 (October 1996): 871-77.

51. Research from multiple medical sources collated by Albert Donnay, executive director, MCS Referral & Resources, July 1998 www.mcsrr.org/factsheets/mcsdisorders.html. For more information: MCS Referral & Resources, 508 Westgate Road, Baltimore, MD 21229; tel: 410-362-6400; fax: 410-362-6401.

52. Albert Donnay, "Overlapping Disorders: Chronic Fatigue Syndrome, Fibromyalgia Syndrome, Multiple Chemical Sensitivity & Gulf War Syndrome," MCS Referral & Resources, 29 May 1997 www.mcsrr.org/factsheets/mcsdisorders.html.

53. Julius Anderson, "Reactions to Carpet Emissions: A Case Series," *Journal of Nutritional and Environmental Medicine* 7 (1997): 177-185.

54. Bake-outs have been tested on commercial buildings. It has been found that the best results are obtained when the interior is heated to at least 90°F and kept there for several days (about three days); a one-day bake-out is usually not long enough to release the maximum VOCs possible through this technique. Even so, overall release of VOCs is not necessarily high. The average obtained over several tests was twenty percent to thirty percent (based on measuring fifteen to twenty of the most abundant indoor VOCs), but one building achieved a ninety-four percent reduction, and another had a sixty percent reduction of concentrations; another had an initial VOC decrease of sixty-five

percent one day after the bake-out, but this had declined to only six percent after a month. See John R. Girman, "Volatile Organic Compounds and Building Bake-Out," in *Occupational Medicine—State of the Art Reviews* 4 (October-December 1989): 695-712.

55. Information Technology Specialists, Inc. REED (Residential Energy Efficiency Database), Site 4, Box 16, RR1, Carvel, Alberta, Canada T0E 0H0; tel: 780-829-3594; fax: 780-892-3598; e-mail: info@its-canada.com; website: www.its-canada.com/reed.

56. John Bower, *The Healthy House* (Bloomington, Ind.: The Healthy House Institute, 1997): 536.

57. Annie Berthold-Bond, *Better Basics for the Home* (New York: Three Rivers Press, 1999): 52-54.

58. T.J. Kelly et al., "Emission Rates of Formaldehyde from Materials and Consumer Products Found in California Homes," *Environmental Science & Technology* 33 (January 1, 1999): 81.

59. Hal Levin, "Building Materials and Indoor Air Quality," in *Occupational Medicine—State of the Art Reviews* 4 (October-December 1989): 667-693.

60. John R. Girman, "Volatile Organic Compounds and Building Bake-Out," in *Occupational Medicine—State of the Art Reviews* 4 (October-December 1989): 695-712.

61. D. B. Teculescu et al., "Sick-Building Symptoms in Office Workers in Northeastern France: A Pilot Study," *Int Arch Occup Environmental Health* 71 (July 1998): 353-56.

62. J. Bourbeau et al., "Prevalence of the Sick Building Syndrome Symptoms in Office Workers Before and After Being Exposed to a Building with an Improved Ventilation System," *Occupational Environmental Medicine* 53 (March 1996): 204-210.

63. C.S. Li, C.W. Hsu, and M.L. Tai, "Indoor Pollution and Sick Building Syndrome Symptoms Among Workers in Day-Care Centers," *Archives of Environmental Health* 52 (May-June 1997): 200-207.

64. D. Vincent et al., "Ventilation System, Indoor Air Quality, and Health Outcomes in Parisian Modern Office Workers," *Environmental Research* 75 (November 1997): 100-12.

65. B. Thriene et al., "Man-Made Mineral Fibre Boards in Buildings—Health Risks Caused by Quality Deficiencies," *Toxicology Letters* 88 (November 1996): 299-303.

66. G.H. Wan and C.S. Li, "Dampness and Airway Inflammation and Systemic Symptoms in Office Building Workers," *Archives of Environmental Health* 54 (January-February 1999): 58-63.

67. J.J. McGrath et al., "Continually Measured Fungal Profiles in Sick Building Syndrome," *Current Microbiology* 38 (January 1999): 33-36.

68. J.D. Cooley, et al., "Correlation Between the Prevalence of Certain Fungi and Sick Building Syndrome," *Occupational Environmental Medicine* 55 (September 1998): 579-84.

69. D. Menzies et al., "Effect of a New Ventilation System on Health and Well-Being of Office Workers," *Archives of Environmental Health* 52 (September/October 1997): 360-367.

70. "Fungi Suspected 'Culprit' in 'Sick Building Syndrome," Georgia Tech Alumni Association www.alumni.gatech.edu/news/topics/sum96/RealFungus.html.

71. W.J. Kowalski and William Bahnfleth, "Airborne Respiratory Diseases and Mechanical Systems for Control of Microbes," Pennsylvania State University, Architectural Engineering Department, July 1988 www.engr.psu.edu/www/dept/arc/server/wjk/ardtie.html.

72. "Molds in the Environment," Centers for Disease Control and Prevention-National Center for Environmental Health Factsheet, 3 April 1997 www.cdc.gov/nceh/pubcatns/facts/molds/molds.htm.

73. Eckardt Johanning, M.D., "Hazardous Molds in Homes and Offices: Stachybotrys atra and Others . . ." Enviro Village Library, Acumen Technologies, 1997 www.envirovillage.com/Papers.

74. "Fungi Suspected 'Culprit' in 'Sick Building Syndrome,'" Georgia Tech Alumni Association www.alumni.gatech.edu/news/topics/sum96/RealFungus.html.

75. W.J. Kowalski, and William Bahnfleth, Ph.D., P.E., "Airborne Respiratory Diseases and Mechanical Systems for Control of Microbes," Pennsylvania State University, Architectural Engineering Department July 1998 www.engr.psu.edu/www/dept/arc/server/wjk/ardtie.html.

76. "Negative Ions: Vitamins of the Air?" Don Strachan and Jim Karnstedt, *New Realities*, reprinted on Library-Electrocorp website: www.net-gain.com/electrocorp.

77. Research data compiled as "Medical Studies" by The IonAir Company; website: www.purifyonline.com/studies_chart.html.

78. Virginia Peart, "Indoor Air Quality in Florida: Houseplants to Fight Pollution," Fact Sheet HE 3208, Florida Cooperative Extension Service, University of Florida, April 1993.

79. B.C. Wolverton, "Removal of Formaldehyde from Sealed Experimental Chambers by Azalea, Poinsettia, and Dieffenbachia," Research Report No. WES/100/01-91/005 January 1991, published by Wolverton Environmental Products, 514 Pine Grove Road, Picayune, MS 39466; website: www.wolvertonenvironmental.com.

80. Data on trichloroethylene and benzene air filtration from Plants for Clean Air Council, 3458 Godspeed Road, Davidsonville, MD 21035; fax: 410-956-9039; website: www.plants4cleanair.org.

81. Data drawn from these sources: "Clean Air Plants & Sick Building Syndrome," interiorlandscape.com, 1997. W. Prescod, "More Indoor Plants as Air Purifiers," *Pappus* 11:4 (1992). United States Environmental Protection Agency, "Sick Building Syndrome," Air and Radiation, Indoor Air Facts, 4, 1991. B.C. Wolverton, *Interior*

Landscape Plants and Their Role in Improving Indoor Air Quality (Picayune, Miss.:, Wolverton Environmental Services, 1990).

82. B.C. Wolverton, Ph.D. and John Wolverton, "Improving Indoor Air Quality Using Orchids and Bromeliads," Wolverton Environmental Services (514 Pine Grove Road, Picayune, MS 39466) December 1991 www.wolvertonenvironmental.com.

83. "Hydroculture: The Cure for 'Sick Building Syndrome,'" and from information published by Inter Urban Water Farms Online (3638 University Avenue, Suite 225, Riverside, CA 92501; tel: 909-342-7947; fax: 909-342-7984. This is a good source for information about hydroponics.

84. B.C. Wolverton and John Wolverton, "Interior Plants and Their Role in Indoor Air Quality: An Overview," Research Report # WES/100/06-92-008, Wolverton Environmental Services. C. Wolverton and John Wolverton, "Plants and Soil Microorganisms: Removal of Formaldehyde, Xylene, and Ammonia from the Indoor Environment," *Journal of the Mississippi Academy of Sciences* 38 (August-September 1993). Virginia I. Lohr and Caroline H. Pearson-Mims, "Particulate Matter Accumulation on Horizontal Surfaces in Interiors: Influence of Foliage Plants," *Atmospheric Environment* 30:14 (1996).

85. "The Breathing Wall from Genetron," *TFM On-line (Today's Facility Manager)*, 6 September 1999 www.tfmgr.com.

86. Bower, *The Healthy House*, 501.

87. "Biological Effects of Ionizing Radiation (BEIR) VI Report: 'The Health Effects of Exposure to Indoor Radon,' Executive Summary," The National Academy of Sciences, 19 February 1998 www.epa.gov/iaq/radon/beirvi1.html.

88. Melatonin, a hormone produced by the pea-sized, light-sensitive pineal gland in the center of the brain, regulates the body's internal clock, or circadian rhythm, which determines the twenty-four-hour sleep-wake cycle. Low melatonin levels have been associated with sleeping disturbances and light-related conditions such as SAD. With aging, the peak in melatonin secretion is about one hour later than normal (normal peak secretion time is about 2 a.m.), and the maximum peak of melatonin is only one-half the level of young adults.

89. Nicholas Harmon, "Lose Those Winter Blues with Verilux's Newest Full Spectrum Lighting," press release, 4 November 198 www.ergolight.com.

90. "SAD Info," Light Therapy Products; website: www.light therapyproducts.com.

91. Overuse of light therapy is possible and may produce side effects if overused for four to six weeks. The symptoms include irritability, agitation, eye strain, and fatigue. About one percent of users are prone to mania from consistent overuse.

92. Alfred J. Lewy, M.D., "Treating Chronobiologic Sleep and Mood Disorders with Bright Light," *Psychiatric Annals* 17 (October 1987).

93. "Tests Prove Children Do Better in School with Full Spectrum, Visually-Efficient Lighting," press release, Verilux, 13 May 1998 www.ergolight.com.

94. John Downing, O.D., Ph.D., F.C.S.O., "Clinical EEG and Neurophysiological Case Studies in Ocular Light Therapy," in *Light Years Ahead: The Illustrated Guide to Full Spectrum and Colored Light in Mindbody Healing*, ed. Brian J. Breiling (Berkeley: Celestial Arts,1996): 133-164.

95. Sheri Lundstrom, "Light Therapy a 'Natural prozac' for Winter Depression, *Twin City Wellness*, November 1997, reprinted at www.lighttherapyproducts.com.

96. *The Seventh Generation Guide to a Toxic-Free Home* (Burlington, Vt. Seventh Generation, n.d.): 11.

97. "Just the FAQs: Answers to Frequently Asked Questions about Petroleum and Household Cleaners," Seventh Generation, 16 June 1998 www.seventhgen.com/petrol.htm.

98. Julia Kendall, "Chemicals Found in Fabric Softeners by U.S. Environmental Protection Agency (EPA)," 1995 www.immune web.org/articles/fabricsoftener.html.

99. Julia Kendall, "Twenty Most Common Chemicals in Thirty-One Fragrance Products [Based on a] 1991 EPA Study," Environmental Health Network (n.d.) www.users.lmi.net/wilworks.

100. Julia Kendall, "Making Sense of Scents," collated scientific research (n.d.) www.ourlittleplace.com/scents.html.

101. Damon Franz and Holly Prall, "Smelling Good but Feeling Bad," *E Magazine*, XI (January-February 2000).

102. Debra Lynn Dadd, *Home Safe Home: Protecting Yourself and Your Family from Everyday Toxics and Harmful Household Products* (New York: Jeremy P. Tarcher/Putnam, 1997): 281-282.

Chapter 11

1. Larry Sang, *The Principles of Feng Shui*, 2d ed. (Monterey Park, Calif.: American Feng Shui Institute, 1996). For more information about feng shui training, class schedules, and books, contact: American Feng Shui Institute, 108 North Ynez, Suite 202, Monterey Park, CA 91754; tel: 626-571-2757; fax: 626-571-2065; e-mail: fsinfo@amfengshui.com; website: www.amfengshui.com.

2. Thomas Lee, "Temporal Location Theory, Kan Yu (Feng Shui)—An Ancient Chinese Theory on Site Location" (paper presented at GeoInformatics '95 conference, The Association of Chinese Professionals in Geographic Information System, Hong Kong, 1995), published at http://home.hkstar.com/~starvsn/fsgeoinf.html.

3. Thomas Lee, "Kan Yu—The Book of Change Concept in Environmental and Architectural Planning" (paper presented at "Greening to the Blue" conference, Yale University, New Haven, 1996), published at http://home.hkstar.com/~starvsn/kyyale.html.

4. Sophia Tang Shaul and Chris Shaul, "Why Feng Shui?" 168 Feng Shui Advisors website, June 1998 www.168fengshui.com.

5. Here are more examples of the yin/yang polarity. Yin: passive, cold, death, winter, female, night, even numbers, moon, water; yang: active, hot, life, summer, male, day, odd numbers, sun, fire.

6. In Chinese philosophy, the five elements are wood, fire, earth, metal, and water. In contrast, the Western philosophical tradition originally accorded five also, but differently: earth, water, fire, air, and ether (for space); later, the fifth element, ether, was relegated to the metaphysicians while the chemists tended to deal with only the first four. The Chinese elements have to be understood with a fair degree of "poetic license," in the sense that they do not mean that, literally, trees and branches are the wood element, or that steel and iron are the sole expression of the metal element. The Chinese elements of wood and metal partake in some degree of the qualities of the Western elements of ether and air. The Chinese elements are assigned many qualities, including direction, time of year, yin or yang shadings, and their own trigram.

7. Sophia Tang Shaul and Chris Shaul, "The Five Elements, Part One," 168 Feng Shui Advisors website, 1999 www.168fengshui.com.

8. Terah Kathryn Collins, *The Western Guide to Feng Shui* (Carlsbad, Calif.: Hay House, 1996): 63.

9. Stanley Aaga Bartlett, "Feng Shui for Lightworkers: Feng Shui and the Spirit of Change," *Planet Lightworker,* 1999 www.planetlightworker.com.

10. Ibid.

11. Willy Schrödter, quoting Eira Hellberg in *History of Energy Transference* (York Beach, Maine: Samuel Weiser, 1999): 118.

12. Willy Schrödter, quoting Paul Sedir, in *History of Energy Transference*, 120.

13. Carol Bridges, "The Bones of Your Home," in *The Feng Shui Anthology: Contemporary Earth Design*, ed. Jami Lin (Miami: Earth Design, Inc., 1997): 400.

14. Karen Kingston, *Creating Sacred Space with Feng Shui* (New York: Broadway Books, 1997): 30.

15. Schrödter, History of Energy Transference, 124.

16. Carol Bridges, "The Bones of Your Home," 401.

17. Stanley Bartlett, "Feng Shui for Lightworkers: Part III, Getting Rid of Density and Creating Light Centers," *Planet Lightworker, 1999* www.planetlightworker.com.

18. Kingston, *Creating Sacred Space with Feng Shui*, 95-98.

19. Angel Thompson, *Feng Shui. How to Achieve the Most Harmonious Arrangement of Your Home and Office* (New York: St. Martins Griffin, 1996): 34.

20. Lillian Too, *Feng Shui Fundamentals: Health* (Rockport, Mass.:Element Books, 1997): 47.

21. Nancilee Wydra, *Feng Shui. The Book of Cures* (Lincolnwood, Ill.: Contemporary Books, 1996): 134.

22. Simon Brown, *Practical Feng Shui* (London: Ward Lock, 1997): 62.

23. Thompson, *Feng Shui*, 83.

24. Sarah Rossbach, *Interior Design with Feng Shui* (New York: Arkana/Penguin Books, 1991): 21-22.

25. Thompson, *Feng Shui*, 38-39.

26. Collins, *The Western Guide to Feng Shui*, 44.

27. Stanley Bartlett, "Feng Shui for Lightworkers: Part II, Practical/Physical Aspects of Feng Shui," *Planet Lightworker,* 1999 www.planetlightworker.com.

28. Collins, *The Western Guide to Feng Shui*, 41.

29. Kirsten M. Lagatree, *Feng Shui. Arranging Your Home to Change Your Life* (New York: Villard Books, 1996): 29.

30. Rossbach, *Interior Design with Feng Shui*, 84.

31. Lagatree, *Feng Shui. Arranging Your Home to Change Your Life*, 40.

32. The flat spiral dielectric resonator is available through Stanley Bartlett.

33. Thompson, *Feng Shui*, 101.

34. Collins, *The Western Guide to Feng Shui*, 82-86.

35. Richard Webster, *101 Feng Shui Tips for the Home* (St. Paul, Minn.: Llewellyn Publications, 1998): 93-97.

36. George Birdsall, *The Feng Shui Companion: A User-Friendly Guide to the Ancient Art of Placement* (Rochester, Vt.: Destiny Books, 1997): 117-118.

37. The reader should bear in mind that feng shui encompasses a great deal more than what I have surveyed in this chapter. It has a more complex model of energy influences, timing, and location, and a copious amount of practical solutions for all aspects of our environment. What I've presented in this chapter, is merely a précis of what is possible, in terms both of analysis and remedy, as well as the range of thinking available from practitioners.

38. Jenny Liu, "Sick House, Sick People," 1998 www.spiritweb.org.

Chapter 12

1. Jane Thurnell-Read, *Geopathic Stress. How Earth Energies Affect Our Lives* (Rockport, Mass.: Element Books, 1995): 2.

2. Information provided by Dulwich Health at www.dulwich health.uk.com.

3. Ionizing radiation consists of high-energy rays capable of taking electrons out of molecules and forming ions in the substances through which it passes, thereby producing genetic mutations that can lead to cancer. Examples include X-rays, mammography, and other non-nuclear medical sources such as radiation therapy, used in conventional cancer treatment, and food irradiation, used to sterilize foods. An ion is an atom, or group of atoms, that has a negative or positive charge *as a result* of having lost or gained one or more electrons. Ionizing radiation can break atomic bonds and affect chromosomes, thereby making gene changes. Nonionizing radiation does not possess enough energy to remove electrons from atoms. This makes it unable to alter genes.

4. Gustav Freiherr von Pohl, *Earth Currents. Causative Factor of Cancer and Other Diseases* (Stuttgart, Germany: Frech-Verlag, 1983): 11, 12, 13, 22, 33.

5. J.M. Gobet, "Geobiology—The Holistic House," (n.d.) www.earth transitions.com/articles/geobiology.htm.

6. Serotonin is a neurotransmitter involved in many key body functions (and can produce problems when its levels are off), such as hunger and appetite regulation, sleep induction, cardiovascular activity, motor activity, respiration, control of body temperature, perception and moods and mood disorders (depression). Deficiencies or imbalances in serotonin levels are associated with violence, aggressive behavior, suicide, schizophrenia, and Parkinson's, among other health problems.

7. Melatonin, a hormone produced by the pea-sized, light-sensitive pineal (pronounced pie-NEEL) gland in the center of the brain, regulates the body's internal clock, or circadian rhythm, which determines the twenty-four-hour sleep-wake cycle. With aging, the peak in melatonin secretion is about one hour later than normal (normal peak secretion time is about 2 a.m.), and the maximum peak of melatonin is only one-half the level of young adults. Low melatonin levels have been associated with sleeping disturbances and light-related conditions such as seasonal affective disorder (SAD). Eating vitamin- and mineral-rich foods and increasing your exposure to bright light can improve the body's natural melatonin production.

8. Alf Riggs, "Harmful Effects from Earth Radiation & Electrical Fields," http://whale.to/Earth_Radiation/Riggs1.html.

99. Hans Nieper, M.D., "Modern Medical Cancer Therapy Following the Decline of Toxic Chemotherapy," *Townsend Letter for Doctors & Patients*, November 1996, 88-89. *Dr. Nieper's Revolution in Technology, Medicine and Society* (MIT, Oldenburg, 1985): 206, 222. Lecture notes from Professional Medical Seminar, Los Angeles, California, July 4, 1986, 13-15, 22, 28 (From A. Keith Brewer International Science Library, Richland Center, WI; tel: 608-647-6513; fax: 608-647-6797; e-mail: drbrewer@mwt.net; website: www.mwt.net/

~drbrewer/other.htm). See also Hans Alfred Nieper, et al., *The Curious Man: The Life and Works of Dr. Hans Nieper* (Garden City Park, N.Y.: Avery Publishing Group, 1998).

10. Anthony Scott-Morley, "Geopathic Stress: The Reason Why Therapies Fail?" *Journal of Alternative Medicine*, May 1985.

11. D. Freshwater, "Geopathic Stress," *Complement Ther. Nurs. Midwifery* 3 (December 1997): 160-2.

12. Kathe Bachler, "Noxious Earth Energies and Their Influence on Human Beings" (talk given in 1987), published at http://whale.to/Earth_Radiation/Bachler.htm. See also Kathe Bachler, *Discoveries of a Dowser* (n.p.: Veritas, 1981) and *Earth Radiation* (Manchester, U.K.: Wordmasters, Ltd., 1989).

13. In some senses, the presence of a geopathogenic zone and what it dictates for bedroom arrangement may have to take priority over what a feng shui analysis reveals about the mouth of *qi* and the optimal flow of *qi* through a bedroom. It is possible of course, that when you move the bed out of the toxic zone you also move it into the healthy *qi* zone. It is also possible to consult a professional who is skilled in both disciplines.

14. Christopher Bird, quoting Herbert Douglas, in *The Divining Hand. The 500-Year-Old Mystery of Dowsing* (Black Mountain, N.C.: New Age Press, 1979): 268-269.

15. Bird, *The Divining Hand*, 273.

16. Alf Riggs, "Myalgic Encephalomyelitis" http://www.simnet.is/vgv/jardarur.htm.

17. Thurnell-Read, *Geopathic Stress*, 63-64.

18. Tom Passey and Robert D. Egby, "Is the Place Where You Sleep Making You Sick?" http://members.spree.com/achievers/page11.htm. Egby is a professional "hypnoanalyst" and director of the Center for Inner Healing and Meditation Studies. P.O. Box 1494, Hightstown, NJ 08520; tel: 609-581-2415.

19. Chuck Pettis, *Secrets of Sacred Space: Discover and Create Places of Power* (St. Paul, Minn.: Llewellyn Publications, 2000): 87.

20. Samuel Sagan, M.D., *Entity Possession. Freeing the Energy Body of Negative Influences* (Rochester, Vt.: Destiny Books, 1997), 98,106-7. See his website at: www.clairvision.org. Dr. Sagan's Clairvision School in Sydney, Australia, offers courses in developing sensitivity to land energies and energy qualities of homes.

21. Dr. Sagan recommends leaving a food offering for the bhutas you are removing. It is well known that entities have food cravings—usually for sugar, chocolate, heavy fried foods, and meats—and inspire or compel their hosts to overconsume these foods. In his practice of bhuta-suddhi ("entity purification" or cleansing of the elemental energy layer, the one just beyond the physical), he puts out a sugar cube or two, offering it to the entities; at the end of the ritual, he wraps

the cube (or sweet, if he used something else sugary) in a leaf and buries it. A certain portion of the energy essence (or at least the debris remaining from the ritual clearing) of the entity adheres to the sugar and is thus removed from the scene.

22. Patrick MacManaway, "A Definition of Geomancy," MAG E-zine, Mid-Atlantic Geomancy, Winter Solstice 1996 www.geomancy.org/ezines/ezine_4/ezine_4c.html.

23. In Dr. MacManaway's usage of the term a ley line is a narrow track of dowsable Earth energy that usually runs in straight lines and upon which in Europe old churches are oriented. Ley lines are not the same thing as a geopathogenic zone, although they can have strong effects on one's state of mind and to a lesser extent, upon one's physiology. Within circles of dowsers, there is disagreement whether a ley line is the track of subtle telluric energy (more recent definition), or is merely a straight line of alignment between ancient structures, such as old churches, standing stones, and other megalithic structures, but one which has no discernible energy (old definition). "Pre-Reformation English and European churches will always have an energy ley line running down their long axis, which is the same pattern as you find in temple space in much of the world," says Dr. MacManaway.

24. Ernest Hartmann, M.D., (1915-1992) practiced medicine in Eberbach, Germany, for over forty years. In 1961, he created the Institute for Geobiology and served for almost thirty years as its chairman.

25. Manfred Curry, M.D., lived from 1899-1953.

26. David Cowan and Rodney Girdlestone, *Safe as Houses? Ill Health and Electro-Stress in the Home* (Bath, England: Gateway Books, 1996): 124.

27. Blanche Merz, *Points of Cosmic Energy* (Saffron Walden, England: C.W. Daniel Company, 1987): 17-20.

28. J.M. Gobet, "Geobiology—The Holistic House," (n.d.) www.earthtransitions.com/articles/geobiology.htm.

29. Reshad Field, *Here to Heal* (Shaftesbury, U.K.: Element Books, 1985): 81, 88-89.

30. Joan McFarlane, "Dowsing Geopathogenic, Electromagnetic, and Other Irritation Zones" http://members.tripod.com/Reid_J/Joan.htm.

31. Mary K. Kuhner, "Useful Ritual Techniques," 22 August 1996, posted on soc.religion.paganism (internet newsgroup), University of Washington at Seattle, by mkkuhner@phylo.genetics.washington.edu.

32. William Bloom, *Psychic Protection. Creating Positive Energies for People and Places* (London, England: Judy Piatkus Publishers, 1996): 65-66.

33. Rescue Remedy is a formula originally developed in the 1930s by English physician Edward Bach. It contains the essences of five flowers, including Star of Bethlehem (for trauma and shock), clematis

(for a tendency to pass out into unconsciousness), cherry plum (for being on the verge of a breakdown), impatiens (for irritability and tension), and rock rose (for frozen terror and panic). The combination produces a first aid effect on an overly charged emotional body. Rescue Remedy is available in the United States from Belson Bach USA, 100 Research Drive, Wilmington, MA 01887; tel: 978-988-3833; fax: 508-988-0223. For more about Bach flower remedies, see these websites: www.bachflower.com; www.nelsonbach.com; www.bachcentre.com. The same formula is also available as Five Flower Formula, made by Flower Essence Society, P.O. Box 459, Nevada City, CA 95959; tel: 800-736-9222 or 530-265-9163; fax: 530-265-0584; e-mail: mail@flowersociety.org; website: www.flowersociety.org.

34. William Bloom, *Psychic Protection. Creating Positive Energies for People and Places* (London: Judy Piatkus Publishers, 1996): 126-7.

35. Bloom, *Psychic Protection,* 16.

36. From information provided by Geomack Products under "Alternative Health Practitioners" www.geomack.force9.co.uk/geo0.7.html.

37. Samuel Sagan, M.D., *Awakening the Third Eye* (Roseville, Australia: Clairvision, 1997): 173-180.

Index

4-phenylcyclohexene, 427, 429
9th Report on Carcinogens, 2000, 13

AAL Reference Laboratories, Inc., 122
Ace Pump Corp., 156
acetone, 455, 472
N-acetyl-cysteine, 221
Acremonium spp., 443
activated charcoal, 233-234
activated intermediates, 69
Affinity Labelling Technologies, 131
aging, 64-65
Agrippa, Henry Cornelius, 354
Air Check, Inc., 461
air conditioning, 439-440
air filters, 445-448
air pollution
   illness correlated with, 37-41
   major pollutants, 37, 39
   mortality rates and, 40-41
   See also indoor air
Air Quality Research, 444
airborne pesticides, 29
AirChek, 461
Aireox Activated Carbon Air Purifier, 446
AirFilters.net, 447
Alaska Northern Lights, 465
albumin, 118, 237
aldehyde detoxification pathway, 77-78
alginate, 311-312
aliphatic hydrocarbon solvents, 17
allergies
   Candida albicans and, 305
   food
      eliminating, 134-135
      identifying, 132
      symptoms of, 131-132
      tests for, 132-135
      wheat, 133
   from air pollution, 40
   from genetically modified foods, 173
   triggers of, 12
alpha-lipoic acid, 221
alpha-terpineol, 471
ALS (amyotrophic lateral sclerosis), 49
Alternaria, 442, 443
Alzheimer's disease, 12, 48, 49
Amelung, Wolfgang, 458
American Academy of Biological Dentistry, 312
American cheese, 54
American Institute of Reboundology, 272
American Society of Dowsers, 499
amino acid conjugation, 71
amino acids, 71, 116, 221
Amjo Corp., 465
Amjo Sunrise light boxes, 465
ammonia, 410, 457
amyotrophic lateral sclerosis (ALS), 49
anaphylaxis, 50
Anderson Laboratories, 434
Anderson, Richard, 427
Anderson, Rosalind, 427, 473
androgens, 87
anemia, 12
angina, 524
anti-idiotype allergen, 173
antibiotic resistance, 173, 304-305
antibiotics in livestock feed, 51-52
antimony, test for, 113-114
antioxidants

action of, 66
   as cleansing support, 221
   blood test for, 118
   defined, 65, 116
   nutrient, 66
   plant, 66
anxiety reduction, 198-200, 349-351
Apollo Light Systems, 465
Aqua-Stream shower water filter, 154, 156
Arctic, pollution in, 3, 55
Arise & Shine Cleanse Thyself program, 250-251
aromaSpa, 282-283
aromatherapy, 198
arsenic
   effects on body, 32, 564n46
   levels considered safe, 32
   levels in drinking water, 32
   test for, 113-114
arthritis
   dental focal infection and, 317
   emotional problems and, 328-329
   geopathic stress and, 526
   trigger of, 12
Ashtar Natural Dead Sea Products, 379
aspartame (NutraSweet), 48, 176
Aspergillus, 440, 442, 443
aspirin, 71
asthma, 12, 14, 39-40, 50
atrazine, 31-32
Aura-Soma International Academy of Colour Therapeutics, 394
Aura-Soma Products, Ltd., 394
Aura-Soma USA Inc., 394
auras
   damaged, 355-356, 372-375
   detecting toxins in, 376
   detoxification methods
      requesting a cleansing, 369-370
      salting energy centers, 359-362
      using pomanders, 391-394
      using psychic methods, 375-376
   entities and, 365-369
   ill-health and, 362-364
   nature and characteristics of, 353-355, 357-358
   of the unhealthy, 358-359
   professional detoxification, 375-376
   protecting, 388-389
autoimmune disease, 12
automobile emissions, 37, 565n55
autonomic nervous system, 586n113
Ayurveda, 239-240, 590n51
azaleas, 454

B-vitamins, test for, 115-117
Ba-Gua, 479-484
baby food, contaminated, 51
Bach, Edward, 336
Bach Flower Remedies, 336
Bachler, Kathe, 524
bacteria
   antibiotic-resistant, 52
   sizes of, 445
bagels, 54
bake-outs, 435, 609n54
Baldwin, William J., 368, 369
Ballentine, Rudolf, 60
Barrie, Stephen, 59, 137, 220
Bartlett Designs, 488
Bartlett, Stanley Aaga, 483-490
Bassett Aromatherapy, 201

bathrooms, 512-515
baths
   body-detoxifying, 284-286
   chlorine from, 33-34
   relaxation, 198
   spirit-detoxifying, 377-380, 382-384
Batmanghelidj, F., 137
Bau-biologie, 410-411, 413
BDCM (bromodichloromethane), 147
bedding, 473-474
bedrooms, 509-512
beds, 520-528, 530, 541
beech remedy, 343
beets, 217-218
Befit Enterprises, 448
Bell, Iris, 8
Bennett, Peter, 59, 137, 220
bentonite, 234-236, 285
benzaldehyde, 472
benzene
   from carpets, 429
   health problems associated with, 146
   incidence in humans, 24
   plants which absorb, 454, 455
   sources of, 410
   symptoms produced by, 410
benzoate(s), 50, 71
benzopyrene, 410
benzyl acetate, 471
benzyl alcohol, 471
benzyl butyl phthalate, 25
berberine, 257-258
Berger, Ruth, 355
Bergsmann, Otto, 522
Berkeley Psychic Institute, 391
Bernard, Claude, 119
Berthold-Bond, Annie, 436, 474
Beta-BHC (benzene hexachloride), 16
beta-carotene, test for, 118
Bieler's broth, 214
Bifidobacterium bifidum, 261, 263
bile, 587n3
bile lubricants, 220
bilirubin, test for, 118
Bio-Fighter Anti-Microbial UV Light System, 448
BioCalex, 320-321
biochemical defenses, test for, 118
BioDemocracy and Organic Consumers Assoc., 174, 177
biodetoxification, 93
Biofeedback Instrument Corporation, 203
biological dentistry, 597n1
Biological Technologies International, Inc., 121
Biological Terrain Assessment, 112, 119-120, 121
BioProbe, Inc., 321
biotransformation, 67
birds, 8
Birdsall, George, 514
bismuth, test for, 114-115
bitter melon, 259-260
blackberry remedy, 351
bladder cancer, 13, 148, 149
Blastocystis hominus, 253
Blaylock, Russell L., 48
bleeding heart remedy, 343
blood levels of toxins, mothers and infants, 16
blood pressure, 596n16
blood tests

comparisons with known patterns/standards, 115
   nutrient and toxic element, 113-115
Bloom, William, 380, 549
Bock, Kenneth, 60
borage remedy, 343
boron, test for, 113-114
botulinum, 180
bovine growth hormone (BGH), 176-177
bowel movement frequency, 231
Bower, John, 411
Bower, Lynn Marie, 411, 413, 456
brain cancer, 105, 150
brain symptoms, 8
Braly, James, M.D., 131
bread, cracked wheat, 54
breast cancer
   Baby Boomer mortality, 47
   case of, 290-291
   dental problems and, 289
   nuclear counties mortality, 45
   organochlorine compounds and, 80, 467
   X-ray-caused, 181
breast-feeding, 3
breast milk, 44
Breathing Wall, 458-459
Breiner, Mark A., 314
BRI. *See* building-related illness
Bridges, Carol, 493
bright light therapy, 464, 612n91
Brite Lite IV light box, 465
bromodichloromethane (BDCM), 147, 148
bronchitis, 13
Brown, Simon, 503
Browning, John M., 391
building-related illness (BRI)
   defined, 401
   symptoms of, 401
   See also indoor air; sick building syndrome
bulimia case, 335
burdock, 216-217
butter, 54
buttercup remedy, 350
butyl cellosolve, 471

cadmium, test for, 113-114
calcium, test for, 113-114
calendula remedy, 344
California wild rose remedy, 345, 351
camphor, 471
cancer
   childhood, 80
   daily development of, 105
   geopathic stress and, 520-524, 526
   rates, and nuclear radiation, 47-48
   triggers of, 12
   See also specific types of cancer
Candida albicans
   and intestinal dysbiosis, 128
   allergies and, 305
   cleansing toxins from, 233-234
   defined, 599n32
   FOS and, 266
Canyon Dudleya remedy, 348
Carbon Based Corporation, 120
carbon dioxide, 403, 407, 455
carbon monoxide, 37, 438, 453-455
carbon tetrachloride, 146
carcinogens, 12-13
Care 2000 Air Purifier, 448-449

carmine dye, 50
carpets
    'bake-outs' of new, 435
    benzene from, 429
    cleaning, 435
    dangers of new, 426, 428-429
    Environmental Protection
        Agency, 427
    gas emissions from, 427-428
    house dust and, 430
    neurotoxicity of, 428
    'new carpet' smell, 427
    old, 430
    sub-acute reactions to, 430
    symptoms in humans from,
        428-429
    symptoms in mice from, 428
    testing for toxicity, 434
    use in U.S., 426-427
    wool, 436-437
carrots, 28
Carson, Rachel L., *xxi*
cascara sagrada, 245-246
cataracts, 12, 526
cats, 529
cauliflower mosaic virus, 172-173
cavitations
    dangers of, 294-295, 314-315
    debridement of, 317-318
    defined, 294, 313
    incidence of, 314
Cayce, Edgar, 225
CDSA (Comprehensive Digestive
    Stool Analysis), 128, 131
CellMate Blood Test Report, 115,
    120
Center for Food Safety, 179, 183
central nervous system (CNS) dis-
    orders, 13, 19-20
chakras, 359
charcoal water filtration, 151
cheddar cheese, 54
cheeseburgers, 54
chemical sensitivity. *See* multiple
    chemical sensitivities (MCS)
chemicals
    commercially used, 13
    household, logging exposure to,
        22-24
    industrial, 13, 24, 25
    'organic,' 470-471
Chernobyl, 46, 47
chickens, 52
children
    air pollution and, 39-40
    behavior problems, 83
    DMSA administration to, 309
    geopathic stress and, 524-525
    infants
        atrazine in, 32
        DBCP in, 31
        dioxin in, 44
        hypothyroidism in, 46
        L. acidophilus for, 263
        underweight newborns, 47
    neurological disorders in, 81-83
    sexual maturation, 87-88
    susceptibility of, 90
chloral hydrate, 77-78
chlordane
    amounts in home building, 412
    effects of, 79, 89, 412-413
    foods found in, 54
    incidence in foods, 53
    levels in homes, 412
chlordecone, 238-239
chlorella, 237-239
chlorinated hydrocarbon pesti-
    cides, 17
chlorine, 42-43, 144, 566n68
chlorine absorption by the body,
    33-34
chlorine chemistry, 45
chlorine industry, 566n72

chloroform, 141, 146, 147, 410,
    471
chloropyrifos, 90
cholesterol, 243, 591-59
cholinesterase, 90
chronic fatigue syndrome
    case of, 106
    chemicals associated with, 80
    coincident with fibromyalgia,
        14-15, 433
    coincident with MCS, 14-15,
        433
    geopathic stress and, 526-527,
        536
    MCS and, 431-432
    mercury and, 107
    toxicity and, 79
cilantro, 308
circulating immune complexes
    (CIC), 74, 374
Cladosporium, 442
Clarus Products International, 424
Clean Air Plant System, 457-458
cleansing
    auras
        requesting a cleansing, 369-
            370
        salting energy centers, 359-
            362
        using pomanders, 391-394
        using psychic methods, 375-
            376
    intestinal, 232-247
    whole body, 267-286
    See also liver cleansing; detoxi-
        fication
clear cell cancer, 89
ClearWave digital clock, 425
Clifford Consulting and Research,
    323
Clifford Materials Reactivity
    Testing, 322-323
clofibric acid, 34-35
Clorox, 165-166
clutter, 486-488
cochineal extract, 50
Cody, Pierre, 526
coffee, 137
Colborn, Theo, 2-3, 4, 91-92
Colin Campbell & Sons Ltd., 434
Collins, Terah Kathryn, 483, 507
colon. *See* intestinal tract
colon cancer
    chlorinated water and, 149
    diet associated with, 228-229
    fecal free radicals and, 229-230
    fiber-rich diets preventing, 229
    slow transit times and, 228-229
    THM levels and, 148
colon cleansers, 232-247
colonics, 232
Committee for Nuclear
    Responsibility, 184
Comprehensive Digestive Stool
    Analysis, 128, 131
Comprehensive Parasitology
    Profile, 129-130, 131
Comtech Research, 452
Comtech Research IG-033A ion-
    izer, 453
conjugation, 70
consensus reality, 195
constipation, 73, 227
consumer products
    advice on, 474
    assessing, 469
    chemicals used in, 469-470
    common toxic, 471-474
    potentially toxic, 21, 468
copper toxicity, 293
core pictures, 372-374, 390
Corsello, Serafina, 227
Cram, Jeffrey R., 425
cramps, 50

Crinnion, Walter J., N.D., 78, 79, 84
cruciferous vegetables, 211-212,
    587-92
Cryptosporidia, 253, 255
Cryptosporidium parvum,
    578n7
Crystal Enterprises, 447
Culturelle, 264, 266
Curry-Hartmann Grid, 540-546
Curry, Manfred, 542
cutting *qi*, 499-504
cytochrome P450
    defined, 67-68
    function of, 110
    nutrients needed by, 68
    vulnerability to mercury, 110
Czech Republic, 41

Dadd, Debra Lynn, 429, 456, 474
dairy products, 176-179
DAMS (Dental Amalgam Mercury
    Syndrome), 313
dandelion root, 219
dawn simulators, 467-468
DBCP (dibromochloropropane),
    31
DDE
    (dichlorodiphenyldichloroethyl-
    ene), 16, 80
DDT (dichlorodiphenyl-
    trichloroethane)
    immune damage from, 78-79
    in children, 24
    in fish, 4, 43
    in foods, 53-54
    incidence in chemically sensi-
        tive patients, 16
    spread of, 4
death rates
    from chemical exposures, 13
    infectious disease, 13-14
dehydration, 137-139
dental
    composites, 322
    fluorosis, 159-160
    foci, 289-290
    infections, 576n8
Dental Amalgam Mercury
    Syndrome (DAMS), 313
dental material biocompatibility,
    321-324
dental mercury amalgam fillings
    alloy composition, 296
    annual use, 296
    antibiotic-resistant bacteria
        and, 304-305
    controversy over, 295-296, 297
    mercury levels per number of,
        302-303
    mercury release rates from, 300
    multiple sclerosis patients with,
        300-301
    outgassing from, 297-298
    removal of
        assessing need for, 306-307
        case study of, 108-109
        cautions during, 307
        incorrect, 294
        nutritional support for, 313
        patient satisfaction after, 307
        problems prompting, 307
        symptom reduction after,
            301-302
        timing of, 312
    toxicity of, 106-108
    urinary mercury per number of,
        303
dentists, 108, 295, 301-302
depression
    case of entities and, 366-367
    electromagnetic fields and, 420
    flower essences for, 345-346
    nature of, 344

toxicity and, 17
trans-fatty acids and, 186
DES (diethylstilbestrol), 89
detoxification
    aura
        requesting a cleansing, 369-
            370
        salting energy centers, 359-
            362
        using pomanders, 391-394
        using psychic methods, 375-
            376
    benefits of, 94-99, 208-209, 557-
        559
    defined, *xxii-xxiii*, 93-94, 96
    global consequences of, 97-98
    importance of, *xxv*, 94
    liver as primary organ for, 67
    nutrients supporting, 220-221
    phases of, 67-73
    shaking for, 380-381
    spiritual, 387-390, 394-396
    whole body, 267-286
    See also colon cleansers; liver
        cleansing
Detoxification Profile, 122
detoxification program compo-
    nents, 92-93
detoxification system, maladapta-
    tion of, 77-79
Developmental Natural Resources,
    286
developmental neurotoxicants, 83-
    84
Diamond, John, 326
diarrhea, 50
dibutyl phthalate, 25
dieldrin
    basics of, 572n37
    breast cancer and, 87
    daily dietary intake of, 54
    residues in foods, 53
Dientamoeba fragilis, 253
diesel engine exhaust, 39
diet
    assessing, 10
    high-fiber, 229, 230
    low-fiber, 228-229
    meat, 228-230
diethyl phthalate, 25
digestive tract symptoms, 8
dill pickles, 54
dioxin, 3, 44-45, 55
dizziness, 90
DMPS (2,3-dimercaptopropane-1-
    sulfonic acid), 126, 310-311,
    575-3
DMSA (dimercaptosuccinic acid),
    126, 309, 310
DNA repair enzymes, test for, 118
doctors, 7
Doctor's Data, 120, 130
Donner, Florinda, 325
Douglas, Herbert, 526
Downing, John, 466
dowsing, therapeutic, 533-535
Dr. Gauss, 423
Dragon River Herbals, 308, 311
drainage pipes, energy
    homes to earth, 549-551
    people to earth, 387-389
drinking water
    chlorinated
        carcinogenic effects, 147-150
        organochlorine byproducts
            from 42-43, 141-143
        reproductive problems and,
            144-147
        usage of, 33
    consumption of, 140
    fluoridated
        cancer and, 160-161
        cavity reduction and, 158-
            159

dental fluorosis from, 159-160
extent of, 156-157
inception of, 157
lead levels and, 83
typical fluoride concentrations, 157
personal care product residues in, 35-36
pharmaceutical drug residues in, 34-36
untreated, VOCs in, 577n5
See also water (tap)
dry cleaning solvent case, 18-19
Duehring, Cindy, 430
Dulwich Health, 554
Dursban, 90
dust, 430
Dust Fighter 95 filter, 447-448
Dust Free, 447
dysbiosis
defined, 127-128, 252, 577n9
problems from, 128, 253, 254
dyspepsia, 138-139

ear symptoms of toxicity, 9
Earth acupuncture, 545-546
Earth Essentials, 237
Earth Partnership, Inc., 168
Earthrise Nutritionals, Inc., 237
East Germany, 40
Edelson, Stephen B., M.D., 92-93
Egby, Robert D., 529
EI (environmental illness), 14-16, 74-75
Electrocorp, 452
electrodermal screening (EDS), 111-112, 575n4
electrolytes, 278, 596n14
electromagnetic field, 606n26
electropollution
action of, 420-421
body-shielding devices, 424-425
cases involving, 421-422
detecting, 415
exposure reduction devices, 423-424
field strengths per source, 418
hot spots, 419
low-frequency, 420
measuring devices, 423
symptoms due to, 419, 420
ElectroStatic Air Filter, 447
electrostatic air filters, 447-448
E.L.F.-Zone Gauss Meter, 423
emotional symptoms of toxicity, 10
emotions, toxic, 333
endocrine system
disruptors, 572n36
glands in, 84
symptoms of damage to, 84-85
endometriosis, 44
Endosulfan, 16, 167
endotoxins, 62
Energeia, 553-554
energy cords
cutting, 385-387
defined, 384-385
energy level symptoms, 9
energy refreshing, 490-495
energy toxins, 362-369, 384-387
energy wells, 555-556
Entamoeba histolytica, 253
entities
cases of, 366-367
defined, 365-366
food cravings of, 617n21
points of residence, 363, 368
symptoms of, 368-369
environment, toxins in, 2-5, 26
environmental estrogens
concentrations in body, 88
defined, 86
effects of, 86, 91-92
fetal susceptibilities to, 88-89, 91

illnesses linked with, 87-88
marine life affected by, 88
multiplicity of, 89-90
sources of, 86, 88
Environmental Health Center, 78, 570n14
Environmental Health Information Service, 12-13
Environmental Health Network, 472
environmental illness (EI), 14-16, 74-75
Environmental Lighting Concepts, 465
Environmental Management, Inc., 164
environmental medicine, 76
enzymatic activity test, 119-120
enzymes
defined, 68
liver, action on toxins, 68
mixed function oxidative, 67-68
epilepsy, 365
Epsom salt, 198, 284, 585n108
Epstein, Samuel, 177
estrogen, 88
estrogenicity, 89
ethyl acetate, 455, 471
Everpure, Inc., 155
Everpure water filters, 152, 155
EWG (Environmental Working Group), 29
excitotoxins, 48-49
exercise, 270-272
exotoxins, 62
expelling mudra, 493
extracellular connective tissue matrix, 60
eye symptoms, 8

facial paralysis, 524
facility managers, and SBS, 409
Fagan, John B., 171
Farin, Jacob, 208, 216
fasting
benefits of, 189
frequency of, 191
mental, 193-197
precautions, 190-191
some drinks for, 191-193
water, 193
fatty acids
basics of, 575n5
defined, 184
functions of, 186
saturated, 184-85
test for, 115-117
unsaturated, 185
fear and flower essence therapy, 349-351
feces
free radical generation in, 229-230
tests of, 127-129, 130
Feldman, Jay, 90
feng shui
basics of, 477-479, 484, 615n37
conflicts with geopathogenic zones, 617
evaluation tool for, 479-484
Feng Shui Warehouse, 505
fertilizers, toxic components of, 30
fetuses, 88-89, 91, 303
FIA (Functional Intracellular Analysis), 117, 120
fibroids, uterine, 327, 367
fibromyalgia
chronic fatigue and, 14-15, 433
defined, 608n46
emotional problems and, 329
MCS and, 14-15, 431-432, 433
pesticides and, 12
Fife, Bruce, 190, 278
Finlandia Sauna, 281-282, 283
fish, 4, 43

Fit vegetable wash, 166-167
five elements, 614n6
Five Flower Formula remedy, 347-348, 618n33
flatulence, 233
Flotation REST, 201-204, 586n112
Flower Essence Society, 352, 424
flower essence therapy
basics of, 336-338, 341-342, 351-352
case study, 338-341
emotion-essences summary, 341
for anxiety/fear, 349-351
for depression, 344-346
for EMF stress, 425-426
for hostility, 342-344
for stress/tension, 347-349
fluoridated water. *See* drinking water, fluoridated
fluoride
adult daily intake of, 163
ill effects of, 161-163
industrial emissions, 163, 580n36
removing from tap water, 163-164
source of, 580n35
See also drinking water, fluoridated
Fluoride-X filter, 164
fluorosilicic acid, 580n35
food additives, 50
foods
contaminants of, 53
dairy products, 176-179
DDT-laden, 54
genetically modified
avoiding, 174-176
commercially prepared (list), 174-175
crops containing GMOs, 169
dangers of, 171-173
public's view of, 173-174
heptachlor-laden, 54
irradiated
dangers of, 180-184
energy sources used for, 179
exposures allowed on, 181
inception of, 179
labelling of, 179-180
nutritional deficits of, 180
POP-laden, 54
testing for GMOs in, 170-171
formaldehyde
case history involving, 19
hypersensitives and, 439
monitors, 444
plants which absorb, 454
products contained in, 471
'safe' level of, 439
sources of, 410, 411, 429, 438
symptoms produced by, 410
toxicity symptoms of, 438
FOS (fructo-oligosaccharides), 265-266
fragrances, 472-473
free radicals
action of, 63
defined, 62-63, 421, 607n32
effects of, 63
fecal, 229-230
sources of, 62, 68-69, 120
test for, 115-117
front door area *qi*, 506-509
fructo-oligosaccharides (FOS), 265-266
full spectrum lights, 465-467
Functional Intracellular Analysis (FIA), 117
fungi, 440, 441, 442-443
furnishings, 495
Fusarium, 442, 443

General Ecology, Inc., 154
Genetic ID, Inc., 170-171, 177

Genetically Engineered Food Alert, 177
genetically modified organisms (GMO)
crops containing (list), 169
cross-species examples, 169-170
defined, 168-169
See also foods, genetically modified
Genetron Systems, Inc., 458
Genox Corporation, 122
gentian remedy, 346
Geo Group, 532
geocancerology, 541
Geomack Products, 554
geomancy
case studies employing, 536-540
defined, 533
geopathic stress
biochemical factors and, 522
defined, 518-520, 524
devices for clearing spaces of, 551-554
effects of, 524, 535
entities and, 530-532
health problems near, 521-523
indicators of, 528-529
neutralizing, 545-546, 617n13
women's estrogen cycle and, 527
ghost-busting, 495-499
Giardia lambia, 253, 255
ginger root, 217
gingival crevicular fluid, 576n8
Gittleman, Ann Louise, 254
gliadin, 133
global distillation, 4-5
Global Environment Technologies, 154
glucuronidation, 71
glutamate, 49
glutathione, 69, 70, 213
glutathione conjugation, 70
glutathione peroxidase, test for, 118
glutathione S-transferase, 70
gluten, 133
glycine, 221
GMOs. *See* genetically modified organisms
Goffman, John W., 181
golden ear drops remedy, 344
golden sponge, 381, 387
golf courses, 22
Gould, Jay, 45, 46
Grant, Lucinda, 417
grapes, 28
Great Smokies Diagnostic Laboratory, 122, 131
green drink, 193
Greenberg, Robert C., 119-120
greens, 216
Grossman, Terry, 139
grounding cords
homes to earth, 549-551
people to earth, 387-389
growth periods, 377-378
GTC Nutrition Company, 266
Guirdham, Arthur, M.D., 364
gutta percha alternative, 320-321

Haas, Elson M., 93-94, 191
Hailey, Boyd, 315
hair analysis test, 123-124, 130
hair-pulling case, 331-332
Hall, Judy, 384
Halpern, Steven, 204
hamburger, 54
Harman, Denham, 65
Harmon, Nicholas, 464
Harrison, Lewis, 192
Hartmann, Ernest, 515
Hathaway, Warren E., 466
headaches
case of entities and, 367
chloropyrifos and, 90

excitotoxins and, 48
geopathic stress and, 539
tartrazine and, 50
triggers of, 12
Healing Center, 554
Health Mate Sauna, 280-281, 283
Healthy Home Test Kit, 444
Healthy House Institute, 411, 413
healthy living resources, 78
heart problems, 9, 524
heat depuration, 93
heavy metals
found in tap water, 142
poisoning from, 107
testing feces for, 128-129
testing hair for, 123-124
testing urine for, 124-125
Hellberg, Eira, 491
Hendricksen Natürlich, 434, 437
HEPA air filters, 445-448
heptachlor, 53, 54
heptachlor epoxide, 16
herbicide exposure case, 19-20
Heron, Silena, 254
Herxheimer reaction, 244, 377, 591-62
hexachlorobenzene, 16, 53, 79
hives, 50
Hobbs, Christopher, 224
Hodgson, Michael, 407
Hoffman, David, 220
Holistic Dental Association, 312
holly remedy, 342
Holyk, Peter, 104, 112
homes
bathroom considerations, 512-515
bed location in, 523-527
bedroom considerations, 509-512
chlordane in, 412
clutter in, 486-488
construction, 411-412
design and arrangement, 484-486
energy flow evaluation, 479-483
energy imbalance costs, 515-517
energy of, 485-486
energy refreshing of, 490-495
environmental assessments of, 414-417, 444
front door area qi, 506-509
furnishings, 495
geopathic zone testing for, 528-530, 532
ghost-busting, 495-499
lights in, 494
location of. See geopathic stress
neighboring homes' influences, 499-504
painting interior, 488-490
room detoxification, 546-548
underground water near, 518-522, 526-527, 535
hormones (fed to livestock), 53
hormones (human)
central, 84
defined, 84
thyroid T4, 85
hostility and flower essence therapy, 342-344
hot flashes case, 333-334
houseplants as air filters, 453-459
Huebner, Friedrich Markus, 354
Huggins, Hal, 291, 299, 311
human milk, 3
humic water, 147
humidifiers, 443, 445
Hussar, Christopher, 294
HVP (hydrolyzed vegetable protein), 48
hydrocarbons, 410
hydrochloric acid dumping, 33
hydrogen fluoride dumping, 33
hydrogenated fats, 184
hydrolyzed vegetable protein

(HVP), 48
hydroponic plants, 455-456
hyperactivity, 50
hypertension, 12
hypnotherapy, 331-333
hypochondriacs, 7, 8
'hypochondriasis,' 75
hypoglycemia, 48
hypothyroidism, 46

ice cream, 54
IGF-1 (insulin-like growth factor), 176-178
illness
chronic, 11-12
environmental, 7-8
rate from workplace exposures, 13
immune system
anti-cancer capability of, 105
intestines as part of, 227
overloaded, 60, 73
pesticides and, 29-30
response to toxins in blood, 74
spiritual, 389-390
Immuno 1 Bloodprint test, 132-134, 135
Immuno Laboratories, 135
immunoglobulins, 132, 592n68
impatiens remedy, 348
indian pink remedy, 348-349
Individualized Optimal Nutrition (ION) test, 115-117, 120
indoor air
carbon monoxide in, 438
chemicals found in, 438, 439
chlordane in, 412-413
damp, 439, 440, 441
dust in, 440-441
factors affecting, 438
filtering
with houseplants, 453-459
with machines, 445-448
formaldehyde in, 438-439
fungi in, 440, 441, 442-443
ionizing, 449-453
molds in, 440, 442-443, 444-445
organochlorines in, 34
pollutant sources, 438
productivity and, 442
purifying, 448-449
sick building syndrome and, 403-405, 440
infants. See under children
Infinity Heavenly Horsetail, 436
insulin-like growth factor (IGF-1), 176-178
International Academy of Oral Medicine and Toxicology, 312
International Dental Health Foundation, 312
intestinal tract
bacteria in
beneficial, 127-128, 252
harmful, 252
basics of, 225-226, 227-228
colon
average American male, 231
cleansers for, 232-247
diseased, 230
nature and function of, 226-227
transit times in, 227, 228
leaky, 74, 129, 209
length of, 73
mucoid plaque in, 247-249
parasites in, 129-130, 131
small intestine, 225-226
stagnation symptoms, 231
toxicity of, 73-74
See also parasites
Inuit, 4
ion generators, 449-453
ION (Individualized Optimal

Nutrition) test, 115-117, 120
ion levels, 450-451, 526
IonAir Company, 452
IonAir Wein VI-2000 High Density Negative Ion Generator, 452-453
ionizing radiation, 616n3
ions
defined, 449
negative, 449, 451-452
positive, 451
iron, test for, 113-114

Jainism, 394-395
Janov, Arthur, 334
Jarro-Dophilus, 264-265, 266
Jarrow Formulas, 266
Jenny, S., 522
Jensen, Barnard, 230
joints, 8, 90

Kaminski, Patricia, 335-341, 352
Kan Yu, 477
Kane, Patricia, 185
Karagulla, Shafica, M.D., 358
Kaufman, Richard C., 234
KDF shower water filter, 155, 156, 580n32
Kellogg, John Harvey, 228
Kendall, Julia, 471
kidney inflammation, 524
Kilner, Walter, 357
kinesiological muscle testing, 111, 529
King James Medical Laboratory, 120, 130
Klinghardt, Dietrich, 305
Knishinsky, Ran, 235
Kron, Jacquelin, 193

Lactobacillus acidophilus, 261, 262-264
Lake Baikal, 4
lakes, 4
Lange, Susan, 407
lasagna with meat, 54
laxative types, 240
lead, 37, 114, 444
lead poisoning, 82-83, 106-107
leaky gut syndrome, 74
learning disorders, 48
LeGant, Leon S., 371-376
lemon juice, 218
LessEMF Inc., 424
lethargy, 535, 536
leukemia, 13, 80, 291-292
Levin, Norman, 328
ley lines, 618n23
Lichtenberg, H., 298
light therapy, 464, 612n91
lightning, 536
lights
dawn simulators, 467-468
feng shui of, 494
full-spectrum
fluorescent tubes, 465-466
light boxes, 464-465
light bulbs, 467
partial spectrum, 465-466
Lilly, John C., 586n112
limonen, 471
linalool, 471
lindane, 80
ling energies, 485, 492, 496-499, 534
lipid peroxides, 63, 116, 121
liquid clay. See bentonite
Liquid Needle Rebalancer, 286
Liu, Jenny, 515
liver
backlogged, 209-210
cleansing frequency, 210
common toxicity of, 209
function of, 67, 68, 208
overloaded, 69, 408
test for health of, 122
liver cleansers

commercial, 212-213, 222
homemade, 214, 220
liver cleansing
benefits of, 210
castor oil compresses during, 225
flushing
overview of, 222
protocols for, 223-225
foods for, 216-218
frequency recommended, 210
herbs for 218-224
program for 211-215
results to expect, 215-216
living space. See homes
Logan, Karen, 474
logging one's chemical exposures, 22-24
Lord, Richard S., 127
Los Angeles air pollution, 38
Lotz, K.E., 522
love-lies-bleeding remedy, 346
Lundstrom, Sheri, 467
lung cancer, 13, 80
lung symptoms, 9, 38-39
lymph, 269, 270
lymphatic system
defined, 268, 269, 270
dysfunctional, 269-270
function of, 268-269
stimulating, 270-272
lymphocytes, viability test for, 117
lymphoma, 13, 80

MacManaway, Patrick, 532-540
Mag-Stop Plates, 424
magnesium
deficiency, 110
metabolic role, 78
tests for, 111, 113-114, 115-117
magnetic fields, 414-415
magnetic shielding material, 423-424
manganese toxicity, 83
manufactured foods, 51
marine life, 88
marine pollution, 88
Masada Marketing Corp., 379
Masters, Roger D., 83
MCS (multiple chemical sensitivities)
CFS, fibromyalgia, and, 14-15
defined, 432
incidence of, 14, 15, 433
VOCs and, 431-434
meditation, 531
Meinig, George, D.D.S., 318
melatonin, 522, 612n88, 616n7
melons, 28
menstrual bleeding, 327
mental symptoms, 9, 17
Merchant, Randal, 238
mercury
absorber of, 305
action of, 303-304
binder of, 308
chelators of, 126, 309-311
conversion to methylmercury, 299-300
dangers of, 296, 299
displacing magnesium, 110
exposure standards, 298-299
nervous system effects from, 305-306
persistence in body, 299
tests for, 113-114, 126
transmission to fetuses, 303
mercury toxicity
cases of, 106-109, 291-294
health problems associated with, 107, 300-301, 574n2
in dentists, 301-302
mood altering effects of, 302-303
sources of, 106-107, 292
studies on rats, 299-300

Metagenics, 216
MetaMetrix Clinical Laboratory, 120
methionine, 221
methyl alcohol, 455
methyl bromide, 29
methylmercury, 54, 55, 299
methylene chloride, 472
Meurmann, J.H., 317
'Mickey Finn,' 77-78
microfiltration water filters, 151-152
micronutrients, testing for, 111
Micropolyspora faeni, 443
microwave pollution, 416
milk thistle, 218-219
mimulus remedy, 349
Mineral Rich, 236, 237
mirrors, 503, 504-505, 508
miscarriage, 44, 144-147
Modi, Shakuntala, 362, 369
molds, 440, 442-443, 444-445
molecular medicine, 574n51
molybdenum, test for, 113-114
Mom's Veggiewash, 167-168
monobutyl phthalate, 25
monosodium glutamate (MSG), 48
Monsanto, 170, 176
montmorillonite. *See* bentonite
Mother & Others, 179
mountain pride remedy, 350-351
moving between homes, 533-534
Mowrey, Daniel B., 246
MSG (monosodium glutamate), 48
mucoid plaque, 247-249
multiple chemical sensitivities
    (MCS)
    chemicals in people with, 16
    proof of, 76
    toxicity and, 14, 15
    VOCs and, 431-434
multiple sclerosis, 300-301, 523
MuMetal, 423
muscle symptoms, 8
muscle testing, 111, 530
music therapy, 204-206
mustard remedy, 345-346

Nambudripad Allergy Elimination
    Technique, 112, 134-135
Nambudripad, Devi S., 134, 135
nasal symptoms, 9
National Human Adipose Tissue
    Survey, 24
National Toxicology Program, 12-13
natural killer cells, 105, 574n1
Natural Solutions Environmental,
    Inc., 156
Nature's Carpet, 434, 436-437
naturopathy, 587n1
nausea, 90
neck, nape of, 604n18
Needak Manufacturing, 272
Needak Soft-Bounce rebounder, 272
negative ion generators, 449-453
negative ions, 449, 451-452
neighbor pacification, 504-506
neighboring homes' influences, 499-
    504
nervous system
    autonomic, 586n113
    central, disorders of, 13, 19-20
    mercury and, 305-306
    peripheral, 599n34
    sympathetic, 599n36
Nestle, Marion, 173
neurological disorders, 48-49, 81, 90
neuropeptides, 330-331
neurosis, 335
NF Formulas, 216
Nickel, David J., 292-293
nickel, test for, 114-115
Nieper, Hans, 523
Nirvana Safe Haven, 154, 448
nitrites, 50
nitrogen dioxide, 37, 40
nitrogen oxide, 453

nitrosamines, 50
Noetic Field Therapy, 391
nonionizing radiation, 616n3
nonyl-phenol-ethoxylate, 471
Nordic Naturals, 311
North Star 10,000 Bright Light Box,
    465
Northeast Center for Environmental
    Medicine, 78
Northrup, Christiane, 333
nuclear counties, 45
nuclear power plants, 47
nuclear weapons testing, 45-46
NutraFlora, 266
NutraSweet (aspartame), 48, 176
nutrients, intracellular, 111
nutritional deficiencies, 106

OCCs (organochlorine compounds).
    See organochlorines
Olestra, 50
oral
    bacterial populations, 315
    diseases and heart problems,
        316, 317
    focal infections, 316-317
    toxicity symptoms, 9
    toxicity tests, 126-127, 131
orchids, 455
Oregon grape remedy, 342-343
Organic Crop Improvement Assn.,
    179
Organiclean E-Commerce Division,
    168
Organiclean Fruit and Vegetable
    Wash, 166, 168
organochlorines
    average dietary intake of, 53-54
    bodily damage from, 44-45
    defined, 41
    formation of, 42
    half-lives of, 566n69
    in dolphins, 43
    in humans, 43-44
    multiple, in blood, 79
    persistence of, 43, 566n69,
        568n93
    sources of, 42
Ott, John Nash, 465
Ott-Lite, 465
outgassing
    of carpets, 430
    from dental mercury amalgam
        fillings, 297-298
ovarian cancer case, 332-333
Owens, Kagan, 90
oxidation, 62-63, 66
Oxidative Protection Screen test,
    120-121, 122
oxidative stress, 63, 64-65, 121
Oxidative Stress Profile, 121-122
OxyClean Air Filter, 447
Oxystat, 222, 223
ozone, 37

Pacific Northwest Laboratory, 420
Packed Blood Cell Elements Profile,
    113-114, 120
packed red blood cell intracellular
    analysis, 111, 113-114
paint exposure case, 18
painting home interiors, 488-490
Pantox Laboratories, 121
Pantox Profile, 118, 121
Paragon shower water filter, 154,
    156
Paragon Water Systems, 156
Paraquat, 235
parasites
    action of, 253
    arthropod, 253
    formula for purging, 258-259
    incidence of, 255-257
    symptoms from, 253-255
    test for, 129-130, 131

treatments for, 257-261
    worms, 253
Parkinson's disease
    excitotoxins and, 48, 49
    pesticide exposure and, 30
    triggers of, 12
particulate matter, as air pollutant,
    37, 39
Passey, Tom, 529
pathological detoxifiers, 69
patient evaluation, 111-112
PBBs (polybrominated biphenyls),
    24, 85
PBTs (persistent, bioaccumulative,
    toxic substances), 53
4-PC (4-phenylcyclohexene), 427,
    429
PCBs (polychlorinated biphenyls)
    amount produced worldwide, 3
    banning of, 3
    in dolphins, 43
    in humans, 3, 24, 44
    thyroid function and, 85-86
    uses of, 85-86
peanut butter, 54
peanuts, 54
Penicillium, 441, 443
penstemon remedy, 350
pentane, 471
perchloroethylene, 471
perfumes, 472-473
periodontal disease, 315-316
peripheral nervous system, 599n34
persistent organic pollutants. *See*
    POPs
Pert, Candace, 330
pesticides
    airborne, 29
    annual market for, 22
    California agricultural use of, 27-
        28
    cancer and, 80
    'drift' from, 28, 29
    exposure case, 20
    household, 21-22
    in house dust, 430
    licensed agricultural, 27
    proportion not reaching target,
        31
    proscription in schools, 573n47
    residue levels in humans, 17
    usage rates, 21-22, 27-28
    water contamination from, 31-32,
        34
Pettis, Chuck, 530
pH, intracellular, test for, 119-120
Phase I detoxification
    action of, 67, 68
    defined, 67
    enzymes involved in, 67-68
    nutrients needed for, 69
    substances blocking, 70
    triggering substances, 69
Phase II detoxification
    defined, 70
    nutrients needed for, 72
    pathways in, 70-72
phenols, 471
phosphorus, test for, 113-114
phthalates in urine, 25
Phyto-Pro, 213
Pi-Square SunUp dawn simulator,
    467
pickles, 54
Pierrakos, John C., 357
pineal function, 540
pizza, pepperoni, 54
Pizzorno, Joseph, 70, 256
Planetary Formulas, 223
PLH Products, 283
"poison arrows," cutting *qi*, 499-504
Polari Tea, 224
polychlorinated biphenyls. *See*
    PCBs

polycyclic aromatic hydrocarbons,
    430
polyurethane, 438
polyurethane foam, 474
polyvinyl chloride (PVC), 80-81
pomanders, 391-394
POPs (persistent organic pollu-
    tants), 3-4, 43, 53
positive ions, 451
potassium, test for, 113-114
potato chips, 54
potatoes, 170
p,p-DDE, 24
prebiotics, 265-266
Prestige Publishing, 78
Price, Weston A., 319
ProAlgen, 311
probiotics, 261-265
produce
    cleaning, 165
    organically grown, 174
    washes for, 165-168
Professional House Doctors, 444
prostate cancer
    case of, 290
    dental problems and, 289
    rates of, 47
proteins, metal-binding, test for, 118
Psenner, Roland, 4
Pseudomonas aeruginosa, 443
psyllium husks and seeds, 241-245
Public Citizen, 183, 184
pumpkin pie, 54
pumpkin seeds, 260-261
Pur Recovery Engineering, 154
Pur water filters, 151, 154
Pure-Pro USA Corp., 155
Pure-Pro water filters, 153, 155
PVC (polyvinyl chloride), 80-81
pyrethroids, 90-91

qi, 476-479
    cutting, 499-504
QLink, 424-425

radiation
    effects of, 46-48
    ionizing, 616n3
    radioactive fallout, 45-46
    radiolytic products, 181-182
RadiTech, 551-553, 554
radon
    assessing homes for, 461
    dangers of, 459-460
    deaths attributed to, 460
    mode of entry, 438, 459
    residential levels of, 460
    sources of, 459
    U.S. concentration maps, 461
raisins, 54
Rancho Seco nuclear plant, 47
Randolph, Theron, 75
Rau, Thomas, 289
Rea, William J., 16, 75, 78, 432
Real Goods, 154
ReboundAIR rebounder, 272
rebounding, 270-272
rectal cancer, 149, 150
redox, 66
reduction, 66
relaxation suggestions, 197-206
reproductive problems, 144-147
Rescue Remedy, 347-348, 618n33
resistivity, intracellular, test for, 119-
    120
restricted environmental stimulation
    therapy (REST), 201-204, 586-
    112
reverse osmosis water filters, 152-
    153
Riccioli, Joseph, 331
Riggs, Alf, 526
Riversong, Michael, 413-417
Rogers, Sherry, 7, 8, 76-77, 78
root canals, 313-314, 318-321

Rossbach, Sarah, 505
Roundup, 235
Roundup Ready, 170
Royal Center of Advanced Medicine, 311
Royal, Daniel F., 311, 313

SAD (seasonal affective disorder), 462-464
Safe Zone filters, 446
Sagan, Samuel, 365, 369, 531, 555
salmonella, 52
Samadhi Tank Company, 203
sauna units, 280-284
saunas, 278-280, 283-284, 596n15
SBS. See sick building syndrome
scarlet monkeyflower remedy, 349-350
Schrödter, Willy, 492
Scientific Consulting Service, 260
scleranthus remedy, 348
scotch broom remedy, 345
Scott-Morley, Anthony, 523-524
scrubs, 273-275, 381-382
Seagull IV X-1 water filters, 151-152, 154
seals, and POPs in body fat, 4
seasonal affective disorder (SAD), 462-464
Sedir, Paul, 491
seizures, 48
serotonin, 467-468, 522, 535, 616n6
Seventh Generation, 472
sexual maturation, 87-88
shaking, 380-381
Sharan, Farida, 274-275
Shaul, Chris, 480
Shaul, Sophia Tang, 480
Shelter Ecology, 472
Shelton, Bruce, 305
Sherman, Janette D., 18, 22
shower water filters, 154-155
showers, chlorine exposure in, 33-34
sick building syndrome (SBS)
    air quality and, 403-405
    defined, 400-401
    dust and, 440-441
    incidence of, 402-406
    stress and, 405
    symptoms of, 401-402
    toxin sources surrounding, 409, 410
    women and, 406
    See also building-related illness; indoor air
silicofluoride, 83
Silver, Helene, 223
Simontacchi, Carol, 50-51
skin
    brushing, 273-274
    scrubs for, 274-275
    symptoms, 9
smectite. See bentonite
smog, 37-38
solvents, 17, 18-19
sour cream, 54
soy products, 170-171
soybeans, 170, 171
Special Provocative Mercury Test, 126, 130
SpectraCell Laboratories, 120
spider plants, 453
spiritual
    antioxidant, 389-390
    detoxification, 387-390, 394-396
    guide, 373-374
    toxins, 370-376
Sprite Slim-Line shower water filter, 155, 156
St. John's wort remedy, 345
Stachybotrys atra, 441
Stachybotrys chartarum, 442
Stangle, Jacob, 521-522

star tulip remedy, 349
steam distillation, 163-164
Steingraber, Sandra, 33
Steven Halpern's Inner Peace Music, 206
sticky monkeyflower remedy, 350
stomach cancer, 80
stool tests, 127-129, 130
strawberries, 28
stress
    flower essence therapy for, 347-349
    relieving, 198-200
    types of, 199-200
    See also geopathic stress
strokes, 48, 524
strontium-90, 47
styrene, 429
sulfation, 72
sulfur dioxide, 37
sulfuric acid dumping, 33
Sun-Pure Water Purifier, 154, 155
sunflower remedy, 350
SunRizr dawn simulator, 467
Sunshine Tropical Foliage, 458
superoxide dismutase, test for, 118
sweet chestnut remedy, 346
sympathetic nervous system, 599n36
symptoms
    per organ or organ system, 8-10
    vague, 6-7
Synercid, 52

Tagamet, 61
Tanalbit, 259, 260
Tart, Charles, 195
tartrazine, 50
teeth-brushing, 316
tension and flower essence therapy, 347-349
Ternes, Thomas A., 35
TerraFlo CBLX water filter, 151, 154
testicular cancer, 80-81
tests available, body nutrients and toxins, 113-135
tetrachloroethylene, 16-17
Thermoactinomycetes vulgaris, 443
ThinkTank International, 203
THMs. See trihalomethanes
Thompson, Angel, 500
Thornton, Joe, 41
Three Mile Island, 47
throat symptoms, 9, 13
Thurnell-Read, Jane, 528
thyroid gland
    function of, 567n74, 571n32
    incidence of malfunctioning, 85
    PCBs and, 85-86
thyroid hormones
    T3, 86
    T4, 85
Tierra, Michael, 223
tinnitus, 524
toluene
    asthma and, 473
    basics of, 570n12
    benzoates as block to cleansing of, 71
    houseplants which absorb, 454
    incidence in fat tissue, 24
    incidence in fragrances, 473
toluene diisocyanate, 474
tomatoes, 28
Too, Lillian, 501
tooth extractions, 294
TOPAS (Toxicity Prescreening Assay), 127
Total Antioxidant Status test, 118, 120
total environmental load, 76
Total Shield, 424
toxaphene, 53

toxic bowel, 228, 230
toxic load, tests for, 123-135
toxic substances
    annual dumping of, 5
    carcinogenic, 12
'toxic triggers,' 12
Toxicant-Induced Loss of Tolerance, 432
toxicity
    as disease, 12
    assessment criteria, 8-11
    degrees of, 109
    effects of, xxii, 12
    gradual development of, 6, 17
    long-term, 12, 104
    mistaken as fatigue, 7
    unrelieved, 78
toxins
    blood levels of, in mothers and infants, 16
    buildup in environment, 2
    defined, 94
    energy, 362-369, 384-387
    exposures to, versus body levels of, 81
    fat-soluble, 3, 24
    human milk, 3
    incidence in humans, 2, 24-25, 106
    indoor sources of, 409, 410
    levels in body, 58-59
    migration of, 2, 4-5
    non-chemical, 94
    'safe' levels of, 469
    spiritual, 370-376
    toxics versus, 561n6
    types of, 62
    ubiquity of, xxi-xxii, 2-5
toxoplasmosis, 257
Trace Mineral Systems, 130
trampolining, 270-272
trans-fatty acids
    avoiding consumption of, 188
    consumption statistics, 188
    dangers of, 186-188
    defined, 185
    history of, 185
    nature of, 186
transgenic, 169
transit times, 227, 228, 242
trauma, unresolved, 543
trees, 529, 540
trichloroethane, 42
trichloroethylene, 410, 454, 455
Trifield Meter, 423
trigrams, 479-481
trihalomethanes (THMs)
    carcinogenic effects of, 147-150
    defined, 141
    levels considered acceptable, 141
    modes of ingestion, 143
    reproductive effects of, 144-147
Triphala, 239-241
tubulin, 306
twitching, 524

Ultra Clear, 212-213, 216
ultraviolet light air purification, 448-449
ultraviolet purification water filters, 153-154
uranium, 114-115, 459
uric acid, test for, 118
urine
    color of, 139
    mercury in, 303
    phthalates in, 25
    testing for heavy metals, 124-125
Urine Elements Profiles, 124-125, 130

van Benschoten, M.M., O.M.D., 293-294
vanadium, test for, 113-114
Variel Health International, 283

ventilation systems, 20, 403-404, 409
Verilux, 466, 467
Video Operator Distress Syndrome, 453
villi, intestinal, 226
Vilsbiburg, Germany, 520-521
Viracin, 259, 260
Virginiamycin, 52
virus sizes, 445
Vita-Lite, 466-467
Vitamin C, test for, 118
Vitamin E, test for, 118
Vitamin Research Products, 266
VOCs (volatile organic compounds), 28-29, 141-143
    examples of, 431
    houseplants as absorbers of, 453-455
    human-made, 430
    in blood, 433
    indoor levels of, 431
    in tap water, 141-143
    natural sources of, 431
    sources of, 28-29, 141-143, 431
von Pohl, Gustav Freiherr, 520, 524

Walker, Morton, 300, 303
water consumption
    benefit of, 94
    best times for, 139
    inadequate, 137-139
    indicator of adequate, 139-140
    minimum recommended, 139
water contamination, 31-33, 34, 140-143
water filter types, 151-154
water filtration, 150
water, stagnant, 531
water (tap)
    chlorination of, 141
    contaminants in, 140-143
    reproductive problems from, 144-147
    See also drinking water
Waterman, Robert D., 391
Waterwise, Inc., 164
WaveGuide, 420
Webster, Richard, 514
weight symptoms, 9
    whacks, auric, 372
white blood cell counts, 30
Whole Blood Elements Profile, 114-115, 120
willow remedy, 343
Wolverton, B.C., 456
women
    colon cancer in, 148, 149
    endocrine disruptors and, 87
    health problems and geopathic stress, 527, 535
    pregnant and nursing, 54
    sick building syndrome in, 406
    See also breast cancer
World Resources Institute, 29
Wydra, Nancilee, 502

X-rays, 181
xenobiotics, 2
xenoestrogens. See environmental estrogens
xylene, 17, 410, 455

Yarnell, Eric, 254
yarrow remedy, 348
Yarrow Special Formula remedy, 347, 425
Yerba Prima, Inc., 237
Yerba Santa remedy, 346
yin/yang polarities, 614n5

Zestron Ionair ionizers, 452
zinc, test for, 113-114
zinnia remedy, 343

Hampton Roads Publishing Company

. . . for the evolving human spirit

Hampton Roads Publishing Company
publishes books on a variety of subjects,
including metaphysics, health, integrative medicine,
visionary fiction, and other related topics.

For a copy of our latest catalog, call toll-free
(800) 766-8009, or send your name and address to:

Hampton Roads Publishing Company, Inc.
1125 Stoney Ridge Road
Charlottesville, VA 22902

e-mail: hrpc@hrpub.com
www.hrpub.com